Contents

Preface

NCLEX-RN Pediatric Nursing Made Incredibly Easy is really two books in one. The first is designed to provide you with a detailed review of essential nursing concepts, nursing diagnoses, and clinical information you need to pass the NCLEX-RN. The second provides hundreds of challenging questions, answers, and detailed rationales following the NCLEX 2010 test plan. The content review section follows the same chapter structure as the Q&A section to help you organize your study.

The content section is presented in the appealing and effective style of the *Incredibly Easy* series. Its humor encourages you to relax and have fun while learning. You will also find these valuable features in every chapter of the review:
- **Brush up on key concepts** provides an overview of anatomy and physiology.
- **Cheat sheets** provide you with a concise overview of key signs and symptoms, test results, treatments, and interventions of common diseases. Use this feature to quickly review the material you will cover in depth in the *Polish up on client care* section.
- **Keep abreast of diagnostic tests** highlights the most important tests for the disorders being discussed, including pertinent nursing actions you will need to perform to ensure client safety—a key area of NCLEX-RN testing.
- **Polish up on client care** provides a thorough review of disorders with a focus on the expected nursing care. Starting with a description of the problem, this section also covers causes, assessment findings, diagnostic test results, nursing diagnoses, treatments, and drug therapy for each disorder. Key interventions and their rationales are also provided.

In addition to your nursing knowledge, your test-taking skills can help you pass the exam. This book introduces you to the NCLEX-RN exam structure and covers techniques that will help you learn how to read test questions and understand what they are really asking—skills that are vital to NCLEX success. You also have access to study strategies, such as scheduling study time, maintaining your concentration, and finding the right study space.

Questions, Questions, and More Questions

The more you become accustomed to the styles and types of questions that may be asked, the more successful you will be on the actual exam, and that's a special strength of this book. You will find *Pump up on practice questions* at the end of each chapter, and in addition you will find an entire second section of the book featuring hundreds of additional questions. The easy-to-use format features questions on the left and answers on the right side of the same page. The questions help you assess and remember what you've just reviewed and determine areas in which you might need further review. Detailed rationales for both correct and incorrect answers are provided, and each answer provides information on the client needs category, the cognitive level of the question, and the nursing process. Helpful hints are scattered throughout the practice questions. These hints greatly increase your ability to determine the correct answer, retain important content information, and learn essential test-taking strategies. In addition, the graphics keep you focused and help build your confidence.

Be proud of your accomplishments and of your decision to prepare yourself well for the NCLEX-RN. You've worked hard to come this far. Now it's time to prepare, to practice, to build your confidence, and to succeed!

Part I   Getting ready

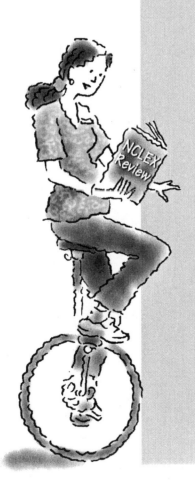

1 Preparing for the NCLEX®

NCLEX basics

Passing the National Council Licensure Examination (NCLEX®) is an important landmark in your career as a nurse. The first step on your way to passing the NCLEX is to understand what it is and how it's administered.

NCLEX structure

The *NCLEX* is a test written by nurses who, like most of your nursing instructors, have an advanced degree and clinical expertise in a particular area. Only one small difference distinguishes nurses who write NCLEX questions: They're trained to write questions in a style particular to the NCLEX.

If you've completed an accredited nursing program, you've already taken numerous tests written by nurses with backgrounds and experiences similar to those of the nurses who write for the NCLEX. The test-taking experience you've already gained will help you pass the NCLEX. So your NCLEX review should be just that — a review. (For eligibility and immigration requirements for nurses from outside of the United States, see *Guidelines for international nurses,* page 4.)

What's the point of it all?
The NCLEX is designed for one purpose: namely, to determine whether it's appropriate for you to receive a license to practice as a nurse. By passing the NCLEX, you demonstrate that you possess the minimum level of knowledge necessary to practice nursing safely.

Mix 'em up
In nursing school, you probably took courses that were separated into such subjects as pharmacology, nursing leadership, health assessment, adult health, pediatric, maternal-neonatal, and psychiatric nursing. In contrast, the NCLEX is integrated, meaning that different subjects are mixed together.

As you answer NCLEX questions, you may encounter clients in any stage of life, from neonatal to geriatric. These clients — clients, in NCLEX lingo — may be of any background, may be completely well or extremely ill, and may have any disorder.

Client needs, front and center
The NCLEX draws questions from four categories of client needs that were developed by the *National Council of State Boards of Nursing* (NCSBN), the organization that sponsors and manages the NCLEX. *Client needs categories* ensure that a wide variety of topics appear on every NCLEX examination.

The NCSBN developed client needs categories after conducting a practice analysis of new nurses. All aspects of nursing care observed in the study were broken down into four main categories, some of which were broken down further into subcategories. (See *Client needs categories,* page 5.)

The whole kit and caboodle
The categories and subcategories are used to develop the *NCLEX test plan,* the content guidelines for the distribution of test questions. Question-writers and the people who put the NCLEX together use the test plan and client needs categories to make sure that a full spectrum of nursing activities is covered in the examination. Client needs categories appear in most NCLEX review and question-and-answer books, including this one. As a test-taker, you don't have to concern yourself with client needs categories. You'll see those categories for each question and answer in this book, but they'll be invisible on the actual NCLEX.

Guidelines for international nurses

To become eligible to work as a registered nurse in the United States, you'll need to complete several steps. In addition to passing the NCLEX® examination, you may need to obtain a certificate and credentials evaluation from the Commission on Graduates of Foreign Nursing Schools (CGFNS®) and acquire a visa. Requirements vary from state to state, so it's important that you first contact the Board of Nursing in the state where you want to practice nursing.

CGFNS CERTIFICATION PROGRAM

Most states require that you obtain CGFNS certification. This certification requires:
• review and authentication of your credentials, including your nursing education, registration, and licensure
• passing score on the CGFNS Qualifying Examination of nursing knowledge
• passing score on an English language proficiency test.

To be eligible to take the CGFNS Qualifying Examination, you must complete a minimum number of classroom and clinical practice hours in medical-surgical nursing, maternal-infant nursing, pediatric nursing, and psychiatric and mental health nursing from a government-approved nursing school. You must also be registered as a first-level nurse in your country of education and currently hold a license as a registered nurse in some jurisdiction.

The CGFNS Qualifying Examination is a paper and pencil test that includes 260 multiple-choice questions and is administered under controlled testing conditions. Because the test is designed to predict your likelihood of successfully passing the NCLEX-RN examination, it's based on the NCLEX-RN test plan.

You may select from three English proficiency examinations—Test of English as a Foreign Language (TOEFL®), Test of English for International Communication (TOEIC®), or International English Language Testing System (IELTS). Each test has different passing scores, and the scores are valid for up to 2 years.

CGFNS CREDENTIALS EVALUATION SERVICE

This evaluation is a comprehensive report that analyzes and compares your education and licensure with U.S. standards. It's prepared by CGFNS for a state board of nursing, an immigration office, employer, or university. To use this service you must complete an application, submit appropriate documentation, and pay a fee.

More information about the CGFNS certification program and credentials evaluation service is available at *www.cgfns.org*.

VISA REQUIRED

You can't legally immigrate to work in the United States without an occupational visa (temporary or permanent) from the United States Citizenship and Immigration Services (USCIS). The visa process is separate from the CGFNS certification process, although some of the same steps are involved. Some visas require prior CGFNS certification and a *VisaScreen*™ Certificate from the International Commission on Healthc are Professions (ICHP). The VisaScreen program involves:
• credentials review of your nursing education and current registration or licensure
• successful completion of either the CGFNS certification program or the NCLEX-RN to provide proof of nursing knowledge
• passing score on an approved English language proficiency examination.

After you successfully complete all parts of the *VisaScreen* program, you'll receive a certificate to present to the USCIS. The visa granting process can take up to one year.

You can obtain more detailed information about visa applications at *www.uscis.gov*.

Testing by computer

Like many standardized tests today, the NCLEX is administered by computer. That means you won't be filling in empty circles, sharpening pencils, or erasing frantically. It also means that you must become familiar with computer tests, if you aren't already. Fortunately, the skills required to take the NCLEX on a computer are simple enough to

Client needs categories

Each question on the NCLEX is assigned a category based on client needs. This chart lists client needs categories and subcategories and the percentages of each type of question that appears on an NCLEX examination.

Category	Subcategories	Percentage of NCLEX questions
Safe and effective care environment	• Management of care • Safety and infection control	16% to 22% 8% to 14%
Health promotion and maintenance		6% to 12%
Psychosocial integrity		6% to 12%
Physiological integrity	• Basic care and comfort • Pharmacological and parenteral therapies • Reduction of risk potential • Physiological adaptation	6% to 12% 13% to 19% 10% to 16% 11% to 17%

allow you to focus on the questions, not the keyboard.

Q&A

When you take the test, depending on the question format, you'll be presented with a question and four or more possible answers, a blank space in which to enter your answer, a figure on which you'll identify the correct area by clicking the mouse on it, a series of charts or exhibits you'll use to select the correct response, items you must rearrange in priority order by dragging and dropping them in place, an audio recording to listen to in order to select the correct response, or a question and four graphic options.

Feeling smart? Think hard!

The NCLEX is a *computer-adaptive test*, meaning that the computer reacts to the answers you give, supplying more difficult questions if you answer correctly, and slightly easier questions if you answer incorrectly. Each test is thus uniquely adapted to the individual test-taker.

A matter of time

You have a great deal of flexibility with the amount of time you can spend on individual questions. The examination lasts a maximum of 6 hours, however, so don't waste time. If you fail to answer a set number of questions within 6 hours, the computer will determine that you lack minimum competency.

Most students have plenty of time to complete the test, so take as long as you need to get the question right without wasting time. But remember to keep moving at a decent pace to help you maintain concentration.

Difficult Items = Good news

If you find as you progress through the test that the questions seem to be increasingly difficult, it's a good sign. The more questions you answer correctly, the more difficult the questions become.

Some students, though, knowing that questions get progressively harder, focus on the degree of difficulty of subsequent questions to try to figure out if they're answering questions correctly. Avoid the temptation to do this, as this may get you off track.

Free at last!

The computer test finishes when one of the following events occurs:

• You demonstrate minimum competency, according to the computer program, which

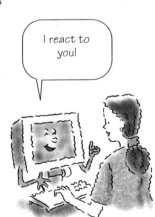

I react to you!

does so with 95% certainty that your ability exceeds the passing standard.
- You demonstrate a lack of minimum competency, according to the computer program.
- You've answered the maximum number of questions (265 total questions).
- You've used the maximum time allowed (6 hours).

Unlocking the NCLEX mystery

In April 2004, the NCSBN added alternate-format items to the examination. However, most of the questions on the NCLEX are four-option, multiple-choice items with only one correct answer. Certain strategies can help you understand and answer any type of NCLEX question.

Alternate formats

The first type of alternate-format item is the *multiple-response question*. Unlike a traditional multiple-choice question, each multiple-response question has one or more correct answers for every question, and it may contain more than four possible answer options. You'll recognize this type of question because it will ask you to select *all* answers that apply — not just the best answer (as may be requested in the more traditional multiple-choice questions).

All or nothing

Keep in mind that, for each multiple-response question, you must select at least one answer and you must select all correct answers for the item to be counted as correct. On the NCLEX, there is no partial credit in the scoring of these items.

Don't go blank!

The second type of alternate-format item is the *fill-in-the-blank* question. These questions require you to provide the answer yourself, rather than select it from a list of options. You will perform a calculation and then type your answer (a number, without any words, units of measurements, commas, or spaces) in the blank space provided after the question. Rules for rounding are included in the question stem if appropriate. A calculator button is provided so you can do your calculations electronically.

Mouse marks the spot!

The third type of alternate-format item is a question that asks you to identify an area on an illustration or graphic. For these *"hot spot" questions*, the computerized exam will ask you to place your cursor and click over the correct area on an illustration. Try to be as precise as possible when marking the location. As with the fill-in-the-blanks, the identification questions on the computerized exam may require extremely precise answers in order for them to be considered correct.

Click, choose, and prioritize

The fourth alternate-format item type is the *chart/exhibit* format. For this question type, you'll be given a problem and then a series of small screens with additional information you'll need to answer the question. By clicking on the tabs on screen, you can access each chart or exhibit item. After viewing the chart or exhibit, you select your answer from four multiple-choice options.

Drag n' drop

The fifth alternate-format item type involves prioritizing actions or placing a series of statements in correct order using a *drag-and-drop* (ordered response) technique. To move an answer option from the list of unordered options into the correct sequence, click on it using the mouse. While still holding down the mouse button, drag the option to the ordered response part of the screen. Release the mouse button to "drop" the option into place. Repeat this process until you've moved all of the available options into the correct order.

Now hear this!

The sixth alternate-format item type is the *audio item* format. You'll be given a set of headphones and you'll be asked to listen to an

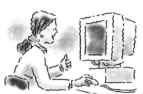

The harder it gets, the better I'm doing.

audio clip and select the correct answer from four options. You'll need to select the correct answer on the computer screen as you would with the traditional multiple-choice questions.

Picture perfect
The final alternate-format item type is the *graphic option* question. This varies from the exhibit format type because in the graphic option, your answer choices will be graphics such as ECG strips. You'll have to select the appropriate graphic to answer the question presented.

The standard's still the standard
The NCSBN hasn't yet established a percentage of alternate-format items to be administered to each candidate. In fact, your exam may contain only one alternate-format item. So relax; the standard, four-option, multiple-choice format questions constitute the bulk of the test. (See *Sample NCLEX questions*, pages 8 to 10.)

Understanding the question

NCLEX questions are commonly long. As a result, it's easy to become overloaded with information. To focus on the question and avoid becoming overwhelmed, apply proven strategies for answering NCLEX questions, including:
- determining what the question is asking
- determining relevant facts about the client
- rephrasing the question in your mind
- choosing the best option or options before entering your answer.

DETERMINE WHAT THE QUESTION IS ASKING
Read the question twice. If the answer isn't apparent, rephrase the question in simpler, more personal terms. Breaking down the question into easier, less intimidating terms may help you to focus more accurately on the correct answer.

Give it a try
For example, a question might be, "A 74-year-old client with a history of heart failure is admitted to the coronary care unit with pulmonary edema. He's intubated and placed on a mechanical ventilator. Which parameters should the nurse monitor closely to assess the client's response to a bolus dose of furosemide (Lasix) I.V.?"

The options for this question — numbered from 1 to 4 — might include:
1. Daily weight
2. 24-hour intake and output
3. Serum sodium levels
4. Hourly urine output

Hocus, focus on the question
Read the question again, ignoring all details except what's being asked. Focus on the last line of the question. It asks you to select the appropriate assessment for monitoring a client who received a bolus of furosemide I.V.

DETERMINE WHAT FACTS ABOUT THE CLIENT ARE RELEVANT
Next, sort out the relevant client information. Start by asking whether any of the information provided about the client isn't relevant. For instance, do you need to know that the client has been admitted to the coronary care unit? Probably not; his reaction to I.V. furosemide won't be affected by his location in the hospital.

Determine what you do know about the client. In the example, you know that:
- he just received an I.V. bolus of furosemide, a crucial fact
- he has pulmonary edema, the most fundamental aspect of the client's underlying condition
- he's intubated and placed on a mechanical ventilator, suggesting that his pulmonary edema is serious
- he's 74 years old and has a history of heart failure, a fact that may or may not be relevant.

REPHRASE THE QUESTION
After you've determined relevant information about the client and the question being asked, consider rephrasing the question to make it more clear. Eliminate jargon and put the question in simpler, more personal terms. Here's how you might rephrase the question in the example: "My client has pulmonary edema. He requires intubation and

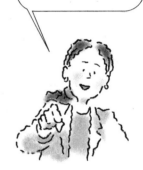

Focusing on what the question is really asking can help you choose the correct answer.

(Text continues on page 10.)

Sample NCLEX questions

Sometimes, getting used to the format is as important as knowing the material. Try your hand at these sample questions and you'll have a leg up when you take the real test!

Sample four-option, multiple-choice question

A client's arterial blood gas (ABG) results are as follows: pH, 7.16; $Paco_2$, 80 mm Hg; Pao_2, 46 mm Hg; HCO_3^-, 24 mEq/L; Sao_2, 81%. These ABG results represent which condition?

1. Metabolic acidosis
2. Metabolic alkalosis
3. Respiratory acidosis
4. Respiratory alkalosis

Correct answer: 3

Sample multiple-response question

A nurse is caring for a 45-year-old married woman who has undergone hemicolectomy for colon cancer. The woman has two children. Which concepts about families should the nurse keep in mind when providing care for this client?

Select all that apply:
1. Illness in one family member can affect all members.
2. Family roles don't change because of illness.
3. A family member may have more than one role at a time in the family.
4. Children typically aren't affected by adult illness.
5. The effects of an illness on a family depend on the stage of the family's life cycle.
6. Changes in sleeping and eating patterns may be signs of stress in a family.

Correct answer: 1, 3, 5, 6

Sample fill-in-the-blank calculation question

An infant who weighs 8 kg is to receive ampicillin 25 mg/kg I.V. every 6 hours. How many milligrams should the nurse administer per dose? Record your answer using a whole number.

_____ milligrams

Correct answer: 200

Sample hot spot question

A client has a history of aortic stenosis. Identify the area where the nurse should place the stethoscope to best hear the murmur.

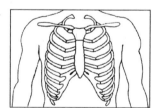

Correct answer:

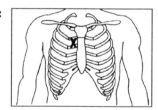

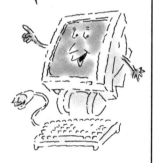
I can be ambivalent. More than one answer may be correct.

Sample NCLEX questions *(continued)*

Sample exhibit question

A 3-year old child is being treated for severe status asthmaticus. After reviewing the progress notes (shown below), the nurse should determine that this client is being treated for which condition?

Progress notes	
9/1/10	Pt. was acutely restless, diaphoretic, and with dyspnea at 0530. Dr. T.
0600	Smith notified of findings at 0545 and ordered ABG
	analysis. ABG drawn from R radial artery. Stat results as follows: pH
	7.28, Paco₂ 55 mm Hg, HCO₃⁻ 26 mEg/L. Dr. Smith
	with pt. now. ———————— J. Collins, RN.

1. Metabolic acidosis
2. Respiratory alkalosis
3. Respiratory acidosis
4. Metabolic alkalosis

Correct answer: 3

Sample drag-and-drop (ordered response) question

When teaching an antepartal client about the passage of the fetus through the birth canal during labor, the nurse describes the cardinal mechanisms of labor. Place these events in the sequence in which they occur. Use all options:

1. Flexion	
2. External rotation	
3. Descent	
4. Expulsion	
5. Internal rotation	
6. Extension	

Correct answer:

3. Descent
1. Flexion
5. Internal rotation
6. Extension
2. External rotation
4. Expulsion

(continued)

Sample NCLEX questions (continued)

Sample audio item question

Listen to the audio clip. What sound do you hear in the bases of this client with heart failure?

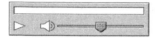

1. Crackles
2. Rhonchi
3. Wheezes
4. Pleural friction rub

Correct answer: 1

Sample graphic option question

Which electrocardiogram strip should the nurse document as sinus tachycardia?

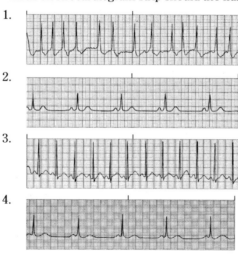

Correct answer: 1

---

mechanical ventilation. He's 74 years old and has a history of heart failure. He received an I.V. bolus of furosemide. What assessment parameter should I monitor?"

CHOOSE THE BEST OPTION

Armed with all the information you now have, it's time to select an option. You know that the client received an I.V. bolus of furosemide, a diuretic. You know that monitoring fluid intake and output is a key nursing intervention for a client taking a diuretic, a fact that eliminates options 1 and 3 (daily weight and serum sodium levels), narrowing the answer down to option 2 or 4 (24-hour intake and output or hourly urine output).

Can I use a lifeline?

You also know that the drug was administered by I.V. bolus, suggesting a rapid effect. (In fact, furosemide administered by I.V. bolus takes effect almost immediately.)

Monitoring the client's 24-hour intake and output would be appropriate for assessing the effects of repeated doses of furosemide. Hourly urine output, however, is most appropriate in this situation because it monitors the immediate effect of this rapid-acting drug.

Key strategies

Regardless of the type of question, four key strategies will help you determine the correct answer for each question. These strategies are:
- considering the nursing process
- referring to Maslow's hierarchy of needs
- reviewing client safety
- reflecting on principles of therapeutic communication.

Nursing process

One of the ways to answer a question is to apply the nursing process. Steps in the nursing process include:
- assessment
- diagnosis
- planning
- implementation
- evaluation.

First things first
The nursing process may provide insights that help you analyze a question. According to the nursing process, assessment comes before analysis, which comes before planning, which comes before implementation, which comes before evaluation.

You're halfway to the correct answer when you encounter a four-option, multiple-choice question that asks you to assess the situation and then provides two assessment options and two implementation options. You can immediately eliminate the implementation options, which then gives you, at worst, a 50-50 chance of selecting the correct answer. Use the following sample question to apply the nursing process:

A client returns from an endoscopic procedure during which he was sedated.

Before offering the client food, which action should the nurse take?
1. Assess the client's respiratory status.
2. Check the client's gag reflex.
3. Place the client in a side-lying position.
4. Have the client drink a few sips of water.

Assess before intervening
According to the nursing process, the nurse must assess a client before performing an intervention. Does the question indicate that the client has been properly assessed? No, it doesn't. Therefore, you can eliminate options 3 and 4 because they're both interventions.

That leaves options 1 and 2, both of which are assessments. Your nursing knowledge should tell you the correct answer — in this case, option 2. The sedation required for an endoscopic procedure may impair the client's gag reflex, so you would assess the gag reflex before giving food to the client to reduce the risk of aspiration and airway obstruction.

Final elimination
Why not select option 1, assessing the client's respiratory status? You might select this option but the question is specifically asking about offering the client food, an action that wouldn't be taken if the client's respiratory status was at all compromised. In this case, you're making a judgment based on the phrase, "Before offering the client food." If the question was trying to test your knowledge of respiratory depression following an endoscopic procedure, it probably wouldn't mention a function — such as giving food to a client — that clearly occurs only after the client's respiratory status has been stabilized.

Maslow's hierarchy

Knowledge of Maslow's hierarchy of needs can be a vital tool for establishing priorities on the NCLEX. Maslow's theory states that physiologic needs are the most basic human needs of all. Only after physiologic needs have been met can safety concerns be addressed. Only after

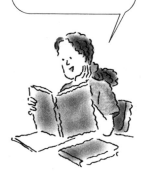

Say it 1,000 times: Studying for the exam is fun... studying for the exam is fun...

safety concerns are met can concerns involving love and belonging be addressed, and so forth. Apply the principles of Maslow's hierarchy of needs to the following sample question:

A client complains of severe pain 2 days after surgery. Which action should the nurse perform first?

1. Offer reassurance to the client that he will feel less pain tomorrow.
2. Allow the client time to verbalize his feelings.
3. Check the client's vital signs.
4. Administer an analgesic.

Phys before psych

In this example, two of the options — 3 and 4 — address physiologic needs. Options 1 and 2 address psychosocial concerns. According to Maslow, physiologic needs must be met before psychosocial needs, so you can eliminate options 1 and 2.

Final elimination

Now, use your nursing knowledge to choose the best answer from the two remaining options. In this case, option 3 is correct because the client's vital signs should be checked before administering an analgesic (assessment before intervention). When prioritizing according to Maslow's hierarchy, remember your ABCs — airway, breathing, circulation — to help you further prioritize. Check for a patent airway before addressing breathing. Check breathing before checking the health of the cardiovascular system.

One caveat...

Just because an option appears on the NCLEX doesn't mean it's a viable choice for the client referred to in the question. Always examine your choice in light of your knowledge and experience. Ask yourself, "Does this choice make sense for this client?" Allow yourself to eliminate choices — even ones that might normally take priority — if they don't make sense for a particular client's situation.

Client safety

As you might expect, client safety takes high priority on the NCLEX. You'll encounter

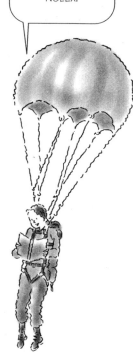

Client safety takes a high priority on the NCLEX.

many questions that can be answered by asking yourself, "Which answer will best ensure the safety of this client?" Use client safety criteria for situations involving laboratory values, drug administration, activities of daily living, or nursing care procedures.

Client first, equipment second

You may encounter a question in which some options address the client and others address the equipment. When in doubt, select an option relating to the client; never place equipment before a client.

For example, suppose a question asks what the nurse should do first when entering a client's room where an infusion pump alarm is sounding. If two options deal with the infusion pump, one with the infusion tubing, and another with the client's catheter insertion site, select the one relating to the client's catheter insertion site. Always check the client first; the equipment can wait.

Therapeutic communication

Some NCLEX questions focus on the nurse's ability to communicate effectively with the client. Therapeutic communication incorporates verbal or nonverbal responses and involves:

- listening to the client
- understanding the client's needs
- promoting clarification and insight about the client's condition.

Room for improvement

Like other NCLEX questions, those dealing with therapeutic communication commonly require choosing the best response. First, eliminate options that indicate the use of poor therapeutic communication techniques, such as those in which the nurse:

- tells the client what to do without regard to the client's feelings or desires (the "do this" response)
- asks a question that can be answered "yes" or "no," or with another one-syllable response
- seeks reasons for the client's behavior
- implies disapproval of the client's behavior
- offers false reassurances

- attempts to interpret the client's behavior rather than allow the client to verbalize his own feelings
- offers a response that focuses on the nurse, not the client.

Ah, that's better!

When answering NCLEX questions, look for responses that:
- allow the client time to think and reflect
- encourage the client to talk
- encourage the client to describe a particular experience
- reflect that the nurse has listened to the client, such as through paraphrasing the client's response.

Avoiding pitfalls

Even the most knowledgeable students can get tripped up on certain NCLEX questions. (See *A tricky question*, page 14.) Students commonly cite three areas that can be difficult for unwary test-takers:

 knowing the difference between the NCLEX and the "real world"

 delegating care

knowing laboratory values.

NCLEX versus the real world

Some students who take the NCLEX have extensive practical experience in health care. For example, many test-takers have worked as licensed practical nurses or nursing assistants. In one of those capacities, test-takers might have been exposed to less than optimum clinical practice and may carry those experiences over to the NCLEX.

However, the NCLEX is a textbook examination — not a test of clinical skills. Take the NCLEX with the understanding that what happens in the real world may differ from what the NCLEX and your nursing school say should happen.

Don't take shortcuts

If you've had practical experience in health care, you may know a quicker way to perform a procedure or tricks to get by when you don't have the right equipment. Situations such as staff shortages may force you to improvise. On the NCLEX, such scenarios can lead to trouble. Always check your practical experiences against textbook nursing care, taking care to select the response that follows the textbook.

Delegating care

On the NCLEX, you may encounter questions that assess your ability to delegate care. Delegating care involves coordinating the efforts of other health care workers to provide effective care for your client. On the NCLEX, you may be asked to assign duties to:
- licensed practical nurses or licensed vocational nurses
- direct-care workers, such as certified nursing assistants and personal care aides
- other support staff, such as nutrition assistants and housekeepers.

In addition, you'll be asked to decide when to notify a physician, a social worker, or another hospital staff member. In each case, you'll have to decide when, where, and how to delegate.

Shoulds and shouldn'ts

As a general rule, it's okay to delegate actions that involve stable clients or standard, unchanging procedures. Bathing, feeding, dressing, and transferring clients are examples of procedures that can be delegated.

Be careful not to delegate complicated or complex activities. In addition, don't delegate activities that involve assessment, evaluation, or your own nursing judgment. On the NCLEX and in the real world, these duties fall squarely on your shoulders. Make sure that you take primary responsibility for assessing and evaluating the client and for making decisions about the client's care. Never hand off those responsibilities to someone with less training.

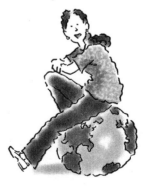

Remember, this is an exam, not the real world.

Normal laboratory values

- Blood urea nitrogen: 8 to 25 mg/dl
- Creatinine: 0.6 to 1.5 mg/dl
- Sodium: 135 to 145 mmol/L
- Potassium: 3.5 to 5.5 mEq/L
- Chloride: 97 to 110 mmol/L
- Glucose (fasting plasma): 70 to 110 mg/dl
- Hemoglobin
  Male: 13.8 to 17.2 g/dl
  Female: 12.1 to 15.1 g/dl
- Hematocrit
  Male: 40.7% to 50.3%
  Female: 36.1% to 44.3%

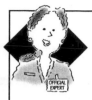

Advice from the experts

A tricky question

The NCLEX occasionally asks a particular kind of question called the "further teaching" question, which involves client-teaching situations. These questions can be tricky. You'll have to choose the response that suggests the client has *not* learned the correct information. Here's an example:

37. A client undergoes a total hip replacement. Which statement by the client indicates he requires further teaching?
1. "I'll need to keep several pillows between my legs at night."
2. "I'll need to remember not to cross my legs. It's such a bad habit."
3. "The occupational therapist is showing me how to use a 'sock puller' to help me get dressed."
4. "I don't know if I'll be able to get off that low toilet seat at home by myself."

The option you should choose here is 4 because it indicates that the client has a poor understanding of the precautions required after a total hip replacement and that he needs further teaching. Remember: If you see the phrase further teaching or further instruction, you're looking for a wrong answer by the client.

Calling in reinforcements

Deciding when to notify a physician, a social worker, or another hospital staff member is an important element of nursing care. On the NCLEX, however, choices that involve notifying the physician are usually incorrect. Remember that the NCLEX wants to see you, the nurse, at work.

If you're sure the correct answer is to notify the physician, though, make sure the client's safety has been addressed before notifying a physician or another staff member. On the NCLEX, the client's safety has a higher priority than notifying other health care providers.

Knowing laboratory values

Some NCLEX questions supply laboratory results without indicating normal levels. As a result, answering questions involving laboratory values requires you to have the normal range of the most common laboratory values memorized to make an informed decision (See *Normal laboratory values*.)

2 Strategies for success

Study preparations

If you're like most people preparing to take the NCLEX®, you're probably feeling nervous, anxious, or concerned. Keep in mind that most test takers pass the first time around.

Passing the test won't happen by accident, though; you'll need to prepare carefully and efficiently. To help jump-start your preparations:

- determine your strengths and weaknesses
- create a study schedule
- set realistic goals
- find an effective study space
- think positively
- start studying sooner rather than later.

Strengths and weaknesses

Most students recognize that, even at the end of their nursing studies, they know more about some topics than others. Because the NCLEX covers a broad range of material, you should make some decisions about how intensively you'll review each topic.

Make a list
Base those decisions on a list. Divide a sheet of paper in half vertically. On one side, list topics you think you know well. On the other side, list topics you feel less secure about. Pay no attention if one side is longer than the other. When you're done studying, you'll feel strong in every area.

Where the list comes from
To make sure your list reflects a comprehensive view of all the areas you studied in school, look at the contents page in the front of this book. For each topic listed, place it in the "know well" column or "needs review" column. Separating content areas this way shows immediately which topics need less study time and which need more time.

Scheduling study time

Study when you're most alert. Most people can identify a period of the day when they feel most alert. If you feel most alert and energized in the morning, for example, set aside sections of time in the morning for topics that need a lot of review. Then you can use the evening to study topics for which you just need some refreshing. The opposite is true as well; if you're more alert in the evening, study difficult topics at that time.

What you'll do, when
Set up a basic schedule for studying. Using a calendar or organizer, determine how much time remains before you'll take the NCLEX. (See *2 to 3 months before the NCLEX,* page 16.) Fill in the remaining days with specific times and topics to be studied. For example, you might schedule the respiratory system on a Tuesday morning and the GI system that afternoon. Remember to schedule difficult topics during your most alert times.

Keep in mind that you shouldn't fill each day with studying. Be realistic and set aside time for normal activities. Try to create ample study time before the NCLEX and then stick to the schedule. Allow some extra time in the schedule in case you get behind or come across a topic that requires extra review.

Set goals you can meet
Part of creating a schedule means setting goals you can accomplish. You no doubt studied a great deal in nursing school, and by now you have a sense of your own capabilities. Ask yourself, "How much can I cover in a day?" Set that amount of time aside and

To-do list

2 to 3 months before the NCLEX

With 2 to 3 months remaining before you plan to take the examination, take these steps:
• Establish a study schedule. Set aside ample time to study but also leave time for social activities, exercise, family or personal responsibilities, and other matters.
• Become knowledgeable about the NCLEX-RN, its content, the types of questions it asks, and the testing format.
• Begin studying your notes, texts, and other study materials.
• Answer some NCLEX practice questions to help you diagnose strengths and weaknesses as well as to become familiar with NCLEX-style questions.

then stay on task. You'll feel better about yourself — and your chances of passing the NCLEX — when you meet your goals regularly.

Study space

Find a space conducive to effective learning and then study there. Whatever you do, don't study with a television on in the room. Instead, find a quiet, inviting study space that:
• is located in a quiet, convenient place, away from normal traffic patterns
• contains a solid chair that encourages good posture (Avoid studying in bed; you'll be more likely to fall asleep and not accomplish your goals.)
• uses comfortable, soft lighting with which you can see clearly without eye strain
• has a temperature between 65° and 70° F
• contains flowers or green plants, familiar photos or paintings, and easy access to soft, instrumental background music.

Accentuate the positive
Consider taping positive messages around your study space. Make signs with words of encouragement, such as, "You can do it!" "Keep studying!" and "Remember the goal!" These upbeat messages can help keep you going when your attention begins to waver.

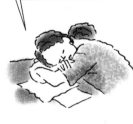

Approach your studying with enthusiasm, sincerity, and determination.

Maintaining concentration

When you're faced with reviewing the amount of information covered by the NCLEX, it's easy to become distracted and lose your concentration. When you lose concentration, you make less effective use of valuable study time. To stay focused, keep these tips in mind:
• Alternate the order of the subjects you study during the day to add variety to your study. Try alternating between topics you find most interesting and those you find least interesting.
• Approach your studying with enthusiasm, sincerity, and determination.
• Once you've decided to study, begin immediately. Don't let anything interfere with your thought processes once you've begun.
• Concentrate on accomplishing one task at a time, to the exclusion of everything else.
• Don't try to do two things at once, such as studying and watching television or conversing with friends.
• Work continuously without interruption for a while, but don't study for such a long period that the whole experience becomes grueling or boring.
• Allow time for periodic breaks to give yourself a change of pace. Use these breaks to ease your transition into studying a new topic.

- When studying in the evening, wind down from your studies slowly. Don't progress directly from studying to sleeping.

Taking care of yourself

Never neglect your physical and mental well-being in favor of longer study hours. Maintaining physical and mental health are critical for success in taking the NCLEX. (See *4 to 6 weeks before the NCLEX*.)

A few simple rules
You can increase your likelihood of passing the test by following these simple health rules:
- Get plenty of rest. You can't think deeply or concentrate for long periods when you're tired.
- Eat nutritious meals. Maintaining your energy level is impossible when you're under-nourished.
- Exercise regularly. Regular exercise, preferably 30 minutes daily, helps you work harder and think more clearly. As a result, you'll study more efficiently and increase the likelihood of success on the all-important NCLEX.

Memory powers, activate!
If you're having trouble concentrating but would rather push through than take a break, try making your studying more active by reading out loud. Active studying can renew

your powers of concentration. By reading review material out loud to yourself, you're engaging your ears as well as your eyes — and making your studying a more active process. Hearing the material out loud also fosters memory and subsequent recall.

You can also rewrite in your own words a few of the more difficult concepts you're reviewing. Explaining these concepts in writing forces you to think through the material and can jump-start your memory.

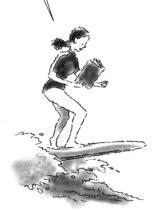

> Kowabonga! Regular exercise helps you work harder and think more clearly.

Study schedule

When you were creating your schedule, you might have asked yourself, "How long should I study? One hour at a stretch? Two hours? Three?" To make the best use of your study time, you'll need to answer those questions.

Optimum study time

Consider studying in 20- to 30-minute intervals with a short break in-between. You remember the material you study at the beginning and end of a session best and tend to remember less material studied in the middle of the session. The total length of time in each study session depends on you and the amount of material you need to cover.

To-do list

4 to 6 weeks before the NCLEX

With 4 to 6 weeks remaining before you plan to take the examination, take these steps:
- Focus on your areas of weakness. That way, you'll have time to review these areas again before the test date.
- Find a study partner or form a study group.
- Take a practice test to gauge your skill level early.
- Take time to eat, sleep, exercise, and socialize to avoid burnout.

To-do list

1 week before the NCLEX

With 1 week remaining before the NCLEX examination, take these steps:
- Take a review test to measure your progress.
- Record key ideas and principles on note cards or audiotapes.
- Rest, eat well, and avoid thinking about the examination during nonstudy times.
- Treat yourself to one special event. You've been working hard, and you deserve it!

To thine own self be true

So what's the answer? It doesn't matter as long as you determine what's best for you. At the beginning of your NCLEX study schedule, try study periods of varying lengths. Pay close attention to those that seem more successful.

Remember that you're a trained nurse who is competent at assessment. Think of yourself as a client, and assess your own progress. Then implement the strategy that works best for you.

Studying getting dull? Get creative and liven it up.

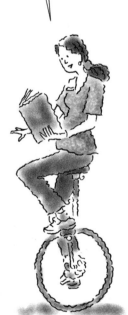

Finding time to study

So does that mean that short sections of time are useless? Not at all. We all have spaces in our day that might otherwise be dead time. (See *1 week before the NCLEX.*) These are perfect times to review for the NCLEX but not to cover new material because, by the time you get deep into new material, your time will be over. Always keep some flash cards or a small notebook handy for situations when you have a few extra minutes.

You'll be amazed how many short sessions you can find in a day and how much reviewing you can do in 5 minutes. The following occasions offer short stretches of time you can use for studying:
- eating breakfast
- waiting for, or riding on, a train or bus
- waiting in line at the bank, post office, bookstore, or other places
- using exercise equipment, such as a treadmill.

Creative studying

Even when you study in a perfect study space and concentrate better than ever, studying for the NCLEX can get a little, well, dull. Even people with terrific study habits occasionally feel bored or sluggish. That's why it's important to have some creative tricks in your study bag to liven up your studying during those down times.

Creative studying doesn't have to be hard work. It involves making efforts to alter your study habits a bit. Some techniques that might help include studying with a partner or group and creating flash cards or other audiovisual study tools.

Study partners

Studying with a partner or group of students (3 or 4 students at most) can be an excellent way to energize your studying. Working with a partner allows you to test each other on the material you've reviewed. Your partner can give you encouragement and motivation. Perhaps most important, working with a partner can provide a welcome break from solitary studying.

What to look for in a partner

Exercise some care when choosing a study partner or assembling a study group. A partner who doesn't fit your needs won't help you make the most of your study time. Look for a partner who:

• possesses similar goals to yours. For example, someone taking the NCLEX at approximately the same date who feels the same sense of urgency as you do might make an excellent partner.

• possesses about the same level of knowledge as you. Tutoring someone can sometimes help you learn, but partnering should be give-and-take so both partners can gain knowledge.

• can study without excess chatting or interruptions. Socializing is an important part of creative study but, remember, you still have to pass the NCLEX — so stay serious!

Audiovisual tools

Using flash cards and other audiovisual tools fosters retention and makes learning and reviewing fun.

Flash Gordon? No, it's Flash Card!

Flash cards can provide you with an excellent study tool. The process of writing material on a flash card will help you remember it. In addition, flash cards are small and easily portable, perfect for those 5-minute slivers of time that show up during the day.

Creating a flash card should be fun. Use magic markers, highlighters, and other colorful tools to make them visually stimulating. The more effort you put into creating your flash cards, the better you'll remember the material contained on the cards.

Other visual tools

Flowcharts, drawings, diagrams, and other image-oriented study aids can also help you learn material more effectively. Substituting images for text can be a great way to give your eyes a break and recharge your brain. Remember to use vivid colors to make your creations visually engaging.

Hear's the thing

If you learn more effectively when you hear information rather than see it, consider recording key ideas using a handheld tape recorder. Recording information helps promote memory because you say the information aloud when taping and then listen to it when playing it back. Like flash cards, tapes are portable and perfect for those short study periods during the day. (See *The day before the NCLEX*.)

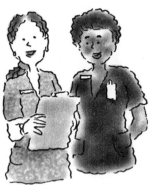

It wasn't easy finding a partner who has the same study habits I do.

To-do list

The day before the NCLEX

With 1 day before the NCLEX examination, take these steps:

• Drive to the test site, review traffic patterns, and find out where to park. If your route to the test site occurs during heavy traffic or if you're expecting bad weather, set aside extra time to ensure prompt arrival.

• Do something relaxing during the day.

• Avoid concentrating on the test.

• Eat well and avoid dwelling on the NCLEX during nonstudy periods.

• Call a supportive friend or relative for some last-minute words of encouragement.

• Get plenty of rest the night before and allow plenty of time in the morning.

To-do list

The day of the NCLEX

On the day of the NCLEX examination, take these steps:
• Get up early.
• Wear comfortable clothes, preferably with layers you can adjust to fit the room temperature.
• Leave your house early.
• Arrive at the test site early with required paperwork in hand.
• Avoid looking at your notes as you wait for your test computer.
• Listen carefully to the instructions given before entering the test room.

Good luck!

> Practice questions provide an excellent means of marking your progress.

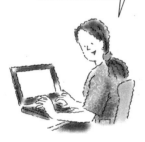

Practice questions

Practice questions should be an important part of your NCLEX study strategy. Practice questions can improve your studying by helping you review material and familiarizing yourself with the exact style of questions you'll encounter on the NCLEX.

Practice at the beginning
Consider working through some practice questions as soon as you begin studying for the NCLEX. For example, you might try a few of the questions that appear at the end of each chapter in this book.

If you do well, you probably know the material contained in that chapter fairly well and can spend less time reviewing that particular topic. If you have trouble with the questions, spend extra study time on that topic.

I'm getting there
Practice questions can also provide an excellent means of marking your progress. Don't worry if you have trouble answering the first few practice questions you take; you'll need time to adjust to the way the questions are asked. Eventually you'll become accustomed to the question format and begin to focus more on the questions themselves.

If you make practice questions a regular part of your study regimen, you'll be able to notice areas in which you're improving. You can then adjust your study time accordingly.

Practice makes perfect
As you near the examination date, you should increase the number of NCLEX practice questions you answer at one sitting. This will enable you to approximate the experience of taking the actual NCLEX examination. Note that 75 questions is the minimum number of questions you'll be asked on the actual NCLEX examination. By gradually tackling larger practice tests, you'll increase your confidence, build test-taking endurance, and strengthen the concentration skills that enable you to succeed on the NCLEX. (See *The day of the NCLEX.*)

Part II   Review

Brush up on key concepts

Growth and development are fundamental concepts in pediatric nursing. Each developmental stage presents unique client care challenges in such areas as nutrition, language, safety education, medication administration, and pain management.

You can review the major points of this chapter by consulting the *Cheat sheet* on page 24.

An infant's developmental milestones

A child is considered an infant from the time he's born until age 1. During this time, development is marked by five major periods:
- the neonatal period (up to 28 days)
- 1 to 4 months
- 5 to 6 months
- 7 to 9 months
- 10 to 12 months.

NEONATAL PERIOD
The neonatal period covers the time from birth to age 28 days.

Reflexes reign
During this period, you'll note these findings:
- Head and chest circumferences are approximately equal.
- Behavior is under reflex control.
- Extremities are flexed.
- Vision is poor (the neonate fixates momentarily on light).
- Hearing and touch are well developed.
- When prone, the neonate can lift the head slightly off the bed.

Rapid pulse and respiration
- Normal pulse rate ranges from 110 to 160 beats/minute.
- Normal respiratory rate is 32 to 60 breaths/minute.
- Respirations are irregular and use the diaphragm and abdominal muscles.
- The neonate is an obligate nose breather.

Hot and cold
- Normal blood pressure is 82/46 mm Hg.
- Temperature regulation is poor.

1 TO 4 MONTHS
At age 3 months, the most primitive reflexes begin to disappear, except for the protective and postural reflexes (blink, parachute, cough, swallow, and gag reflexes), which remain for life. The infant reaches out voluntarily but is uncoordinated.

Heads up
The posterior fontanel closes by 2 to 3 months of age. In addition, the infant:
- begins to hold up his head
- begins to put hand to mouth
- develops binocular vision
- cries to express needs
- smiles (the instinctual smile appears at 2 months and the social smile at 3 months)
- laughs in response to the environment (at 4 months).

5 TO 6 MONTHS
At 5 to 6 months, birth weight doubles. In addition, the infant:
- rolls over from stomach to back
- cries when the parent leaves
- attempts to crawl when prone
- voluntarily grasps and releases objects.

7 TO 9 MONTHS
At 7 to 9 months, the infant can self-feed crackers and a bottle. When physically and

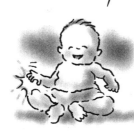

Ha, ha. That's a good one. At 4 months, I laugh in response to the environment.

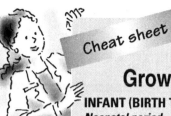

Growth and development refresher

INFANT (BIRTH TO AGE 1)

Neonatal period
- Behavior is under reflex control.
- Extremities are flexed.
- Normal pulse rate ranges from 110 to 160 beats/minute.
- Normal respiratory rate is 32 to 60 breaths/minute. Respirations are irregular and use the diaphragm and abdominal muscles; the neonate is an obligate nose breather.
- Normal blood pressure is 82/46 mm Hg.
- Temperature regulation is poor.

1 to 4 months
- The posterior fontanel closes.
- The infant begins to hold up his head.
- The infant cries to express needs.

5 to 6 months
- The infant rolls over from stomach to back.
- The infant cries when the parent leaves.

7 to 9 months
- The infant sits alone with assistance.
- The infant creeps on the hands and knees the with belly off the floor.
- The infant verbalizes all vowels and most consonants but speaks no intelligible words.
- Fear of strangers appears to peak during the 8th month.

10 to 12 months
- The infant holds onto furniture while walking (cruising) at age 10 months, walks with support at age 11 months, and stands alone and takes first steps at age 12 months.
- The infant says "mama" and "dada" and responds to own name at age 10 months; he can say about five words but understands many more.

TODDLER (AGES 1 TO 3)
- Normal pulse rate is 100 beats/minute.
- Normal respiratory rate is 26 breaths/minute.
- Normal blood pressure is 99/64 mm Hg.
- Separation anxiety arises.
- The child is toilet-trained; day dryness is achieved between ages 18 months and 3 years and night dryness between ages 2 and 5.

PRESCHOOL CHILD (AGES 3 TO 5)
- Normal pulse rate ranges from 90 to 100 beats/minute.
- Normal respiratory rate is 25 breaths/minute.
- Normal blood pressure ranges from 85/60 to 90/70 mm Hg.
- The child may express fear of mutilation or intrusion of his body, animal noises, new experiences, and the dark.

SCHOOL-AGE CHILD (AGES 5 TO 12)
- Normal pulse rate ranges from 75 to 115 beats/minute.
- Normal blood pressure ranges from 106/69 to 117/76 mm Hg.
- Normal respiratory rate ranges from 20 to 25 breaths/minute.
- The child plays with peers, initially prefers friends of the same sex, develops a first true friendship, and develops a sense of belonging, cooperation, and compromise.
- The child learns to read and spell.
- Accidents are a major cause of death and disability during this period.

ADOLESCENT (AGES 12 TO 18)
- The adolescent experiences puberty-related changes in body structure and psychosocial adjustment.
- Peers influence behavior and values.
- Vital signs approach adult levels.

emotionally ready, the infant can be weaned. The infant understands the word "no." Efforts to enforce discipline are appropriate at this time. Fear of strangers appears to peak during the 8th month. Attempts to assess breath and heart sounds should be made while the mother holds the infant.

Sit, creep, and prespeak
In addition, the infant:
- sits alone with assistance

Infants and nutrition

Here's a rundown of primary nutrition guidelines for a child's first year of life:
- Begin with formula (containing iron) or breast milk; give no more than 30 oz (887 ml) of formula each day.
- Iron supplements may be necessary after 4 months.
- No solid foods should be given for the first 6 months.
- Provide rice cereal as the first solid food; follow with other cereals (except wheat-based products).
- Yellow and green vegetables may be given at 8 to 9 months.
- Provide noncitrus fruits at 6½ to 8 months, followed by citrus fruits late in the first year.
- Give junior foods or soft table foods after 9 months.

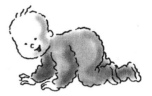

> Goo goo. Ga ga. (Translation: I verbalize all vowels and most consonants but don't articulate intelligible words.)

- creeps on the hands and knees with the belly off the floor
- verbalizes all vowels and most consonants but doesn't articulate intelligible words.

10 TO 12 MONTHS

At 10 to 12 months, birth weight triples and birth length increases about 50%. The anterior fontanel normally closes between ages 9 and 18 months. In addition, the infant:
- may walk while holding onto furniture (cruising) at age 10 months
- walks with support at age 11 months, and stands alone and takes first steps at age 12 months
- says "mama" and "dada" and responds to own name at age 10 months
- can say about five words but understands many more
- is ready to be weaned from the bottle and breast. (See *Infants and nutrition*.)

Toddler developmental milestones

The toddler period includes ages 1 to 3. This is a slow growth period with a weight gain of 4 to 9 lb (2 to 4 kg) over 2 years.

Vital measurements
- Normal pulse rate is 100 beats/minute.
- Normal respiratory rate is 26 breaths/minute.
- Normal blood pressure is 99/64 mm Hg.

Me, myself, and I
The toddler exhibits the following behavioral and psychological characteristics:
- egocentricity
- frequent temper tantrums, especially when confronted with the conflict of achieving autonomy and relinquishing dependence on others
- follows the parent wherever he or she goes
- experiences separation anxiety
- lacks the concept of sharing
- prefers solitary play and has little interaction with others; this progresses to parallel play (toddler plays alongside but not with another child).

Look, Ma
The toddler:
- plants his feet wide apart and walks by age 15 months
- climbs stairs at 21 months, runs and jumps by age 2, and rides a tricycle by age 3
- uses at least 400 words as well as two- to three-word phrases and comprehends many more (by age 2)
- uses about 11,000 words (by age 3)
- undergoes toilet training; day dryness should be achieved between ages 18 months and 3 years and night dryness between ages 2 and 5.

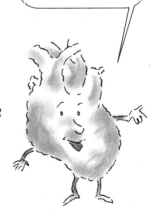

> I mellow with age. At ages 1 to 3, my rate is 100 beats/minute. By ages 3 to 5, it may slow to 90 beats/minute.

Preschool developmental milestones

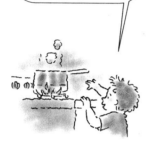

Look out. Accidents are the major cause of school-age disability.

The preschool period encompasses ages 3 to 5. Slow growth continues during this period. Birth length doubles by age 4.

Vital measurements
• Normal pulse rate ranges from 90 to 100 beats/minute.
• Normal respiratory rate is 25 breaths/minute.
• Normal blood pressure ranges from 85/60 to 90/70 mm Hg.

Facing fear
The child may begin to express fear. Anticipate the child's fear of mutilation or intrusion of his body, animal noises, new experiences, and the dark. Provide adhesive bandages for cuts because the child may fear losing blood. Using dolls for role-playing may reduce the preschool child's anxiety.

Playtime progress
The child:
• exhibits parallel play, associative play, and group play in activities with few or no rules and independent play accompanied by sharing or talking
• develops a body image
• may count but not understand what numbers mean
• may recognize some letters of the alphabet
• dresses without help but may be unable to tie shoes
• speaks in grammatically correct, complete sentences
• gets along without parents for short periods.

School-age developmental milestones

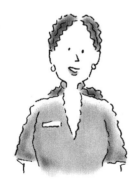

As the child moves into adolescence, nutritional needs increase significantly — remember, most eating disorders emerge during adolescence.

The school-age years are defined as ages 5 to 12.

Beat, blood, breath
• Normal pulse rate ranges from 75 to 115 beats/minute.
• Normal blood pressure ranges from 106/69 to 117/76 mm Hg.
• Normal respiratory rate ranges from 20 to 25 breaths/minute.

Watch out
• Accidents are a major cause of death and disability during this period.
• Height increases about 2" (5 cm) a year, and weight doubles between ages 6 and 12.
• The first primary tooth is displaced by a permanent tooth at age 6, and permanent teeth erupt by age 12 except for final molars.
• Vision matures by age 6.

Best friends forever
The child:
• engages in cooperative play
• plays with peers, initially prefers friends of the same sex, develops a first true friendship, and develops a sense of belonging, cooperation, and compromise
• develops concepts of time and place, cause and effect, reversibility, conversation, and numbers
• learns to read and spell
• engages in fantasy play and daydreaming.

Adolescent developmental milestones

Ages 12 to 18 encompass the adolescent period. Adolescence is a period of rapid growth characterized by puberty-related changes in body structure and psychosocial adjustment.

What's happening to me?
During adolescence, these changes are noted:
• Vital signs approach adult levels.
• Peers influence behavior and values.
• Nutritional needs increase significantly.

Ch..ch..changes

Other milestones in adolescent development include:

• increased ability to engage in abstract thinking and to analyze, synthesize, and use logic

• increased attraction to the opposite sex (or same sex)

• breast development in females (the first sign of puberty; begins at about age 9 with the bud stage; may be asymmetrical)

• the onset of menses in females (between ages 8 and 16; possibly irregular initially)

• testicular enlargement in males (the first sign of puberty).

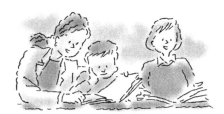

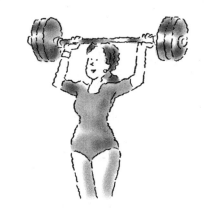

Pump up on practice questions

1. A parent brings a 19-month-old toddler to the clinic for a well-child checkup. When palpating the toddler's fontanels, the nurse should expect to find:

    1. closed anterior fontanel and open posterior fontanel.

    2. open anterior fontanel and closed posterior fontanel.

    3. closed anterior and posterior fontanels.

    4. open anterior and posterior fontanels.

Answer: 3. By age 18 months, the anterior and posterior fontanels should be closed. The diamond-shaped anterior fontanel normally closes between ages 9 and 18 months. The triangular posterior fontanel normally closes between ages 2 and 3 months.

➡ NCLEX keys

Client needs category: Health promotion and maintenance

Client needs subcategory: None

Cognitive level: Knowledge

2. A nurse is instructing a mother about the nutritional needs of her full-term, breast-feeding infant age 2 months. Which response shows that the mother understands the infant's dietary needs?

    1. "We won't start any new foods now."

    2. "We'll start the baby on skim milk."

3. "We'll introduce cereal into the diet now."
4. "We should add new fruits to the diet one at a time."

Answer: 1. Because breast milk provides all the nutrients that a full-term infant needs for the first 6 months, the parents shouldn't introduce new foods into the infant's diet at this point. They shouldn't provide skim milk because it doesn't have sufficient fat for infant growth. The parents also shouldn't provide solid foods, such as cereal and fruit, before age 6 months because the infant's GI tract doesn't tolerate them well.

➡ *NCLEX keys*
Client needs category: Health promotion and maintenance
Client needs subcategory: None
Cognitive level: Application

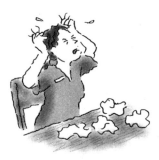

3. A nurse is teaching the parents of a 6-month-old infant about usual growth and development. Which statements about infant development are true? Select all that apply.
1. A 6-month-old infant has difficulty holding objects.
2. A 6-month-old infant can usually roll from prone to supine and supine to prone positions.
3. A teething ring is appropriate for a 6-month-old infant.
4. Stranger anxiety usually peaks at age 12 to 18 months.
5. Head lag is commonly noted in infants at age 6 months.
6. Lack of visual coordination usually resolves by age 6 months.

Answer: 2, 3, 6. Gross motor skills of the 6-month old infant include rolling from front to back and back to front. Teething usually begins around age 6 months and, therefore, a teething ring is appropriate. Visual coordination is usually resolved by age 6 months. At age 6 months, fine motor skills include purposeful grasps. Stranger anxiety normally peaks at age 8 months. A 6-month-old infant should have good head control and no longer display head lag when pulled up to a sitting position.

➡ *NCLEX keys*
Client needs category: Health promotion and maintenance
Client needs subcategory: None
Cognitive level: Application

4. A preschooler is admitted to the hospital the day before scheduled surgery. This is the child's first hospitalization. Which action will best help reduce the child's anxiety about the upcoming surgery?
1. Begin preoperative teaching immediately.
2. Describe preoperative and postoperative procedures in detail.
3. Give the child dolls and medical equipment to play out the experience.
4. Explain that the child will be put to sleep during surgery and won't feel anything.

Answer: 3. By playing with medical equipment and acting out the experience with dolls, the preschooler can begin to reduce anxiety. The nurse should schedule teaching shortly before surgery because preschoolers have little concept of time and because a delay between teaching and surgery may increase anxiety by giving the child time to worry. Detailed explanations are inappropriate for this developmental stage and may promote anxiety. The nurse should avoid such phrases as "put to sleep" because they might have a negative meaning to the child.

➡ *NCLEX keys*
Client needs category: Psychosocial integrity
Client needs subcategory: None
Cognitive level: Application

5. Before a well checkup in the pediatrician's office, an 8-month-old infant is sitting contentedly on the mother's lap, chewing a toy. When preparing to examine this infant, which step should the nurse do first?

1. Obtain body weight.
2. Auscultate heart and breath sounds.
3. Check pupillary response.
4. Measure the head circumference.

Answer: 2. Heart and lung auscultation shouldn't distress the infant, so it should be done early in the assessment. Placing a tape measure on the infant's head, shining a light in the eyes, or undressing the infant before weighing may cause distress, making the rest of the examination more difficult.

➡ *NCLEX keys*
Client needs category: Health promotion and maintenance
Client needs subcategory: None
Cognitive level: Application

6. A nurse is teaching a mother who plans to discontinue breast-feeding after 5 months. The nurse should advise her to include which food in her infant's diet?

1. Iron-rich formula and baby food
2. Whole milk and baby food
3. Skim milk and baby food
4. Iron-rich formula only

Answer: 4. The American Academy of Pediatrics recommends that infants at age 5 months should receive iron-rich formula and that they shouldn't receive solid food — even baby food— until age 6 months. The Academy doesn't recommend whole milk until age 12 months or skim milk until after age 2 years.

➡ *NCLEX keys*
Client needs category: Health promotion and maintenance
Client needs subcategory: None
Cognitive level: Application

7. A mother tells the nurse that her 22-month-old child says "no" to everything. When scolded, the toddler becomes angry and starts crying loudly, but then immediately wants to be held. What should the nurse tell the mother?

1. "The toddler isn't effectively coping with stress."
2. "The toddler's need for affection isn't being met."
3. "This is normal behavior for a 2-year-old child."
4. "This behavior suggests the need for counseling."

Answer: 3. Because toddlers are confronted with the conflict of achieving autonomy yet relinquishing the much-enjoyed dependence on the affection of others, their negativism is a necessary assertion of self-control. Therefore, this behavior is a normal part of the child's growth and development. Nothing about the behavior indicates that the child is under stress, isn't receiving sufficient affection, or requires counseling.

➡ *NCLEX keys*
Client needs category: Health promotion and maintenance
Client needs subcategory: None
Cognitive level: Application

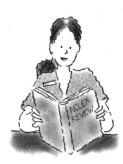

8. A mother asks the nurse how she will know when her son is entering puberty. The nurse tells the mother to watch for which sign?

1. Appearance of pubic hair
2. Appearance of axillary hair
3. Testicular enlargement
4. Nocturnal emissions

Answer: 3. Testicular enlargement signifies the onset of puberty in the male adolescent. Then sexual development progresses, causing the appearance of pubic hair and axillary hair and the onset of nocturnal emissions.

Client needs category: Health promotion and maintenance
Client needs subcategory: None
Cognitive level: Application

9. A nurse is teaching the parents of a school-age child. Which teaching topic should take priority?
1. Accident prevention
2. Keeping a night light on to allay fears
3. Normalcy of fears about body integrity
4. Encouraging the child to dress without help

Answer: 1. Accidents are the major cause of death and disability during the school-age years. Therefore accident prevention should take priority when teaching parents of school-age children. Preschool children are afraid of the dark, have fears concerning body integrity, and should be encouraged to dress without help (with the exception of tying shoes), but none of these should take priority over accident prevention.

Client needs category: Health promotion and maintenance
Client needs subcategory: None
Cognitive level: Analysis

10. A mother brings her infant to the pediatrician's office for his 2-week-old checkup. The nurse is evaluating whether the mother has understood teaching points discussed during a previous visit. Which statement indicates that further teaching is needed?
1. "I don't understand why my baby doesn't look at me."
2. "I know I should keep my baby's nasal passages clear."
3. "I should limit my baby's exposure during bath time."
4. "I should cover my baby's head when he's wet or cold."

Answer: 1. Further teaching is indicated if the mother states that she doesn't understand why her 2-week-old infant doesn't look at her. The infant at this period of development has poor vision, is only able to fixate on light momentarily, and can't distinguish objects. The 2-week-old infant should have his nasal passages kept clear because he's an obligate nose breather, he should have limited exposure at bath time, and he should have his head covered when he's wet or cold.

Client needs category: Health promotion and maintenance
Client needs subcategory: None
Cognitive level: Analysis

Reviewing this chapter was good preparation for the pediatric chapters ahead. Good luck!

4 Cardiovascular system

Brush up on key concepts

The cardiovascular system consists of the heart and central and peripheral blood vessels. A child's cardiovascular system closely resembles that of an adult. The system's main functions are to pump and circulate blood throughout the body.

At any time, you can review the major points of this chapter by consulting the *Cheat sheet* on pages 32 and 33.

Communication breakdown

A child may have congenital heart defects that impair the movement of blood between the heart's chambers. For example, some congenital heart defects cause a **left-to-right shunt,** in which increased pressure on the left side of the heart forces blood back to the right side. This can lead to tissue hypertrophy on the right side and increased blood flow to the lungs.

Not closed

The blood vessels surrounding the heart may also suffer congenital defects. Soon after birth, the ductus arteriosus (located between the aorta and the pulmonary artery) normally closes. If it doesn't, the infant may experience **patent ductus arteriosus,** in which blood shunts from the aorta to the pulmonary artery. If a large patent ductus arteriosus remains uncorrected, pressure within the pulmonary arteries may increase dramatically and cause blood to flow from the right side of the heart to the left, eventually leading to heart failure.

Keep abreast of diagnostic tests

The most important tests used to diagnose cardiovascular disorders include cardiac catheterization and echocardiography.

Cardiac cath

In **cardiac catheterization,** a catheter is inserted into an artery or vein (in the arm or leg) and advanced to the heart. This procedure is used to:
* evaluate ventricular function
* measure heart pressures
* measure the blood's oxygen saturation level.

Nursing actions

Before the procedure
* Explain the procedure to the child and parents.
* Describe the sensations the child will experience.
* Weigh the child.
* Check the child's color, pulse rate, blood pressure, and temperature of extremities.
* Check the child's activity level.
* Prepare the child based on his developmental level. Show where the catheter is inserted. Make a security object (for example, a teddy bear or toy) available.

After the procedure
* Keep the affected extremity immobile after catheterization to prevent hemorrhage.
* Keep the catheter site clean and dry, and monitor for hematoma formation.
* Monitor peripheral pulses, temperature, and the color of the affected extremity.
* Compare postcatheterization assessment data to precatheterization baseline data, comparing all four extremities.

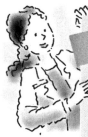

Cheat sheet

Cardiovascular system refresher

ACYANOTIC HEART DEFECTS

Key signs and symptoms
- Congested cough
- Diaphoresis
- Fatigue
- Machinelike heart murmur (in patent ductus arteriosus)
- Mild cyanosis (if the condition leads to right-sided heart failure)
- Respiratory distress
- Tachycardia
- Tachypnea
- Poor oral intake

Key test results
- Echocardiography and cardiac catheterization confirm the type of defect.

Key treatments
- Cardiac glycoside: digoxin (Lanoxin)
- Diuretic: furosemide (Lasix)
- Surgical repair

Key interventions
- Monitor vital signs, pulse oximetry, and intake and output.
- Assess cardiovascular and respiratory status.
- Take the apical pulse for 1 minute before giving digoxin, and withhold the drug if the heart rate is below 100 beats/minute.
- Monitor fluid status, enforcing fluid restrictions as appropriate.

CYANOTIC HEART DEFECTS

Key signs and symptoms
- Clubbing
- Cyanosis
- History of poor feeding
- Poor weight gain
- Failure to thrive
- Irritability
- Tachycardia
- Tachypnea

Key test results
- Arterial blood gas shows diminished arterial oxygen saturation.

Key treatments
- For transposition of the great vessels or arteries: corrective surgery (called *arterial switch*) performed in the first few days of life
- For tetralogy of Fallot: complete repair or palliative treatment with Blalock-Taussig anastomosis; client's age at repair depends on the degree of pulmonic stenosis
- For hypoplastic left-heart syndrome: surgical repair in three stages (Norwood procedure I, II, and III)
- For truncus arteriosis: Norwood procedure I, II, and III

Key interventions
- Assess cardiovascular and respiratory status.
- Monitor vital signs and pulse oximetry
- Monitor intake and output.
- Administer prophylactic antibiotics.

HEART FAILURE

Key signs and symptoms
- Fussiness
- Lethargy
- Poor feeding
- Poor weight gain

Key test results
- Chest X-ray shows fluid in lungs and possible consolidation.
- Echocardiogram may show decreased or increased cardiac output and poor filling.
- Exercise stress test (in children older than 4) indicates poor activity tolerance.

Key treatments
- Diuretics: furosemide (Lasix), metolazone (Zaroxolyn)
- Cardiac glycoside: digoxin (Lanoxin)
- Inotropic agents: dopamine, dobutamine
- Surgery, if caused by congenital defect
- Extracorporeal membrane oxygenation, in severe cases

Key interventions
- Assess cardiovascular status, including vital signs and hemodynamic variables.
- Assess respiratory status and oxygenation.

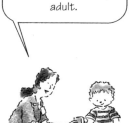

A child's cardiovascular system closely resembles that of an adult.

Cardiovascular system refresher (continued)

HEART FAILURE (CONTINUED)
- Keep the child in semi-Fowler's position.
- Administer oxygen.
- Weigh the child daily.

HYPERTROPHIC CARDIOMYOPATHY
Key signs and symptoms
- Heart failure, in infants
- Murmur, third heart sounds
- Sudden cardiac death
- Syncope, with exertion

Key test results
- Electrocardiogram (ECG) shows left ventricular hypertrophy and nonspecific changes.

Key treatments
- Dual chamber pacing
- Beta-adrenergic blockers: propranolol (Inderal), nadolol (Corgard), metoprolol (Lopressor)
- Calcium channel blockers: verapamil (Calan), diltiazem (Cardizem)
- Diuretics: furosemide (Lasix), spirolactone

Key interventions
- Monitor ECG.
- Assess cardiovascular status, vital signs, and hemodynamic variables.

- Administer oxygen and medications, as prescribed.

RHEUMATIC FEVER
Key signs and symptoms
Major rheumatic fever
- Carditis
- Chorea
- Erythema marginatum (temporary, disk-shaped, nonpruritic, reddened macules that fade in the center, leaving raised margins)
- Polyarthritis
- Subcutaneous nodules

Key test results
- Erythrocyte sedimentation rate is increased.
- Electrocardiogram shows prolonged PR interval.

Key treatments
- Bed rest during fever and until sedimentation rate returns to normal
- Antibiotic: penicillin to prevent additional damage from future attacks

Key interventions
- Monitor vital signs and intake and output.

- Ensure adequate intake (I.V. and oral) to compensate for blood loss during the procedure, nothing-by-mouth status, and diuretic action of some dyes used.

Heart mapping
Echocardiography is a noninvasive test used to evaluate the size, shape, and motion of cardiac structures by recording the echoes of ultrasonic waves of those structures.

Nursing actions
- Explain the procedure to the child and parents.
- Explain to the child and parents that the child may have to lie on his left side, inhale and exhale slowly, or hold his breath at intervals during the test.

Polish up on client care

Major pediatric cardiovascular disorders include acyanotic heart defects, cyanotic heart defects, heart failure, hypertrophic cardiomyopathy, and rheumatic fever. (See *From high to low,* page 34.)

Acyanotic heart defects

In an acyanotic defect, blood is usually shunted from the left (oxygenated) side to the right (unoxygenated) side of the heart. Acyanotic defects include:
- **aortic stenosis** — a narrowing or fusion of the aortic valves, interfering with left ventricular outflow

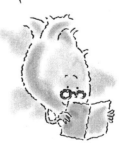

Well, I'll be. Mild cyanosis can occur in an acyanotic heart defect.

From high to low

When cardiac anomalies involve communication — movement of blood through a common opening — between chambers, blood flows from areas of high pressure to areas of low pressure. For example, a left-to-right shunt may result when increased pressure on the left side of the heart causes increased blood flow to the right.

DEFECTS THAT DON'T INVOLVE CHAMBERS
In defects that don't involve the cardiac chambers, blood can also flow from high-pressure to low-pressure areas. In patent ductus arteriosus, for instance, the ductus arteriosus (located between the aorta and pulmonary artery) remains open after birth. This opening causes blood to shunt from the aorta to the pulmonary artery.

• **atrial septal defect** — a defect stemming from a patent foramen ovale or the failure of a septum to develop completely between the atria
• **coarctation of the aorta** — a narrowing of the aortic arch, usually distal to the ductus arteriosus beyond the left subclavian artery
• **patent ductus arteriosus** — a defect resulting from the failure of the ductus to close, causing shunting of blood to the pulmonary artery
• **pulmonary artery stenosis** — a narrowing or fusing of valve leaflets at the entrance of the pulmonary artery, interfering with right ventricular outflow
• **ventricular septal defect** — a defect occurring when the ventricular septum fails to complete its formation between the ventricles, resulting in a left-to-right shunt

CAUSES
• Defects between structures that inhibit blood flow to the system or alter pulmonary resistance
• Defects in the septa that lead to a left-to-right shunt

ASSESSMENT FINDINGS
• Congested cough
• Diaphoresis
• Fatigue
• Frequent respiratory infections
• Hepatomegaly
• Machinelike heart murmur (in patent ductus arteriosus)
• Mild cyanosis (if the condition leads to right-sided heart failure)

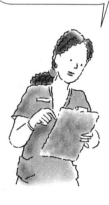

Echocardiography and cardiac catheterization distinguish the various acyanotic heart defects.

• Poor growth and development as a result of increased energy expenditure for breathing
• Poor oral intake
• Respiratory distress
• Tachycardia
• Tachypnea

DIAGNOSTIC TEST RESULTS
Echocardiography and cardiac catheterization confirm the type of defect.
• In **aortic stenosis,** echocardiography shows left ventricular hypertrophy and prominent pulmonary vasculature. Cardiac catheterization helps determine the degree of shunting and the extent of pulmonary vascular disease.
• In **atrial septal defect,** echocardiography shows enlargement of the right atrium and ventricle and prominent pulmonary vasculature. Cardiac catheterization shows right atrial blood that's more oxygenated than superior vena cava blood. It also helps determine the degree of shunting and the extent of pulmonary vascular disease.
• In **coarctation of the aorta,** echocardiography shows left ventricular hypertrophy, wide ascending and descending aorta, and prominent collateral circulation. Cardiac catheterization shows affected collateral circulation and pressures in the right and left ventricles.
• In **patent ductus arteriosus,** echocardiography shows prominent pulmonary vasculature and enlargement of the left ventricle and aorta. Cardiac catheterization helps determine the extent of pulmonary vascular disease and shows an oxygen content higher in the pulmonary artery than in the right ventricle.

- In **pulmonary artery stenosis,** echocardiography shows right ventricular hypertrophy. Cardiac catheterization provides evidence of the degree of shunting.
- In **ventricular septal defect,** echocardiography may be normal for small defects or show cardiomegaly with a large left atrium and ventricle. In a large defect, echocardiography may show prominent pulmonary vasculature. Cardiac catheterization helps determine the size and exact location of ventricular septal defect and the degree of shunting.

NURSING DIAGNOSES
- Anxiety
- Decreased cardiac output
- Impaired gas exchange
- Delayed growth and development

TREATMENT
- **Aortic stenosis:** surgery (valvulotomy or commissurotomy)
- **Atrial septal defect:** surgery to patch the hole (mild defects may close spontaneously) or balloon umbrella device inserted in an opening in the cardiac catheterization laboratory.
- **Coarctation of the aorta:** inoperable if the coarctation is proximal to the ductus arteriosus—a stent is placed in cardiac catheterization laboratory; closed heart resection if the coarctation is distal to the ductus arteriosus
- **Patent ductus arteriosus:** ligation of the patent ductus arteriosus in a closed-heart operation
- **Pulmonary artery stenosis:** open-heart surgery to separate the pulmonary valve leaflets
- **Ventricular septal defect:** as a last resort, permanent correction with a patch later when the heart is larger (spontaneous closure of the ventricular septal defect may occur in some children by age 3) or pulmonary artery banding to prevent heart failure

Drug therapy
- Cardiac glycoside: digoxin (Lanoxin)
- Diuretic: furosemide (Lasix)
- Anti-inflammatory agent: indomethacin (Indocin) to achieve pharmacologic closure

(in patent ductus arteriosus) during the neonatal period only
- Prophylactic antibiotics to prevent endocarditis

INTERVENTIONS AND RATIONALES
- Explain the heart defect and answer any questions *to prepare the child for cardiac catheterization or surgery.*
- Monitor vital signs, pulse oximetry, and intake and output *to assess renal function and detect change.*
- Assess cardiovascular and respiratory status *to detect early signs of decompensation.*
- Take the apical pulse for 1 minute before giving digoxin and hold the drug if the heart rate is below 100 beats/minute *to prevent toxicity.*
- Monitor fluid status, enforcing fluid restrictions as appropriate *to prevent fluid overload.*
- Weigh the child daily *to determine fluid overload or deficit.*
- Organize physical care and anticipate the child's needs *to reduce the child's oxygen demands.*
- Give an infant high-calorie formula. Give a child high-calorie, easy-to-chew, and easy-to-digest foods *to maintain adequate nutrition and decrease oxygen demands.*
- Maintain normal body temperature *to prevent cold stress.*
- Raise the head of the bed or place the infant in an infant car seat *to ease breathing.*

Teaching topics
- Preparing the child and parents for the sights and sounds of the intensive care unit
- Explanation of the disorder and treatment plan
- Medication use and possible adverse effects

Cyanotic heart defects

Cyanotic heart defects result in unoxygenated blood or a mixture of oxygenated and unoxygenated blood being shunted through the cardiovascular system. This shunting can lead to left-sided heart failure, decreased oxygen supply to the body, and the development of

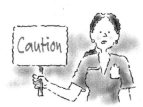

Remember to take an apical pulse for 1 minute before giving digoxin. You're checking for bradycardia, which is a rate below 100 beats/minute for infants.

Caution

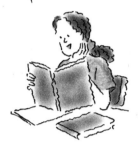

If I keep studying, there won't be anything "defective" about my knowledge of cardiovascular defects.

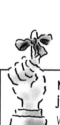

Memory jogger

When a child has a cyanotic heart defect, check for the 4 C's:

Cyanosis, especially increasing with crying

Crabbiness or irritability

Clubbing of digits

Crouching, or squatting, which increases systemic venous return, shunts blood from the extremities to the head and trunk, and decreases cyanosis.

collateral circulation. Cyanotic heart defects include:

- **transposition of the great vessels or arteries** — a defect in which the aorta arises from the right ventricle, the pulmonary artery arises from the left ventricle, and the position of the coronary arteries is also reversed
- **tetralogy of Fallot** — a defect consisting of pulmonary artery stenosis, ventricular septal defect, hypertrophy of the right ventricle, and an overriding aorta
- **hypoplastic left-heart syndrome** — a defect consisting of aortic valve atresia, mitral atresia or stenosis, diminutive or absent left ventricle, and severe hypoplasia of the ascending aorta and aortic arch
- **truncus arteriosis** — a defect in which there's incomplete division of the common great vessel.

CAUSES
- Any condition that increases pulmonary vascular resistance
- Structural defects

ASSESSMENT FINDINGS
- Clubbing
- Cyanosis
- History of poor feeding
- Poor weight gain
- Diaphoresis when feeding (infants)
- Failure to thrive
- Increasing dyspnea, cyanosis, and tachypnea during the first few days after birth; without treatment, heart failure after closure of the ductus (in hypoplastic left-heart syndrome)
- Irritability
- Tachycardia
- Tachypnea

DIAGNOSTIC TEST RESULTS
- Arterial blood gas analysis shows diminished arterial oxygen saturation.
- Cardiac catheterization results confirm the diagnosis through visualization of defects and measurement of oxygen saturation level.

NURSING DIAGNOSES
- Impaired gas exchange
- Anxiety
- Decreased cardiac output

TREATMENT
For transposition of the great vessels or arteries, several therapies are possible, including:
- corrective surgery (called *arterial switch*) to redirect blood flow by switching the position of the major blood vessels; performed in the first few days of life
- palliative surgery to provide communication between the chambers.

For tetralogy of Fallot, the physician can use:
- complete repair or palliative treatment to increase blood flow to the lungs by bypassing pulmonic stenosis (Blalock-Taussig anastomosis of the right pulmonary artery to the right subclavian artery); age at repair depends on the degree of pulmonic stenosis
- oxygen therapy
- repair of ventricular septal defect and stenosis (may be done in stages).

For hypoplastic left-heart syndrome, surgical repair is done in three stages (Norwood procedure I, II, and III).

For truncus arteriosis, several options include:
- medical management of heart failure
- surgical re-creation of the pulmonary trunk
- corrective surgery to repair ventricular septal defect
- Norwood procedure I, II, and III. (Without surgery, death occurs in early infancy.)

Drug therapy
- Opioid analgesic: morphine during tet spell
- Beta-adrenergic blocker: propranolol (Inderal)
- Prostaglandin E to keep the ductus arteriosus patent

INTERVENTIONS AND RATIONALES
- Assess cardiovascular and respiratory status *to detect early signs of compromise.*
- Monitor vital signs and pulse oximetry *to detect hypoxia.*
- Monitor intake and output *to assess renal status.*
- Provide oxygen, when necessary, *to compensate for impaired oxygen exchange.*

• Provide the infant with high-calorie formula *to meet nutritional needs.*
• Anticipate needs and prevent distress *to decrease oxygen demands on the child.*
• Use a preemie nipple *to decrease the energy needed for sucking.*
• Provide adequate hydration *to prevent sequelae of polycythemia.*
• Administer prophylactic antibiotics *to prevent endocarditis.*
• Provide thorough skin care *to prevent skin breakdown.*
• Prepare the child for cardiac catheterization *to decrease anxiety.*

Teaching topics
• Explanation of the disorder and treatment plan
• Preparing the child and parents for the sights and sounds of the intensive care unit
• Explaining the difference between palliative and corrective procedures

Heart failure

Heart failure occurs when the heart can't pump enough blood to meet the body's metabolic needs.

CAUSES
• Congenital defect, such as atrial septal defect, ventricular septal defect, or tetralogy of Fallot
• Infection, causing myocarditis
• Anemia
• Viral infection
• Medications such as chemotherapeutic agents

ASSESSMENT FINDINGS
• Fussiness
• Lethargy
• Diaphoresis
• Poor feeding
• Poor weight gain

DIAGNOSTIC TEST RESULTS
• Chest X-ray shows fluid in lungs and possible consolidation.
• Echocardiogram may show decreased or increased cardiac output and poor filling.
• Exercise stress test (in children older than 4) indicates poor activity tolerance.

NURSING DIAGNOSES
• Decreased cardiac output
• Excess fluid volume
• Impaired gas exchange

TREATMENT
• Oxygen therapy, possibly requiring intubation and mechanical ventilation
• Surgery, if caused by congenital defect
• Left ventricular assist device
• Extracorporeal membrane oxygenation, in severe cases

Drug therapy
• Diuretics: furosemide (Lasix), metolazone (Zaroxolyn)
• Cardiac glycoside: digoxin (Lanoxin)
• Inotropic agents: dopamine, dobutamine

INTERVENTIONS AND RATIONALES
• Assess cardiovascular status, vital signs, and hemodynamic variables *to detect signs of reduced cardiac output.*
• Assess respiratory status and oxygenation *to detect increasing fluid in the lungs and respiratory failure.*
• Keep the child in semi-Fowler's position *to increase chest expansion and improve ventilation.*
• Administer medications, as prescribed, *to enhance cardiac performance and reduce excess fluids.*
• Administer oxygen *to enhance arterial oxygenation.*
• Measure and record intake and output; *intake greater than output may indicate fluid retention.*
• Monitor laboratory studies *to detect electrolyte imbalances, renal failure, and impaired cardiac circulation.*
• Provide suctioning, if necessary, and assist with turning, coughing, and deep breathing *to prevent pulmonary complications.*
• Restrict oral fluids because *excess fluids can worsen heart failure.*
• Weigh the child daily.

Teaching topics
• Explanation of the disorder and treatment plan
• Medications and possible adverse effects
• Limiting sodium intake
• Increasing caloric need to meet metabolic requirements
• Recognizing signs and symptoms of fluid overload

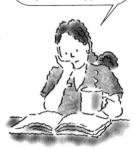

Infants with cyanotic defects have less energy for sucking; use a preemie nipple.

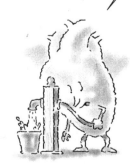

Argh! Sometimes I just can't pump enough to meet demand!

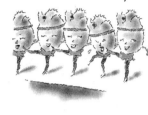

C'mon ladies...
you don't want your
myocardium to get
flabby! And a one,
and a two...

Hypertrophic cardiomyopathy

In cardiomyopathy, the myocardium (middle muscular layer) around the left ventricle becomes flabby, altering cardiac function and resulting in decreased cardiac output. Increased heart rate and increased muscle mass compensate in early stages; however, in later stages, heart failure develops.

There are three types of cardiomyopathy: dilated, obstructive, and hypertrophic; hypertrophic is the most common type seen in children. In hypertrophic cardiomyopathy, the hypertrophied left ventricle can't relax and fill properly.

CAUSES
- Congenital
- Genetic link under consideration

ASSESSMENT FINDINGS
- Heart failure, in infants
- Palpitations
- Murmur, third heart sounds
- Syncope, with exertion
- Sudden cardiac death

DIAGNOSTIC TEST RESULTS
- Chest X-ray shows cardiomegaly and pulmonary congestion.
- Electrocardiogram (ECG) shows left ventricular hypertrophy and nonspecific changes.
- Echocardiogram shows decreased myocardial function.

NURSING DIAGNOSES
- Decreased cardiac output
- Impaired gas exchange
- Activity intolerance

TREATMENT
- Dual chamber pacing
- Septal alcohol ablation
- Surgery (when medication fails): heart transplant or ventricular myotomy

Drug therapy
- Antiarrhythmics
- Anticoagulant: warfarin (Coumadin)
- Beta-adrenergic blockers: propranolol (Inderal), nadolol (Corgard), metoprolol (Lopressor)

- Calcium channel blockers: verapamil (Calan), diltiazem (Cardizem)
- Diuretics: furosemide (Lasix), spirolactone

INTERVENTIONS AND RATIONALES
- Monitor ECG *to detect arrhythmias and ischemia.*
- Assess cardiovascular status, vital signs, and hemodynamic variables *to detect heart failure.*
- Monitor respiratory status *to detect evidence of heart failure, such as dyspnea and crackles.*
- Administer oxygen and medications, as prescribed, *to improve oxygenation and cardiac output.*
- Monitor and record intake and output *to detect fluid volume overload.*
- Keep the child in semi-Fowler's position *to enhance gas exchange.*
- Maintain bed rest *to reduce oxygen demands on the heart.*
- Monitor laboratory results *to detect abnormalities, such as hypokalemia, from the use of diuretics.*

Teaching topics
- Explanation of the disorder and treatment plan
- Medications and possible adverse effects
- Early signs and symptoms of heart failure
- Monitoring pulses and blood pressure
- Avoiding straining during bowel movements
- Contacting the Children's Cardiomyopathy Foundation

Rheumatic fever

Rheumatic fever is an inflammatory disease of childhood. It first occurs 1 to 3 weeks after a group A beta-hemolytic streptococcal infection and may recur. Rheumatic fever results in antigen-antibody complexes that ultimately destroy heart tissue.

Rheumatic heart disease refers to the cardiac effects of rheumatic fever and includes pancarditis (inflammation of the heart muscle, heart lining, and sac around the heart) during the early acute phase and chronic heart valve disease later.

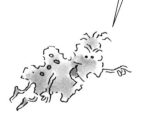

In rheumatic fever, antibodies manufactured to combat streptococci react and produce lesions at specific tissue sites, especially in the heart and joints.

CAUSES
- Production of antibodies against group A beta-hemolytic *Streptococcus*
- Untreated or improperly treated group A beta-hemolytic *Streptococcus* infection (1% to 5% of children infected with *Streptococcus* develop rheumatic fever)

ASSESSMENT FINDINGS
The Jones criteria for assessing major rheumatic fever include:
- carditis
- chorea
- erythema marginatum (temporary, disk-shaped, nonpruritic, reddened macules that fade in the center, leaving raised margins)
- polyarthritis
- subcutaneous nodules.
    The Jones criteria for assessing minor rheumatic fever include:
- arthralgia
- evidence of a *Streptococcus* infection
- fever
- history of rheumatic fever
- new-onset murmur.

DIAGNOSTIC TEST RESULTS
- Antistreptolysin-O titer is elevated.
- Erythrocyte sedimentation rate is increased.
- ECG shows a prolonged PR interval.

NURSING DIAGNOSES
- Decreased cardiac output
- Impaired gas exchange
- Imbalanced nutrition: Less than body requirements

TREATMENT
- Bed rest during fever and until sedimentation rate returns to normal

Drug therapy
- Analgesic: aspirin for arthritis pain
- Antibiotic: penicillin to prevent additional damage from future attacks (taken until age 20 or for 5 years after the attack, whichever is longer)

INTERVENTIONS AND RATIONALES
- Monitor vital signs and intake and output *to detect fluid volume overload or deficit.*
- Institute safety measures for chorea; maintain a calm environment, reduce stimulation, avoid the use of forks or glass, and assist in walking *to prevent injury.*
- Provide appropriate passive stimulation *to maintain growth and development.*
- Provide emotional support for long-term convalescence *to help relieve anxiety.*
- Use sterile technique in dressing changes and standard precautions *to prevent reinfection.*

Teaching topics
- Explanation of the disorder and treatment plan
- Medication use and possible adverse effects
- Understanding the need to inform health care providers of existing medical conditions
- Signs and symptoms of aspirin toxicity (tinnitus, bruising, bleeding gums)

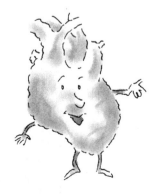

Effective treatment eliminates strep infection, relieves symptoms, and prevents recurrence, reducing the chance I'll suffer permanent damage.

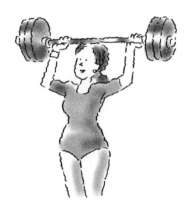

Pump up on practice questions

1. A child returns to his room after a cardiac catheterization. Which nursing intervention is most appropriate?
  1. Maintain the child on bed rest with no further activity restrictions.
  2. Maintain the child on bed rest with the affected extremity immobilized.
  3. Allow the child to get out of bed to go to the bathroom, if necessary.
  4. Allow the child to sit in a chair with the affected extremity immobilized.

Answer: 2. The child should be maintained on bed rest with the affected extremity immobilized after cardiac catheterization to prevent hemorrhage. Allowing the child to move the affected extremity while on bed rest, allowing the child bathroom privileges, or allowing the child to sit in a chair with the affected extremity immobilized places the child at risk for hemorrhage.

➠ NCLEX keys
Client needs category: Physiological integrity
Client needs subcategory: Reduction of risk potential
Cognitive level: Application

2. A child is scheduled for echocardiography. The nurse is providing teaching to the child's mother. Which statement by the mother about echocardiography indicates the need for further teaching?

  1. "I'm glad my child won't have an I.V. catheter inserted for this procedure."
  2. "I'm glad my child won't need to have dye injected into him before the procedure."
  3. "How am I going to explain to my son that he can't have anything to eat before the test?"
  4. "I know my child may need to lie on his left side and breathe in and out slowly during the procedure."

Answer: 3. Echocardiography is a noninvasive procedure used to evaluate the size, shape, and motion of various cardiac structures. Therefore, it isn't necessary for the client to have an I.V. catheter inserted, dye injected, or nothing by mouth, as would be the case with a cardiac catheterization. The child may need to lie on his left side and inhale and exhale slowly during the procedure.

➠ NCLEX keys
Client needs category: Physiological integrity
Client needs subcategory: Reduction of risk potential
Cognitive level: Analysis

3. An infant with a ventricular septal defect is receiving digoxin (Lanoxin). Which intervention by the nurse is most appropriate before digoxin administration?
  1. Take the infant's blood pressure.
  2. Check the infant's respiratory rate for 1 minute.
  3. Check the infant's radial pulse for 1 minute.
  4. Check the infant's apical pulse for 1 minute.

Answer: 4. Before administering digoxin, the nurse should check the infant's apical pulse for 1 minute. Checking the radial pulse may be inaccurate. Checking the blood pressure and respiratory rate isn't necessary before digoxin administration because the medication doesn't affect these parameters.

➠ NCLEX keys
Client needs category: Physiological integrity
Client needs subcategory: Pharmacological and parenteral therapies
Cognitive level: Application

4. A nurse checks an infant's apical pulse before digoxin (Lanoxin) administration and finds that the pulse rate is 90 beats/minute. Which action is most appropriate for the nurse?

1. Withhold the digoxin and notify the physician.
2. Administer the digoxin and notify the physician.
3. Administer the digoxin and document the infant's pulse rate.
4. Withhold the digoxin and document the infant's pulse rate.

Answer: 1. The nurse should withhold the digoxin and notify the physician because an apical pulse below 100 beats/minute in an infant is considered bradycardic. The nurse should also document her findings and interventions in the medical record. Administering the drug to a bradycardic infant could further decrease his heart rate and compromise his status. Withholding the drug and not notifying the physician could compromise the existing treatment plan.

➡ *NCLEX keys*
Client needs category: Physiological integrity
Client needs subcategory: Pharmacological and parenteral therapies
Cognitive level: Application

5. A child has been diagnosed with rheumatic fever. Which statement by the mother indicates an understanding of rheumatic fever?

1. "I should avoid giving my child aspirin for the arthritic pain."
2. "It's very upsetting that my child must take penicillin until he's 20 years old."
3. "I need to wear a gown, gloves, and mask to stay in my child's room."
4. "I don't know how I'll be able to keep my child away from his sister when he gets home."

Answer: 2. Rheumatic fever is an acquired autoimmune-complex disorder that occurs 1 to 3 weeks after an infection of group A beta-hemolytic streptococci, in many cases as a result of strep throat that hasn't been treated with antibiotics. To prevent additional heart damage from future attacks, the child must take penicillin or another antibiotic until the age of 20 or for 5 years after the attack, whichever is longer. Children shouldn't be given aspirin because it may result in Reye's syndrome. Rheumatic fever isn't contagious, so isolation precautions aren't necessary.

➡ *NCLEX keys*
Client needs category: Physiological integrity
Client needs subcategory: Reduction of risk potential
Cognitive level: Analysis

6. A nurse is caring for a child with a cyanotic heart defect. Which signs should the nurse expect to observe?

1. Cyanosis, hypertension, clubbing, and lethargy
2. Cyanosis, hypotension, crouching, and lethargy
3. Cyanosis, irritability, clubbing, and crouching
4. Cyanosis, confusion, clonus, and crouching

Answer: 3. The child with a cyanotic heart defect has cyanosis along with crabiness (irritability), clubbing of the digits, and crouching or squatting. The child with cyanotic heart defect doesn't typically have hypertension, lethargy, confusion, or clonus.

➡ *NCLEX keys*
Client needs category: Physiological integrity
Client needs subcategory: Physiological adaptation
Cognitive level: Comprehension

7. A nurse is caring for an infant with tetralogy of Fallot. Which drug should the nurse anticipate administering during a tet spell?

1. Propranolol (Inderal)
2. Morphine
3. Meperidine (Demerol)
4. Furosemide (Lasix)

Answer: 2. The nurse should anticipate administering morphine during a tet spell to decrease the associated infundibular spasm. Propranolol may be administered as a preventive measure in an infant with tetralogy of Fallot but isn't administered during a tet spell. Furosemide and meperidine aren't appropriate agents for an infant experiencing a tet spell.

Client needs category: Physiological integrity
Client needs subcategory: Pharmacological and parenteral therapies
Cognitive level: Analysis

8. An infant is diagnosed with patent ductus arteriosus. Which drug should the nurse anticipate administering to attempt to close the defect?
1. Digoxin (Lanoxin)
2. Prednisone
3. Furosemide (Lasix)
4. Indomethacin (Indocin)

Answer: 4. Indomethacin is administered to an infant with patent ductus arteriosus in the hope of closing the defect. Digoxin and furosemide may be used to treat the symptoms associated with patent ductus arteriosus, but they don't achieve closure. Prednisone isn't used to treat the condition.

Client needs category: Physiological integrity
Client needs subcategory: Pharmacological and parenteral therapies
Cognitive level: Application

9. An infant age 2 months has a tentative diagnosis of congenital heart defect. During physical assessment, the nurse notes that the infant has a pulse rate of 168 beats/minute and a respiratory rate of 72 breaths/minute. In which position should the nurse place the infant?
1. Upright in an infant seat
2. Lying on the back
3. Lying on the abdomen
4. Sitting in high Fowler's position

Answer: 1. Because these signs suggest development of respiratory distress, the nurse should position the infant with the head elevated at a 45-degree angle to promote maximum chest expansion. This can be accomplished by placing the infant in an infant seat. Placing an infant flat on the back or abdomen or in high Fowler's position could increase respiratory distress by preventing maximum chest expansion.

Client needs category: Physiological integrity
Client needs subcategory: Physiological adaptation
Cognitive level: Application

10. An infant with a congenital cyanotic heart defect has a complete blood count drawn, revealing an elevated red blood cell (RBC) count. Which condition do these findings indicate?
1. Anemia
2. Dehydration
3. Jaundice
4. Hypoxia compensation

Answer: 4. A congenital cyanotic heart defect alters blood flow through the heart and lungs, which produces hypoxia. To compensate for this, the body increases the oxygen-carrying capacity by increasing RBC production, which causes the hemoglobin level and hematocrit to increase. The hemoglobin level and hematocrit are typically decreased in anemia. Altered electrolyte levels and other laboratory values provide better evidence of dehydration. An elevated hemoglobin level and hematocrit aren't associated with jaundice.

Client needs category: Physiological integrity
Client needs subcategory: Physiological adaptation
Cognitive level: Analysis

5 Respiratory system

Brush up on key concepts

The primary function of the respiratory system is to distribute air to the alveoli in the lungs, where gas exchange takes place. Gas exchange includes:
• the addition of oxygen (O_2) to pulmonary capillary blood
• the removal of carbon dioxide (CO_2) from pulmonary capillary blood.

At any time, you can review the major points of this chapter by consulting the *Cheat sheet* on pages 44 and 45.

Upper and lower
The parts of the respiratory system include the **upper airway** and the **lower airway.**

The upper airway includes the:
• epiglottis
• nasopharynx
• oropharynx
• larynx.

The lower airway includes the:
• trachea
• bronchi
• bronchioles
• alveoli.

Take a deep breath
Breathing delivers inspired gas to the lower respiratory tract and alveoli. Contraction and relaxation of the respiratory muscles move air into and out of the lungs. Here are some important aspects of the breathing process:
• **Ventilation** begins with the contraction of the inspiratory muscles: The diaphragm (the major muscle of respiration) descends while the external intercostal muscles move the rib cage upward and outward.

• Air then enters the lungs in response to the pressure gradient between the atmosphere and the lungs.
• The lungs adhere to the chest wall and diaphragm because of the vacuum created by negative pleural pressure.
• As the thorax expands, the lungs also expand, causing a decrease in pressure in the lungs.
• The accessory muscles of inspiration, which include the scalene and sternocleidomastoid muscles, raise the clavicles, upper ribs, and sternum.
• To reach the capillary lumen, O_2 diffuses across the alveolocapillary membrane into the blood.
• Normal expiration is passive; the inspiratory muscles cease to contract, and the elastic recoil of the lungs causes the lungs to contract.
• These actions increase the pressure in the lungs above atmospheric pressure, moving air from the lungs to the atmosphere.

Air system under construction
A **child's respiratory tract** differs anatomically from an adult's in ways that predispose the child to many respiratory problems. A child's respiratory tract differs from an adult's in the following ways:
• Lungs aren't fully developed at birth.
• Alveoli continue to grow and increase in size through age 8.
• A child's respiratory tract has a narrower lumen than an adult's until age 5; the narrow airway makes the young child prone to airway obstruction and respiratory distress from inflammation, mucus secretion, or a foreign body.
• Elastic connective tissue becomes more abundant with age in the peripheral part of the lung.
• A child's respiratory rate decreases as body size increases.

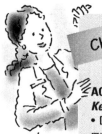

Cheat sheet

Respiratory refresher

ACUTE RESPIRATORY FAILURE
Key signs and symptoms
- Decreased respiratory excursion, accessory muscle use, retractions
- Difficulty breathing, shortness of breath, dyspnea, tachypnea, orthopnea
- Fatigue
- Fussiness
- Grunting

Key test results
- Arterial blood gas (ABG) levels show hypoxia, acidosis, alkalosis, and hypercapnia.

Key treatments
- Oxygen (O_2) therapy, intubation, and mechanical ventilation
- Analgesic: morphine
- Bronchodilators: terbutaline, aminophylline, theophylline; via nebulizer: albuterol, ipratropium
- Steroids: hydrocortisone, methylprednisolone

Key interventions
- Assess respiratory status.
- Administer O_2.
- Provide suctioning; assist with turning, coughing, and deep breathing; perform chest physiotherapy and postural drainage.
- Maintain bed rest.

ASTHMA
Key signs and symptoms
- Diaphoresis
- Dyspnea
- Prolonged expiration with an expiratory wheeze; in severe distress, possible inspiratory wheeze
- Unequal or decreased breath sounds
- Use of accessory muscles

Key test results
- O_2 saturation via pulse oximetry may show decreased O_2 saturation.
- ABG measurement may show increased partial pressure of arterial carbon dioxide from respiratory acidosis.

Key treatments
- Short-acting bronchodilators (inhaled beta$_2$-adrenergic agonists): albuterol (Proventil-HFA, Ventolin), levalbuterol (Xopenex)

Key interventions
- Assess respiratory and cardiovascular status.
- Monitor vital signs.
During an acute attack
- Allow the child to sit upright; provide moist O_2, if necessary.
- Monitor vital signs.

BRONCHOPULMONARY DYSPLASIA
Key signs and symptoms
- Atelectasis
- Crackles, rhonchi, wheezes
- Dyspnea
- Sternal retractions

Key test results
- Chest X-ray reveals pulmonary changes (bronchiolar metaplasia and interstitial fibrosis).

Key treatments
- Chest physiotherapy
- Ventilatory support and oxygen

Key interventions
- Assess respiratory and cardiovascular status.
- Monitor vital signs, pulse oximetry, and intake and output.

CROUP
Key signs and symptoms
- Barking, brassy cough or hoarseness sometimes described as a "seal bark" cough
- Inspiratory stridor with varying degrees of respiratory distress

Key test results
- Laryngoscopy may reveal inflammation and obstruction in epiglottal and laryngeal areas.
- Neck X-ray shows areas of upper airway narrowing and edema in subglottic folds.

Key treatments
- Cool humidification during sleep with a cool mist tent or room humidifier
- Inhaled racemic epinephrine and corticosteroids such as methylprednisolone sodium succinate
- Tracheostomy, O_2 administration

Key interventions
- Monitor vital signs and pulse oximetry readings.
- Administer O_2 therapy and maintain the child in a cool mist tent, if needed.

Respiratory refresher *(continued)*

CYSTIC FIBROSIS
Key signs and symptoms
- History of a chronic, productive cough and recurrent respiratory infections
- Parents' report of a salty taste on the child's skin

Key test results
- Sweat test using pilocarpine iontophoresis is greater than 60 mEq/L.

Key treatments
- Oral pancreatic enzyme replacement with pancrelipase (Pancrease)

Key interventions
- Assess respiratory and cardiovascular status.
- Administer pancreatic enzymes with meals and snacks.
- Encourage breathing exercises and perform chest physiotherapy two to four times per day.

EPIGLOTTIDITIS
Key signs and symptoms
- Difficult and painful swallowing
- Increased drooling
- Restlessness
- Stridor

Key test results
- Lateral neck X-ray shows an enlarged epiglottis.

Key treatments
- Possible emergency endotracheal intubation or a tracheotomy
- Oxygen therapy or cool mist tent
- Parenteral antibiotics: 10-day course according to the causative organism

Key interventions
- Monitor vital signs and pulse oximetry.
- Assess respiratory and cardiovascular status.
- Don't inspect the oropharynx if epiglottiditis is suspected.

RESPIRATORY SYNCYTIAL VIRUS
Key signs and symptoms
- Sternal retractions, nasal flaring
- Tachypnea
- Increased mucus production

Key test results
- Bronchial mucus culture shows respiratory syncytial virus (RSV).

Key treatments
- Humidified O_2
- I.V. fluids (with severe infection)

Key interventions
- Monitor vital signs and pulse oximetry.
- Assess respiratory and cardiovascular status.
- Administer humidified O_2 therapy.
- Monitor for signs and symptoms of dehydration. Administer and maintain I.V. therapy.

SUDDEN INFANT DEATH SYNDROME
Key signs and symptoms
- Death occurring during sleep without noise or struggle

Key test results
- Autopsy is the only way to diagnose sudden infant death syndrome (SIDS).

Key treatments
- If the child can be resuscitated (near-SIDS): monitoring

Key interventions
- Let the parents touch, hold, and rock the infant, and allow them to say good-bye to the infant.

Keep abreast of diagnostic tests

Here are the most important tests used to diagnose respiratory disorders, along with common nursing interventions associated with each test.

Check the gas
Arterial blood gas (ABG) analysis is used to assess gas exchange:
- Decreased partial pressure of arterial oxygen (PaO_2) may indicate hypoventilation, ventilation-perfusion mismatch, or shunting of blood away from gas exchange sites.
- Increased partial pressure of arterial carbon dioxide ($PaCO_2$) reflects hypoventilation or marked ventilation-perfusion mismatch.
- Decreased $PaCO_2$ reflects increased alveolar ventilation.
- Changes in pH may reflect metabolic or respiratory dysfunction.

Nursing actions
Before the procedure
- Explain the procedure to the parents and child.

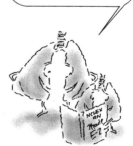

It says here that a decreased PaO_2, along with an increased $PaCO_2$, may indicate hypoventilation or ventilation-perfusion mismatch.

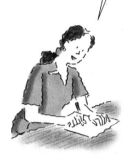

Hmmm. ABG analysis helps to assess gas exchange: pH, $Paco_2$, and Pao_2. Pulse oximetry is used to measure O_2 saturation only.

• Check arterial circulation before making the arterial puncture.

After the procedure
• After the sample is obtained, apply firm pressure to the arterial site.
• Keep the sample on ice, and transport it immediately to the laboratory.
• Assess the puncture site for bleeding or hematoma formation.

Oxygen observation
Pulse oximetry is a painless alternative to ABG analysis for measuring O_2 saturation only. This test may be less effective in jaundiced children or those with dark skin.

Nursing actions
• Explain the procedure to the parents and child.
• Place the oximeter on a site with adequate circulation, such as the finger, toe, or nose.
• Periodically rotate sites to prevent skin breakdown and pressure ulcers.
• Ensure that pulse readings from the site used for oximetry correlate with the child's heart rate before performing oximetry.

Lung function
Pulmonary function tests are used to measure lung volume, flow rates, and compliance. Pulmonary function test results may not be accurate if the young child has difficulty following directions.

Nursing actions
• Explain the procedure to the child and his parents.
• Instruct the child and his parents that he should have only a light meal before the test.
• Tell the parents to withhold bronchodilators and intermittent positive-pressure breathing therapy.
• Just before the test, tell the child to void and loosen tight clothing.

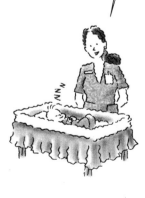

Sleeping like a baby? Not so for neonates and infants who breathe through their nose and develop nasal congestion. In this age-group, it can cause respiratory distress.

Chest check
Chest X-rays show such conditions as atelectasis, pleural effusion, infiltrates, pneumothorax, lesions, mediastinal shifts, and pulmonary edema.

Nursing actions
• Explain the procedure to the parents and child.
• Ensure adequate protection by covering the child's gonads and thyroid gland with a lead apron.

Polish up on client care

Major pediatric respiratory disorders include acute respiratory failure, asthma, bronchopulmonary dysplasia, croup, cystic fibrosis, epiglottiditis, respiratory syncytial cirus (RSV) and sudden infant death syndrome (SIDS).

For information about special respiratory treatments for pediatric patients, see *Respiratory assistance for children.*

Acute respiratory failure

In acute respiratory failure, the respiratory system can't adequately supply the body with the O_2 it needs or adequately remove CO_2. The frequency of acute respiratory failure is higher in infants and young children than in adults. This is due to several situations:
• Neonates and infants breathe through the nose until age 6 months because of the proximity of the epiglottis to the nasopharynx. Nasal congestion can lead to significant respiratory distress in this age-group.
• The small size of the airway allows for less room for edema or swelling.
• Infants and young children have a large tongue that fills a small oropharynx.
• The epiglottis is larger and more horizontal to the pharyngeal wall in children than in adults.
• Infants and young children have a narrow subglottic area. A small amount of subglottic edema can lead to clinically significant narrowing, increased airway resistance, and increased work of breathing.
• In slightly older children, adenoidal and tonsillar lymphoid tissue is prominent and can contribute to airway obstruction.

Management moments

Respiratory assistance for children

The oxygen tent, the cool mist tent, the nasal cannula, and chest physiotherapy are specialized treatments for pediatric respiratory disorders. Here are the nursing actions associated with each treatment.

OXYGEN TENT
• Keep the plastic sides down and tucked in; because oxygen is heavier than air, oxygen loss is greater at the bottom of the tent.
• Keep the plastic away from the child's face.
• Prevent the use of toys that produce sparks or friction.
• Frequently assess oxygen concentration.
• To return the child to a tent, put the tent sides down, turn on the oxygen, wait until the oxygen is at the prescribed concentration, and then place the child in the tent.

COOL MIST TENT (CROUP TENT)
• Explain that the cool mist thins mucus, facilitating expectoration.
• Provide the same care as with an oxygen tent.
• Expect the child to be fearful if the mist obscures vision.
• Encourage the use of transitional objects in the tent, except for stuffed toys, which may become damp and promote bacterial growth.
• Keep the child dry by changing bed linens and pajamas frequently.

• Maintain a steady body temperature.
• Teach the parents about cool mist vaporizers for home use; tell them to clean the vaporizers frequently to prevent organisms from being sprayed into the air.

NASAL CANNULA
• Remove nasal secretions from the end of tubing frequently.
• Administer saline nose drops or nasal spray to moisten passages.
• Remove cannula and moisten nares every 8 hours to prevent skin breakdown.

CHEST PHYSIOTHERAPY
• Perform at least 30 minutes before meals.
• Use a cupped hand over a covered rib cage for 2 to 5 minutes on the five major positions (upper anterior lobes, upper posterior lobes, lower posterior lobes, and right and left sides) for a maximum of 30 minutes; for infants, preformed rubber percussors are available.
• Avoid physiotherapy during acute bronchoconstriction (for example, asthma) or airway edema (for example, croup) to prevent mucus plugs from loosening and causing airway obstruction.
• Administer aerosol-nebulized medications immediately before percussion and postural drainage.

CAUSES
• RSV
• Infection
• Atelectasis
• Acute respiratory distress syndrome
• Abdominal or thoracic surgery
• Anesthesia
• Bronchopulmonary dysplasia
• Congential heart defect
• Meningitis
• Muscular dystrophy
• Encephalitis
• Pneumonia
• Ingestion of toxic substance

ASSESSMENT FINDINGS
• Decreased respiratory excursion, accessory muscle use, retractions
• Difficulty breathing, shortness of breath, dyspnea, tachypnea, orthopnea

• Nasal flaring
• Fatigue
• Fussiness
• Grunting
• Adventitious breath sounds (crackles, rhonchi, wheezing)
• Cough, sputum production
• Cyanosis
• Change in mentation
• Tachycardia

DIAGNOSTIC TEST RESULTS
• ABG levels show hypoxia, acidosis, alkalosis, and hypercapnia.
• Chest X-ray shows pulmonary infiltrates, interstitial edema, and atelectasis.
• Lung scan shows ventilation-perfusion ratio mismatch.

NURSING DIAGNOSES
• Activity intolerance

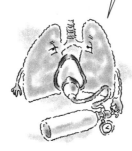

Oxygen can help reduce hypoxemia and relieve respiratory distress!

- Impaired gas exchange
- Ineffective peripheral tissue perfusion
- Ineffective airway clearance
- Anxiety
- Ineffective breathing pattern

TREATMENT
- Chest physiotherapy, postural drainage, incentive spirometry
- Humidity to liquefy secretions
- Inhaled nitric oxide
- O_2 therapy, intubation, and mechanical ventilation

Drug therapy
- Analgesic: morphine
- Bronchodilators: terbutaline, aminophylline, theophylline; via nebulizer: albuterol, ipratropium
- Steroids: hydrocortisone, methylprednisolone
- Exogenous surfactant: calfactant (Infasurf)
- Histamine-2 blockers: famotidine (Pepcid), ranitidine (Zantac), nizatidine (Axid)
- Antibiotics: according to sensitivity of causative organism

INTERVENTIONS AND RATIONALES
- Assess respiratory status *to detect early signs of compromise and hypoxemia.*
- Monitor and record intake and output *to detect fluid volume excess, which may lead to pulmonary edema.*
- Track laboratory values. Report deteriorating ABG levels, such as a fall in PaO_2 levels and rise in $PaCO_2$ levels. *Low hemoglobin and hematocrit levels reduce oxygen-carrying capacity of the blood.*
- Monitor pulse oximetry *to detect a drop in arterial O_2 saturation.*
- Monitor and record vital signs. *Tachycardia and tachypnea may indicate hypoxemia.*
- During steroid therapy, monitor blood glucose level every 6 to 12 hours using a blood glucose meter *to detect hyperglycemia caused by steroid use.*
- Administer O_2 *to reduce hypoxemia and relieve respiratory distress.*
- Monitor mechanical ventilation *to prevent complications and optimize PaO_2.*
- Provide suctioning; assist with turning, coughing, and deep breathing; and perform chest physiotherapy and postural drainage.

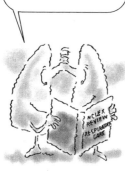

Asthma typically causes prolonged expiration with an expiratory wheeze. However, during severe distress, you may hear an inspiratory wheeze.

- Maintain bed rest.
- Keep the child in semi-Fowler's or high Fowler's position *to promote chest expansion and ventilation.*
- Administer medications as prescribed *to treat infection, dilate airways, and reduce inflammation.*

Teaching topics
- Explanation of the disorder and treatment plan
- Recognizing the early signs and symptoms of respiratory difficulty
- Performing deep-breathing and coughing exercises and incentive spirometry
- Drug therapy

Asthma

Asthma is a reversible, chronic, diffuse, inflammatory disease that produces the following effects:
- increased resistance to airflow
- decreased expiratory flow rates
- smooth-muscle bronchospasm
- increased mucus secretion leading to airway obstruction and air trapping.

CAUSES
- Hyperresponsiveness of the lower airway (may be idiopathic or intrinsic; may be caused by a hyperresponsive reaction to an allergen, exercise, or environmental change)

ASSESSMENT FINDINGS
During an attack
- Increased anteroposterior diameter of chest
- Altered cerebral function (with severe attack)
- Pulsus paradoxus (with moderate to severe attack)
- Diaphoresis
- Tachypnea
- Dyspnea
- Chest tightness
- Tachycardia
- Exercise intolerance
- Fatigue and apprehension
- Agitation
- Prolonged expiration with an expiratory wheeze; in severe distress, possible inspiratory wheeze
- Coarse crackles

- Unequal or decreased breath sounds
- Use of accessory muscles
- Talking in words, not sentences

DIAGNOSTIC TEST RESULTS
- Oxygen saturation via pulse oximetry may show decreased O_2 saturation.
- ADG measurement may show increased $Paco_2$ from respiratory acidosis.
- Skin test identifies the source of the allergy.
- Sputum analysis rules out respiratory infection.
- Exercise challenge (for children younger than age 6) identifies respiratory-induced symptoms and reversibility with aerosolized bronchodilators.

NURSING DIAGNOSES
- Anxiety
- Fear
- Impaired gas exchange
- Ineffective airway clearance

TREATMENT
- Chest physiotherapy (after edema has abated)
- Parenteral fluids to thin mucus secretions
- Oxygen therapy

Status asthmaticus
- Oxygen therapy with possible endotracheal intubation and mechanical ventilation

Drug therapy
Quick relief
- Short-acting bronchodilators (inhaled beta$_2$-adrenergic agonists): albuterol (Proventil-HFA, Ventolin), levalbuterol (Xopenex)

Long-term control
- Inhaled corticosteroid: beclomethasone
- Oral corticosteroid: prednisone
- Long-acting bronchodilator: salmeterol (Serevent)
- Methylxanthene: theophylline
- Mast cell stabilizer: cromolyn (Intal)
- Leukotriene modifier: montelukast (Singulair)

Status asthmaticus
- Corticosteroid: methylprednisolone

INTERVENTIONS AND RATIONALES
- Assess respiratory and cardiovascular status. *Tachycardia, tachypnea, and decreased breath sounds signal worsening respiratory status.*
- Monitor vital signs *to detect changes and prevent complications.*
- Assess the nature of the child's cough (hacking, unproductive progressing to productive), especially at night in the absence of infection. *Early detection and treatment may prevent complications.*
- Modify the environment to avoid an allergic reaction; remove the offending allergen. *Allergens can trigger an asthma attack.*
- Rinse the child's mouth after he inhales medication *to promote comfort and prevent irritation to the oral mucosa.*
- For exercise-induced asthma, give prophylactic treatments of beta-adrenergic blockers or cromolyn 10 to 15 minutes before the child exercises. *Premedication before exercise may prevent an asthma attack.* (See *Living with asthma.*)

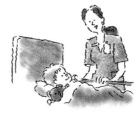

Assess the nature of the child's cough, especially at night. Early detection and treatment can prevent complications.

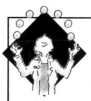

Management moments

Living with asthma

Encourage the parents of a child with asthma to help the child lead as normal a life as possible. Stress the importance of not restricting activities. Encourage participation in exercise and sports. Explain that aerobic activities, such as swimming, running, and brisk walking, increase the efficiency of the body's oxygen use. Prophylactic use of medication typically allows participation in almost any activity, even those that typically precipitate an attack.

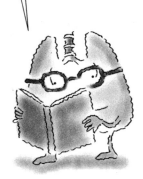

During an acute attack, allow the child to sit upright to ease breathing. Also provide moist oxygen, if necessary.

• For status asthmaticus or severe asthma attack, provide appropriate respiratory support *to prevent complications.*

During an acute attack

• Allow the child to sit upright *to promote chest expansion and ease breathing;* provide moist oxygen, if necessary. *Moist oxygen promotes mobilization of secretions.*
• Monitor vital signs *to detect signs of impending respiratory failure and cardiac decompensation.*
• Monitor the urine for glucose if the child is receiving corticosteroids *to detect early signs of hyperglycemia.*
• Administer inhaled medications through a metered-dose inhaler, and monitor peak flow rates. *Peak flow rates indicate the degree of lung impairment.*
• Maintain a calm environment; provide emotional support and reassurance *to decrease anxiety and decrease oxygen demands.*
• Monitor the effectiveness of drug therapy. *Failure to respond to drugs during an acute attack can result in status asthmaticus.*

Teaching topics

• Explanation of the disorder and treatment plan
• Medication use and possible adverse effects
• Breathing exercises to increase ventilatory capacity
• Proper use of inhalers
• Avoiding smoking areas
• Identifying and avoiding triggers

Bronchopulmonary dysplasia

Bronchopulmonary dysplasia is a chronic lung disease that begins in infancy. It occurs in neonates who require ventilatory support with high positive airway pressure and oxygen in the first 2 weeks of life. Infants at risk may be born prematurely or may have a respiratory disorder.

In this disorder, an acute insult to the neonate's lungs, such as respiratory distress syndrome, pneumonia, or meconium aspiration, requires positive-pressure ventilation

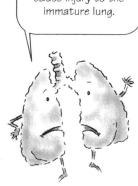

Oxygen may cause injury to the immature lung.

and a high concentration of oxygen over time. These therapies result in tissue and cellular injury to the immature lung.

CONTRIBUTING FACTORS

• Damage to the bronchiolar epithelium (from hyperoxia and positive pressure)
• Difficulty clearing mucus from the lungs
• Illness, such as respiratory distress syndrome, pneumonia, or meconium aspiration
• Oxygen toxicity from administration of a high concentration of oxygen and long-term assisted ventilation
• Possible genetic factors
• Prematurity

ASSESSMENT FINDINGS

• Atelectasis
• Crackles, rhonchi, wheezes
• Delayed development
• Dyspnea
• Hypoxia without ventilator assistance
• Fatigue
• Delayed muscle growth
• Pallor
• Circumoral cyanosis
• Prolonged capillary filling time
• Respiratory distress
• Right-sided heart failure
• Sternal retractions
• Weight loss or difficulty feeding

DIAGNOSTIC TEST RESULTS

• ABG analysis reveals hypoxemia.
• Chest X-ray reveals pulmonary changes (bronchiolar metaplasia and interstitial fibrosis).

NURSING DIAGNOSES

• Delayed growth and development
• Imbalanced nutrition: Less than body requirements
• Impaired gas exchange

TREATMENT

• Chest physiotherapy
• Ventilatory support and oxygen
• Enteral or total parenteral nutrition
• Supportive measures to enhance respiratory function

Drug therapy
- Bronchodilator: albuterol (Proventil-HFA) to counter increased airway resistance
- Corticosteroid: dexamethasone therapy to reduce inflammation
- Diuretic: furosemide (Lasix)

INTERVENTIONS AND RATIONALES
- Assess respiratory and cardiovascular status. *Monitoring is essential because children with bronchopulmonary dysplasia are susceptible to lower respiratory tract infections, hypertension, and respiratory failure.*
- Monitor vital signs, pulse oximetry, and intake and output *to assess and maintain adequate hydration, which is necessary to liquefy secretions and detect early signs of respiratory compromise.*
- Provide adequate time for rest *to decrease oxygen demands.*
- Provide chest physiotherapy *to mobilize secretions that interfere with oxygenation.*
- Administer medications as ordered *to improve pulmonary function and improve oxygenation.*
- Provide a quiet environment. *Unnecessary noise or activity may increase the child's anxiety and cause respiratory distress.*

Teaching topics
- Explanation of the disorder and treatment plan
- Medication use and possible adverse effects
- Visiting and becoming involved in the child's care, especially if the child requires lengthy hospitalization

Croup

Croup is a group of related upper airway respiratory syndromes that commonly affect toddlers. It includes acute spasmodic laryngitis, acute obstructive laryngitis, and acute laryngotracheobronchitis.

CAUSES
- Adenoviruses
- Bacteria (pertussis and diphtheria)
- Influenza viruses
- Measles virus
- Parainfluenza viruses
- RSV

ASSESSMENT FINDINGS
- Barking, brassy cough or hoarseness, sometimes described as a "seal bark" cough
- Condition usually begins at night and during cold weather and frequently recurs
- Crackles and decreased breath sounds (indicate that the condition has progressed to the bronchi)
- Increased dyspnea and lower accessory muscle use
- Inspiratory stridor with varying degrees of respiratory distress
- Onset sudden or gradual

DIAGNOSTIC TEST RESULTS
- If bacterial infection is the cause, throat cultures may identify the organisms and their sensitivity to antibiotics as well as rule out diphtheria.
- Laryngoscopy may reveal inflammation and obstruction in epiglottal and laryngeal areas.
- Computed tomography scan of the neck helps differentiate among croup, epiglottiditis, and noninfection.
- Neck X-ray shows areas of upper airway narrowing and edema in subglottic folds and rules out the possibility of foreign body obstruction as well as masses and cysts.

NURSING DIAGNOSES
- Anxiety
- Fear
- Hyperthermia
- Ineffective airway clearance
- Ineffective breathing pattern
- Risk for imbalanced fluid volume

TREATMENT
- Clear liquid diet to keep mucus thin
- Cool humidification during sleep with a cool mist tent or room humidifier
- Rest from activity
- Tracheostomy, O_2 administration

Drug therapy
- Antipyretic: acetaminophen (Tylenol)
- Antibiotics if the cause is bacterial

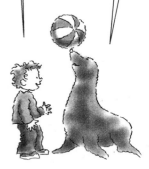

We may sound alike, but one of us has croup...

...and one of us is just asking for applause.

• Inhaled racemic epinephrine and cortico-steroids such as methylprednisolone sodium succinate to alleviate severe respiratory distress

INTERVENTIONS AND RATIONALES
• Assess respiratory and cardiovascular status *to detect any indications that the obstruction is worsening.*
• Monitor vital signs and pulse oximetry readings *to detect early signs of respiratory compromise.*
• Administer O_2 therapy and maintain the child in a cool mist tent, if needed. *Cool mist helps liquefy secretions.*
• Administer medications, as ordered, and note their effectiveness *to maintain or improve the child's condition.*
• Prop the infant in a car seat or with a pillow; position an older child in Fowler's position *to ease respiratory effort.*
• Provide emotional support for the parents *to decrease anxiety.*
• Provide age-appropriate activities for the child confined to the mist tent *to ease anxiety.*
• Monitor for rebound obstruction when administering racemic epinephrine; *the drug's effects are short term and may result in rebound obstruction.*

Teaching topics
• Explanation of the disorder and treatment plan
• Medication use and possible adverse effects
• Humidification method
• Importance of hydration
• Signs and symptoms of complications
• Keeping the child calm to ease respiratory effort and conserve energy

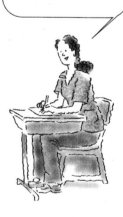

Parents may report a salty taste on the child's skin. In cystic fibrosis, the child's sweat contains two to five times the normal levels of sodium and chloride.

Cystic fibrosis

Cystic fibrosis is a generalized dysfunction of the exocrine glands that affects multiple organ systems. This disorder is characterized by:
• airway obstruction caused by the increased production of thick, tenacious mucus

• little or no release of pancreatic enzymes (lipase, amylase, and trypsin).

Transmitted as an autosomal recessive trait, cystic fibrosis is one of the most common inherited diseases in children. The disease occurs equally in both sexes. With improvements in treatment over the past decade, the average life expectancy has risen dramatically. The clinical effects may become apparent soon after birth or take years to develop.

CAUSES
• Autosomal recessive mutation of gene on chromosome 7

ASSESSMENT FINDINGS
• Bulky, greasy, foul-smelling stools that contain undigested food
• Distended abdomen and thin arms and legs from steatorrhea
• Failure to thrive from malabsorption
• History of a chronic, productive cough and recurrent respiratory infections
• Meconium ileus in the neonate from a lack of pancreatic enzymes
• Parents' report of a salty taste on the child's skin
• Voracious appetite from undigested food lost in stools

DIAGNOSTIC TEST RESULTS
• Chest X-ray indicates early signs of obstructive lung disease.
• Sweat test using pilocarpine iontophoresis is greater than 60 mEq/L.
• Stool specimen analysis indicates the absence of trypsin.
• Deoxyribonucleic acid testing shows presence of the delta F 508 cystic fibrosis gene.
• Serum albumin is decreased.

NURSING DIAGNOSES
• Imbalanced nutrition: Less than body requirements
• Impaired gas exchange
• Risk for infection
• Ineffective airway clearance
• Delayed growth and development

TREATMENT
- Chest physiotherapy
- Nebulization and breathing exercises several times a day
- Postural drainage
- Heart-lung transplant
- High-protein formula, if needed

Drug therapy
- Mucolytic (dornase alfa [Pulmozyme]), bronchodilator, or antibiotic nebulizer inhalation treatment before chest physiotherapy
- I.V. antibiotics for a *Pseudomonas* infection when the infection interferes with daily functioning
- Oral pancreatic enzyme replacement with pancrelipase (Pancrease)
- Multivitamins twice per day, especially fat-soluble vitamins A, D, E, and K

INTERVENTIONS AND RATIONALES
- Assess respiratory and cardiovascular status *for early detection of hypoxia.*
- Monitor vital signs and intake and output *to detect dehydration, which may worsen respiratory status.*
- Monitor pulse oximetry readings *to detect early signs of hypoxia.*
- Administer pancreatic enzymes with meals and snacks *to aid digestion and absorption of nutrients.*
- Provide high-calorie, high-protein foods with added salt *to replace sodium loss and promote normal growth.*
- Encourage breathing exercises and perform chest physiotherapy two to four times per day *to mobilize secretions, maintain lung capacity, and increase oxygenation.*
- Encourage physical activity *to promote normal development.*

Teaching topics
- Explanation of the disorder and treatment plan
- Medication use and possible adverse effects
- Chest physiotherapy
- Signs and symptoms of infection or complications

- Avoiding cough suppressants and antihistamines because the child must be able to cough and expectorate
- Genetic counseling for the family

Epiglottiditis

Epiglottiditis, a potentially life-threatening infection, causes inflammation and edema of the epiglottis, a lidlike cartilaginous structure overhanging the entrance to the larynx and serving to prevent food from entering the larynx and trachea while swallowing. Epiglottiditis is most common among preschoolers.

CAUSES
- Bacterial *Haemophilus influenzae* (most common causative organism)
- Pneumococci and group A beta-hemolytic streptococci

ASSESSMENT FINDINGS
- Cough
- Difficult and painful swallowing
- Extending the neck in a sniffing position
- Fever
- Increased drooling
- Irritability
- Lower rib retractions
- Pallor
- Rapid pulse rate
- Rapid respirations
- Refusal to drink
- Restlessness
- Sore throat
- Stridor
- Tripod sitting position
- Use of accessory muscles

DIAGNOSTIC TEST RESULTS
- Lateral neck X-ray shows an enlarged epiglottis.
- Direct laryngoscopy shows a swollen, beefy epiglottis.

NURSING DIAGNOSES
- Fear
- Deficient fluid volume
- Anxiety

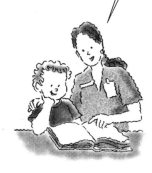

Key assessment findings for epiglottiditis: difficulty swallowing, increased drooling, restlessness, and stridor.

- Ineffective airway clearance
- Ineffective breathing pattern

TREATMENT
- Possible emergency endotracheal intubation or a tracheotomy
- Oxygen therapy or a cool mist tent
- I.V. fluid to prevent dehydration

Drug therapy
- Parenteral antibiotics: 10-day course according to the causative organism

INTERVENTIONS AND RATIONALES
- Monitor vital signs and pulse oximetry *to detect changes in oxygenation.*
- Assess respiratory and cardiovascular status *to determine the severity of the child's condition and prevent respiratory failure or arrest.*
- Don't inspect the oropharynx if epiglottiditis is suspected *because of the risk of occluding the airway.*
- Allow the child to sit on a parent's lap; *sitting on a parent's lap makes breathing easier and decreases anxiety.*
- Have equipment ready for a tracheotomy or intubation. *Emergency intubation and tracheotomy equipment should be on hand in case complete obstruction occurs.*
- Provide humidified oxygen therapy and a cool mist tent. *Humidified oxygen prevents secretions from thickening.*
- Administer medications as ordered *to treat infection and improve respiratory function.*
- Provide emotional support for the child and family *to decrease anxiety.*

Teaching topics
- Explanation of the disorder and treatment plan
- Medication use and possible adverse effects
- Importance of beginning *H. influenzae* immunization at age 2 months

Respiratory syncytial virus

RSV is a lower respiratory infection that's spread by respiratory secretions rather than droplets. It's the leading cause of lower respiratory infections in infants and young children and typically affects infants younger than age 6 months in the winter and spring. Mortality in this age-group is 1% to 6%.

CAUSES
- RSV

ASSESSMENT FINDINGS
- Sternal retractions, nasal flaring
- Tachypnea
- Thick mucus
- Nasal congestion
- Increased mucus production
- Watery drainage from the eyes
- Coughing
- Malaise
- Fever
- Dyspnea
- Sore throat
- Wheezes, rhonchi, crackles

DIAGNOSTIC TEST RESULTS
- Bronchial mucus culture shows RSV.
- Serum RSV antibody titers are elevated.

NURSING DIAGNOSES
- Impaired gas exchange
- Ineffective airway clearance
- Ineffective breathing pattern
- Fear
- Activity intolerance

TREATMENT
- Oral hydration, if possible
- Cool mist tent
- Humidified oxygen
- I.V. fluids (with severe infection)
- Rest periods when fatigued

Drug therapy
- Antiviral agent: ribavirin (Virazole)
- Antiviral immunoglobulin: palivizumab (Synagis) administered prophylactically to high-risk patients to prevent RSV infection

INTERVENTIONS AND RATIONALES
- Monitor vital signs and pulse oximetry *to determine oxygenation needs and to detect deterioration or improvement in the child's condition.*

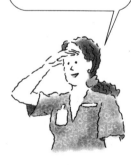

Key findings in RSV: sternal retractions and tachypnea.

- Assess respiratory and cardiovascular status. *Tachycardia may result from hypoxia or the effects of bronchodilator use.*
- Use gloves, gowns, and aseptic hand washing as secretion precautions *to prevent the spread of infection.*
- Administer chest physiotherapy after edema has abated. *Chest physiotherapy helps loosen mucus that may be blocking small airways.*
- Administer humidified oxygen therapy *to liquefy secretions and reduce bronchial edema.*
- Monitor for signs and symptoms of dehydration. Administer and maintain I.V. therapy *to promote hydration and replace electrolytes.*

Teaching topics
- Explanation of the disorder and treatment plan
- Review of medications, dosages, and adverse reactions
- Providing adequate nutrition and hydration
- Importance of humidified environment
- Avoiding people with cold symptoms
- Preventing the spread of infection

Sudden infant death syndrome

SIDS is the sudden death of an infant in which a postmortem examination fails to confirm the cause of death. The peak age is 3 months; 90% of cases occur before age 6 months, especially during the winter and early spring months.

Children who are diagnosed with SIDS are typically described as healthy with no previous medical problems. They're usually found dead sometime after being put down to sleep.

CAUSES
- Possibly viral
- Hypoxia theory
- Apnea theory
- Possible clostridium botulism toxin
- Possibly associated with diphtheria, tetanus, and pertussis vaccines

- Higher incidence with parents who smoke

ASSESSMENT FINDINGS
- History of low birth weight
- History of siblings with SIDS
- Previous near-SIDS event
- Death occurring during sleep without noise or struggle

DIAGNOSTIC TEST RESULTS
- Autopsy is the only way to diagnose SIDS. Autopsy findings indicate pulmonary edema, intrathoracic petechiae, and other minor changes suggesting chronic hypoxia and rules out suffocation and aspiration as a cause of death.

NURSING DIAGNOSES
- Impaired gas exchange
- Impaired spontaneous ventilation

TREATMENT
- None
- If the child can be resuscitated, it's called an *acute life-threatening event* (near-SIDS) and monitoring of the child is initiated.

Drug therapy
- If resuscitation is attempted, drugs are administered according to Pediatric Advanced Life Support protocols; drug therapy may include epinephrine, atropine and, after ABG analysis, sodium bicarbonate, if appropriate.

INTERVENTIONS AND RATIONALES
- Because the infant can't be resuscitated, focus your interventions on providing emotional support for the family. Keep in mind that grief may be coupled with guilt. Allow them to express their feelings. *Parents need to express feelings to prevent dysfunctional grieving.*
- Let the parents touch, hold, and rock the infant, if desired, and allow them to say goodbye to the infant *to facilitate the grieving process.*
- Contact appropriate spiritual support *to help the parents cope with grief.*

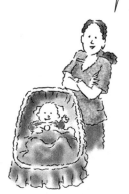

Research indicates a decreased incidence of SIDS in infants maintained in a supine position.

- Provide literature on SIDS and support groups; suggest psychological support for the surviving children *to help prevent maladaptive emotional responses to loss, to promote a realistic perspective on the tragedy, and to promote coping.*
- Act as an advocate for the parents if a police investigation is performed *to provide support.*

Teaching topics

- Explanation of the disorder as a reason for infant death
- Preparing the family for how the infant will look and feel if members touch and hold him
- Providing information on end-of-life procedures

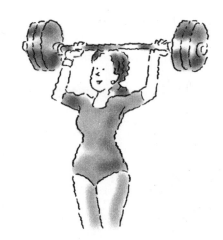

Pump up on practice questions

1. A parent brings her child to the pediatrician's office because of difficulty breathing and a "barking" cough. These signs are associated with which of the following conditions?
1. Cystic fibrosis
2. Asthma
3. Epiglottiditis
4. Croup

Answer: 4. A "seal bark" cough and difficulty breathing indicate croup. Cystic fibrosis produces a chronic productive cough and recurrent respiratory infections. Asthma may cause prolonged expiration with an expiratory wheeze on auscultation, dyspnea, and accessory muscle use. Epiglottiditis results in increased drooling, difficulty swallowing, tachypnea, and stridor.

➡ NCLEX keys

Client needs category: Physiological integrity
Client needs subcategory: Physiological adaptation
Cognitive level: Analysis

2. A woman with a child who awakes at night with a "barking" cough asks the nurse for advice. The nurse should instruct the mother to:
1. take the child in the bathroom, turn on the shower, and let the room fill with steam.

2. bring the child to the emergency department immediately.
3. notify the pediatrician immediately.
4. call emergency medical services to transport the child to the hospital for an emergency tracheotomy.

Answer: 1. The nurse should instruct the mother to take her child into the bathroom, close the door, turn on the shower's hot-water spigot full-force, and sit with the child as the room fills with steam; this should decrease laryngeal spasm. Epiglottiditis is a potentially life-threatening infection that causes inflammation and edema of the epiglottis. If a child demonstrates symptoms associated with epiglottiditis, not croup (increased drooling, stridor, tachypnea), the mother should notify the pediatrician immediately and call the emergency medical services to transport the child to the hospital; emergency tracheotomy may be necessary. Taking the child to the hospital by herself could jeopardize the child's condition if that condition deteriorates en route.

➡ *NCLEX keys*
Client needs category: Physiological integrity
Client needs subcategory: Reduction of risk potential
Cognitive level: Application

3. A child with croup is placed in a cool mist tent. Which statement should the nurse include when teaching the mother about this type of therapy?
1. "You won't be able to touch your child while he's in the cool mist tent."
2. "The cool mist is necessary because it will thin the child's mucus, making it easier to expectorate."
3. "You can bring in your child's favorite stuffed animal to comfort him while he's in the cool mist tent."
4. "You can bring in any of your child's favorite toys so he can play while he's in the cool mist tent."

Answer: 2. The mother should be taught the purpose of the cool mist tent, which is to thin mucus and facilitate expectoration. The mother is able to touch her child while he's in the cool mist tent. She should be encouraged to bring in toys for the child to play with but to avoid stuffed toys, which may become damp and promote bacterial growth, and toys that produce sparks or friction.

➡ *NCLEX keys*
Client needs category: Physiological integrity
Client needs subcategory: Reduction of risk potential
Cognitive level: Application

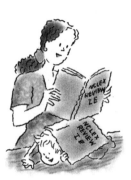

4. A physician orders chest physiotherapy for a child. The nurse shouldn't perform chest physiotherapy when the child is experiencing:
1. a productive cough.
2. retained secretions.
3. acute bronchoconstriction.
4. hypoxia.

Answer: 3. The nurse shouldn't administer chest physiotherapy during episodes of acute bronchoconstriction or airway edema (loosening mucus plugs could cause airway obstruction). Chest physiotherapy aids the elimination of secretions and reexpansion of lung tissue. Successful treatment with chest physiotherapy produces improved breath sounds, improved oxygenation, and increased sputum production and airflow. Therefore, it should be performed when a productive cough, retained secretions, or hypoxia is present.

➡ *NCLEX keys*
Client needs category: Physiological integrity
Client needs subcategory: Reduction of risk potential
Cognitive level: Application

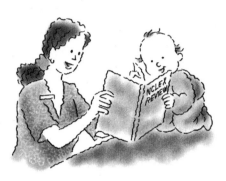

5.   A nurse is caring for a 17-year-old female client with cystic fibrosis who has been admitted to the hospital to receive I.V. antibiotic and respiratory treatment for exacerbation of a lung infection. The client has questions about her future and the consequences of the disease. Which statements about the course of cystic fibrosis are true? Select all that apply.
1.   Breast development is commonly delayed.
2.   The client is at risk for developing diabetes.
3.   Pregnancy and child-bearing aren't affected.
4.   Normal sexual relationships can be expected.
5.   Only males carry the gene for the disease.
6.   By age 20, the client can probably decrease the frequency of respiratory treatment.

Answer: 1, 2, 4. Cystic fibrosis delays growth and the onset of puberty. Children with cystic fibrosis tend to be smaller than average size and develop secondary sex characteristics later in life. In addition, clients with cystic fibrosis are at risk for developing diabetes mellitus because the pancreatic duct becomes obstructed as pancreatic tissues are destroyed. Clients with cystic fibrosis can expect to have normal sexual relationships, but fertility becomes difficult because thick secretions obstruct the cervix and block sperm entry. Males and females carry the gene for cystic fibrosis. Pulmonary disease commonly progresses as the client ages, requiring additional (not fewer) respiratory treatments.

➡ *NCLEX keys*
Client needs category: Physiological integrity
Client needs subcategory: Physiological adaptation
Cognitive level: Analysis

6.   Which test result is a key finding in the child with cystic fibrosis?
1.   Chest X-ray that reveals interstitial fibrosis
2.   Neck X-ray showing areas of upper airway narrowing
3.   Lateral neck X-ray revealing an enlarged epiglottis
4.   Positive pilocarpine iontophoresis sweat test

Answer: 4. A child with cystic fibrosis has a positive pilocarpine iontophoresis sweat test. The child sweats normally, but this sweat contains two to five times the normal levels of sodium and chloride. Chest X-ray findings that reveal bronchiolar metaplasia and interstitial fibrosis are associated with bronchopulmonary dysplasia. A neck X-ray that reveals upper airway narrowing and edema in the subglottic folds indicates croup. A lateral neck X-ray that reveals an enlarged epiglottis indicates epiglottiditis.

➡ *NCLEX keys*
Client needs category: Physiological integrity
Client needs subcategory: Reduction of risk potential
Cognitive level: Knowledge

7. When communicating with the grieving family after a death from sudden infant death syndrome (SIDS), the nurse should:

1. instruct the parents to place other infants on their backs to sleep.
2. stress that the death isn't the parents' fault.
3. stress that an autopsy must be done to confirm diagnosis.
4. stress that the parents are still young and can have more children.

Answer: 2. It's most important for the nurse to stress that death from SIDS isn't predictable or preventable and that it isn't the parents' fault. Although it's important to inform the parents that an autopsy is necessary, that's secondary. Instructing the parents to place other infants on their backs to sleep implies that the parents did something wrong to cause the infant's death. Stressing that the parents are still young and can have other children minimizes their grief.

➡ *NCLEX keys*
Client needs category: Psychosocial integrity
Client needs subcategory: None
Cognitive level: Application

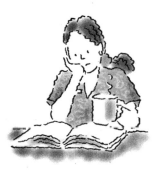

8. A 12-year-old with asthma suddenly becomes short of breath. How should a nurse position the child?

1. Dorsal recumbent position
2. Lithotomy position
3. Semi-Fowler's position
4. Sims' position

Answer: 3. The nurse should position the child in semi-Fowler's position (or sitting at about 45 degrees) because it facilitates lung expansion. The dorsal recumbent position doesn't ease the work of breathing.

The lithotomy position is normally used for gynecologic examinations. Sims' position is a lateral position with the top leg flexed toward the chest; this position inhibits lung expansion.

➡ *NCLEX keys*
Client needs category: Physiological integrity
Client needs subcategory: Basic care and comfort
Cognitive level: Application

9. A nurse is teaching the parents of a child with cystic fibrosis. The nurse should teach the parents to:

1. discourage their child from being physically active.
2. administer pancreatic enzymes after meals and snacks.
3. avoid administering cough suppressants.
4. have their child avoid salt intake.

Answer: 3. The parents of a child with cystic fibrosis should be taught to avoid administering cough suppressants and antihistamines to their child. Administration of these drugs interferes with the child's ability to cough and expectorate. The parents should encourage the child to be physically active. Pancreatic enzymes should be administered with meals and snacks, not after meals. Salt shouldn't be avoided; the child with cystic fibrosis has an increased salt loss.

➡ *NCLEX keys*
Client needs category: Physiological integrity
Client needs subcategory: Reduction of risk potential
Cognitive level: Application

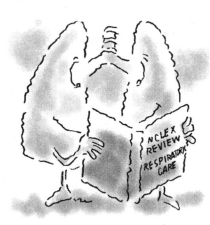

10. Which is the most appropriate nursing diagnosis for the child with epiglottiditis?
  1. *Anxiety related to separation from the parent*
  2. *Decreased cardiac output related to bradycardia*
  3. *Ineffective airway clearance related to laryngospasm*
  4. *Impaired gas exchange related to noncompliant lungs*

Answer: 3. Epiglottiditis is a life-threatening emergency that results from laryngospasm and edema. Therefore, ineffective airway clearance is the most appropriate diagnosis for this child. Anxiety related to separation shouldn't apply because the child doesn't need to be separated from the parent. The child will most likely be tachycardiac, not bradycardiac, unless respiratory failure ensues. The child has impaired gas exchange from impeded airflow, not from a noncompliant lung.

➡ *NCLEX keys*
Client needs category: Physiological integrity
Client needs subcategory: Physiological adaptation
Cognitive level: Analysis

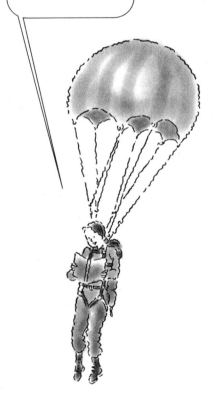

Take a breath, and then get ready to jump into the next chapter.

6 Hematologic & immune systems

Brush up on key concepts

The hematologic and immune systems consist of blood and blood-forming tissues and structures, such as the lymph nodes, thymus, spleen, and tonsils. Reviewing the functions of these systems and the development of a child's immune response lays the groundwork for effective care.

At any time, you can review the major points of this chapter by consulting the *Cheat sheet* on pages 62 and 63.

What blood does
The functions of blood include:
• regulating body temperature by transferring heat from deep within the body to small vessels near the skin
• providing cell nutrition by carrying nutrients from the GI tract to the tissues and removing waste products by transporting them to the lungs, kidneys, liver, and skin for excretion
• defending against foreign antigens by transporting leukocytes and antibodies to the sites of infection, injury, and inflammation
• transporting hormones from endocrine glands to various parts of the body
• maintaining acid-base balance
• carrying oxygen to tissues and removing carbon dioxide.

Each little component does its part
Blood is composed of several components. These include:
• **erythrocytes** (red blood cells [RBCs]), which carry oxygen to the tissues and remove carbon dioxide
• **leukocytes** (white blood cells [WBCs]), which include lymphocytes, monocytes, and granulocytes; these participate in the immune response
• **thrombocytes** (platelets), which contribute to clotting
• **plasma** (the fluid part of blood), which carries antibodies and nutrients to tissues and carries wastes away.

It's common
Communicable diseases and **infections** are commonly seen during the time a child's immune system develops. Over time, a child receives protection from communicable diseases either naturally or artificially.

It's natural
• **Natural (innate) immunity** is present at birth. Examples of natural immunity include barriers against disease, such as skin and mucous membranes, and bacteriocidal substances of body fluids, such as intestinal flora and gastric acidity.
• In **naturally acquired active immunity,** the immune system makes antibodies after exposure to disease. It requires contact with the disease.
• In **naturally acquired passive immunity,** no active immune process is involved. The antibodies are passively received through placental transfer by immunoglobulin G (the smallest immunoglobulin) and breast-feeding (colostrum).

It's artificial
Artificially acquired immunity can be active or passive. In **artificially acquired active immunity,** medically engineered substances are ingested or injected to stimulate the immune response against a specific disease. Immunizations are an example of this kind of immunity.

In **artificially acquired passive immunity,** antibodies are injected without

(Text continues on page 64.)

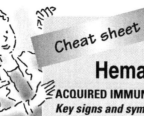

Hematologic & immune refresher

ACQUIRED IMMUNODEFICIENCY SYNDROME
Key signs and symptoms
- Failure to thrive
- Mononucleosis-like prodromal symptoms
- Night sweats
- Recurring diarrhea
- Weight loss

Key test results
- CD4+ T-cell count measures the severity of immunosuppression.
- Enzyme-linked immunosorbent assay and Western blot are positive for human immunodeficiency virus (HIV) antibody.
- Polymerase chain reaction detects HIV deoxyribonucleic acid.

Key treatments
- Antibiotic therapy according to sensitivity of infecting organisms
- Antiviral agent: zidovudine (Retrovir)
- Monthly gamma globulin administration

Key interventions
- Monitor vital signs and intake and output
- Monitor developmental progress at regular intervals.
- Assess respiratory and neurologic status.
- Maintain standard precautions.

HEMOPHILIA
Key signs and symptoms
- Multiple bruises without petechiae
- Prolonged bleeding after circumcision, immunizations, or minor injuries

Key test results
- Partial thromboplastin time (PTT) is prolonged (for both types).
Hemophilia A
- Factor VIII assay is 25% of normal or less.
Hemophilia B
- Factor IX assay is deficient.
- Baseline coagulation results are similar to those of hemophilia A but with normal factor VIII.

Key treatments
- Avoiding I.M. injections

Hemophilia A
- Cryoprecipitated antihemophilic factor (AHF), lyophilized AHF, or both
- Desmopressin (Stimate)
Hemophilia B
- Factor IX concentrate

Key interventions
- Monitor vital signs and intake and output.
- When bleeding occurs:
  - elevate the affected extremity above the heart
  - immobilize the site to prevent clots from dislodging
  - apply pressure to the site for 10 to 15 minutes to stop bleeding
  - decrease anxiety to lower the child's heart rate.

IRON DEFICIENCY ANEMIA
Key signs and symptoms
- Fatigue, listlessness
- Increased susceptibility to infection
- Pallor
- Tachycardia
- Numbness and tingling of the extremities
- Vasomotor disturbances

Key test results
- Hemoglobin, hematocrit, and serum ferritin levels are low.
- Serum iron levels are low, with high binding capacity.

Key treatments
- Oral preparation of iron (Fer-In-Sol) or a combination of iron and ascorbic acid (which enhances iron absorption)

Key interventions
- Administer iron before meals with citrus juice. (Iron is best absorbed in an acidic environment.)
- Give liquid iron through a straw to prevent staining the child's skin and teeth; for infants, administer by oral syringe toward the back of the mouth.
- Don't give iron with milk products because these products may interfere with absorption.

Hematologic & immune refresher *(continued)*

LEUKEMIA

Key signs and symptoms
- Fatigue
- Sudden onset of high fever
- Lymphadenopathy
- Pallor
- Petechiae and ecchymosis
- Liver or spleen enlargement

Key test results
- Blast cells appear in the peripheral blood.
- Blast cells may be as high as 95% in the bone marrow.
- Initial white blood cell count may be less than 10,000/µl at the time of diagnosis in a child with acute lymphocytic leukemia between ages 3 and 7.

Key treatments
- Stem cell transplantation
- Chemotherapy: vincristine, high-dose cytarabine (Cytosaru), and daunorubicin (Cerubidine); intrathecal chemotherapy usually with methotrexate
- Radiation therapy

Key interventions
- Provide pain relief, as ordered, and document its effectiveness and adverse effects.
- Monitor vital signs and intake and output.
- Inspect the skin frequently.
- Provide nursing measures to ease adverse effects of radiation and chemotherapy.

REYE SYNDROME

Key signs and symptoms
- Stage 5: seizures, loss of deep tendon reflexes, flaccidity, respiratory arrest (death is usually a result of cerebral edema or cardiac arrest)

Key test results
- Blood test results show elevated serum ammonia levels; serum fatty acid and lactate levels are also elevated.
- Coagulation studies reveal prolonged prothrombin time and PTT.
- Liver biopsy shows fatty droplets distributed through cells.
- Liver function studies show aspartate aminotransferase and alanine aminotransferase are elevated to twice normal levels.

Key treatments
- Endotracheal intubation and mechanical ventilation
- Osmotic diuretic: mannitol

Key interventions
- Monitor vital signs and pulse oximetry.
- Assess cardiac, respiratory, and neurologic status.
- Monitor fluid intake and output.
- Monitor blood glucose levels.

- Maintain seizure precautions.
- Keep the head of the bed at a 30-degree angle.
- Assess pulmonary artery catheter pressure.
- Administer blood products as necessary.
- Administer medications, as ordered, and monitor for adverse effects.
- Maintain a hypothermia blanket as needed, and monitor temperature every 15 to 30 minutes while in use.
- Check for loss of reflexes and signs of flaccidity.

SICKLE CELL ANEMIA

Key signs and symptoms
- In infants and toddlers, colic and splenomegaly
- In preschoolers, hypovolemia, shock, and pain at the site of vaso-occlusive crisis
- In school-age children and adolescents, enuresis, extreme pain at the site of crisis, and priapism

Key test results
- More than 50% hemoglobin S indicates sickle cell disease; a lower level of hemoglobin S indicates sickle cell trait.

Key treatments
- Hydration with I.V. fluid administration
- Transfusion therapy as necessary
- Treatment for acidosis as necessary
- Analgesic: morphine

Key interventions
- Monitor vital signs and intake and output.
- Administer pain medications and note their effectiveness.

THALASSEMIA

Key signs and symptoms
- Jaundice
- Anemia, commonly severe
- Bone abnormalities
- Failure to thrive

Key test results
- Complete blood count shows lowered red blood cell (RBC) and hemoglobin levels, microcytosis, and elevated reticulocyte count.
- Folate level will be decreased.

Key treatments
- Mostly supportive
- Transfusion to raise hemoglobin level; care must be used not to cause iron overload

Key interventions
- Monitor for signs and symptoms of transfusion reaction after RBC transfusions.
- Encourage genetic counseling for the child's parents.

stimulating the immune response. Examples include tetanus antitoxin, hepatitis B immune globulin, and varicella zoster immune globulin.

Keep abreast of diagnostic tests

Here are the most important tests used to diagnose hematologic and immunologic disorders, along with common nursing interventions associated with each test.

Not my type?
Blood typing is used to determine the antigens present in a patient's RBCs. A reaction with standardized sera indicates the presence of specific antigens.

Nursing actions
• Explain the procedure to the child and family.
• Handle the sample gently to prevent hemolysis.
• Apply pressure to the venipuncture site to prevent hematoma or bleeding.

Tuning into the immune system
Laboratory studies, such as **CD4+ T-cell count** and **enzyme-linked immunosorbent assay (ELISA),** are used to assess immunosuppression.

Nursing actions
• Explain the procedure to the child and family.
• Handle the sample gently to prevent hemolysis.
• Apply pressure to the venipuncture site to prevent hematoma or bleeding.

Clot measure
A **coagulation study** tests a blood sample to analyze platelet function, platelet count, prothrombin time (PT), International Normalized Ratio, partial thromboplastin time (PTT), coagulation time, and bleeding time.

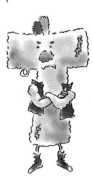

Be gentle with me. CD4+ T-cell counts measure the severity of immunosuppression. Handle the sample gently to prevent hemolysis.

Nursing actions
• Explain the procedure to the child and family.
• Note the child's current drug therapy before procedure.
• Check the venipuncture site for bleeding after the procedure.

A look at the liver
Liver function studies measure levels of hepatic enzymes, such as aspartate aminotransferase (AST) and alanine aminotransferase (ALT).

Nursing actions
• Explain the procedure to the child and family.
• After the test, check the venipuncture site for bleeding.

Polish up on client care

Major pediatric hematologic and immune disorders include acquired immunodeficiency syndrome (AIDS), hemophilia, iron deficiency anemia, leukemia, Reye syndrome, sickle cell anemia, and thalassemia.

Acquired immunodeficiency syndrome

In AIDS, the human immunodeficiency virus (HIV) attacks helper T cells. AIDS may be spread through sexual contact or percutaneous or mucous membrane exposure to needles or other sharp instruments contaminated with blood or bloody body fluid (for example, in I.V. drug abuse). Transmission may also occur between mother and infant during pregnancy or as a result of breastfeeding.

HIV has a much shorter incubation period in children than in adults. In adults, the incubation period may last 10 years or more. By contrast, children who receive the virus by placental transmission are usually HIV-positive by age 6 months and develop clinical signs by age 3.

Because of passive antibody transmission, all infants born to HIV-infected mothers test positive for antibodies to the HIV virus up to about age 18 months. Confirmation of diagnosis during this time requires detection of the HIV antigen.

CAUSES
- Contact with contaminated blood or bloody body fluid
- Infected parent via the birth process or breast-feeding

CONTRIBUTING FACTORS
- Drug use
- Sexual activity

ASSESSMENT FINDINGS
- Failure to thrive
- Lymphadenopathy
- Mononucleosis-like prodromal symptoms
- Neurologic impairment, such as loss of motor milestones and behavioral changes
- Night sweats
- Recurrent opportunistic infections
- Recurring diarrhea
- Weight loss

DIAGNOSTIC TEST RESULTS
- CD4+ T-cell count measures the severity of immunosuppression.
- Culture and sensitivity tests reveal infection with opportunistic organisms.
- ELISA and Western blot are positive for HIV antibody.
- Polymerase chain reaction (PCR) test detects HIV deoxyribonucleic acid (preferred test for children younger than age 18 months).

NURSING DIAGNOSES
- Risk for infection
- Anxiety
- Fear
- Interrupted family processes
- Ineffective protection
- Imbalanced nutrition: Less than body requirements
- Deficient fluid volume

TREATMENT
- Blood administration, if necessary
- Follow-up laboratory studies
- High-calorie diet provided in small, frequent meals
- I.V. fluids to maintain hydration
- Nutrition supplements, if necessary
- Parenteral nutrition, if necessary

Drug therapy
- Antibiotic therapy according to sensitivity of the infecting organisms
- Antiviral agent: zidovudine (Retrovir)
- Monthly gamma globulin administration
- Prophylactic antibiotic therapy with co-trimoxazole (Bactrim) to prevent *Pneumocystis carinii* pneumonia
- Routine immunizations (however, "live" vaccines, such as measles-mumps-rubella, varicella, and the nasal flu vaccine [FluMist] aren't recommended for HIV-infected children)

INTERVENTIONS AND RATIONALES
- Monitor vital signs and intake and output *to detect tachycardia, dyspnea, hypertension, or decreased urine output, which may indicate fluid volume deficit or electrolyte imbalance.*
- Monitor developmental progress at regular intervals *to detect changes in level of functioning and, as appropriate, adapt activity program.*
- Provide appropriate play activities *to promote development.*
- Encourage fluid intake *to prevent dehydration.*
- Assess respiratory and neurologic status *to detect early signs of compromise.*
- Maintain standard precautions *to prevent the spread of infection.*
- Administer medications as ordered *to help boost immune response and prevent opportunistic infections.*
- Provide psychosocial support. *An AIDS diagnosis is devastating for the child and his family.*
- Assess the child's support system and provide referrals. *The child may have no one to care for him.*

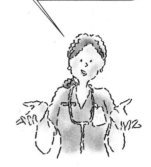

As with adults, children with AIDS exhibit nonspecific signs and symptoms.

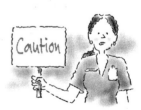

Children with HIV or AIDS and their families must maintain strict personal hygiene.

Caution

Teaching topics

- Explanation of the disorder and treatment plan
- Medication use and possible adverse effects
- Controlling infection in the home using sanitary measures
- Avoiding the consumption of raw or under-cooked meats
- Avoiding swimming in a lake or river
- Avoiding contact with young farm animals
- Understanding risk factors from pets (especially cats)
- Recognizing the signs and symptoms of infection and getting immediate treatment
- Practicing safer sex, if appropriate

Hemophilia

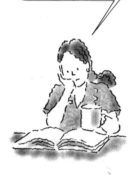

A classic sign of hemophilia: prolonged bleeding after minor injuries.

Hemophilia results from a deficiency in one of the coagulation factors.

The types of hemophilia are:
- hemophilia A (also called *factor VIII deficiency* or *classic hemophilia*), the most common type (75% of all cases)
- hemophilia B (also called *factor IX deficiency* or *Christmas disease*)

Hemophilia is an X-linked recessive disorder. The inheritance pattern is described here:
- If the father has the disorder and the mother doesn't, all daughters will be carriers but sons won't have the disease.
- If the mother is a carrier and the father doesn't have hemophilia, each son has a 50% chance of getting hemophilia and each daughter has a 50% chance of being a carrier.
- If the mother is a carrier and the father has hemophilia, the daughter will inherit the disease, but this situation is extremely rare.

CAUSES
- Genetic inheritance

ASSESSMENT FINDINGS
- Bleeding into the throat, mouth, and thorax
- Hemarthrosis; refusal to move affected joint
- Multiple bruises without petechiae
- Peripheral neuropathies from bleeding near peripheral nerves
- Prolonged bleeding after circumcision, immunizations, or minor injuries

DIAGNOSTIC TEST RESULTS
- PTT is prolonged (for both types).

Hemophilia A
- Factor VIII assay is 25% of normal or less.

Hemophilia B
- Factor IX assay is deficient.
- Baseline coagulation results are similar to those of hemophilia A but with normal factor VIII.

NURSING DIAGNOSES
- Acute pain
- Ineffective protection
- Risk for deficient fluid volume
- Risk for injury

TREATMENT
- Blood transfusion, if necessary
- Avoiding I.M. injections
- Promoting vasoconstriction during bleeding episodes by applying ice, pressure, and hemostatic agents

Drug therapy
- Aminocaproic acid (Amicar)
Hemophilia A
- Cryoprecipitated antihemophilic factor (AHF), lyophilized AHF, or both
- Desmopressin (Stimate)
Hemophilia B
- Factor IX concentrate

INTERVENTIONS AND RATIONALES
- Monitor vital signs and intake and output *to assess renal status and monitor for fluid overload or dehydration.*
- Assess cardiovascular status and check for signs of bleeding; *fever, tachycardia, or hypotension may indicate hypovolemia.*
- Measure the joint's circumference and compare it to that of an unaffected joint *to assess for bleeding into the joint, which may lead to hypovolemia.*
- Note swelling, pain, or limited joint mobility. *Changes may indicate progressive decline in function.*

- Assess for joint degeneration from repeated hemarthroses *to detect extent of damage.*
- Pad toys and other objects in the child's environment *to promote child safety and prevent bleeding.*
- Recommend protective headgear, soft foam Toothettes, soft toothbrush, and stool softeners as appropriate *to prevent bleeding.*
- Discourage abnormal weight gain, *which increases the load on joints.*

When bleeding occurs
- Elevate the affected extremity above the heart *to decrease circulation to the affected area and promote venous return.*
- Immobilize the site *to prevent clots from dislodging.*
- Apply pressure to the site for 10 to 15 minutes *to stop bleeding.*
- Decrease anxiety *to lower the child's heart rate.*
- Apply ice to the site *to promote vasoconstriction.*

To treat hemarthrosis
- Immobilize the affected extremity; elevate it in a slightly flexed position *to prevent further injury.*
- Decrease pain and anxiety *to lower the child's heart rate and minimize blood loss.*
- Avoid excessive handling or weight bearing for 48 hours *to prevent bleeding and to rest the site.*
- Begin mild range-of-motion exercises after 48 hours *to facilitate absorption and prevent contractures.*

Teaching topics
- Explanation of the disorder and treatment plan
- Meticulous dental care
- Medication use and possible adverse effects
- Genetic counseling for the parents
- Encouraging non-contact sports

Iron deficiency anemia

The most common nutritional anemia during childhood, iron deficiency anemia is characterized by poor RBC production. Insufficient body stores of iron lead to:
- depleted RBC mass
- decreased hemoglobin concentration (hypochromia)
- decreased oxygen-carrying capacity of blood.

Most commonly, iron deficiency anemia occurs when the child experiences rapid physical growth, low iron intake, inadequate iron absorption, or loss of blood. Peak incidence is at 12 to 18 months.

CAUSES
- Blood loss secondary to drug-induced GI bleeding (from anticoagulants, aspirin, steroids) or due to heavy menses, hemorrhage from trauma, GI ulcers, or cancer
- Inadequate dietary intake of iron (less than 1 to 2 mg/day), which may occur following prolonged unsupplemented breast-feeding or during periods when the body is stressed, such as rapid growth in children and adolescents; may also occur from excessive consumption of cow's milk rather than iron-fortified foods.
- Iron malabsorption, as in chronic diarrhea, partial or total gastrectomy, and malabsorption syndromes, such as celiac disease and pernicious anemia
- Intravascular hemolysis-induced hemoglobinuria or paroxysmal nocturnal hemoglobinuria
- Mechanical erythrocyte trauma caused by a prosthetic heart valve or vena cava filters

ASSESSMENT FINDINGS
Anemia progresses gradually, and many children are initially asymptomatic, except for symptoms of an underlying condition. Children with advanced anemia display the following symptoms:
- dyspnea on exertion
- fatigue
- headache
- inability to concentrate
- irritability
- listlessness
- pallor
- increased susceptibility to infection
- tachycardia.

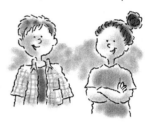

Anemia can follow periods of stress, such as times of rapid growth.

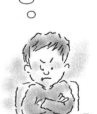

I wish liver wasn't so good for me.

In cases of chronic iron deficiency anemia, children display the following symptoms:
- cracks in corners of the mouth
- dysphagia
- neuralgic pain
- numbness and tingling of the extremities
- smooth tongue
- spoon-shaped, brittle nails
- vasomotor disturbances.

DIAGNOSTIC TEST RESULTS
- Bone marrow studies reveal depleted or absent iron stores and normoblastic hyperplasia.
- Hemoglobin, hematocrit, and serum ferritin levels are low.
- Mean corpuscular hemoglobin is decreased in severe anemia.
- RBC count is low, with microcytic and hypochromic cells. (In early stages, RBC count may be normal, except in infants and children.)
- Serum iron levels are low, with high binding capacity.

NURSING DIAGNOSES
- Activity intolerance
- Imbalanced nutrition: Less than body requirements
- Fatigue
- Impaired gas exchange
- Constipation

TREATMENT
- Increased iron intake (for children and adolescents) by adding foods rich in iron to the diet, or (for infants) adding iron supplements

Drug therapy
- Oral preparation of iron (Fer-In-Sol) or a combination of iron and ascorbic acid (which enhances iron absorption)
- Vitamin supplement: cyanocobalamin (vitamin B_{12}) if intrinsic factor is lacking
- Iron supplement: iron dextran (INFeD) if additional therapy is needed

INTERVENTIONS AND RATIONALES
- Carefully assess a child's drug history. *Certain drugs, such as pancreatic enzymes and vitamin E, may interfere with iron metabolism and absorption.*
- Provide passive stimulation; allow frequent rest; give small, frequent feedings; and elevate the head of the bed *to decrease oxygen demands.*
- Implement proper hand washing *to decrease the risk of infection.*
- Provide foods high in iron (liver, dark leafy vegetables, and whole grains) *to replenish iron stores.*
- Administer iron before meals with citrus juice. *Iron is best absorbed in an acidic environment.*
- Give liquid iron through a straw *to prevent staining the child's skin and teeth.* For infants, administer by oral syringe toward the back of the mouth.
- Don't give iron with milk products. *Milk products may interfere with iron absorption.*
- Monitor bowel patterns *to detect constipation.*
- Be supportive of the family and keep them informed of the child's status *to decrease anxiety.*

Teaching topics
- Explanation of the disorder and treatment plan
- Medication use and possible adverse effects
- Keeping iron supplements safely stored out of the child's reach at home
- Brushing teeth after iron administration
- Reporting reactions to iron supplementation, such as nausea, vomiting, diarrhea, constipation, fever, or severe stomach pain (may require a dosage adjustment)
- Understanding that iron supplements can affect bowel patterns and turn stools tarry black in color

Leukemia

Leukemia is the abnormal, uncontrolled proliferation of WBCs. In leukemia, WBCs are produced so rapidly that immature cells (blast cells) are released into the circulation. These blast cells are nonfunctional, can't fight infection, and are formed continuously without

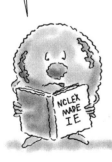

Blast it. In leukemia, I can't get the nutrition I need!

respect to the body's needs. This proliferation robs healthy cells of sufficient nutrition.

In children, the most common type of leukemia is acute lymphocytic leukemia (ALL). This type of leukemia is marked by extreme proliferation of immature lymphocytes (blast cells). In adolescents, acute myelogenous leukemia is more common and is believed to result from a malignant transformation of a single stem cell.

CAUSES AND CONTRIBUTING FACTORS
- Chemical exposure and viruses
- Chromosomal disorders
- Down syndrome
- Ionizing radiation

ASSESSMENT FINDINGS
Clinical findings for leukemia may appear with surprising abruptness in children with few, if any, warning signs. The following are common assessment findings of leukemia:
- blood in urine, stool, or emesis
- bone and joint pain
- decrease in all blood cells when bone marrow undergoes atrophy (leads to anemia, bleeding disorders, and immunosuppression)
- fatigue
- history of infections
- lassitude
- sudden onset of high fever
- lymphadenopathy
- pallor
- pathologic fractures when bone marrow undergoes hypertrophy
- petechiae and ecchymosis
- poor wound healing and oral lesions
- liver or spleen enlargement.

DIAGNOSTIC TEST RESULTS
- Blast cells appear in the peripheral blood (where they normally don't appear).
- Blast cells may be as high as 95% in the bone marrow (they're normally less than 5%) as measured by marrow aspiration in the posterior iliac crest (the sternum can't be used in children).
- Initial WBC count may be less than 10,000/µl at the time of diagnosis in a child with ALL between ages 3 and 7. (This child has the best prognosis.)

- Lumbar puncture indicates whether leukemic cells have crossed the blood-brain barrier.

NURSING DIAGNOSES
- Ineffective protection
- Acute or chronic pain
- Risk for infection
- Anxiety
- Fear
- Interrupted family processes

TREATMENT
- Hematopoietic stem cell transplant: stem cells are harvested and then returned to the recipient; stem cells can also be obtained from a sibling or a donor pool
- High-protein, high-calorie, bland diet
- I.V. fluids as necessary
- Oxygen therapy, if needed
- Radiation therapy
- Transfusion therapy as needed

Drug therapy
- Analgesics
- Antiemetic: ondansetron (Zofran)
- Chemotherapy: vincristine, high-dose cytarabine (Cytosaru), and daunorubicin (Cerubidine); intrathecal chemotherapy, usually with methotrexate
- Corticosteroid: prednisone (Deltasone)

INTERVENTIONS AND RATIONALES
- Monitor vital signs and intake and output *to determine fluid volume deficit and renal status.*
- Monitor for signs of infection. *Children with leukemia are highly susceptible to infection.*
- Give special attention to mouth care *to prevent infection and bleeding.*
- Inspect the skin frequently *to assess for skin breakdown.*

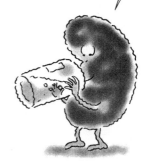

Increased fluid intake helps to flush chemotherapeutic drugs through the kidneys.

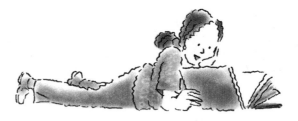

Stem cells may be transfused from a twin or another HLA-identical donor.

- Give increased fluids *to flush chemotherapeutic drugs through the kidneys.*
- Provide a "neutropenic diet" — a high-protein, high-calorie, bland diet with no raw fruits or vegetables. *Eliminating raw fruits and vegetables helps prevent infection. A diet meeting the child's caloric requirements helps ensure that the child's maintenance and growth needs are met.*
- Discourage keeping any live plants in the room *to prevent introduction of bacteria.*
- Provide pain relief, as ordered, and document its effectiveness and adverse effects. *Analgesics depress the central nervous system (CNS), thereby reducing pain.*
- Monitor the CNS *to assess for changes such as confusion that may result from cerebral damage.*
- Provide nursing measures to ease the adverse effects of radiation and chemotherapy *to promote comfort and encourage adequate nutritional intake.*

Teaching topics
- Explanation of the disorder and treatment plan
- Avoiding crowds, people with infection or illness, pets, and raw fruits and vegetables
- Medication use and possible adverse effects
- Adjusting to changes in body image
- Contacting support groups
- Recognizing the signs and symptoms of infection and the need to seek immediate medical attention

Reye syndrome

Reye syndrome is an acute illness that causes fatty infiltration of the liver, kidneys, brain, and myocardium. It can lead to hyperammonemia, encephalopathy, and increased intracranial pressure (ICP).

CAUSES
- Acute viral infection, such as upper respiratory tract, type B influenza, or varicella (Reye syndrome almost always follows within 1 to 3 days of infection)
- Concurrent aspirin use (high incidence)

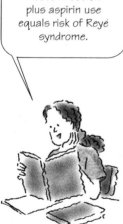

Acute infection plus aspirin use equals risk of Reye syndrome.

ASSESSMENT FINDINGS
Reye syndrome develops in five stages. The severity of signs and symptoms varies with the degree of encephalopathy and cerebral edema:
- Stage 1: vomiting, lethargy, hepatic dysfunction
- Stage 2: hyperventilation, delirium, hyperactive reflexes, hepatic dysfunction
- Stage 3: coma, hyperventilation, decorticate rigidity, hepatic dysfunction
- Stage 4: deepening coma, decerebrate rigidity, large fixed pupils, minimal hepatic dysfunction
- Stage 5: seizures, loss of deep tendon reflexes, flaccidity, respiratory arrest (death is usually a result of cerebral edema or cardiac arrest)

DIAGNOSTIC TEST RESULTS
- Blood test results show elevated serum ammonia levels; serum fatty acid and lactate levels are also increased.
- Cerebrospinal fluid (CSF) analysis shows WBC less than 10/µl; with coma, there's increased CSF pressure.
- Coagulation studies reveal prolonged PT and PTT.
- Liver biopsy shows fatty droplets uniformly distributed throughout cells.
- Liver function studies show AST and ALT elevated to twice normal levels.

NURSING DIAGNOSES
- Decreased intracranial adaptive capacity
- Ineffective thermoregulation
- Risk for imbalanced fluid volume
- Risk for injury

TREATMENT
- Craniotomy
- Endotracheal intubation and mechanical ventilation to control partial pressure of arterial carbon dioxide levels
- Enteral or parenteral nutrition as needed
- Exchange transfusion
- Induced hypothermia
- Transfusion of fresh frozen plasma
- I.V. fluids

Drug therapy
- Osmotic diuretic: mannitol
- Vitamin: phytonadione
- Ammonia detoxicants: sodium phenylacetate and sodium benzoate (Ammonul)

INTERVENTIONS AND RATIONALES
- Monitor ICP with a subarachnoid screw or other invasive device *to closely assess for increased ICP.*
- Monitor vital signs and pulse oximetry *to determine oxygenation status.*
- Assess cardiac, respiratory, and neurologic status *to evaluate the effectiveness of interventions and monitor for complications such as seizures.*
- Monitor fluid intake and output *to prevent fluid overload.*
- Monitor blood glucose levels *to detect hyperglycemia or hypoglycemia and prevent complications.*
- Maintain seizure precautions *to prevent injury.*
- Keep the head of the bed at a 30-degree angle *to decrease ICP and promote venous return.*
- Assess pulmonary artery catheter pressures *to assess cardiopulmonary status.*
- Maintain oxygen therapy, which may include intubation and mechanical ventilation, *to promote oxygenation and maintain thermoregulation.*
- Administer blood products as necessary *to increase oxygen-carrying capacity of the blood and prevent hypovolemia.*
- Administer medications, as ordered, and monitor for adverse effects *to detect complications.*
- Maintain a hypothermia blanket as needed and monitor temperature every 15 to 30 minutes while in use *to prevent injury and maintain thermoregulation.*
- Check for loss of reflexes and signs of flaccidity *to determine the degree of neurologic involvement.*
- Provide good skin and mouth care and range-of-motion exercises *to prevent alteration in skin integrity and promote joint motility.*
- Provide postoperative craniotomy care, if necessary, *to promote wound healing and prevent complications.*

- Be supportive of the family and keep them informed of the child's status *to decrease anxiety.*

Teaching topics
- Explanation of the disorder and treatment plan
- Medication use and possible adverse effects
- Avoiding aspirin products
- Explaining all procedures and nursing care measures to family
- Referring family to support groups as indicated

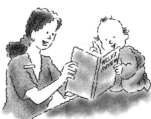

To prevent Reye syndrome, use nonsalicylate analgesics and antipyretics.

Sickle cell anemia

In sickle cell anemia, a defect in the hemoglobin molecule changes the oxygen-carrying capacity and shape of RBCs. The altered hemoglobin molecule is referred to as *hemoglobin S.* In this disorder, RBCs acquire a sickle shape.

The child may experience periodic, painful attacks called *sickle cell crises.* A sickle cell crisis may be triggered or intensified by:
- dehydration
- deoxygenation
- acidosis.

CAUSES
- Genetic inheritance (sickle cell anemia is an autosomal recessive trait; the child inherits the gene that produces hemoglobin S from two healthy parents who carry the defective gene)

ASSESSMENT FINDINGS
Assessment findings vary with the age of the child. Before age 4 months, symptoms are rare (because fetal hemoglobin prevents excessive sickling).

In infants and toddlers
- Colic from pain caused by an abdominal infarction
- Dactylitis or pain in the hands and feet caused by sickling and resulting in decreased blood flow to the hands and feet
- Splenomegaly from sequestered RBCs

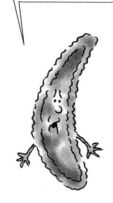

Red blood cells become sickle-shaped. Oh my.

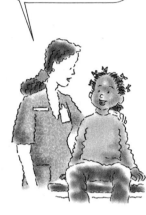

Findings for sickle cell anemia vary with age. For example, the spleen is enlarged in a young child. As the child grows, the spleen atrophies.

In preschoolers
• Hypovolemia and shock from sequestration of large amounts of blood in the spleen
• Pain at the site of vaso-occlusive crisis

In school-age children and adolescents
• Delayed growth and development and delayed sexual maturity
• Enuresis
• Extreme pain at the site of crisis
• History of pneumococcal pneumonia and other infections due to atrophied spleen
• Poor healing of leg wounds from inadequate peripheral circulation of oxygenated blood
• Priapism

DIAGNOSTIC TEST RESULTS
• Laboratory studies show hemoglobin level is 6 to 9 g/dl (in a toddler).
• More than 50% hemoglobin S indicates sickle cell disease; a lower level of hemoglobin S indicates sickle cell trait.
• RBCs are crescent-shaped and prone to agglutination.

NURSING DIAGNOSES
• Ineffective peripheral tissue perfusion
• Impaired gas exchange
• Acute pain

TREATMENT
• Bed rest
• Hydration with I.V. fluid administration (may be increased to 3 L/day during crisis)
• Short-term oxygen therapy (long-term oxygen decreases bone marrow activity, further aggravating anemia)
• Transfusion therapy as necessary
• Treatment for acidosis as necessary

Drug therapy
• Analgesic: morphine
• Antineoplastic: hydroxyurea (Droxia)
• Antibiotics: prophylaxis until age 6 to prevent bacterial septicemia
• Vaccine: pneumococcal vaccine

INTERVENTIONS AND RATIONALES
• Administer pain medication and note their effectiveness *to promote comfort.*

• Assess cardiovascular, respiratory, and neurologic status. *Tachycardia, dyspnea, or hypotension may indicate fluid volume deficit or electrolyte imbalance. Change in level of consciousness may signal neurologic involvement.*
• Assess for symptoms of acute chest syndrome from sickling of cells in the lung *to identify early complications.*
• Assess vision *to monitor for retinal complications.*
• Encourage the child to receive the pneumococcal vaccine *to prevent infection.*
• Give large amounts of oral or I.V. fluids *to prevent fluid volume deficit and prevent complications.*
• Teach the child relaxation techniques *to decrease the child's stress level.*
• Maintain the child's normal body temperature *to prevent stress and maintain adequate metabolic state.*
• Monitor vital signs and intake and output *to assess renal function and hydration status.*
• Provide proper skin care *to prevent skin breakdown.*
• Reduce the child's energy expenditure *to improve oxygenation.*
• Remove tight clothing *to prevent inadequate circulation.*
• Suggest family screening and initiate genetic counseling *to identify possible carriers of the disease.*

Teaching topics
• Explanation of the disorder and treatment plan
• Medication use and possible adverse effects
• Avoiding activities that promote a crisis, such as excessive exercise, mountain climbing, or deep sea diving
• Avoiding high altitudes
• Seeking early treatment of illness to prevent dehydration
• Avoiding aspirin use, which enhances acidosis and promotes sickling

Thalassemia

Thalassemia is characterized by a defective synthesis in the polypeptide chains necessary for hemoglobin production. RBC synthesis is also impaired.

β-thalassemia is the most common form of this disorder. It results from defective beta polypeptide chain synthesis and occurs in three clinical forms: major, intermedia, and minor.

The resulting anemia's severity depends on whether the patient is homozygous or heterozygous for the thalassemic trait. *Thalassemia major* and *thalassemia intermedia* result from homozygous inheritance or the partially dominant autosomal gene responsible for the trait. *Thalassemia minor* results from heterozygous inheritance of the same gene. Thalassemia is most common in people with Mediterranean ancestry, but also occurs in blacks and people from southern China, southeast Asia, and India.

Children with thalassemia major seldom survive to adulthood; children with thalassemia intermedia develop normally into adulthood, although puberty is usually delayed. Those with thalassemia minor can expect a normal life span.

CAUSES
- Genetic

ASSESSMENT FINDINGS
All types
- Jaundice
- Hepatomegaly
- Frequent infections
- Anemia, often severe
- Anorexia
- Bleeding tendencies
- Splenomegaly
- Bone abnormalities
- Failure to thrive

Thalassemia major
- Large head
- Mongoloid features
- Small body

DIAGNOSTIC TEST RESULTS
- Complete blood count shows lowered RBC and hemoglobin levels, microcytosis, and elevated reticulocyte count.
- Folate level is decreased.

- Peripheral blood smear shows target cells, microcytes, pale RBCs, and marked anisocytosis.
- X-ray may show osteoporosis.

NURSING DIAGNOSES
- Risk for injury
- Activity intolerance
- Ineffective protection

TREATMENT
- Mostly supportive
- Transfusion to raise hemoglobin level; care must be used not to cause iron overload
- Bone marrow transplant: showing early success

Drug therapy
- No iron supplements (they're contraindicated)
- Antibiotics: to treat infections
- Folic acid supplements

INTERVENTIONS AND RATIONALES
- Monitor for signs and symptoms after RBC transfusions *to help detect possible transfusion reaction.*
- Administer medications, as prescribed, *to help support the child.*
- Encourage genetic counseling for the parents *because thalassemia is a genetic condition.*

Teaching topics
- Explanation of the disorder and treatment plan
- Medication use and possible adverse effects
- Avoiding products that contain iron
- Recognizing signs and symptoms of hepatitis and iron overload
- Encouraging non-contact sports

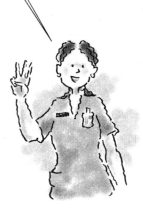

There are three types of β-thalassemia: major, intermedia, and minor.

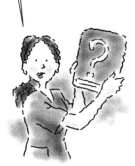

What does an X-ray show with thalassemia? Sometimes, it reveals osteoporosis.

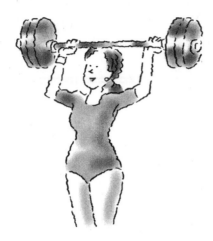

Pump up on practice questions

1. A nurse is taking a history from the mother of a child suspected of having Reye syndrome. The history reveals the use of several medications. Which medication might be implicated in the development of Reye syndrome?

1. Phenytoin (Dilantin)
2. Furosemide (Lasix)
3. Phytonadione
4. Aspirin

Answer: 4. Aspirin use has been implicated in the development of Reye syndrome in children with a history of recent acute viral infection. Phenytoin, furosemide, and phytonadione aren't associated with the development of Reye syndrome.

➡ NCLEX keys
Client needs category: Physiological integrity
Client needs subcategory: Reduction of risk potential
Cognitive level: Application

2. A 3-year-old child has been hospitalized in a vaso-occlusive crisis. To manage the pain associated with this crisis, the nurse should perform which intervention?

1. Apply moist heat and administer analgesics based on pain assessment.
2. Apply ice compresses to the affected areas and initiate range-of-motion exercises.
3. Elevate the affected areas and administer analgesics.
4. Provide a cooling blanket and administer acetaminophen (Tylenol).

Answer: 1. The major clinical feature of sickle cell anemia is pain from a vaso-occlusive crisis. Moist heat is applied to promote tissue oxygenation. Cold should be avoided because it promotes vasoconstriction and sickling. Analgesics should be administered based on the child's pain level, and aren't limited to acetaminophen.

➡ NCLEX keys
Client needs category: Physiological integrity
Client needs subcategory: Basic care and comfort
Cognitive level: Application

3. A nurse is teaching the mother of a child with sickle cell anemia. Which statement by the mother indicates a need for further teaching?

1. "My child can't possibly have sickle cell anemia. He's 4 months old, and he has never been sick before."
2. "I know my child should receive a pneumococcal vaccine when the doctor suggests."
3. "I know I should call the pediatrician immediately if my child begins to vomit."

4. "I know I should try to keep my child's body temperature normal by keeping him away from fluctuations in temperature."

Answer: 1. Further teaching is indicated if the mother states that her child can't have sickle cell anemia because he's 4 months old and has never been sick before. Symptoms of sickle cell anemia rarely appear before age 4 months because the predominance of fetal hemoglobin prevents excessive sickling. The child should receive a pneumococcal vaccine when appropriate. The mother should notify the physician if the child vomits so that treatment can be initiated to prevent dehydration, which can precipitate crisis. Changes in body temperature may also trigger crisis and should be avoided.

➡ *NCLEX keys*
Client needs category: Physiological integrity
Client needs subcategory: Reduction of risk potential
Cognitive level: Analysis

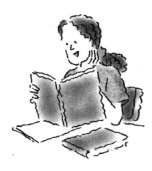

4. A nurse is teaching a mother about the benefits of breast-feeding her infant. Which type of immunity is passed on to the infant during breast-feeding?
1. Natural immunity
2. Naturally acquired active immunity
3. Naturally acquired passive immunity
4. Artificially acquired active immunity

Answer: 3. Naturally acquired passive immunity is received through placental transfer and breast-feeding. Natural immunity is present at birth. Naturally acquired active immunity occurs when the immune system makes antibodies after exposure to disease. Artificially acquired immunity occurs when medically engineered substances are ingested or injected to stimulate the immune response against a specific disease (immunizations).

➡ *NCLEX keys*
Client needs category: Health promotion and maintenance
Client needs subcategory: Safety and infection control
Cognitive level: Application

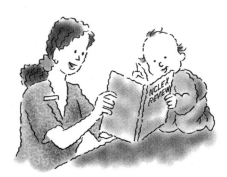

5. Which nursing interventions should a nurse anticipate when caring for a child in acute sickle cell crisis? Select all that apply.
1. Maintaining adequate hydration
2. Providing adequate pain control
3. Assessing family education needs
4. Encouraging healthy eating habits
5. Monitoring vital signs frequently
6. Attending to the child's play needs

Answer: 1, 2, 5. Because the child is in acute crisis, maintaining adequate hydration, providing pain control, and monitoring vital signs frequently are priority points of care. After the child's condition is stabilized, the nurse can then evaluate family learning needs, encourage healthy eating habits, and attend to the child's play needs.

➡ *NCLEX keys*

Client needs category: Physiological integrity
Client needs subcategory: Basic care and comfort
Cognitive level: Application

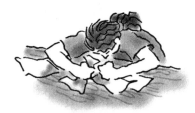

6. A nurse is providing dietary teaching for the mother of a child with iron deficiency anemia. Which iron-rich foods should the nurse instruct the mother to include in her child's diet?
1. Liver, dark leafy vegetables, and whole grains
2. Dark leafy vegetables, chicken, and whole grains
3. Whole grains, citrus fruit, and yogurt
4. Citrus fruit, liver, and whole grains

Answer: 1. The mother should be instructed to give her child iron-rich foods, such as liver, dark leafy vegetables, and whole grains. Chicken is a good source of protein, but it isn't high in iron. Citrus fruits aid iron absorption but aren't high in iron. Yogurt is a good source of calcium but isn't high in iron.

➡ *NCLEX keys*

Client needs category: Physiological integrity
Client needs subcategory: Basic care and comfort
Cognitive level: Application

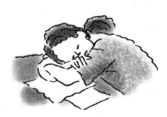

7. A nurse is teaching a child with sickle cell anemia and the child's mother about activities that may promote a vaso-occlusive crisis. Which activity is acceptable for this child?
1. Skiing
2. Mountain climbing
3. Deep sea diving
4. Bowling

Answer: 4. A child with sickle cell anemia should be instructed to avoid activities that promote a crisis, such as excessive exercise, mountain climbing, or deep sea diving. Extremes in temperature can also promote a crisis, so skiing should be avoided. Mountain climbing and deep sea diving may expose the child to altered atmospheric pressures and a deoxygenated state. These conditions can lead to a sickle cell crisis.

➡ *NCLEX keys*

Client needs category: Physiological integrity
Client needs subcategory: Reduction of risk potential
Cognitive level: Application

8. A neonate experiences prolonged bleeding after his circumcision and has multiple bruises without petechiae. These assessment findings suggest which condition?
  1. Iron deficiency anemia
  2. Hemophilia
  3. Sickle cell anemia
  4. Leukemia

Answer: 2. Signs of hemophilia include prolonged bleeding after circumcision, immunizations, or minor injuries; multiple bruises without petechiae; peripheral neuropathies from bleeding near peripheral nerves; bleeding into the throat, mouth, and thorax; and hemarthrosis. Some of the signs associated with iron deficiency anemia include dyspnea on exertion, fatigue, and listlessness. Signs and symptoms associated with sickle cell anemia include pain at the site of occlusion, poor healing of leg wounds, priapism, enuresis, and delayed growth and sexual maturity. Signs and symptoms associated with leukemia include history of infections, lymphadenopathy, hematuria, hematemesis, blood in stools, petechiae, and ecchymosis.

➡ *NCLEX keys*
Client needs category: Physiological integrity
Client needs subcategory: Reduction of risk potential
Cognitive level: Application

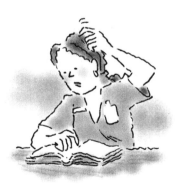

9. A child is admitted to the pediatric floor with hemophilia. The nurse encourages fantasy play and participation in his care. This developmental approach is most appropriate for which pediatric age-group?
  1. The school-age child (ages 5 to 12)
  2. The preschool child (ages 3 to 5)
  3. The toddler (ages 1 to 3)
  4. The adolescent (ages 12 to 18)

Answer: 1. School-age children engage in fantasy play and daydreaming. Therefore, it's appropriate for the nurse to encourage this type of play for the hospitalized child. The school-age child is also able to participate in his care. Doll play is helpful for the preschool hospitalized child. The toddler enjoys push-pull toys and games of peek-a-boo. The adolescent can engage in role playing in various situations.

➡ *NCLEX keys*
Client needs category: Health promotion and maintenance
Client needs subcategory: None
Cognitive level: Application

10. A nurse is providing instructions to the parents of an infant recovering from a sickle cell crisis. Which instruction should the nurse include in her teaching?
  1. "Discontinue administration of all antibiotics."
  2. "Keep the child isolated from all family members."
  3. "Restrict the child's nighttime fluids."
  4. "Make sure you hold the thermometer tightly under the arm."

Answer: 4. Infants with sickle cell anemia have altered immune function and are highly susceptible to bacterial sepsis. A fever in a child with sickle cell anemia is a medical emergency that requires prompt evaluation. The child should receive antibiotics until he is at least 5 years old. The infant should be isolated from persons with a known illness, but there's no reason to isolate him from all family members. Hydration is necessary for hemodilution and the prevention of sickling.

➡ *NCLEX keys*
Client needs category: Physiological integrity
Client needs subcategory: Reduction of risk potential
Cognitive level: Analysis

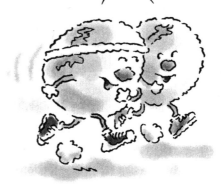

We bet this chapter got your blood pumping. Now it's on to the next one.

7 Neurosensory system

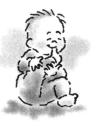

In time, my earliest, reflex-driven responses are replaced by motor responses that are under conscious control.

Brush up on key concepts

The **central nervous system** (CNS) is the body's communication network. It receives sensory stimuli through the five senses and either perceives, integrates, interprets, or retains the stimulus in memory. In an infant, early responses are primarily reflexive; the infant learns to discriminate stimuli and bring motor responses under conscious control. Language helps the older child improve and increase perception. In pediatric patients, flaccid muscles usually indicate a CNS disorder.

At any time, you can review the major points of this chapter by consulting the *Cheat sheet* on pages 80 to 82.

Upward, then downward
In children younger than age 3, the **ear canal** is directed upward. In older children, the ear canal is directed downward and forward. A child's **hearing** develops as follows:
- Sound discrimination is present at birth.
- By ages 5 to 6 months, the infant can localize sounds presented on a horizontal plane and begins to imitate selected sounds.
- By ages 7 to 12 months, the infant can localize sounds in any plane.
- By age 18 months, the child can hear and follow a simple command without visual cues.

Children who have difficulty with language development by age 18 months should have their hearing evaluated.

First, just alert
At birth, **visual function** is limited to alertness to visual stimuli 8" to 12" (20.5 to 30.5 cm) from the eyes. Normal newborns already have a blink reflex. After that, these findings are noted:

- Tear glands begin to secrete within the first 2 weeks of life.
- Transient strabismus (deviation of the eye) is a normal finding in the first few months.
- An infant can fixate on an object and follow a bright light or toy by ages 5 to 6 weeks.
- An infant can reach for objects at varying distances at ages 3 to 4 months.
- Vision reaches 20/20 when the child is about 4 years old.

Keep abreast of diagnostic tests

Here are the most important tests used to diagnose pediatric neurosensory disorders, along with common nursing interventions associated with each test.

Head check
A **basic assessment of cerebral function** includes:
- level of consciousness
- communication
- mental status.

3-D pics
Computed tomography (CT) scanning is a test process that produces three-dimensional images. It can be invasive (if contrast medium is used) or noninvasive.

Nursing actions
- Explain the purpose of the test to the parents and child.
- Make sure that the child holds still during the test.
- Make sure that written, informed consent has been obtained.

(Text continues on page 82.)

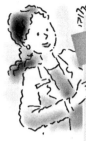

Neurosensory refresher

ATTENTION DEFICIT HYPERACTIVITY DISORDER

Key signs and symptoms
- Decreased attention span
- Difficulty organizing tasks and activities
- Easily distracted

Key test results
- Complete psychological, medical, and neurologic evaluations rule out other problems.

Key treatments
- Behavioral modification and psychological therapy
- Amphetamines: methylphenidate (Ritalin), dextroamphetamine (Dexedrine), amphetamine with dextroamphetamine (Adderall), lisdexamfetamine dimesylate (Vyvanse)

Key interventions
- Give one simple instruction at a time.
- Formulate a schedule for the child.
- Reduce environmental stimuli.

CEREBRAL PALSY

Key signs and symptoms
- Abnormal muscle tone and coordination (the most common associated problem)
- Other symptoms specific to cerebral palsy type

Key test results
- Neuroimaging studies determine the site of brain impairment.
- Cytogenic studies (genetic evaluation of the child and other family members) rule out other potential causes.
- Metabolic studies rule out other causes.

Examination findings
- Infant has difficulty sucking or keeping the nipple or food in his mouth.
- Infant seldom moves voluntarily or has arm or leg tremors with voluntary movement.
- Infant crosses legs when lifted from behind rather than pulling them up or "bicycling" like a normal infant.

Key treatments
- Braces or splints and special appliances, such as adapted eating utensils and a low toilet seat with arms, to help child perform activities independently
- Range-of-motion (ROM) exercises to minimize contractures
- Muscle relaxants or neurosurgery to decrease spasticity, if appropriate

Key interventions
- Assist with locomotion, communication, and educational opportunities.
- Divide tasks into small steps.
- Perform ROM exercises if the child is spastic.

DOWN SYNDROME

Key signs and symptoms
- Mild to moderate retardation
- Short stature with pudgy hands
- Simian crease
- Small head with slow brain growth
- Upward slanting eyes

Key test results
- Amniocentesis allows prenatal diagnosis.

Key treatments
- Treatment for coexisting conditions — congenital heart problems, vision defects, or hypothyroidism

Key interventions
- Provide activities and toys appropriate for the child.
- Set realistic, reachable, short-term goals; break tasks into small steps.
- Provide stimulation and communicate at a level appropriate to the child's mental age rather than chronological age.

HYDROCEPHALUS

Key signs and symptoms
- High-pitched cry
- Rapid increase in head circumference and full, tense, bulging fontanels (before cranial sutures close); bulging forehead

A *Cheat sheet*. Way cool.

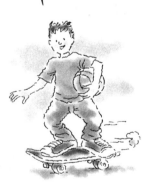

Neurosensory refresher (continued)

HYDROCEPHALUS (CONTINUED)
Key test results
• Skull X-rays show thinning of the skull with separation of the sutures and widening of the fontanels.

Key treatments
• Ventriculoperitoneal shunt insertion: to allow cerebrospinal fluid (CSF) to drain from the lateral ventricle in the brain to the peritoneal cavity
• Antiepileptics for seizures: carbamazepine (Tegretol), phenobarbital (Luminal), diazepam (Valium), phenytoin (Dilantin)

Key interventions
• Monitor vital signs and intake and output.
• Assess neurologic status.
• After the shunt is inserted, position the child on the side of the body opposite from where the shunt is located.
• Lay the child flat.
• If the caudal end of the shunt must be externalized because of infection, keep the bag at ear level.

MENINGITIS
Key signs and symptoms
• Nuchal rigidity that may progress to opisthotonos
• Positive Brudzinski's sign (the child flexes the knees and hips in response to passive neck flexion)
• Positive Kernig's sign (inability to extend the leg when the hip and knee are flexed)

Key test results
• Lumbar puncture shows increased CSF pressure, cloudy color, increased white blood cell count and protein level, and decreased glucose level if meningitis is caused by bacteria.
• Culture and sensitivity of CSF identifies the causative organism.
• Xpert EV test helps distinguish between viral and bacterial meningitis.

Key treatments
• Analgesics to treat the pain of meningeal irritation
• Corticosteroid: dexamethasone (Decadron)
• Droplet precautions (should be maintained until at least 24 hours of effective antibiotic therapy have elapsed; continued isolation recommended for meningitis caused by *Haemophilus influenzae* or *Neisseria meningitidis*)
• Antibiotics (based on results of CSF culture and sensitivity): ceftazidime (Fortaz), ceftriaxone (Rocephin)
• Seizure precautions

Key interventions
• Monitor vital signs and intake and output.
• Assess the child's neurologic status frequently.

• Examine the young infant for bulging fontanels, and measure head circumference.

OTITIS MEDIA
Key signs and symptoms
Acute suppurative otitis media
• Fever (mild to very high)
• Pain that suddenly stops (occurs if the tympanic membrane ruptures)
• Severe, deep, throbbing pain (from pressure behind the tympanic membrane)
• Signs of upper respiratory tract infection (sneezing, coughing)
Acute secretory otitis media
• Popping, crackling, or clicking sounds on swallowing or with jaw movement
• Sensation of fullness in the ear
Chronic otitis media
• Cholesteatoma (cystlike mass in the middle ear)
• Decreased or absent tympanic membrane mobility
• Painless, purulent discharge in chronic suppurative otitis media

Key test results
Acute suppurative otitis media
• Otoscopy reveals obscured or distorted bony landmarks of the tympanic membrane.
Acute secretory otitis media
• Otoscopy reveals clear or amber fluid behind the tympanic membrane and tympanic membrane retraction, which causes the bony landmarks to appear more prominent. If hemorrhage into the middle ear has occurred, as in barotrauma, the tympanic membrane appears blue-black.
Chronic otitis media
• Otoscopy shows thickening, decreased mobility of the tympanic membrane and, sometimes, scarring.

Key treatments
Acute suppurative otitis media
• Myringotomy for children with severe, painful bulging of the tympanic membrane
• Antibiotic therapy, usually amoxicillin (Amoxil)
Acute secretory otitis media
• Inflation of the eustachian tube by performing Valsalva's maneuver several times per day, which may be the only treatment required
• Nasopharyngeal decongestant therapy
Chronic otitis media
• Elimination of eustachian tube obstruction

(continued)

Neurosensory refresher (continued)

OTITIS MEDIA (CONTINUED)
- Excision for cholesteatoma
- Mastoidectomy
- Broad-spectrum antibiotics: amoxicillin-clavulanate potassium (Augmentin) or cefuroxime (Ceftin) (in selected situations)

Key interventions
- After myringotomy, maintain drainage flow. Place sterile cotton loosely in the external ear. Change the cotton frequently.
- Watch for and report headache, fever, severe pain, or disorientation.
- After tympanoplasty, reinforce dressings and observe for excessive bleeding from the ear canal.
- Instruct the parents not to feed their infant in a supine position or put him to bed with a bottle.

SEIZURE DISORDERS
Key signs and symptoms
- May experience an aura just before the seizure's onset (reports unusual tastes, feelings, or odors)
- Eyes deviating to a particular side or blinking
- Usually unresponsive during tonic-clonic muscular contractions; may experience incontinence
- Irregular breathing with spasms

Key test results
- EEG results help differentiate epileptic from nonepileptic seizures. Each seizure has a characteristic EEG tracing.

Key treatments
- Antiepileptics: I.V. diazepam (Valium) or lorazepam (Ativan), phenobarbital (Luminal) or fosphenytoin (Cerebyx), phenytoin (Dilantin), valproic acid (Depakote), carbamazepine (Tegretol)
- Rectal diazepam (Diastat) for home management of intractable or prolonged seizures

Key interventions
- Assess neurologic status.
- Stay with the child during a seizure.
- Move the child to a flat surface.
- Place the child on his side.
- Don't try to interrupt the seizure.

SPINA BIFIDA
Key signs and symptoms
Spina bifida occulta
- Dimple or tuft of hair on the skin over the spinal defect
- No neurologic dysfunction (usually), except occasional foot weakness or bowel and bladder disturbances
Meningocele
- No neurologic dysfunction (usually)
- Saclike structure protruding over the spine
Myelomeningocele
- Hydrocephalus
- Permanent neurologic dysfunction (paralysis, bowel and bladder incontinence)

Key test results
- Elevated alpha-fetoprotein levels in the mother's blood may indicate the presence of a neural tube defect.
- Amniocentesis reveals neural tube defect.
- Acetylcholinesterase measurement can be used to confirm the diagnosis.

Key treatments
- Surgery (in meningocele and myelomeningocele)

Key interventions
Before surgery
- Assess for signs of hydrocephalus. Measure head circumference daily. Be sure to mark the spot where the measurement was made.
- Assess for signs of meningeal irritation, such as fever or nuchal rigidity.
After surgery
- Assess for hydrocephalus, which commonly follows surgery. Measure the infant's head circumference as ordered.
- Monitor vital signs often.

More detail
Magnetic resonance imaging (MRI) shows the CNS in greater detail than CT scanning. A noniodinated contrast medium may be used to enhance lesions. Advances in MRI allow visualization of cerebral arteries and venous sinuses without administration of a contrast medium.

Nursing actions
- Explain the procedure to the parents and child.
- If the child has any surgically implanted metal objects (such as pins and clips), notify the radiology department because these may interfere with the picture.
- Make sure the child holds still during the test.

Electric pics

Electroencephalogram (EEG) shows abnormal electrical activity in the brain (such as from a seizure, metabolic disorder, or drug overdose).

Nursing actions

• Explain the purpose of the test to the parents and child.
• Make sure the child holds still during the test.

Wavy reflections

Ultrasonography reveals carotid lesions or changes in carotid blood flow and velocity. High-frequency sound waves reflect the velocity of blood flow, which is then reported as a graphic recording of a waveform.

Nursing actions

• Explain the purpose of the test to the parents and child.
• Make sure the child holds still during the test.

Fluid check

A **lumbar puncture** is the insertion of a needle into the subarachnoid space of the spinal cord, usually between L3 and L4 (or L4 and L5) to allow aspiration of cerebrospinal fluid (CSF) for analysis and measurement of CSF pressure.

Nursing actions

Before the procedure
• Explain the procedure to the parents and child.
• Make sure that written, informed consent has been obtained.
• Keep the child in a side-lying, knee-chest position during the procedure.
After the procedure
• Make sure the child rests for 1 hour or as ordered.

Vessel visualization

In **cerebral arteriography,** also known as *angiography*, a catheter is inserted into an artery — usually the femoral artery — and is indirectly threaded up to the carotid artery.

Then a radiopaque dye is injected, allowing X-ray visualization of the cerebral vasculature.

Nursing actions

Before the procedure
• Explain the procedure to the parents and child.
• Make sure that written, informed consent has been obtained.
• Identify allergies before the test.
• Make sure the child holds still during the test, and monitor him for allergic reaction.
After the procedure
• Immobilize the site after the test, and monitor it for pulses and evidence of bleeding.

Pressure check

Intracranial pressure (ICP) monitoring is a direct, invasive method of identifying trends in ICP. A subarachnoid screw and an intraventricular catheter convert CSF pressure readings into waveforms that are digitally displayed on an oscilloscope monitor. Another option is to insert a fiber-optic catheter in the ventricle, subarachnoid space, subdural space, or the brain parenchyma. Pressure changes are reported digitally or in waveform.

Nursing actions

Before the procedure
• Explain the procedure to the parents and child.
• Make sure that written, informed consent has been obtained.
After the procedure
• Maintain patency of the catheter, and monitor the waveforms. Alert the physician to changes in trends.
• Maintain sterile technique during care of the catheter and monitoring equipment.
• Monitor the site for signs of infection.

Nerve times

Electromyography detects lower motor neuron disorders, neuromuscular disorders, and nerve damage. A needle inserted into selected muscles at rest and during voluntary contraction picks up nerve impulses and measures nerve conduction time.

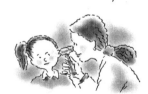

A complete neurologic assessment may require a close look at the eyes, ears, internal structures, fluid pressures, and neural function.

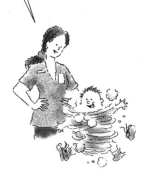

ADHD manifests itself through long-term behaviors that include hyperactivity, impulsiveness, and inattention.

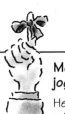

Memory jogger

Here's a tip for remembering diagnostic criteria for ADHD: think of a child who can't **SIT** still.

Seven (age by which symptoms appear)

Impaired social or academic function

Two or more settings

Nursing actions
Before the procedure
- Explain the procedure to the parents and child.
- Check the child's medications for those that may interfere with the test (cholinergics, anticholinergics, skeletal muscle relaxants).
- Make sure that written, informed consent has been obtained.
- Make sure the child holds still during the procedure.

After the procedure
- Monitor the site for infection or bleeding after the procedure.

Ear check
Otoscopic examination allows visualization of the canal and inner structures of the ear.

Nursing actions
- Explain the procedure to the parents and child.
- Use the largest speculum that fits into the ear canal.
- To straighten the ear canal, pull the pinna down and back or out in infants and children younger than age 3. For children older than age 3, the pinna is pulled up and back.

Eye check
Ophthalmoscopic examination helps visualize interior eye structures.

Nursing actions
- Explain the procedure to the parents and child.
- Ensure cooperation during tests by allowing the child to hold a favorite toy, which may decrease anxiety.

Polish up on client care

Major neurologic disorders in pediatric patients are attention deficit hyperactivity disorder (ADHD), cerebral palsy, Down syndrome, hydrocephalus, meningitis, otitis media, seizure disorders, and spina bifida.

Attention deficit hyperactivity disorder

ADHD, previously called *attention deficit disorder*, includes the following long-term behaviors:
- hyperactivity
- impulsiveness
- inattention.

These manifestations occur in all facets of the child's life and commonly worsen when sustained attention is required such as during school. To qualify as ADHD, behaviors must be present in two or more settings, must be present before age 7, and must result in a significant impairment of social or academic functioning, and the symptoms aren't a result of another mental disorder. Three types of ADHD have been identified based on *Diagnostic and Statistical Manual of Mental Disorders,* Fourth Edition, Text Revision (*DSM-IV-TR*) criteria:
- predominantly inattentive type
- predominantly hyperactive-impulsive type
- combined type.

CAUSES
- Deficit in neurotransmitters (possibly)

ASSESSMENT FINDINGS
- Excessive climbing, running, or talking
- Decreased attention span
- Difficulty organizing tasks and activities
- Difficulty waiting for turns
- Easily distracted
- Failure to give close attention to school work or activity
- Failure to listen when spoken to directly
- Fidgets or squirms in seat
- Frequent forgetfulness; frequently loses things needed for tasks
- Impulsive behavior
- Inability to follow directions

DIAGNOSTIC TEST RESULTS
- Complete psychological, medical, and neurologic evaluations rule out other problems.
- *DSM-IV-TR* criteria is met: Six or more symptoms of inattention, hyperactivity, or impulsiveness have been present for at least

6 months or more and are disruptive or inappropriate for developmental level.

NURSING DIAGNOSES
- Imbalanced nutrition: Less than body requirements
- Risk for impaired parenting
- Risk for injury

TREATMENT
- Behavioral modification and psychological therapy
- Interdisciplinary interventions: pathologic assessment and diagnosis of specific learning needs

Drug therapy
- Amphetamines: methylphenidate (Ritalin), dextroamphetamine (Dexedrine), amphetamine with dextroamphetamine (Adderall), lisdexamfetamine dimesylate (Vyvanse)
- Other medications: imipramine (Tofranil), clonidine (Catapres)

INTERVENTIONS AND RATIONALES
- Monitor growth. *If the child is receiving methylphenidate, growth may be slowed.*
- Give one simple instruction at a time *so the child can successfully complete the task, which promotes self-esteem.*
- Give medications in the morning and at lunch *to avoid interfering with sleep.*
- Ensure adequate nutrition; *medications and hyperactivity may cause increased nutrient needs.*
- Reduce environmental stimuli *to decrease distraction.*
- Formulate a schedule for the child *to provide consistency and routine.*

Teaching topics
- Explanation of the disorder and treatment plan
- Medication use and possible adverse effects
- Allowing the child to expend energy after being in a restrictive environment such as school
- Structuring learning to minimize distractions
- Taking breaks from caregiving to avoid strain

- Teaching important material in the morning (when medication levels peak)

Cerebral palsy

Cerebral palsy is a neuromuscular disorder resulting from damage to or a defect in the part of the brain that controls motor function.

The disorder is most commonly seen in children born prematurely. Cerebral palsy can't be cured; treatment includes interventions that encourage optimum development. Defects are common, including musculoskeletal, neurologic, GI, and nutritional defects as well as other systemic complications (abnormal reflexes, fatigue, growth failure, genitourinary complaints, respiratory infections).

Classifications of cerebral palsy include:
- ataxia type — the least common type; essentially a lack of coordination caused by disturbances in movement and balance
- athetoid type — characterized by involuntary, incoordinate motion with varying degrees of muscle tension (Children with this type of cerebral palsy experience writhing muscle contractions whenever they attempt voluntary movement. Facial grimacing, poor swallowing, and tongue movements cause drooling and poor speech articulation. Despite their abnormal appearance, these children commonly have average or above-average intelligence.)
- spastic type — the most common type; featuring hyperactive stretch in associated muscle groups, hyperactive deep tendon reflexes, rapid involuntary muscle contraction and relaxation, contractions affecting extensor muscles, and scissoring (The child's legs are crossed and the toes are pointed down, so the child stands on his toes.)
- rigidity type — an uncommon type of cerebral palsy characterized by rigid postures and lack of active movement
- mixed type — more than one type of cerebral palsy. (These children are usually severely disabled.)

CAUSES
- Anoxia before, during, or after birth
- Infection
- Trauma (hemorrhage)

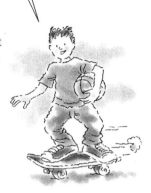

For ADHD, first reduce stimuli during learning times. Then allow the child to expend energy.

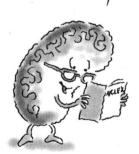

Cerebral palsy arises from a malfunction of motor centers and neural pathways in the brain. Well, I'll be.

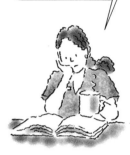

> Abnormal muscle tone and coordination characterize all forms of cerebral palsy.

> Although cerebral palsy can't be cured, treatment encourages the child to reach his full potential.

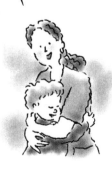

RISK FACTORS
- Low birth weight
- Low Apgar scores at 5 minutes
- Metabolic disturbances
- Seizures

ASSESSMENT FINDINGS
All types
- Abnormal muscle tone and coordination (the most common associated problem)
- Dental anomalies
- Mental retardation of varying degrees in 18% to 50% of cases (most children with cerebral palsy have at least a normal IQ but can't demonstrate it on standardized tests)
- Seizures
- Speech, vision, or hearing disturbances

Ataxic cerebral palsy
- Poor balance and muscle coordination
- Unsteady, wide-based gait

Athetoid cerebral palsy
- Slow state of writhing muscle contractions whenever voluntary movement is attempted
- Facial grimacing
- Poor swallowing
- Drooling
- Poor speech articulation

Rigid cerebral palsy
- Rigid posture
- Lack of active movement

Spastic cerebral palsy
- Hyperactive stretch reflex in associated muscle groups
- Hyperactive deep tendon reflexes
- Rapid involuntary muscle contraction and relaxation
- Contractures affecting the extensor muscles
- Scissoring

Mixed cerebral palsy
- Signs of more than one type of cerebral palsy
- Severely disabled

DIAGNOSTIC TEST RESULTS
- Neuroimaging studies determine the site of brain impairment.
- Cytogenic studies (genetic evaluation of the child and other family members) rule out other potential causes.
- Metabolic studies rule out other causes.

Examination findings
- Infant has difficulty sucking or keeping the nipple or food in his mouth.
- Infant seldom moves voluntarily or has arm or leg tremors with voluntary movement.
- Infant crosses his legs when lifted from behind rather than pulling them up or "bicycling" like a normal infant.
- Infant's legs are difficult to separate, making diaper changing difficult.
- Infant persistently uses only one hand or, as he gets older, uses hands — but not legs — well.

NURSING DIAGNOSES
- Impaired physical mobility
- Delayed growth and development
- Impaired verbal communication

TREATMENT
- High-calorie diet, if appropriate
- Artificial urinary sphincter for the incontinent child who can use hand controls
- Braces or splints and special appliances, such as adapted eating utensils and a low toilet seat with arms, to help the child perform activities independently
- Neurosurgery to decrease spasticity, if appropriate
- Orthopedic surgery to correct contractures
- Range-of-motion (ROM) exercises to minimize contractures

Drug therapy
- Muscle relaxants to decrease spasticity, if appropriate
- Anticonvulsants: phenytoin (Dilantin), phenobarbital (Luminal) to control seizures

INTERVENTIONS AND RATIONALES
- Assist with locomotion, communication, and educational opportunities *to enable the child to attain optimal developmental level.*

- Increase caloric intake for the child with increased motor function *to keep up with increased metabolic needs.*
- Promote age-appropriate mental activities and incentives for motor development *to promote growth and development.*
- Provide rest periods *to promote rest and reduce metabolic needs.*
- Perform ROM exercises if the child is spastic *to maintain proper body alignment and mobility of joints.*
- Provide a safe environment, for example, by using protective headgear or bed pads, *to prevent injury.*
- Divide tasks into small steps *to promote self-care and activity and increase self-esteem.*
- Refer the child for speech, nutrition, and physical therapy *to maintain or improve functioning.*
- Use assistive communication devices if the child can't speak *to promote a positive self-concept.*

Teaching topics
- Explanation of the disorder and treatment plan
- Medication use and possible adverse effects
- Contacting appropriate social service agencies, child development specialist, mental health services, and home care assistance
- Understanding the child's condition and prognosis

Down syndrome

The first disorder researchers attributed to a chromosomal aberration, Down syndrome is characterized by:
- mental retardation
- dysmorphic facial features
- other distinctive physical abnormalities.
(Sixty percent of patients have congenital heart defects, respiratory infections, chronic myelogenous leukemia, and a weak immune response to infection.)

CAUSES
- Genetic nondisjunction, with three chromosomes on the 21st pair (total of 47 chromosomes)

CONTRIBUTING FACTORS
- Maternal age (the older the mother, the greater the risk of genetic nondisjunction)

ASSESSMENT FINDINGS
- Brushfield's spots (marbling and speckling of the iris)
- Flat, broad forehead
- Flat nose and low-set ears
- Hypotonia
- Mild to moderate retardation
- Protruding tongue (because of a small oral cavity)
- Short stature with pudgy hands
- Simian crease (a single crease across the palm)
- Small head with slow brain growth
- Upward slanting eyes

DIAGNOSTIC TEST RESULTS
- Amniocentesis allows prenatal diagnosis. It's recommended for women older than age 34, regardless of a negative family history, or a woman of any age if she or the father carries a translocated chromosome.
- Karyotype shows the specific chromosomal abnormality.

NURSING DIAGNOSES
- Delayed growth and development
- Risk for injury
- Risk for aspiration

TREATMENT
- Treatment for coexisting conditions — congenital heart problems, vision defects, or hypothyroidism
- Skeletal, immunologic, metabolic, biochemical, and oncologic problems treated as per specific problem

Drug therapy
- Megavitamin therapy (controversial) to promote growth and development potential

INTERVENTIONS AND RATIONALES
- Provide activities and toys appropriate for the child *to support optimal development.*
- Set realistic, reachable, short-term goals; break tasks into small steps *to make them easier to accomplish.*

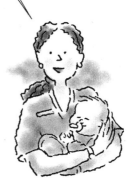

Provide a safe environment for the child with cerebral palsy.

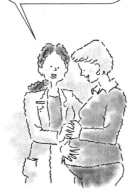

Amniocentesis allows prenatal diagnosis of Down syndrome. It's recommended for any pregnant client older than age 34.

- Use behavior modification, if applicable, *to promote safety and prevent injury to the child and others.*
- Provide stimulation and communicate at a level appropriate to the child's mental age rather than chronological age *to promote a healthy emotional environment.*
- Provide a safe environment *to prevent injury.*
- Mainstream daily routines *to promote normalcy.*

Teaching topics
- Explanation of the disorder and treatment plan
- Contacting early intervention programs
- Contacting support groups for caregivers
- Establishing self-care skills to promote independence

Hydrocephalus

In hydrocephalus, an increase in the amount of CSF occurs in the ventricles and subarachnoid spaces of the brain. The ventricles become dilated because of an imbalance in the rate of production and rate of absorption of CSF. This condition may be congenital or acquired.

In noncommunicating hydrocephalus, an obstruction occurs in the free circulation of CSF, causing increased pressure on the brain or spinal cord. In most cases, congenital hydrocephalus is noncommunicating.

Communicating hydrocephalus involves the free flow of CSF between the ventricles and the spinal theca. Increased pressure on the spinal cord is caused by defective absorption of CSF.

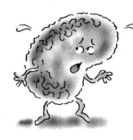

Yikes! In hydrocephalus, an excessive amount of CSF accumulates in the ventricular spaces of the brain.

CAUSES
- Arnold-Chiari malformation (downward displacement of cerebellar components through the foramen magnum into the cervical spinal canal); common in hydrocephalus with spina bifida
- Overproduction of CSF by the choroid plexus
- Scarring, congenital anomalies, or hemorrhage; causes CSF to be absorbed abnormally after it reaches the subarachnoid space (in communicating hydrocephalus)
- Tumors, hemorrhage, or structural abnormalities; block CSF flow, causing fluid to accumulate in the ventricles (in noncommunicating hydrocephalus)

ASSESSMENT FINDINGS
- "Cracked pot" sound when the skull is percussed
- Distended scalp veins
- High-pitched cry
- Inability to support the head when upright
- Irritability or lethargy
- Decreased attention span
- Rapid increase in head circumference and full, tense, bulging fontanels (before cranial sutures close); bulging forehead
- Sunset sign (sclera visible above the iris)
- Widening suture lines
- Vomiting (not related to food intake)

DIAGNOSTIC TEST RESULTS
- Angiography, computed tomography scan, and magnetic resonance imaging differentiate hydrocephalus from intracranial lesions and may demonstrate Arnold-Chiari malformation.
- Light reflects off the opposite side of the skull with skull transillumination.
- Skull X-rays show thinning of the skull with separation of the sutures and widening of the fontanels.

NURSING DIAGNOSES
- Risk for injury
- Delayed growth and development
- Decreased intracranial adaptive capacity

TREATMENT
- Ventriculoperitoneal shunt insertion to allow CSF to drain from the lateral ventricle in the brain to the peritoneal cavity

Drug therapy
- Antiepileptics for seizures: carbamazepine (Tegretol), phenobarbital (Luminal), diazepam (Valium), phenytoin (Dilantin)

INTERVENTIONS AND RATIONALES
- Measure head circumference *to aid in diagnosis of hydrocephalus.*
- Monitor vital signs and intake and output *to assess for fluid volume excess, which can further elevate ICP.*
- Assess neurologic status *to identify changes indicative of increased ICP.*
- After the shunt is inserted, position the child on the side of his body opposite from where it's located *to promote CSF drainage and prevent shunt occlusion.*
- Lay the child flat *to avoid rapid decompression.*
- Observe for signs and symptoms of increased ICP *to prevent complications.*
- Observe for signs of infection. *Signs of shunt infection usually occur within the first month after shunt insertion.*
- If the caudal end of the shunt must be externalized because of infection, keep the bag at ear level *to promote CSF drainage.*
- Support the head when the child is upright *to prevent injury and promote CSF drainage.*
- Provide proper skin care to the head; turn the patient's head frequently *to avoid skin breakdown.*

Teaching topics
- Explanation of the disorder and treatment plan
- Medication use and possible adverse effects
- Recognizing the signs of increasing ICP
- Understanding care required after shunt insertion

Meningitis

Meningitis is an inflammation of the brain and spinal cord meninges. It's most common in infants and toddlers but can occur in other age groups as well. The incidence of meningitis is greatly reduced with routine *Haemophilus influenzae* type B vaccine.

CAUSES
- Viral or bacterial agents, transmitted by the spread of droplets (organisms enter the blood from the nasopharynx or middle ear)

ASSESSMENT FINDINGS
- Nuchal rigidity that may progress to opisthotonos (arching of the back)
- Headache
- Fever
- High-pitched cry
- Irritability
- Delirium
- Coma
- Petechial or purpuric lesions possibly present in bacterial meningitis
- Positive Brudzinski's sign (the child flexes the knees and hips in response to passive neck flexion)
- Positive Kernig's sign (inability to extend the leg when the hip and knee are flexed)
- Projectile vomiting
- Seizures (may occur)

DIAGNOSTIC TEST RESULTS
- Lumbar puncture shows increased CSF pressure, cloudy color, increased white blood cell count and protein level, and decreased glucose level if the meningitis is caused by bacteria.
- Culture and sensitivity of CSF identifies the causative organism.
- Xpert EV test helps distinguish between viral and bacterial meningitis.

NURSING DIAGNOSES
- Decreased intracranial adaptive capacity
- Ineffective breathing pattern
- Risk for injury

TREATMENT
- Droplet precautions (should be maintained until at least 24 hours of effective antibiotic therapy have elapsed; continued precautions recommended for meningitis caused by *H. influenzae* or *Neisseria meningitidis*)
- Hypothermia blanket
- Oxygen therapy may require intubation and mechanical ventilation to induce hyperventilation to decrease ICP
- Seizure precautions
- Treatment for coexisting conditions
- Burr holes to evacuate subdural effusion, if present

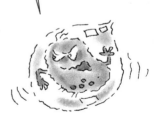

Meningitis is transmitted by the spread of droplets.

Drug therapy

- Analgesics to treat the pain of meningeal irritation
- Corticosteroid: dexamethasone (Decadron)
- Antibiotics (based on results of CSF culture and sensitivity): ceftazidime (Fortaz), ceftriaxone (Rocephin)

INTERVENTIONS AND RATIONALES

- Monitor vital signs and intake and output *to assess for excess fluid volume.*
- Assess the child's neurologic status frequently *to monitor for signs of increased ICP.*
- Provide a dark and quiet environment. *Environmental stimuli can increase ICP or stimulate seizure activity.*
- Maintain seizure precautions *to prevent injury.*
- Administer medications as ordered *to combat infection and decrease ICP.*
- Move the child gently *to prevent a rise in ICP.*
- Maintain isolation precautions as ordered *to prevent the spread of infection.*
- Provide emotional support for the family *to decrease anxiety.*
- Examine the young infant for bulging fontanels, and measure head circumference; *hydrocephalus is a complication that can result from meningitis.*

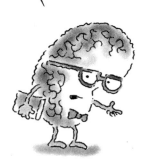

My, oh my... meningitis management mandates meticulous monitoring: Monitor vital signs, intake and output, and neurologic status.

Teaching topics

- Explanation of the disorder and treatment plan
- Medication use and possible adverse effects
- Understanding the importance of isolation and sanitation

Otitis media

Otitis media is inflammation of the middle ear that may be accompanied by infection. The fluid presses on the tympanic membrane, causing pain and leading to possible rupture or perforation. This condition may be chronic or acute and suppurative or secretory.

Acute otitis media is common in children. Its incidence increases during the winter months, paralleling the seasonal increase in

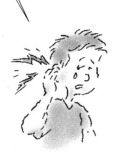

Key clinical fact about acute suppurative otitis media: It HURTS!

nonbacterial respiratory tract infections. With prompt treatment, the prognosis for acute otitis media is excellent; however, prolonged accumulation of fluid in the middle ear cavity causes chronic otitis media and, possibly, perforation of the tympanic membrane.

CAUSES

All types

- Obstructed eustachian tube
- Wider, shorter, more horizontal eustachian tubes and increased lymphoid tissue in children as well as other anatomic anomalies

Suppurative otitis media

- Bacterial infection with pneumococci, *H. influenzae* (the most common cause in children younger than age 6), *Moraxella (Branhamella) catarrhalis,* group A beta-hemolytic streptococci, staphylococci (most common cause in children age 6 or older), or gram-negative bacteria
- Respiratory tract infection, allergic reaction, nasotracheal intubation, or position changes that allow nasopharyngeal flora to reflux through the eustachian tube and colonize the middle ear

Chronic suppurative otitis media

- Recurrent acute otitis episodes
- Infection by resistant strains of bacteria
- Tuberculosis (rarely)

Secretory otitis media

- Barotrauma (pressure injury caused by an inability to equalize pressure between the environment and the middle ear), as occurs during rapid aircraft descent in a person with upper respiratory tract infection or during rapid underwater ascent in scuba diving (barotitis media)
- Obstruction of the eustachian tube secondary to eustachian tube dysfunction from viral infection or allergy, which causes a buildup of negative pressure in the middle ear that promotes transudation of sterile serous fluid from blood vessels in the membrane of the middle ear

Chronic secretory otitis media

- Persistent eustachian tube dysfunction from mechanical obstruction (adenoidal tissue overgrowth or tumors), edema (allergic rhinitis or chronic sinus infection), or inadequate treatment of acute suppurative otitis media

ASSESSMENT FINDINGS
Acute suppurative otitis media
- Bulging and erythema of the tympanic membrane
- Dizziness
- Fever (mild to very high)
- Hearing loss (usually mild and conductive)
- Nausea and vomiting (possibly)
- Pain pattern (pulling the pinna doesn't exacerbate pain)
- Pain that suddenly stops (occurs if the tympanic membrane ruptures)
- Purulent drainage in the ear canal from tympanic membrane rupture
- Severe, deep, throbbing pain (from pressure behind the tympanic membrane)
- Signs of upper respiratory tract infection (sneezing and coughing)
- Tinnitus (ringing in the ears)

Acute secretory otitis media
- Echo heard by the patient when speaking; vague feeling of top-heaviness (caused by accumulation of fluid)
- Popping, crackling, or clicking sounds on swallowing or with jaw movement
- Sensation of fullness in the ear
- Severe conductive hearing loss

Chronic otitis media
- Cholesteatoma (cystlike mass in the middle ear)
- Decreased or absent tympanic membrane mobility
- Painless, purulent discharge in chronic suppurative otitis media
- Thickening and scarring of the tympanic membrane

DIAGNOSTIC TEST RESULTS
Acute suppurative otitis media
- Culture of the ear drainage identifies the causative organism.
- Otoscopy reveals obscured or distorted bony landmarks of the tympanic membrane.
- Pneumatoscopy (pneumatic otoscope) may show decreased tympanic membrane

mobility, but this procedure is painful with an obviously bulging, erythematous tympanic membrane.

Acute secretory otitis media
- Otoscopy reveals clear or amber fluid behind the tympanic membrane and tympanic membrane retraction, which causes the bony landmarks to appear more prominent. If hemorrhage into the middle ear has occurred, as in barotrauma, the tympanic membrane appears blue-black.

Chronic otitis media
- Otoscopy shows thickening, decreased mobility of the tympanic membrane and, sometimes, scarring.
- Pneumatoscopy shows decreased or absent tympanic membrane movement.

NURSING DIAGNOSES
- Acute pain
- Disturbed sensory perception (auditory)
- Hyperthermia

TREATMENT
Acute suppurative otitis media
- Myringotomy for children with severe, painful bulging of the tympanic membrane

Drug therapy
- Antibiotic therapy, usually amoxicillin (Amoxil) (antibiotics must be used with discretion to prevent development of resistant strains of bacteria in children with recurring otitis media)
- Antibiotic: amoxicillin-clavulanate potassium (Augmentin) in areas with a high incidence of beta-lactamase–producing *H. influenzae* and in patients who aren't responding to amoxicillin
- Antibiotic: cefaclor (Ceclor) or co-trimoxazole (Bactrim) for patients allergic to penicillin derivatives
- Prevention: broad-spectrum antibiotics, such as amoxicillin-clavulanate potassium (Augmentin) or cefuroxime (Ceftin) in high-risk clients

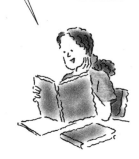

In acute suppurative otitis media, pulling the auricle doesn't worsen the pain.

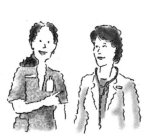

In myringotomy, the physician cuts into the eardrum and gently suctions fluid to relieve pressure.

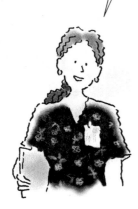

Mastoidectomy is removal of the mastoid process or mastoid cells of the temporal bone.

Acute secretory otitis media
• Concomitant treatment of the underlying cause, such as elimination of allergens, or adenoidectomy for hypertrophied adenoids
• Inflation of the eustachian tube by performing Valsalva's maneuver several times a day, which may be the only treatment required
• Myringotomy and aspiration of middle ear fluid if decongestant therapy fails, followed by insertion of a polyethylene tube into the tympanic membrane for immediate and prolonged equalization of pressure (tube falls out spontaneously after 9 to 12 months)

Drug therapy
• Nasopharyngeal decongestant therapy for at least 2 weeks; sometimes used indefinitely, with periodic evaluation

Chronic otitis media
• Elimination of eustachian tube obstruction
• Excision for cholesteatoma
• Mastoidectomy
• Treatment of otitis externa; myringoplasty and tympanoplasty to reconstruct middle ear structures when thickening and scarring are present

Drug therapy
• Broad-spectrum antibiotic: amoxicillin-clavulanate potassium (Augmentin) or cefuroxime (Ceftin) for exacerbations of otitis media (in selected situations)

INTERVENTIONS AND RATIONALES
• Monitor vital signs *to determine baseline and detect early signs of worsening infection.*
• Watch for and report headache, fever, severe pain, or disorientation *to detect early signs of complications.*
• Administer analgesics, as needed, or recommend applying heat to the ear *to relieve pain.*
• Identify and treat allergies *to prevent recurrences of otitis media.*
• Encourage the child to complete the prescribed course of antibiotic treatment *to prevent reinfection.*
• For children with acute secretory otitis media, watch for and immediately report pain and fever *to detect early signs of secondary infection.*

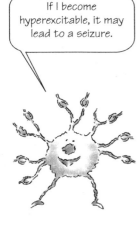

If I become hyperexcitable, it may lead to a seizure.

• Tell the parents to avoid feeding the infant in a supine position or putting him to bed with a bottle *to prevent reflux of nasopharyngeal flora.*
• Encourage the child to perform Valsalva's maneuver several times daily *to promote eustachian tube patency.*
• After myringotomy, maintain drainage flow; place sterile cotton loosely in the external ear *to absorb drainage.* Change the cotton frequently *to prevent infection.*
• After tympanoplasty, reinforce dressings and observe for excessive bleeding from the ear canal *to assess for fluid volume deficit.*

Teaching topics
• Explanation of the disorder and treatment plan
• Medication use and possible adverse effects
• Avoiding blowing the nose or getting the ear wet when bathing
• Instilling nasopharyngeal decongestants properly, if prescribed
• Recognizing upper respiratory tract infections and seeking early treatment
• Returning for follow-up examination after completion of antibiotic therapy

Seizure disorders

A seizure is a sudden, episodic, involuntary alteration in consciousness, motor activity, behavior, sensation, or autonomic function. (See *Classifying seizures.*) Epilepsy is a common, recurrent seizure disorder.

CAUSES
• Excessive neuronal discharges (epilepsy)
• Hyperexcitable nerve cells that surpass the seizure threshold
• Neurons overfiring without regard to stimuli or need

ASSESSMENT FINDINGS
• May experience an aura just before the seizure's onset (the child reports unusual tastes, feelings, or odors)
• Eyes deviating to a particular side or blinking
• Irregular breathing with spasms

Classifying seizures

Seizures can take various forms depending on their origin and whether they're localized to one area of the brain, as occurs in partial seizures, or occur in both hemispheres, as happens in generalized seizures. This chart describes each type of seizure and lists common signs and symptoms.

Type	Description	Signs and symptoms
Partial		
Simple partial	Symptoms confined to one hemisphere	May have motor (change in posture), sensory (hallucinations), or autonomic (flushing, tachycardia) symptoms; no loss of consciousness
Complex partial	Begins in one focal area but spreads to both hemispheres (more common in adults)	Loss of consciousness; aura of visual disturbances; postictal symptoms
Generalized		
Absence (formerly called *petit mal*)	Sudden onset; lasts 5 to 10 seconds; can have 100 daily; precipitated by stress, hyperventilation, hypoglycemia, fatigue; differentiated from daydreaming	Loss of responsiveness but continued ability to maintain posture control and not fall; twitching eyelids; lip smacking; no postictal symptoms
Myoclonic	Movement disorder (not a seizure); seen as the child awakens or falls asleep; may be precipitated by touch or visual stimuli; focal or generalized; symmetrical or asymmetrical	No loss of consciousness; sudden, brief, shocklike involuntary contraction of one muscle group
Clonic	Opposing muscles contract and relax alternately in a rhythmic pattern; may occur in one limb more than others	Mucus production
Tonic	Muscles are maintained in a continuous contracted state (rigid posture)	Variable loss of consciousness; pupils dilate; eyes roll up; glottis closes; possible incontinence; may experience excessive salivation
Tonic-clonic (formerly called *grand mal, major motor*)	Violent total body seizure	Aura; tonic first (20 to 40 seconds); clonic next; postictal symptoms
Atonic	Drop and fall attack; needs to wear protective helmet	Loss of posture tone
Akinetic	Sudden brief loss of muscle tone or posture	Temporary loss of consciousness

(continued)

Classifying seizures *(continued)*

Type	Description	Signs and symptoms
Unclassified		
Febrile	Seizure threshold lowered by elevated temperature; only one seizure per fever; occurs in 4% of population younger than age 5; occurs when temperature is rapidly rising	Lasts less than 5 minutes; generalized, transient, and nonprogressive; doesn't generally result in brain damage; EEG is normal after 2 weeks
Idiopathic	Cause unknown; most common type of pediatric seizures; genetic factors may influence neuronal discharge	Widely variable
Status epilepticus	Prolonged or frequent repetition of seizures without return to baseline; may result in anoxia and cardiac and respiratory arrest.	Consciousness not regained between seizures; lasts more than 30 minutes

- Usually unresponsive during tonic-clonic muscular contractions; may experience incontinence
- May be disoriented to time and place, drowsy, and uncoordinated immediately after seizure

DIAGNOSTIC TEST RESULTS
- EEG results help differentiate epileptic from nonepileptic seizures. Each seizure has a characteristic EEG tracing.

NURSING DIAGNOSES
- Risk for injury
- Ineffective airway clearance
- Disturbed sensory perception (tactile)

TREATMENT
- Drug therapy; if not responsive, ablative therapy
- Supportive until the seizure ends (maintaining airway, protecting from injury)

Drug therapy
- Antiepileptics: I.V. diazepam (Valium) or lorazepam (Ativan), phenobarbital (Luminal) or fosphenytoin (Cerebyx), phenytoin (Dilantin), valproic acid (Depakote), carbamazepine (Tegretol)

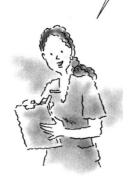

When a seizure occurs, assess neurologic status, move the child to a flat surface, place him on his side, and stay with him.

- Rectal diazepam (Diastat) for home management of intractable or prolonged seizures

INTERVENTIONS AND RATIONALES
- Monitor vital signs *to determine baseline and detect any changes.*
- Assess neurologic status *to monitor for change in neurologic status.*
- Stay with the child during a seizure *to prevent injury.*
- Move the child to a flat surface *to prevent falling.*
- Place the child on his side *to let saliva drain out, ensuring a patent airway.*
- Don't try to interrupt the seizure *to promote safety.*
- Gently support the head and keep the child's hands from inflicting self-harm, but don't restrain *to prevent injury.*
- Don't use tongue blades; *use of tongue blades during seizure activity may cause trauma to the mouth and result in airway obstruction from an aspirated tooth or laryngospasm.*
- Reduce external stimuli. *External stimuli could worsen seizure activity.*
- Loosen tight clothing *to promote comfort.*
- Record seizure activity. *Description of seizure activity helps to diagnose the type, which will aid in developing a treatment plan.*

- Pad the crib or bed *to prevent injury.*
- Monitor serum levels of anticonvulsant medications, such as phenytoin, *to ensure therapeutic levels and prevent toxicity or sub-therapeutic levels.*

Teaching topics
- Explanation of the disorder and treatment plan
- Medication use and possible adverse effects
- Importance of follow-up care
- Instituting safety measures during seizure activity

Spina bifida

Spina bifida is exposure of the spinal cord resulting from a defect of the back bone and spinal cord. It has two main forms. Spina bifida occulta, the more common and less severe form, is characterized by incomplete closure of one or more vertebrae without protrusion of the spinal cord or meninges (membranes covering the spinal cord). Spina bifida cystica, the more severe form, is distinguished by incomplete closure of one or more vertebrae that causes protrusion of the spinal contents in an external sac or cystic lesion.

Spina bifida cystica has two classifications:

myelomeningocele: an external sac that contains meninges, CSF, and a portion of the spinal cord or nerve roots

meningocele: an external sac that contains meninges and CSF.

CAUSES
- Combination of genetic and environmental factors
- Exposure to a teratogen
- Part of a multiple malformation syndrome (for example, chromosomal abnormalities such as trisomy 18 or 13 syndrome)
- Low intake of folic acid by the mother during pregnancy

ASSESSMENT FINDINGS
Spina bifida occulta
- Dimple or tuft of hair on the skin over the spinal defect

- No neurologic dysfunction (usually), except occasional foot weakness or bowel and bladder disturbances
- Port wine nevi (commonly found on the skin over the spinal defect)
- Soft fatty deposits (commonly found on the skin over the spinal defect)
- Trophic skin disturbances (ulcerations, cyanosis)

Meningocele
- No neurologic dysfunction (usually)
- Saclike structure protruding over the spine

Myelomeningocele
- Saclike structure protruding over the spine
- Hydrocephalus
- Permanent neurologic dysfunction (paralysis, bowel and bladder incontinence)
- Possible mental retardation
- Knee contractures
- Clubfoot
- Arnold-Chiari syndrome
- Curvature of the spine

DIAGNOSTIC TEST RESULTS
- Elevated alpha-fetoprotein levels in the mother's blood may indicate the presence of a neural tube defect.
- Amniocentesis reveals neural tube defect.
- Acetylcholinesterase measurement can be used to confirm the diagnosis.
- After birth, spinal X-ray can show the bone defect.
- Fetal karyotype should be done in addition to the biochemical tests because of the association of neural tube defects with chromosomal abnormalities.
- Myelography can differentiate spina bifida from other spinal abnormalities, especially spinal cord tumors.
- Ultrasound may identify the open neural tube or ventral wall defect.

NURSING DIAGNOSES
- Delayed growth and development
- Impaired physical mobility
- Impaired adjustment

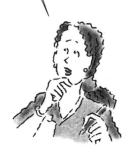

Hmmm. Spina bifida occulta and meningocele rarely cause neurologic dysfunction. However, myelomeningocele may cause permanent problems.

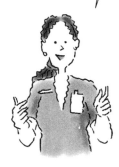

Remember, spina bifida occulta usually requires no treatment. Meningocele and myelomeningocele require surgery.

TREATMENT
- Meningocele: surgical closure of the protruding sac and continual assessment of growth and development
- Myelomeningocele: repair of the sac (doesn't reverse neurologic deficits) and supportive measures to promote independence and prevent further complications
- Spina bifida occulta: usually no treatment

INTERVENTIONS AND RATIONALES
Before surgery
- Hold and cuddle the infant on your lap and position him on his abdomen; handle the infant carefully, and don't apply pressure to the defect *to prevent injury at the site of the defect.*
- Clean the defect, inspect it often, and cover it with sterile dressings moistened with sterile saline solution *to prevent infection.*
- Place the infant in an infant Isolette *to prevent hypothermia.*
- Assess for signs of hydrocephalus. Measure head circumference daily. Be sure to mark the spot where the measurement was made *to ensure accurate readings.*
- Assess for signs of meningeal irritation, such as fever and nuchal rigidity, *to detect signs of meningitis.*
- Provide passive ROM exercises and casting. *To prevent hip dislocation, moderately abduct the hips with a pad between the knees or with sandbags and ankle rolls to prevent hip dislocation.*
- Monitor intake and output. Watch for decreased skin turgor and dryness *to detect dehydration.*

Teaching for spina bifida focuses on coping skills, long-term treatment goals, and signs of complications.

- Provide a diet high in calories and protein *to ensure adequate nutrition.*

After surgery
- Assess for hydrocephalus, which commonly follows surgery. Measure the infant's head circumference as ordered *to detect signs of hydrocephalus and prevent associated complications.*
- Monitor vital signs often *to detect early signs of shock, infection, and increased ICP.*
- Provide wound care and report any signs of drainage, wound rupture, and infection *to promote early treatment and prevent complications.*
- Place the infant in the prone position *to protect and assess the site.*
- If leg casts have been applied to treat deformities, regularly check distal pulses *to ensure adequate circulation.*
- When spina bifida is diagnosed prenatally, refer the prospective parents to a genetic counselor, *who can provide information and support the couple's decisions on how to manage the pregnancy.*

Teaching topics
- Explanation of the disorder and treatment plan
- Handling the infant without applying pressure to the defect
- Coping with the infant's physical problems
- Recognizing early signs of complications, such as hydrocephalus, pressure ulcers, and urinary tract infections
- Maintaining a positive attitude and working through feelings of guilt, anger, and helplessness
- Conducting intermittent catheterization and conduit hygiene
- Bowel training when the child is older
- Recognizing developmental lags (a possible result of hydrocephalus)
- Planning activities appropriate to their child's age and abilities

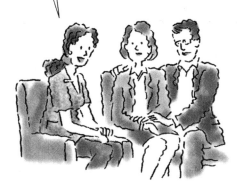

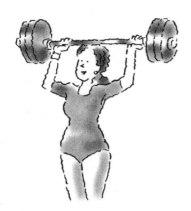

Pump up on practice questions

1. The nurse is assessing a child who may have meningitis. For which of the following assessment findings should the nurse watch?
1. Flat fontanel
2. Irritability, fever, and vomiting
3. Jaundice, drowsiness, and refusal to eat
4. Negative Kernig's sign

Answer: 2. Assessment findings associated with acute bacterial meningitis include irritability, fever, and vomiting along with seizure activity. Fontanels would be bulging as intracranial pressure rises, and Kernig's sign would be present because of meningeal irritation. Jaundice, drowsiness, and refusal to eat may indicate GI disturbance rather than meningitis.

➼ NCLEX keys
Client needs category: Physiological integrity
Client needs subcategory: Physiological adaptation
Cognitive level: Application

2. A nurse is assessing a child who may have a seizure disorder. Which option is a description of an absence seizure?
1. Sudden, momentary loss of muscle tone
2. Minimal or no alteration in muscle tone, with a brief loss of consciousness

3. Muscle tone maintained and child frozen into position
4. Brief, sudden contracture of a muscle or muscle group

Answer: 2. Absence seizures are characterized by a brief loss of responsiveness with minimal or no alteration in muscle tone. They may go unrecognized because the child's behavior changes very little. A sudden loss of muscle tone describes atonic seizures. "Frozen positions" describe akinetic seizures. A brief, sudden contraction of muscles describes a myoclonic seizure.

➼ NCLEX keys
Client needs category: Physiological integrity
Client needs subcategory: Physiological adaptation
Cognitive level: Knowledge

3. A nurse is caring for a child who's experiencing a seizure. Which nursing intervention takes highest priority when caring for this child?
1. Protect the child from injury.
2. Use a padded tongue blade to protect the airway.
3. Shout at the child to end the seizure.
4. Allow seizure activity to end without interference.

Answer: 1. The nurse should identify the seizure type and protect the child from injury. A padded tongue blade should never be used because it can cause damage to the mouth and airway. Shouting will only agitate or confuse the child. Interfering with seizure activity may cause injury to the child. Allowing the seizure activity to end without interference may cause the child injury. The nurse should position the child on his side to ensure a patent airway and place the child on the ground if he's likely to fall and sustain injury.

➼ NCLEX keys
Client needs category: Physiological integrity
Client needs subcategory: Reduction of risk potential
Cognitive level: Analysis

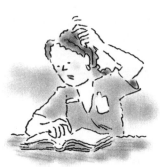

4. A nurse is caring for a 3-year-old child with viral meningitis. Which signs and symptoms should the nurse expect to find during the initial assessment? Select all that apply.
1. Bulging anterior fontanel
2. Fever
3. Nuchal rigidity
4. Petechiae
5. Irritability
6. Photophobia

Answer: 2, 3, 5, 6. Common signs and symptoms of viral meningitis include fever, nuchal rigidity, irritability, and photophobia. A bulging anterior fontanel is a sign of hydrocephalus, which isn't likely to occur in a toddler because the anterior fontanel typically closes by age 24 months. A petechial, purpuric rash may be seen with bacterial meningitis.

➡ NCLEX keys

Client needs category: Physiological integrity
Client needs subcategory: Physiological adaptation
Cognitive level: Application

5. A nurse is caring for an infant with spina bifida. Which assessment findings suggest hydrocephalus?
1. Depressed fontanels and suture lines
2. Deep-set eyes, which appear to look upward only
3. Rapid increase in head size and irritability
4. Motor and sensory dysfunction in the foot and leg

Answer: 3. Hydrocephalus is an increase in the amount of cerebrospinal fluid in the ven-

tricles and subarachnoid spaces of the brain. Assessment findings associated with hydrocephalus include a rapid increase in head size, irritability, suture line separation, and bulging fontanels. The eyes appear to look downward only, with the cornea prominent over the iris (sunset sign). A loss of sensory and motor function is related to the spinal cord defect spina bifida — not hydrocephalus.

➡ NCLEX keys

Client needs category: Physiological integrity
Client needs subcategory: Reduction of risk potential
Cognitive level: Application

6. A nurse is teaching a father whose infant has had several episodes of otitis media. Which statement made by the father indicates that he needs further teaching?
1. "Children who live in homes where family members smoke have fewer infections."
2. "The eustachian tube in infants is shorter and less angled than in older children."
3. "Breast-feeding is one way to help decrease the number of infections."
4. "I wrap him up and always put a hat on him when we go out."

Answer: 1. Children who live in households where smoking occurs have a greater number of respiratory infections that lead to otitis media, not fewer. The other statements about otitis media are correct.

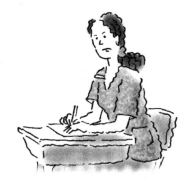

42"

,CI

continued

NCLEX keys
Client needs category: Health promotion and maintenance
Client needs subcategory: None
Cognitive level: Application

7. A school nurse is monitoring several children with attention deficit hyperactivity disorder who are taking methylphenidate (Ritalin). The nurse should conduct monthly follow-up examinations to monitor:

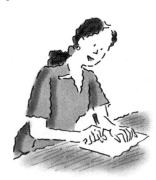

1. whether the child is experiencing dry mouth.
2. whether the child is growing in height.
3. the parent's coping abilities from the child's perspective.
4. when the child is taking the medication.

Answer: 2. Common adverse reactions to methylphenidate include slowed growth in height, sleeplessness, decreased appetite, and crying. Dry mouth is a common adverse reaction to tricyclic antidepressants. Knowing how the parents are coping from the child's perspective may be helpful information but isn't the priority. Knowing when the child takes the medication would be important if the child has problems with sleeplessness.

NCLEX keys
Client needs category: Physiological integrity
Client needs subcategory: Pharmacological and parenteral therapies
Cognitive level: Application

8. A nurse is teaching the mother of a child with attention deficit hyperactivity disorder (ADHD) how to manage the child. Which statement by the mother indicates that she needs further teaching?
1. "I give him only one direction at a time."
2. "I encourage my child to ride his bike after school."
3. "My child enjoys rollerblading with friends."
4. "I have my child do homework right after school."

Answer: 4. Children with ADHD need time to expend their energy after being in a restrictive environment such as school. They need time to participate in activities that they enjoy, such as running, bike riding, or inline skating. Homework should be done later in the evening, not right after school. The other statements indicate effective teaching.

NCLEX keys
Client needs category: Psychosocial integrity
Client needs subcategory: None
Cognitive level: Application

9. A nurse is caring for an infant with spina bifida. Which technique should the nurse anticipate that the physician will use to diagnose hydrocephalus?
1. Measurement of head circumference
2. Skull X-ray showing a thinning skull
3. Angiography revealing hydrocephalus
4. Magnetic resonance imaging (MRI) revealing hydrocephalus

Answer: 1. Measuring head circumference is the most important assessment technique for diagnosing hydrocephalus and is a key part of the routine infant screening. Skull X-rays, angiography, and MRI may be used to confirm the diagnosis.

➡ *NCLEX keys*
Client needs category: Health promotion and maintenance
Client needs subcategory: None
Cognitive level: Application

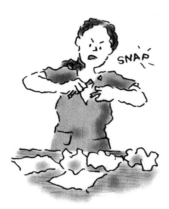

10. A nurse is caring for a child after shunt insertion to relieve hydrocephalus. Which intervention should the nurse perform?
1. Place the child in an upright position.
2. Avoid lying the child on the side where the shunt is located.
3. Place the child in the semi-Fowler position.
4. Place the child in a prone position.

Answer: 2. After the shunt is inserted, the nurse shouldn't lie the child on the side of the body where the shunt is located. The child should lie supine to avoid rapid decompression. The child shouldn't be in an upright, semi-Fowler, or prone position.

➡ *NCLEX keys*
Client needs category: Physiological integrity
Client needs subcategory: Reduction of risk potential
Cognitive level: Application

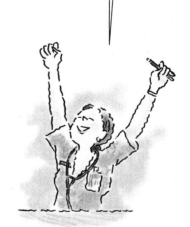

Congratulations! Finishing this chapter shows you have a lot of nerve!

8 Musculoskeletal system

In this chapter, you'll review:

✐ the pediatric musculoskeletal system

✐ tests used to diagnose musculoskeletal disorders

✐ common pediatric musculoskeletal disorders.

Brush up on key concepts

The musculoskeletal system is a complex system of **bones, muscles, ligaments, tendons,** and other **connective tissues.** The functions of the musculoskeletal system include:
- giving the body form and shape
- protecting vital organs
- making movement possible
- storing calcium and other minerals
- providing the site for hematopoiesis (blood cell formation).

At any point, you can review the major points of this chapter by consulting the *Cheat sheet* on pages 102 and 103.

Growing pains
Here are a few facts about the **pediatric musculoskeletal system:**
- Bones and muscles grow and develop throughout childhood.
- Bone lengthening occurs in the epiphyseal plates at the ends of bones; when the epiphyses close, growth stops.
- Bone healing occurs much faster in the child than in the adult because the child's bones are still growing.
- The younger the child, the faster the bone heals.
- Bone healing takes approximately 1 week for every year of life up to age 10.

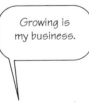

Growing is my business.

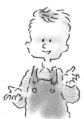

Fractured logic
The most common fractures in the child are **clavicular fractures** and **greenstick fractures:**
- Clavicular fractures may occur during vaginal birth because the shoulders are the widest part of the body.

- Greenstick fractures of the long bones are related to the increased flexibility of the young child's bones. (The compressed side of the bone bends while the side under tension fractures.)

Keep abreast of diagnostic tests

Here are the most important tests used to diagnose musculoskeletal disorders, along with common nursing interventions associated with each test.

Using physical examination to assess the child's musculoskeletal function and ability is also an important element in diagnosis. (See *Assessing musculoskeletal function and ability,* page 104.)

Look inside the joint
Arthroscopy is the visual examination of the interior of a joint with a fiber-optic endoscope.

Nursing actions
- Explain the procedure to the parents and child.
- Make sure that written, informed consent has been obtained.
- Tell the child and his parents that he may need to fast after midnight before the procedure.
- Note allergies because local anesthesia is used.
- Tell the child that he may feel a thumping sensation as the cannula is inserted in the joint capsule.

Soft-tissue sighting
A **computed tomography scan** is used to identify injuries to the soft tissue, ligaments, tendons, and muscles.

(Text continues on page 104.)

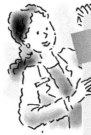

Musculoskeletal refresher

CLUBFOOT
Key signs and symptoms
• Inability to manually correct the deformity (distinguishes true clubfoot from apparent clubfoot)

Key test results
• X-rays show superimposition of the talus and calcaneus and a ladderlike appearance of the metatarsals.

Key treatments
• Correction of the deformity with a series of casts or surgical correction
• Maintenance of correction until the foot gains normal muscle balance
• Close observation of the foot for several years to prevent the deformity from recurring

Key interventions
• Ensure that shoes fit correctly.
• Prepare for surgery, if necessary.

DEVELOPMENTAL HIP DYSPLASIA
Key signs and symptoms
• Increased number of folds on the posterior thigh on the affected side when the child is supine with knees bent
• Appearance of a shortened limb on the affected side
• Restricted abduction of the hips

Key test results
• Barlow's sign: A click is felt when the infant is placed in a supine position with the hips flexed 90 degrees and when the knees are fully flexed and the hip is brought into midabduction.
• Ortolani's click: It can be felt by the fingers at the hip area as the femur head snaps out of and back into the acetabulum. It's also palpable during examination with the child's legs flexed and abducted.
• Positive Trendelenburg's test: When the child stands on the affected leg, the opposite pelvis dips to maintain erect posture.

Key treatments
• Hip-spica cast or corrective surgery (for older children)
• Bryant's traction, if the acetabulum doesn't deepen
• Pavlik harness or casting to keep the neonate's hips and knees flexed and the hips abducted for at least 3 months

Key interventions
• Provide reassurance that early, prompt treatment commonly results in complete correction.
• Reassure the parents that the child will adjust to restricted movement and return to normal sleeping, eating and playing behavior in a few days.

DUCHENNE'S MUSCULAR DYSTROPHY
Key signs and symptoms
• Begins with pelvic girdle weakness, indicated by waddling gait and falling
• Eventual muscle weakness and wasting
• Gowers' sign (use of hands to push self up from floor)

Key test results
• Electromyography typically demonstrates short, weak bursts of electrical activity in the affected muscles.
• Muscle biopsy shows variation in the size of muscle fibers and, in later stages, shows fat and connective tissue deposits, with no dystrophin.

Key treatments
• Physical therapy
• Surgery to correct contractures
• Use of devices, such as splints, braces, trapeze bars, overhead slings, and a wheelchair, to help preserve mobility

Key interventions
• Perform range-of-motion exercises.
• Encourage coughing, deep-breathing exercises, and diaphragmatic breathing.
• Encourage adequate fluid intake, increase dietary fiber, and obtain an order for a stool softener.

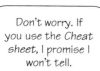

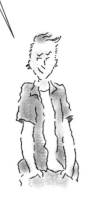

Don't worry. If you use the Cheat sheet, I promise I won't tell.

Musculoskeletal refresher *(continued)*

FRACTURES
Key signs and symptoms
- Pain or tenderness
- Skeletal deformity
- Swelling
- Loss of motor function
- Muscle spasm

Key test results
- X-rays confirm the location and type of fracture.

Key treatments
- Reduction and immobilization of the fracture
- Casting
- Surgery: open reduction and external fixation of the fracture

Key interventions
- Keep the affected extremity in proper body alignment.
- Provide support above and below the fracture site when moving the child.
- Elevate the fracture above the level of the heart.
- Apply ice to the fracture to promote vasoconstriction.
- Monitor pulses distal to the fracture every 2 to 4 hours.
- Assess color, temperature, and capillary refill of the affected extremity.

JUVENILE RHEUMATOID ARTHRITIS
Key signs and symptoms
- Inflammation around joints
- Stiffness, pain, and guarding of affected joints

Key test results
- Hematology reveals an elevated erythrocyte sedimentation rate, a positive antinuclear antibody test, and the presence of rheumatoid factor.

Key treatments
- Heat therapy: warm compresses, baths
- Splint application

Key interventions
- Monitor the joints for deformity.

LEGG-CALVE-PERTHES DISEASE
Key signs and symptoms
- Mild hip, thigh, or knee pain
- Persistent thigh or leg pain
- Shortening of affected leg

Key test results
- Hip X-ray confirms the diagnosis, with the findings based on the stage of the disease.

Key treatments
- Bed rest
- Reduced weight-bearing therapy
- Analgesics: acetaminophen (Tylenol), ibuprofen (Motrin)

Key interventions
- Maintain the child on bed rest.
- Provide stimulation for the child on bed rest.
- Monitor for circulatory or neurologic changes in the leg.

OSGOOD-SCHLATTER DISEASE
Key signs and symptoms
- Aching and pain over tibial tubercle
- Swelling
- Tenderness

Key test results
- X-rays show epiphyseal separation and soft tissue swelling in first 6 months after onset; eventually show bone fragmentation.

Key treatments
- Conservative treatment: designed to decrease stress to affected knee
- Avoiding strenuous exercise for the affected knee
- Analgesics: acetaminophen (Tylenol), ibuprofen (Motrin)

Key interventions
- Monitor the child for circulatory or neurologic changes in the leg.

SCOLIOSIS
Key signs and symptoms
- One shoulder higher than the other
- Uneven waist
- Forward bend test with asymmetry of the trunk or abnormal spinal curve

Key test results
- Spinal X-rays identify the degree of deformity.
- Scoliometer measures the amount of curvature.

Key treatments
- Observation for curves 25 to 40 degrees for a child with completed growth
- Bracing for curves above 25 to 30 degrees in a growing child
- Surgery for curves 40 degrees or greater

Key interventions
- Assess brace fit.
After spinal fusion and insertion of rods
- Turn the child by logrolling only.
- Maintain the child in correct body alignment.
- Maintain the bed in a flat position.

> *Management moments*
>
> ## Assessing musculoskeletal function and ability
>
> To assess a child's musculoskeletal function and ability, perform the following nursing actions:
> • Determine the range of motion.
> • Note the amount of weight the child can bear.
> • Assess gross and fine motor abilities.
> • Note whether both arms and legs are used.
> • Note whether muscle response is brisk and strong.
> • Assess for pain; note whether the child is guarding a body part.
> • Determine the relationship of the child's body size or weight to the defect.
> • Note whether the child has an adequate and even spread of adipose tissue.
> • Note the child's autonomy and independence in terms of mobility and skills.

Nursing actions

• Explain the procedure to the parents and child.
• Make sure written, informed consent has been obtained.
• Tell the child to hold still during the procedure.
• Tell the child that he'll be placed in a tube-like circle for the study and that pictures will be taken of the extremity.

Cross-section check

Magnetic resonance imaging (MRI) allows cross-sectional imaging of bones and joints. MRI, which uses a strong magnetic field and radio waves, has largely replaced arthrography for assessing joint anatomy.

No ionizing radiation is used. MRI studies are also used to assess certain muscle and soft-tissue injuries.

Nursing actions

• Explain the procedure to the parents and child.
• Make sure written, informed consent has been obtained.
• Instruct the child to hold still during the procedure.
• Note whether the child has any metal implants, which may interfere with the study.

Spinal vision

Myelography is an invasive procedure used to evaluate abnormalities of the spinal canal and cord. It entails injection of a radiopaque contrast medium into the subarachnoid space of the spine. Serial X-rays are then used to visualize the progress of the contrast medium as it passes through the subarachnoid space.

Nursing actions

• Explain the procedure to the parents and child.
• Make sure that written, informed consent has been obtained.
• Before the test, check for allergies to the contrast medium.
• If metrizamide (Amipaque) is used as the contrast medium, discontinue phenothiazines 48 hours before the test.
• When the contrast medium is injected, tell the child that he may experience a burning sensation, warmth, headache, salty taste, nausea, and vomiting.
• After the test, have the child sit in his room or lie in bed with his head elevated 60 degrees. He must not lie flat for at least 8 hours.
• Encourage the child to drink extra fluids.
• Check that the child voids within 8 hours after returning to his room.

Hard tissue check

X-rays are probably the most useful diagnostic tool to evaluate musculoskeletal diseases. They can help to identify joint disruption, calcifications, and bone deformities,

> X-rays are excellent! They're a great tool for identifying calcifications, bone deformities, and fractures as well as bone density.

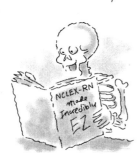

fractures, and destruction as well as measure bone density.

Nursing actions
- Explain the test to the parents and child.
- Tell the child that he must hold still during the X-ray. Cover the genital area with a lead apron.

Polish up on client care

Musculoskeletal disorders in children include clubfoot (talipes), developmental hip dysplasia (dislocated hip), Duchenne's muscular dystrophy, fractures, juvenile rheumatoid arthritis (JRA), Legg-Calve-Perthes disease, Osgood-Schlatter disease, and scoliosis.

Clubfoot

Clubfoot, also known as *talipes,* is a congenital disorder in which the foot and ankle are twisted and can't be manipulated into correct position.

  Clubfoot occurs in these five forms:
- equinovarus: combination of positions
- talipes calcaneus: dorsiflexion, as if walking on one's heels
- talipes equinus: plantar flexion, as if pointing one's toes
- talipes valgus: eversion of the ankles, with the feet turning out
- talipes varus: inversion of the ankles, with the soles of the feet facing each other.

CAUSES
- Arrested development during the 9th and 10th weeks of embryonic life, when the feet are formed
- Deformed talus and shortened Achilles tendon
- Possible genetic predisposition
- Intrauterine positioning

ASSESSMENT FINDINGS
- Deformity usually obvious at birth
- Inability to manually correct the deformity (distinguishes true clubfoot from apparent clubfoot)

DIAGNOSTIC TEST RESULTS
- X-rays show superimposition of the talus and calcaneus and a ladderlike appearance of the metatarsals.

NURSING DIAGNOSES
- Delayed growth and development
- Impaired physical mobility
- Risk for peripheral neurovascular dysfunction

TREATMENT
Treatment is administered in three stages:

  correcting the deformity either with a series of casts to gradually stretch and realign the angle of the foot and, after cast removal, application of a Denis Browne splint at night until age 1 or surgical correction

  maintaining the correction until the foot gains normal muscle balance

  observing the foot closely for several years to prevent the deformity from recurring.

INTERVENTIONS AND RATIONALES
- Assess neurovascular status *to ensure circulation to the foot with the cast in place.*
- Ensure that shoes fit correctly *to promote comfort and prevent skin breakdown.*
- Prepare for surgery, if necessary, *to maintain or promote the healing process and decrease anxiety.*

Teaching topics
- Explanation of the disorder and treatment plan
- Using a blow-dryer on the cool setting to provide relief from itching
- Importance of placing nothing inside the cast
- Keeping corrective devices on as much as possible
- Walking as exercise after surgical repair

Developmental hip dysplasia

Developmental hip dysplasia (dislocated hip) results from an abnormal development of the hip socket. It occurs when the head of the

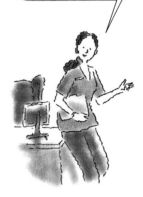

Combos are common. Nearly all cases of talipes are equinovarus, involving a combination of abnormal positions.

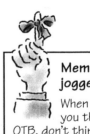

Memory jogger

When you think OTB, don't think Off Track Betting. Instead think of Ortolani, Trendelenburg, and Barlow—all key tests in diagnosing hip dysplasia.

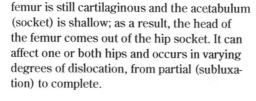

What's the common goal of treatment for developmental hip dysplasia? Enlarging and deepening the socket (acetabulum) through pressure.

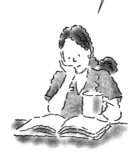

femur is still cartilaginous and the acetabulum (socket) is shallow; as a result, the head of the femur comes out of the hip socket. It can affect one or both hips and occurs in varying degrees of dislocation, from partial (subluxation) to complete.

CAUSES
- Breech delivery
- Fetal position in utero
- Genetic predisposition
- Laxity of the ligaments

ASSESSMENT FINDINGS
- Increased number of folds on the posterior thigh on the affected side when the child is supine with knees bent
- Appearance of a shortened limb on the affected side
- Restricted abduction of the hips

DIAGNOSTIC TEST RESULTS
- Barlow's sign is present: A click is felt when the infant is placed supine with hips flexed 90 degrees, knees fully flexed, and the hip brought into midabduction.
- Ortolani's click is present. It can be felt by the fingers at the hip area as the femur head snaps out of and back into the acetabulum. It's also palpable during examination with the child's legs flexed and abducted.
- Sonography and MRI may be used to assess reduction.
- Trendelenburg's test is positive. When the child stands on the affected leg, the opposite pelvis dips to maintain erect posture.
- Ultrasonography shows the involved cartilage and acetabulum.
- X-rays show the location of the femur head and a shallow acetabulum; X-rays can also be used to monitor progression of the disorder.

NURSING DIAGNOSES
- Delayed growth and development
- Impaired physical mobility
- Risk for impaired skin integrity

TREATMENT
- Hip-spica cast or corrective surgery (for older children)
- Bryant's traction, if the acetabulum doesn't deepen

Here's a hint for early assessment: Duchenne's muscular dystrophy begins with a waddling gait and falling. This indicates pelvic girdle weakness.

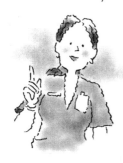

- Pavlik harness or casting to keep the neonate's hips and knees flexed and the hips abducted for at least 3 months

INTERVENTIONS AND RATIONALES
- Assess circulation before application of a cast or traction; after application, have the child wiggle his toes *to detect signs of impaired circulation.* One finger should fit between the child's skin and the cast.
- Provide skin care *to prevent skin breakdown.*
- Provide reassurance that early, prompt treatment commonly results in complete correction *to decrease anxiety.*
- Reassure the parents that the child will adjust to restricted movement and return to normal sleeping, eating, and play in a few days *to ease anxiety.*
- Inspect the skin, especially around bony prominences, *to detect cast complications and skin breakdown.*

Teaching topics
- Explanation of the disorder and treatment plan
- Correctly splinting or bracing the hips
- Receiving frequent checkups
- Coping with restricted movement
- Removing braces and splints while bathing the child and replacing them immediately afterward
- Stressing good hygiene

Duchenne's muscular dystrophy

A genetic disorder (defect on the X chromosome) that occurs only in males, Duchenne's muscular dystrophy (also called *pseudohypertrophic dystrophy*) is marked by muscular deterioration due to a lack of production of dystrophin that progresses throughout childhood. The absence of dystrophin results in breakdown of muscle fibers. Muscle fibers are replaced with fatty deposits and collagen in muscles. There's no known cure. It generally results in death from cardiac or respiratory failure in the late teens or early 20s.

CAUSES
- Sex-linked recessive trait

ASSESSMENT FINDINGS
- Begins with pelvic girdle weakness, indicated by waddling gait and falling
- Cardiac or pulmonary failure
- Decreased ability to perform self-care activities
- Delayed motor development
- Eventual contractures and muscle hypertrophy
- Eventual muscle weakness and wasting
- Gowers' sign (use of hands to push self up from floor)
- Toe-walking

DIAGNOSTIC TEST RESULTS
- Electromyography typically demonstrates short, weak bursts of electrical activity in affected muscles.
- Muscle biopsy shows variations in the size of muscle fibers and, in later stages, shows fat and connective tissue deposits, with no dystrophin.

NURSING DIAGNOSES
- Impaired physical mobility
- Activity intolerance
- Impaired gas exchange

TREATMENT
- High-fiber, high-protein, low-calorie diet
- Physical therapy
- Surgery to correct contractures
- Use of devices, such as splints, braces, trapeze bars, overhead slings, and a wheelchair, to help preserve mobility
- Gene therapy (under investigation to prevent muscle degeneration)

INTERVENTIONS AND RATIONALES
- Perform range-of-motion (ROM) exercises *to promote joint mobility.*
- Provide emotional support to the child and parents *to decrease anxiety and promote coping mechanisms.*
- Initiate genetic counseling *to inform the child and family about passing the disorder on to future children.*
- Encourage coughing, deep-breathing exercises, and diaphragmatic breathing *to maintain a patent airway and mobilize secretions to prevent complications associated with retained secretions.*
- Encourage the use of a footboard or high-topped sneakers and a foot cradle *to increase comfort and prevent footdrop.*
- Encourage adequate fluid intake, increase dietary fiber, and obtain an order for a stool softener *to prevent constipation associated with inactivity.*

Teaching topics
- Explanation of the disorder and treatment plan
- Recognizing early signs of respiratory complications
- Planning a low-calorie, high-protein, high-fiber diet
- Promoting physical activity within limitations of the disorder
- Promoting peer interaction and preventing social isolation

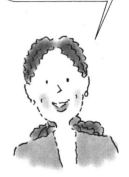

With Duchenne's muscular dystrophy, the goal is to help the child remain as active and independent as possible.

Fractures

A fracture is a break in the bone's integrity. A complete fracture breaks entirely across, resulting in a break in the continuity of the bone. An incomplete fracture extends only partially through the bone, and the bone remains continuous. In a closed or simple fracture, the break doesn't puncture the skin surface, whereas an open or compound fracture punctures through the skin surface.

Common sites of fractures include the long bones of the arms and legs, clavicle, and knee. The outcome usually depends on the severity of the fracture and the treatment provided. Potential complications include the development of fat emboli, improper bone growth, compartment syndrome, and infection.

CAUSES
- Childhood accidents, such as falls and motor vehicle crashes (most common cause)
- Child abuse
- Pathologic conditions

ASSESSMENT FINDINGS
- Pain or tenderness
- Skeletal deformity

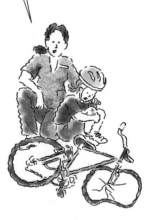

Accidents are the number one cause of fractures in childhood.

Common orthopedic treatments

The use of casts, traction, and braces are common orthopedic treatments.

CASTS

A cast is a hard mold that encases a body part, usually an extremity, to provide immobilization without discomfort.

General cast care

• Turn the child frequently to dry all sides of the cast; use the palms to lift or turn a wet cast to prevent indentations.
• Expose as much of the cast to air as possible to promote drying.
• Assess discomfort in the child because chemical changes in the drying cast cause temperature extremes against the child's skin.
• Maintain a dry cast; wetting the cast softens it and may cause skin irritation.
• Smooth out the cast's rough edges, and petal the edges.
• Assess circulation:
  – Note the capillary refill, color, temperature, and edema of digits.
  – Note the child's ability to wiggle the extremities without tingling or numbness.
• Assess any drainage or foul odor from the cast.
• Prevent small objects or food from falling into the cast.
• Avoid using powder on the skin near the cast; it becomes a medium for bacteria when it absorbs perspiration.

Hip-spica cast care

A hip-spica cast is a body cast extending from the midchest to the legs. The legs are abducted with a bar between them.
• Perform cast care as listed above but with additional measures.
• Line the back edges of the cast with plastic or other waterproof material.
• Keep the cast level but on a slant, with the head of the bed raised (a Bradford frame can be used for this purpose):
  – The body and cast should stay at 180 degrees.
  – The head of the bed is raised on shock blocks or the mattress is raised using a wedge pillow so that the child is on a slant with the head up.
  – Urine and stools drain downward away from the cast.
• Use a mattress firm enough to support the cast; use pillows to support parts of the cast, if needed.
• Reposition frequently to avoid pressure on the skin and the bony prominences; check for pressure as the child grows.

TRACTION

Traction decreases muscle spasms and realigns and positions bone ends by pulling on the distal ends of bones.
• Skin traction pulls indirectly on the skeleton by pulling on the skin with adhesive, moleskin, or elastic bandage.
• Skeletal traction pulls directly on the skeleton with surgically placed pins or tongs.

Traction-related care

• Check that the weights hang free from the bed.
• Monitor for skin irritation, infection at pin sites, and neurovascular response of the extremity.
• Encourage fluids and fiber to prevent constipation.
• Promote pulmonary hygiene using blowing games.
• Provide pain relief through positioning and analgesics.
• Provide stimulation appropriate for the child's age.

Bryant's traction

This skin traction is designed specifically for the lower extremities of the child younger than age 2; the child's body weight provides countertraction. Traction may be followed by application of a hip-spica cast.
• Keep the legs straight and extended 90 degrees toward the ceiling from the trunk (both legs are suspended even if only one is affected).
• Keep the buttocks slightly off the bed to ensure sufficient and continuous traction on the legs.

BRACES

A brace is a plastic shell or metal-hinged appliance that aids mobility and posture.

Brace-related care

• Provide good skin care, especially at the bony prominences.
• Check to ensure accurate fit as the child grows.

Milwaukee brace

This type of brace attempts to slow the progression of spinal curvature of less than 40 degrees until bone growth stops. It can be used until the child reaches skeletal maturity.
• Monitor the use of the brace. It must be worn 20 to 23 hours a day; it may be removed for bathing.

Boston brace

This type of brace functions the same as a Milwaukee brace.
• Make sure the brace extends from the axillary area to the iliac crest.
• Remove the brace for bathing.

- Swelling
- Bony crepitus
- Bruising
- Impaired sensation
- Loss of motor function
- Muscle spasm
- Paralysis
- Paresthesia

DIAGNOSTIC TEST RESULTS

- X-rays confirm the location and type of fracture.

NURSING DIAGNOSES

- Ineffective peripheral tissue perfusion
- Acute pain
- Risk for impaired skin integrity
- Impaired physical mobility

TREATMENT

- Reduction and immobilization of the fracture
- Casting
- Surgery: open reduction and external fixation of the fracture
- Traction, depending on the site of the fracture (see *Common orthopedic treatments*)

Drug therapy

Nonsteroidal anti-inflammatory drug (NSAID): ibuprofen (Motrin)

INTERVENTIONS AND RATIONALES

- Keep the affected extremity in proper body alignment *to promote bone healing and prevent tissue damage.*
- Provide support above and below the fracture site when moving the child *to promote comfort.*
- Monitor pressure areas affected by traction or the child's cast *to prevent impaired tissue perfusion.*
- Elevate the fracture above the level of the heart *to promote venous return and decrease edema.*
- Apply ice to the fracture to promote vasoconstriction, *which inhibits edema and pain.*
- Monitor pulses distal to the fracture every 2 to 4 hours *to assess blood flow to the distal extremity.*
- Assess color, temperature, and capillary refill *to determine whether the affected extremity is adequately perfused.*

- Assess sensation *to determine whether perfusion to the nerves is intact.*
- Assess pain level utilizing pediatric assessment tools and administer analgesia *to provide comfort.*
- Turn and reposition the child every 2 hours *to help relieve skin pressure and prevent skin breakdown.*
- Protect the cast from moisture and petal the edges *to promote healing of the fracture and prevent skin breakdown.*

Teaching topics

- Explanation of the injury and treatment plan
- Caring for a child in cast or traction
- Preventing injury
- Reporting signs of infection or complications

Juvenile rheumatoid arthritis

JRA is an autoimmune disease of the connective tissue. It's characterized by chronic inflammation of the synovia and possible joint destruction. Episodes recur with remissions and exacerbations.

The three main forms of JRA are:
- pauciarticular JRA — asymmetrical involvement of less than five joints, usually affecting large joints such as the knees, ankles, and elbows.
- polyarticular JRA — symmetrical involvement of five or more joints, especially the hands and weight-bearing joints, such as the hips, knees, and feet. Involvement of the temporomandibular joint may cause earache; involvement of the sternoclavicular joint may cause chest pain.
- systemic disease with polyarthritis — involves the lining of the heart and lungs, blood cells, and abdominal organs. Exacerbations may last for months. Fever, rash, and lymphadenopathy may occur.

CAUSES

- Autoimmune response
- Genetic predisposition

ASSESSMENT FINDINGS

- Inflammation around the joints
- Stiffness, pain, and guarding of the affected joints

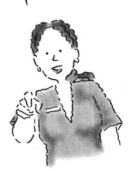

JRA typically involves the joints but can also affect the heart, lungs, liver, and spleen.

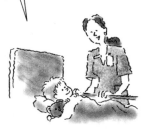

Oh brother! Legg-Calve-Perthes disease occurs most commonly in boys and is seen in families.

DIAGNOSTIC TEST RESULTS

• Hematology reveals an elevated erythrocyte sedimentation rate, a positive antinuclear antibody test, and the presence of rheumatoid factor.
• Slit-lamp evaluation may show iridocyclitis (inflammation of the iris and the ciliary body).

NURSING DIAGNOSES

• Impaired physical mobility
• Chronic pain
• Disturbed body image

TREATMENT

• Heat therapy: warm compresses, baths
• Splint application

Drug therapy

• Low-dose corticosteroids
• Low-dose methotrexate (Trexall) (used as a second-line medication)
• NSAIDs: naproxen (Naprosyn), ibuprofen (Motrin)

INTERVENTIONS AND RATIONALES

• Monitor the joints for deformity *to assess for early changes as a complication of this disease process.*
• Administer medications as prescribed and note the effectiveness *to relieve pain and prevent further joint damage.*
• Assist with exercise and ROM activities *to maintain joint mobility.*
• Apply warm compresses or encourage the child to take a warm bath in the morning *to promote comfort and increase mobility.*
• Apply splints *to maintain position of function and prevent contractures.*
• Provide assistive devices, if necessary, *to encourage the normal performance of daily activities.*

Teaching topics

• Explanation of the disorder and treatment plan
• Medication use and possible adverse effects
• Understanding how stress and climate can influence exacerbations
• ROM exercises

Legg-Calve-Perthes disease

Legg-Calve-Perthes disease is ischemic necrosis that leads to eventual flattening of the head of the femur caused by vascular interruption. Legg-Calve-Perthes disease occurs most commonly in boys ages 4 to 10 and tends to occur in families.

The disease occurs in five stages:
• Growth arrest: avascular phase; may last 6 to 12 months. Early changes include inflammation and synovitis of the hip and ischemic changes in the ossific nucleus of the femoral head.
• Subchondral fracture: Radiographic visualization of the fracture varies with the age of the child at clinical onset and the extent of epiphyseal involvement; may last 3 to 8 months.
• Reabsorption, also called *fragmentation* or *necrosis:* The necrotic bone beneath the subchondral fracture is gradually and irregularly reabsorbed; lasts 6 to 12 months.
• Reossification or healing stage: Ossification of the primary bone begins irregularly in the subchondral area and progresses centrally; takes 6 to 24 months.
• Healed stage, also called *residual stage:* Complete ossification of the epiphysis of the femoral head, with or without residual deformity.

CAUSES

• Unknown
• Theories include trauma, vascular irregularities, increased blood viscosity leading to statis, decreased blood flow

ASSESSMENT FINDINGS

• Mild hip, thigh, or knee pain
• Shortening of affected leg
• Muscle spasm
• Persistent thigh or leg pain
• Muscle atrophy in upper thigh
• Severely restricted abduction and internal rotation of hip

DIAGNOSTIC TEST RESULTS

• Hip X-ray confirms the diagnosis, with the findings based on the stage of the disease.
• MRI helps enhance early diagnosis of necrosis.

NURSING DIAGNOSES
- Impaired physical mobility
- Disturbed body image
- Chronic pain
- Delayed growth and development

TREATMENT
- Bed rest
- Therapy with reduced weight bearing
- Splint, cast, or brace to hold leg in abduction (brace may remain for as long as 18 months)
- Physical therapy after cast removal
- Osteotomy and subtrochanteric derotation: to allow femoral head to return to normal shape (in early stages)

Drug therapy
- Analgesics: acetaminophen (Tylenol), ibuprofen (Motrin)

INTERVENTIONS AND RATIONALES
- Maintain the child on bed rest *to protect the femoral head from further stress and damage.*
- Administer medications, as prescribed, *to reduce the child's pain.*
- Provide stimulation for the child on bed rest *to help promote growth and development.*
- Monitor and record the patient's intake and output and dietary intake. *This helps ensure the child has a diet sufficient for growth without causing excessive weight gain.*
- If the child is in a cast, provide cast care *to help maintain skin integrity.*
- Reposition the child every 2 to 3 hours *to help prevent skin breakdown.*
- Monitor the child for circulatory or neurologic changes in the leg, *which could indicate neurovascular compromise.*
- Provide emotional support to the child and his family.

Teaching topics
- Explanation of the disorder and treatment plan
- Medication use and possible adverse effects
- Following up with physician and therapy appointments
- Importance of socialization

Osgood-Schlatter disease

Osgood-Schlatter disease, also called *osteochondrosis,* is a painful, incomplete separation of the epiphysis of the tibial tubercle from the tibial shaft. This is a common cause of knee pain in adolescents. It's most common in active adolescent boys, but may also be seen in girls ages 10 to 11.

CAUSES
- Trauma before complete fusion of the epiphysis to the main bone
- Locally decreased blood supply
- Genetic factors

ASSESSMENT FINDINGS
- Aching and pain over tibial tubercle
- Swelling
- Tenderness

DIAGNOSTIC TEST RESULTS
- X-rays show epiphyseal separation and soft tissue swelling in first 6 months after onset; eventually show bone fragmentation.
- Bone scan may show increased uptake in area of tibial tuberosity.

NURSING DIAGNOSES
- Impaired physical mobility
- Chronic pain
- Delayed growth and development

TREATMENT
- Conservative: designed to decrease stress to affected knee
- Avoiding strenuous exercise for the affected knee
- Ice application after exercise
- Rest and quadriceps strengthening and hamstring and quadriceps stretching exercises
- Surgery to reposition epiphysis (if conservative methods fail)

Drug therapy
- Analgesics: acetaminophen (Tylenol), ibuprofen (Motrin)

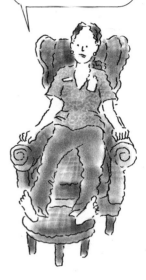

My knees ache from a long day of nursing. Adolescent knee pain could be caused by Osgood-Schlatter disease.

INTERVENTIONS AND RATIONALES

- Monitor the child for circulatory or neurologic changes in the leg, *which could indicate neurovascular compromise.*
- Assess the child for limitations in movement and reposition as needed *to maintain skin integrity.*
- Provide emotional support to the child and family.

Teaching topics

- Explanation of the disorder and treatment plan
- Medication use and possible adverse effects
- Following up with physician and therapy appointments
- Importance of socialization

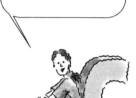

Congenital scoliosis is spinal curvature that occurs before birth.

Scoliosis

Scoliosis is a lateral curvature of the spine. It's commonly identified at puberty and throughout adolescence.

CAUSES

- Congenital: abnormal formation of vertebrae or fused ribs that occurs during prenatal development
- Neuromuscular: scoliosis that occurs as a result of poor muscle control or weakness secondary to another condition, such as cerebral palsy or muscular dystrophy
- Idiopathic: unknown reason for curvature in a previously straight spine

ASSESSMENT FINDINGS

- One shoulder higher than the other
- Tilted pelvis
- Uneven waist
- Backache or lower back pain, especially after prolonged sitting or standing
- Fatigue
- Forward bend test with asymmetry of the trunk or abnormal spinal curve

DIAGNOSTIC TEST RESULTS

- Spinal X-rays identify the degree of deformity.
- Scoliometer measures the amount of curvature.

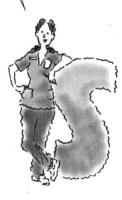

Neuromuscular scoliosis is caused by another condition such as cerebral palsy.

- MRI may identify additional neurologic changes.

NURSING DIAGNOSES

- Delayed growth and development
- Disturbed body image
- Impaired physical mobility

TREATMENT

- Observation for curves 25 to 40 degrees for a child with completed growth
- Bracing for curves above 25 to 30 degrees in a growing child
- Surgery for curves 40 degrees or greater to insert rods or perform spinal fusion

INTERVENTIONS AND RATIONALES

- Provide emotional support *to help the child develop a positive self image.*
- Assess brace fit *to identify pressure areas and skin irritation and to prevent skin breakdown.*

After spinal fusion and insertion of rods

- Monitor vital signs and intake and output *to prevent fluid volume deficit.*
- Turn the child only by logrolling *to prevent injury.*
- Maintain correct body alignment *to promote joint mobility and prevent injury.*
- Maintain the bed in a flat position *to prevent injury and complications.*
- Help the child adjust to altered self-perception *to promote self-esteem and decrease anxiety.*

Teaching topics

- Explanation of the disorder and treatment plan
- Types of braces needed
- Helping the child maintain self-esteem

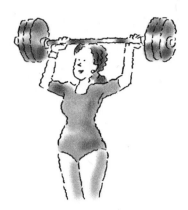

Pump up on practice questions

1. A nurse is caring for a child in traction after a fall. Which action is appropriate when the child is in balanced suspension traction?

1. Increase the weights daily, as ordered.
2. Position the child with his feet against the footboard.
3. Ensure that the weights hang freely.
4. Remove the traction at least three times per day.

Answer: 3. Traction weights must hang freely so that traction and countertraction are properly maintained. The weights aren't increased each day; as the client's muscles relax, the weights may be reduced. To maintain countertraction, position the client in bed so that his feet don't rest against the foot of the bed or against a footboard. Keep the weights in place at all times; neither traction nor the weights are removed until treatment is completed.

➡ *NCLEX keys*
Client needs category: Physiological integrity
Client needs subcategory: Reduction of risk potential
Cognitive level: Application

2. A child must undergo arthroscopy. Teaching about the procedure is effective when the mother states:

1. "I'm glad he won't feel anything during the procedure."
2. "I'm glad he doesn't have to fast before the procedure."
3. "I need to tell the doctor that he's allergic to lidocaine."
4. "I don't need to sign a consent for the procedure."

Answer: 3. Because a local anesthetic is used before the procedure, teaching is effective when the mother states she must make sure that the physician is aware of her child's allergy to lidocaine. The child may feel a thumping sensation as the cannula is inserted in the joint capsule. The child may need to fast after midnight before the procedure. A parent will need to sign a consent form before the procedure.

➡ *NCLEX keys*
Client needs category: Safe and effective care environment
Client needs subcategory: Management of care
Cognitive level: Application

3. A nurse is assessing the hand of a child with a long arm cast. The nail bed blanches white with pressure, and the color doesn't return for 5 seconds. The nurse interprets this finding as indicating:

1. fluid accumulation in the fingers.
2. decreased arterial blood supply.
3. a normal response.
4. venous stasis.

Answer: 2. Blanching with slow return to color (capillary refill) is an indication of decreased arterial blood supply. Normally, the color would return to the client's nail bed in less than 3 seconds. Venous stasis and fluid accumulation don't cause blanching.

➡ *NCLEX keys*
Client needs category: Physiological integrity
Client needs subcategory: Physiological adaptation
Cognitive level: Analysis

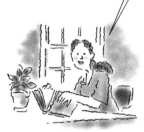

Answer a few *Incredibly Easy* practice questions. Get pumped for the exam!

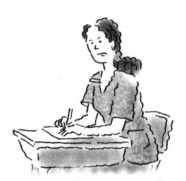

4. An adolescent with scoliosis is fitted for a Milwaukee brace. Which statement made by the client indicates successful teaching?
1. "I'll only have to wear the brace for a few months."
2. "I can take the brace off only for special occasions like the prom."
3. "I can take the brace off for 1 hour per day while I bathe."
4. "The brace will correct the curve if I wear it all the time."

Answer: 3. A Milwaukee brace is used to correct mild scoliosis and needs to be worn approximately 23 hours every day for several months. The brace doesn't correct the curve but prevents the curve from increasing.

➡ *NCLEX keys*
Client needs category: Physiological integrity
Client needs subcategory: Basic care and comfort
Cognitive level: Analysis

5. A child's clubfoot has been placed in a cast. The child develops itching under the cast and asks the nurse for help. The nurse should:
1. use sterile applicators to relieve the itch.
2. apply water under the cast.
3. apply cool air under the cast with a blow-dryer.
4. apply hydrocortisone cream.

Answer: 3. A blow-dryer on the cool setting should be directed toward the itchy area to provide relief. Nothing should be put inside the cast because this can cause further skin irritation. Water would wet the cast and wouldn't be helpful. Hydrocortisone cream can ball up and be irritating, and it would be difficult to apply inside the cast.

➡ *NCLEX keys*
Client needs category: Physiological integrity
Client needs subcategory: Reduction of risk potential
Cognitive level: Application

6. A child has undergone repair of a club-foot and is allowed full activity. The nurse is teaching the child's parents about activities for the child. Which activity would benefit the child most?
1. Walking
2. Playing catch
3. Standing
4. Swimming

Answer: 1. Walking stimulates all of the involved muscles and helps with strengthening. All of the options are good exercises for clubfoot, but walking is the best choice.

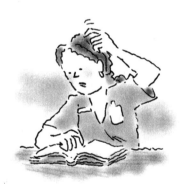

➡ *NCLEX keys*
Client needs category: Physiological integrity
Client needs subcategory: Physiological adaptation
Cognitive level: Application

7. A nurse is doing discharge teaching with a child who has juvenile rheumatoid arthritis (JRA). Which statement indicates that the child and his family understand about exacerbations of JRA?
 1. "I should manage stress carefully and stay in a moderate climate."
 2. "I should avoid dehydration and exposure to cold."
 3. "I should avoid exposure to cold."
 4. "I need to limit my exercise."

Answer: 1. Exacerbations of JRA can be precipitated by exposure to stress and climate. Dehydration and exposure to cold can precipitate vaso-occlusive crisis in the client with sickle cell anemia. Exposure to cold can precipitate an exacerbation of Raynaud's disease. Exercise should be encouraged in the child with JRA.

➤ NCLEX keys
Client needs category: Physiological integrity
Client needs subcategory: Reduction of risk potential
Cognitive level: Application

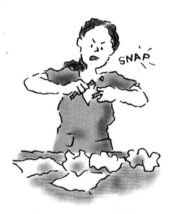

8. A child is admitted with an undiagnosed musculoskeletal condition. Which diagnostic tool is most useful in evaluating a musculoskeletal disorder?
 1. Myelography
 2. Magnetic resonance imaging (MRI)
 3. Computed tomography (CT) scan
 4. X-rays

Answer: 4. X-rays are the most useful diagnostic tool to evaluate musculoskeletal diseases and can be used to help identify joint disruption, bone deformities, calcifications, and bone destruction and fractures as well as to measure bone density. Myelography is an invasive procedure used to evaluate abnormalities of the spinal canal and cord. MRI, a form of cross-sectional imaging using a strong magnetic field and radio waves, has largely replaced arthrography for assessing joint anatomy. A CT scan can be used to identify injuries of soft tissue, ligaments, tendons, and muscles.

➤ NCLEX keys
Client needs category: Physiological integrity
Client needs subcategory: Reduction of risk potential
Cognitive level: Comprehension

9. A nurse is developing a dietary teaching plan for a child with Duchenne's muscular dystrophy. Which elements are most important for the nurse to include in the child's diet?
 1. Lean chicken and brown rice
 2. Chicken breast and refined pasta
 3. Fried chicken and restricted fluids
 4. Chicken breast, brown rice, and supplemental calorie drinks

Answer: 1. A child with muscular dystrophy is prone to constipation and obesity, so dietary intake should include a diet low in calories, high in protein, and high in fiber. Adequate fluid intake should also be encouraged.

➤ NCLEX keys
Client needs category: Physiological integrity
Client needs subcategory: Basic care and comfort
Cognitive level: Analysis

10. A nurse is teaching the mother of a child with scoliosis. The nurse knows that teaching has been successful when the mother makes which statement?

1. "I'm glad my daughter will outgrow this deformity."
2. "I'm afraid that my daughter will feel unattractive because she must wear a brace."
3. "I'll make sure that my daughter doesn't do any stretching exercises that could worsen her spine."
4. "I'm glad my daughter will need to wear a brace for only a short time."

Answer: 2. Teaching is successful when the mother shows concern about her daughter's feelings toward wearing a brace for scoliosis treatment. The brace is uncomfortable and unattractive and may make the child self-conscious about her appearance. The child won't outgrow the deformity. Stretching exercises won't worsen the condition. Brace use is determined on an individual basis, so the duration of treatment will vary.

➡ *NCLEX keys*

Client needs category: Physiological integrity
Client needs subcategory: Reduction of risk potential
Cognitive level: Analysis

Boning up on the pediatric musculoskeletal system before taking the big exam was smart. Now get ready to muscle your way through the next chapter.

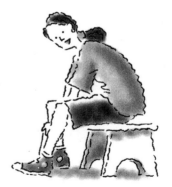

9 Gastrointestinal system

Brush up on key concepts

The GI tract, also known as the **alimentary canal,** consists of a long, hollow, muscular tube that includes several glands and accessory organs. It performs the crucial task of supplying essential nutrients to fuel the other organs and body systems. Because the GI system is so crucial to the rest of the body systems, a problem in this system can quickly affect the overall health, growth, and development of the child.

At any time, you can review the major points of this chapter by consulting the *Cheat sheet* on pages 118 to 120.

GI junior

Characteristics of the pediatric GI system include the following:
- Peristalsis occurs within 2½ to 3 hours of eating in the neonate and extends to 3 to 6 hours in older infants and children.
- Gastric stomach capacity of the neonate is 30 to 60 ml, which gradually increases to 200 to 350 ml by age 12 months and to 1,500 ml as an adolescent.
- The neonatal abdomen is larger than the chest up to ages 4 to 8 weeks, and the musculature is poorly developed.
- The extrusion reflex persists to ages 3 to 4 months (extrusion reflex protects infant from food substances that its system is too immature to digest).
- At age 4 months, saliva production begins and aids in the process of digestion.
- The sucking reflex begins to diminish at age 6 months.
- The neonate has immature muscle tone of the lower esophageal sphincter and low volume capacity of the stomach, which cause the neonate to "spit up" frequently.

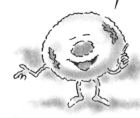

Thanks to the GI tract, I can get a good meal.

- Increased myelination of nerves to the anal sphincter allows for physiologic control of bowel function, usually around age 2.
- The liver's slow development of glycogen storage capacity makes the infant prone to hypoglycemia.
- From ages 1 to 3, composition of intestinal flora becomes more adultlike and stomach acidity increases, reducing the number of GI infections.

Nutrient breakdown

The GI tract breaks down food (carbohydrates, fats, and proteins) into molecules small enough to permeate cell membranes, thus providing cells with the necessary energy to function properly. The GI tract prepares food for cellular absorption by altering its physical and chemical composition. (See *Digestive organs and glands,* page 121.)

Malfunction junction

A malfunction along the GI tract can produce far-reaching metabolic effects, eventually threatening life itself. A common indication of GI problems is referred pain, which makes diagnosis especially difficult.

Keep abreast of diagnostic tests

Here are important tests used to diagnose GI system disorders, along with common nursing interventions associated with each test.

Swallow this

Barium swallow is primarily used to examine the esophagus.

Gastrografin is now used instead of barium for certain patients. Like barium, Gastrografin facilitates imaging through X-rays.

(Text continues on page 120.)

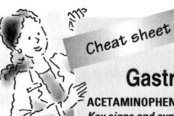

Cheat sheet

Gastrointestinal refresher

ACETAMINOPHEN TOXICITY
Key signs and symptoms
- Diaphoresis
- Nausea and vomiting

Key test results
- Serum aspartate aminotransferase and serum alanine aminotransferase levels become elevated soon after ingestion.

Key treatments
- Gastric lavage or emesis induction with ipecac syrup

Key interventions
- Monitor vital signs and intake and output.
- Assess cardiovascular and GI status.

CELIAC DISEASE
Key signs and symptoms
- Generalized malnutrition and failure to thrive due to malabsorption of protein and carbohydrates
- Steatorrhea and chronic diarrhea due to fat malabsorption
- Weight and height below normal for age-group

Key test results
- Immunoglobulin (Ig) A and IgG anti-tissue transglutaminase antibody test is positive.

Key treatments
- Diet: gluten-free but includes corn and rice products, soy and potato flour, breast milk or soy-based formula, and all fresh fruits

Key interventions
- Monitor growth and development.
- Provide small, frequent, gluten-free meals.

CLEFT LIP AND PALATE
Key signs and symptoms
- Cleft lip: can range from a simple notch on the upper lip to a complete cleft from the lip edge to the floor of the nostril, on either side of the midline but rarely along the midline itself
- Cleft palate without cleft lip: may not be detected until mouth examination or development of feeding difficulties

Key test results
- Prenatal ultrasound may indicate severe defects.

Key treatments
- Cheiloplasty performed between birth and age 3 months to unite the lip and gum edges in anticipation of teeth eruption, providing a route for adequate nutrition and sucking
- Cleft palate repair surgery (staphylorrhaphy); scheduled at about age 18 months to allow for growth of the palate and to be done before the infant develops speech patterns (the infant must be free from ear and respiratory infections)

Key interventions
- Be alert for respiratory distress when feeding.
Before cleft lip repair surgery
- Hold the infant while feeding, and promote sucking between meals.
After cleft lip repair surgery
- Observe for cyanosis as the infant begins to breathe through the nose.
- Keep the infant's hands away from the mouth by using restraints or pinning the sleeves to the shirt; adhesive strips are used to hold the suture line in place.
- Anticipate the infant's needs.
- Place the infant on the right side to prevent aspiration; clean the suture line after each feeding by dabbing it with half-strength hydrogen peroxide or saline solution.
After cleft palate repair surgery
- Position the toddler on the abdomen or side.
- Anticipate edema and a decreased airway from palate closure; this may make the toddler appear temporarily dyspneic; assess for signs of decreased oxygenation.
- Keep hard or pointed objects (utensils, straws, frozen dessert sticks) away from the mouth.

ESOPHAGEAL ATRESIA AND TRACHEO-ESOPHAGEAL FISTULA
Key signs and symptoms
- Sonorous seal bark cough in the delivery room
- Excessive oral secretions and drooling
- Choking when feeding

Gastrointestinal refresher (continued)

ESOPHAGEAL ATRESIA AND TRACHEOESOPHAGEAL FISTULA (CONTINUED)

Key test results
• X-ray confirms esophageal atresia and transesophageal fistula.

Key treatments
• Esophageal atresia repair or tracheoesophageal fistula repair (may be performed immediately or after 2 to 4 months)

Key interventions
• Assess respiratory status.
• Administer I.V. fluids and antibiotics before surgery.
• Keep the neonate warm in an incubator or overhead warmer.
• Maintain continuous suction.

FAILURE TO THRIVE

Key signs and symptoms
• History of feeding problems
• Wasting
• Height, weight, and head circumference less than expected for age

Key test results
• Negative nitrogen balance indicates inadequate intake of protein or calories.

Key treatments
• High-calorie diet
• Parent and child counseling
• Vitamin and mineral supplements

Key interventions
• Properly feed and interact with the child.
• Provide the child with visual and auditory stimulation.
• Provide information on parenting skills.

GASTROENTERITIS

Key signs and symptoms
• Abdominal discomfort
• Diarrhea
• Nausea and vomiting

Key test results
• Stool culture identifies causative bacteria, parasite, or amoebae.

Key treatments
• Increased fluid intake
• I.V. fluid and electrolyte replacement
• Antiemetic: prochlorperazine

Key interventions
• Early intervention with fluid and electrolyte replacement is key.
• Stress hand washing to the child and his family.
• Administer I.V. fluids and medications.

GASTROESOPHAGEAL REFLUX DISEASE

Key signs and symptoms
• Choking or gagging with feeding
• Frequent crying and fussiness
• Frequent or persistent cough
• Frequent or recurrent vomiting

Key test results
• Gastric emptying study shows prolonged emptying time.
• Barium swallow fluoroscopy indicates reflux.
• Esophageal pH probe reveals a low pH, which indicates reflux.

Key treatments
• Positional therapy to help relieve symptoms by decreasing intra-abdominal pressure
• Histamine-2 (H_2) receptor antagonists: ranitidine (Zantac), famotidine (Pepcid)
• Proton-pump inhibitor: esomeprazole (Nexium)

Key interventions
• Encourage the child to eat several small meals during the day to help decrease the pressure on the lower esophageal sphincter.
• Have the parent hold the infant for at least 30 minutes after feeding to reduce intra-abdominal pressure.

INTESTINAL OBSTRUCTION

Key signs and symptoms
• Complete small-bowel obstruction: bowel contents propelled toward mouth (instead of rectum) by vigorous peristaltic waves, along with persistent epigastric or periumbilical pain
• Partial large-bowel obstruction: leakage of liquid stool around the obstruction (common)

Key test results
• With large-bowel obstruction, barium enema reveals a distended, air-filled colon or, in sigmoid volvulus, a closed loop of sigmoid with extreme distention.
• X-rays confirm the diagnosis. Abdominal films show the presence and location of intestinal gas or fluid.

Key treatments
• I.V. therapy to correct fluid and electrolyte imbalances

Key interventions
• Monitor vital signs frequently.
• Assess cardiovascular status; observe the child closely for signs of shock (pallor, rapid pulse, and hypotension).
• Monitor for signs and symptoms of metabolic alkalosis (changes in sensorium; slow, shallow respirations; hypertonic muscles; tetany) or acidosis (dyspnea on exertion, disorientation and, later, deep, rapid breathing, weakness, and malaise).
• Observe for signs and symptoms of secondary infection, such as fever and chills.

(continued)

Gastrointestinal refresher (continued)

LEAD TOXICITY
Key signs and symptoms
- Anorexia, vomiting
- Weight loss

Key test results
- X-rays reveal lead lines near the epiphyseal lines (areas of increased density) of long bones. The thickness of the line shows the length of time the lead ingestion has been occurring.

Key treatments
- Chelating agents: succimer (Chemet) or dimercaprol (BAL In Oil) for a blood lead level greater than 45 mcg/dl.

Key interventions
- Monitor vital signs, intake and output, hydration status, and kidney function.
- Monitor calcium levels (chelating agents also bind with calcium).

PYLORIC STENOSIS
Key signs and symptoms
- Projectile emesis during or soon after feedings, preceded by reverse peristaltic waves (going left to right) but not by nausea (child resumes eating after vomiting)

Key test results
- Ultrasound shows pyloric muscle thickness greater than 4 mm.

Key treatments
- Surgical intervention: pyloromyotomy performed by laparoscopy

Key interventions
- Provide small, frequent, thickened feedings with the head of the bed elevated; burp the child frequently.
- Position the child on his right side.

SALICYLATE TOXICITY
Key signs and symptoms
- High fever
- Petechiae and bleeding tendency

Key test results
- Serum salicylate levels are elevated beyond therapeutic range.

Key treatments
- Gastric lavage
- I.V. fluids
- Alkalinizing agent: sodium bicarbonate

Key interventions
- Administer I.V. fluids.
- Monitor urine pH.
- Assess cardiovascular and GI status.

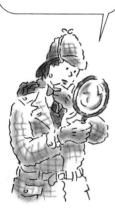

It's alimentary. Barium—or Gastrografin—is swallowed to help visualize the GI tract.

Unlike barium, however, if Gastrografin escapes from the GI tract, it's absorbed by the surrounding tissue. Escaped barium isn't absorbed and can cause complications.

Nursing actions
- Explain the procedure to the child and parents.
- Maintain nothing-by-mouth (NPO) status for 6 to 8 hours before the test.
- Tell the child he must hold still during the X-ray.
- After the test, monitor bowel movements for excretion of barium. Also monitor GI function.

Upper GI imaging
In an **upper GI series,** swallowed barium sulfate proceeds into the esophagus, stomach, and duodenum to reveal abnormalities. The barium outlines stomach walls and delineates ulcer craters and filling defects.

A **small-bowel series,** an extension of the upper GI series, visualizes barium flowing through the small intestine to the ileocecal valve.

Nursing actions
- Explain the procedure to the child and parents.
- Tell the child that he must hold still during the X-ray.
- Make sure the lead apron is properly placed around the genital area.
- After the test, monitor bowel movements for excretion of barium. Also monitor GI function.

Lower GI look
A **barium enema (lower GI series)** allows X-ray visualization of the colon.

Nursing actions
- Explain the procedure to the child and parents.

Digestive organs and glands

Here is a quick rundown of the major organs and glands that facilitate digestion.

SALIVARY GLANDS

The salivary glands provide saliva to moisten the mouth, lubricate food to ease swallowing, and begin food breakdown using the enzyme ptyalin. After food is swallowed, it enters the esophagus and is transported to the stomach.

STOMACH

The stomach is a muscular, saclike organ located between the esophagus and small intestine. Food and fluids enter the stomach and are mixed with stomach secretions. Contractions called *peristalsis* push the food gradually into the small intestine through the pyloric opening at the lower end of the stomach.

INTESTINE

The intestine extends from the pyloric opening to the anus. It's made up of the small and large intestines.
• The small intestine is made up of the duodenum, jejunum, and ileum and is about 20′ (6 m) long. Most digestion takes place in the small intestine; digested food is absorbed through the walls of the small intestine and into the blood for distribution throughout the body.
• The large intestine is about 5′ (1.5 m) long and includes the cecum (and appendix), colon, and rectum. Indigestible food passes into the large intestine, where it's formed into solid feces and eliminated through the rectum.

LIVER

The liver stores and filters blood; secretes bile; processes sugars, fats, proteins, and vitamins; and detoxifies drugs, alcohol, and other substances.

GALLBLADDER

The gallbladder is located beneath the liver and serves as a storage place for bile. Bile is a clear, yellowish fluid that enters the small intestine through bile ducts and aids digestion of fats.

PANCREAS

The pancreas is a large gland located behind the stomach. It secretes digestive enzymes that neutralize stomach acids and break down proteins, carbohydrates, and fats.

• Usually, the child will follow a liquid diet for 24 hours before the test. Bowel preparations are administered before the examination.
• Tell the child that X-rays will be taken on a test table and that he must hold still.
• Cover the genital area with a lead apron during X-ray.

Stool search

A **stool specimen** can be examined for suspected GI bleeding, infection, or malabsorption. Certain tests require several specimens, such as the **guaiac test** for occult blood, a microscopic stool examination for ova and parasites, and tests for fat.

Nursing actions

• Explain the procedure to the child and parents.
• Obtain the specimen in the correct container (the container may need to be sterile or contain preservative).
• Be aware that the specimen may need to be transported to the laboratory immediately or placed in the refrigerator.

Fiber-optic findings

In **esophagogastroduodenoscopy,** insertion of a fiber-optic scope allows direct visual inspection of the esophagus, stomach and, sometimes, duodenum. **Proctosigmoidoscopy** permits inspection of the rectum and

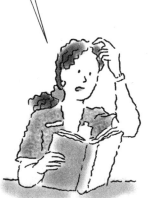

Esophago-gastro-duo-deno-scopy ... No problem!

distal sigmoid colon. **Colonoscopy** allows inspection of the descending, transverse, and ascending colon.

Nursing actions

- Explain the procedure to the child and parents.
- Make sure that written, informed consent has been obtained.
- A mild sedative may be administered before the examination.
- The child may be on NPO status before the procedure (upper GI series).
- The child may be placed on a liquid diet for 24 hours before the examination or require enemas or laxatives until clear (lower GI examinations).

Fluoroscopic findings

Endoscopic retrograde cholangiopancreatography is the radiographic examination of the pancreatic ducts and hepatobiliary tree following the injection of contrast media into the duodenal papilla. It's performed on children with suspected pancreatic disease or obstructive jaundice.

Nursing actions

Before the procedure
- Explain the procedure to the child and parents.
- Make sure that written, informed consent has been obtained.
- Check the child's history for allergies to cholinergics and iodine.
- Administer a sedative, and monitor the child for the drug's effect.

After the procedure
- Monitor the child's gag reflex (the child is kept on NPO status until his gag reflex returns).
- Protect the child from aspiration of mucus by positioning the child on his side.
- Monitor the child for urine retention.

Tube topics

Certain GI disorders require insertion of a **gastric tube** for the following purposes:
- to empty the stomach and intestine
- to aid diagnosis and treatment
- to decompress obstructed areas
- to detect and treat GI bleeding
- to administer medications or feedings.

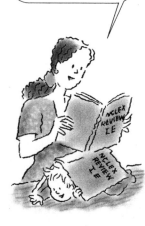

Children who are intubated require diligent oral and nasal care, close monitoring, and emotional support to minimize fear.

Tubes usually inserted through the nose include short nasogastric (NG) tubes (Levin and Salem Sump) and long intestinal tubes (Cantor and Miller-Abbott). The larger Ewald tube is usually inserted orally and is used to empty the stomach.

Nursing actions

- Explain the procedure to the child and parents.
- Maintain accurate intake and output records. Measure gastric drainage every 8 hours; record amount, color, odor, and consistency. When irrigating the tube, note the amount of saline solution instilled and aspirated.
- Monitor for fluid and electrolyte imbalances.
- Provide oral and nasal care. Make sure the tube is secure but isn't causing pressure on the nostrils.
- Anchor the tube to the child's clothing to prevent dislodgment.
- Provide emotional support because many children panic at the sight of a tube. Maintaining a calm, reassuring manner can help minimize the child's fear.

Polish up on client care

Pediatric GI disorders discussed in this chapter include acetaminophen toxicity, celiac disease, cleft lip and palate, esophageal atresia and tracheoesophageal fistula, failure to thrive, gastroenteritis, gastroesophageal reflux disease (GERD), intestinal obstruction, lead toxicity, pyloric stenosis, and salicylate toxicity.

Acetaminophen toxicity

Acetaminophen is an analgesic antipyretic agent that achieves its effect without inhibiting platelet aggregation. Because acetaminophen is an over-the-counter medication commonly found in the home, it's a common cause of poisoning in children.

With acetaminophen toxicity, hepatotoxicity occurs at plasma levels greater than 200 mg/ml at 4 hours after ingestion and greater than 50 mg/ml by 12 hours after ingestion.

CAUSES
• Acetaminophen ingestion beyond the recommended dosage

ASSESSMENT FINDINGS
• Anorexia
• Diaphoresis
• Hypothermia
• Severe hypoglycemia
• Shock
• Oliguria
• Nausea and vomiting
• Pallor
• Right upper quadrant tenderness usually occurring 24 to 48 hours after ingestion; jaundice evident 72 to 96 hours after ingestion
• Hepatic failure, death, or resolution of symptoms occurring 7 to 8 days after ingestion

DIAGNOSTIC TEST RESULTS
• Blood glucose levels are decreased.
• Serum aspartate aminotransferase and serum alanine aminotransferase levels become elevated soon after ingestion.
• Prothrombin time is prolonged.

NURSING DIAGNOSES
• Imbalanced nutrition: Less than body requirements
• Risk for imbalanced fluid volume
• Hypothermia
• Risk for impaired liver function

TREATMENT
• Gastric lavage or emesis induction with ipecac syrup
• Hyperthermia blanket
• I.V. fluid
• Oxygen therapy (intubation and mechanical ventilation may be required)

Drug therapy
• Emetic: ipecac syrup to induce vomiting
• Antidote: acetylcysteine

INTERVENTIONS AND RATIONALES
• Monitor liver function studies *to detect signs of liver damage and to monitor effectiveness of treatment.*
• Monitor vital signs and intake and output. *Tachycardia and decreased urine output may signify dehydration.*

• Assess cardiovascular and GI status *to monitor the effectiveness of treatment.*
• Administer hyperthermia therapy by using a warming blanket, limiting exposure during routine nursing care, and covering the child with warm blankets *to help the child become normothermic.*
• Administer acetylcysteine as ordered *to reduce acetaminophen levels.*

Teaching topics
• Explanation of the disorder and treatment plan
• Storing medication safely and other steps to prevent overdose
• Reading labels carefully (cough and cold preparations may also contain acetominophen)

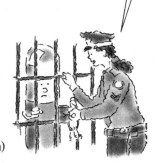

Put it away. Locked medicine storage helps prevent acetaminophen toxicity.

Celiac disease

Celiac disease is an intolerance to gliadin — a gluten protein found in grains, such as wheat, rye, oats, and barley, that causes poor food absorption.

In celiac disease, a decrease in the amount and activity of enzymes in the intestinal mucosal cells causes the villi of the proximal small intestine to atrophy, decreasing intestinal absorption. Celiac disease usually becomes apparent between ages 6 and 18 months.

CAUSES
• Genetic disease that may be triggered by surgery, pregnancy, childbirth, viral infection, or severe emotional stress

ASSESSMENT FINDINGS
• Abdominal distention
• Anorexia
• Generalized malnutrition and failure to thrive due to malabsorption of protein and carbohydrates
• Fatigue
• Bone or joint pain
• Aphthous ulcers
• Itchy rash (dermatitis herpetiform)
• Irritability
• Steatorrhea and chronic diarrhea due to fat malabsorption

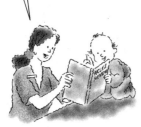

If a child demonstrates malnutrition, steatorrhea, and chronic diarrhea 2 to 4 months after solid foods are introduced, suspect celiac disease.

• Weight and height below normal for age-group

DIAGNOSTIC TEST RESULTS
• Blood chemistry tests reveal hypocalcemia and hypoalbuminemia.
• Hematology reveals decreased hemoglobin level and hypothrombinemia.
• Immunoglobulin (Ig) A and IgG anti-tissue transglutaminase antibody test is positive (not reliable in children younger than age 2).
• IgA and IgG anti-gliadin antibodies are present.
• Intestinal biopsy confirms the diagnosis.
• Stool specimen reveals high fat content.

NURSING DIAGNOSES
• Imbalanced nutrition: Less than body requirements
• Delayed growth and development
• Deficient fluid volume
• Diarrhea

TREATMENT
• Diet: gluten-free but includes corn and rice products, soy and potato flour, breast milk or soy-based formula, and all fresh fruits
• Folate
• Iron (Feosol) supplements
• Vitamins A and D in water-soluble forms

INTERVENTIONS AND RATIONALES
• Provide small, frequent, gluten-free meals *to reduce fatigue and improve nutritional intake.*
• Record the consistency, appearance, and number of stools. *The disappearance of steatorrhea is a good indicator that the child's ability to absorb nutrients is improving.*
• Monitor growth and development *to assess for growth delay and to detect changes in level of functioning* and, as appropriate, plan an activity program for the child.

Teaching topics
• Explanation of the disorder and treatment plan
• Specific foods and formula the child can eat (breads made from rice, corn, soybean, potato, tapioca, sago or gluten-free wheat; dry cereals made with only rice or corn; cornmeal or hominy)

Cleft lip and palate

In cleft lip and palate, the bone and tissue of the upper jaw and palate fail to fuse completely at the midline. The defects may be partial or complete, unilateral or bilateral, and may involve the lip, the palate, or both.

Cleft lip and palate also increase the risk of:
• aspiration because increased open space in the mouth may cause formula or breast milk to enter the respiratory tract
• upper respiratory infection and otitis media, because the increased open space decreases natural defenses against bacterial invasion.

CAUSES
• Congenital defects (in some cases, inheritance plays a role)
• Part of another chromosomal or mendelian abnormality
• Prenatal exposure to teratogens

ASSESSMENT FINDINGS
• Abdominal distention from swallowed air
• Cleft lip: can range from a simple notch on the upper lip to a complete cleft from the lip edge to the floor of the nostril, on either side of the midline but rarely along the midline itself
• Cleft palate: may be partial or complete
• Difficulty swallowing

Note that cleft lip with or without cleft palate is obvious at birth; cleft palate without cleft lip may not be detected until a mouth examination is done or until feeding difficulties develop.

DIAGNOSTIC TEST RESULTS
• Prenatal ultrasonography may indicate severe defects.

NURSING DIAGNOSES
• Imbalanced nutrition: Less than body requirements
• Impaired swallowing
• Risk for aspiration
• Ineffective airway clearance
• Risk for impaired parenting

TREATMENT
- Cheiloplasty performed between birth and age 3 months to unite the lip and gum edges in anticipation of teeth eruption, providing a route for adequate nutrition and sucking
- Cleft palate repair surgery (staphylorrhaphy); scheduled at about age 18 months to allow for growth of the palate and to be done before the infant develops speech patterns (the infant must be free from ear and respiratory infections)
- Long-term, team-oriented care to address speech defects, dental and orthodontic problems, nasal defects, and possible alterations in hearing
- If cleft lip is detected on sonogram while the infant is in utero, possible fetal repair

INTERVENTIONS AND RATIONALES
- Monitor vital signs and intake and output *to determine fluid volume status.*
- Assess respiratory status *to detect signs of aspiration.*
- Assess the quality of the child's suck by determining whether the infant can form an airtight seal around a finger or nipple placed in the infant's mouth *to determine an effective feeding method.*
- Be alert for respiratory distress when feeding *to avoid aspiration.*
- Provide emotional support to the child and parents *to decrease anxiety.*

Preoperative interventions for cleft lip repair
- Feed the infant slowly and in an upright position *to decrease the risk of aspiration.*
- Burp the infant frequently during feeding *to eliminate swallowed air and decrease the risk of emesis.*
- Use gavage feedings *if oral feedings are unsuccessful.*
- Administer a small amount of water after feedings *to prevent formula from accumulating in the cleft and becoming a medium for bacterial growth.*
- Give small, frequent feedings *to promote adequate nutrition and prevent tiring the infant.*
- Hold the infant while feeding and promote sucking between meals. *Sucking is important to speech development.*

Postoperative interventions for cleft lip repair
- Observe for cyanosis as the infant begins to breathe through the nose *to detect signs of respiratory compromise.*
- Keep the infant's hands away from the mouth by using restraints or pinning the sleeves to the shirt; adhesive strips are used to hold the suture line in place *to prevent tension and to maintain an intact suture line.*
- Anticipate the infant's needs *to prevent crying.*
- Use a syringe with tubing to administer foods at the side of the mouth *to prevent trauma to the suture line.*
- Place the infant on the right side *to prevent aspiration;* clean the suture line after each feeding by dabbing it with half-strength hydrogen peroxide or saline solution *to prevent crusts and scarring.*
- Monitor for pain and administer pain medication as prescribed; note the effectiveness of pain medication *to promote comfort.*

Preoperative interventions for cleft palate repair
- Feed the infant with a cleft palate nipple or a Teflon implant *to enhance nutritional intake.*
- Wean the infant from the bottle or breast before cleft palate surgery; *the toddler must be able to drink from a cup.*

Postoperative interventions for cleft palate repair
- Position the toddler on the abdomen or side *to promote a patent airway.*
- Anticipate edema and a decreased airway from palate closure; this may make the toddler appear temporarily dyspneic; assess for signs of decreased oxygenation *to identify airway complications.*
- Keep hard or pointed objects (utensils, straws, frozen dessert sticks) away from the mouth *to prevent trauma to the suture line.*
- Use a cup to feed; don't use a nipple or pacifier *to prevent injury to the suture line.*
- Use elbow restraints *to keep the toddler's hands out of the mouth.*
- Provide soft toys *to prevent injury.*
- Start the toddler on clear liquids and progress to a soft diet; rinse the suture line by giving the toddler a sip of water after each feeding *to prevent infection.*

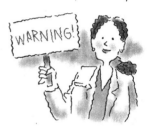

Cleft lip and palate increase the risk of aspiration during feeding as well as the risk of respiratory infection and otitis media.

WARNING!

• Distract or hold the toddler *to try to keep the tongue away from the roof of the mouth.*

Teaching topics

• Explanation of the disorder and treatment options
• Importance of parental involvement (because it results in facial disfigurement, the condition may cause shock, guilt, and grief for the parents and may block parental bonding with the child)
• Need for follow-up speech therapy
• Understanding the child's susceptibility to pathogens and otitis media from the altered position of the eustachian tubes

Esophageal atresia and tracheoesophageal fistula

Esophageal atresia occurs when the proximal end of the esophagus ends in a blind pouch; food can't enter the stomach through the esophagus.

Tracheoesophageal fistula occurs when a connection exists between the esophagus and the trachea. It may result in the reflux of gastric juice after feeding; this can allow acidic stomach contents to cross the fistula, irritating the trachea.

Esophageal atresia and tracheoesophageal fistula occur in many combinations and may be associated with other defects. Esophageal atresia with tracheoesophageal fistula is the most common of these conditions. Esophageal atresia alone is the second most common of these conditions.

Esophageal atresia with tracheoesophageal fistula occurs when either:
• the distal end of the esophagus ends in a blind pouch and the proximal end of the esophagus is linked to the trachea via a fistula
• the proximal end of the esophagus ends in a blind pouch and the distal portion of the esophagus is connected to the trachea via a fistula.

Other birth defects may coexist and should be assessed at birth.

CAUSES
• Unknown

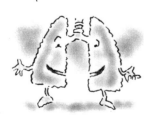

Remember me? Preventing respiratory complications is key to postoperative care in esophageal atresia and tracheoesophageal fistula repair.

ASSESSMENT FINDINGS
• Sonorous seal bark cough in the delivery room
• Excessive oral secretions and drooling
• Choking when feeding
• Regurgitation of undigested formula immediately after feeding; possible respiratory distress and cyanosis if secretions are aspirated
• Abdominal distention (with tracheoesophageal fistula)

DIAGNOSTIC TEST RESULTS
• NG tube doesn't pass because of obstruction 4" to 5" (10 to 12.5 cm) from the neonate's nostrils.
• X-ray confirms esophageal atresia and transesophageal fistula.

NURSING DIAGNOSES
• Imbalanced nutrition: Less than body requirements
• Risk for infection
• Risk for impaired parenting
• Ineffective breathing pattern

TREATMENT
• Gastrostomy tube (PEG tube) insertion and feedings
• Esophageal atresia repair or tracheoesophageal fistula repair (may be performed immediately or after 2 to 4 months)

INTERVENTIONS AND RATIONALES
• Monitor vital signs to detect tachycardia and tachypnea, *which could indicate hypoxemia.*
• Assess respiratory status. *Poor respiratory status may result in hypoxemia.*
• Administer I.V. fluids and antibiotics before surgery *to promote stability.*
• Position the infant with his head elevated to 30 degrees *to decrease reflux at the distal esophagus.*
• Keep the neonate warm in an incubator or overhead warmer *to maintain temperature.*
• Maintain continuous suction *to remove secretions.*
• Suction as needed *to stimulate cough and clear airways.*

After gastrostomy

• Keep the PEG tube open and suspended above the child *for release of gas.*

• If feeding the child through a gastrostomy tube after surgery, anticipate abdominal distention from air; keep the child upright during and after feedings *to reduce the chance of refluxed stomach contents and aspiration pneumonia,* and keep the tube open and elevated before and after feedings.

• Administer gastrostomy feedings only by gravity flow — not a feeding pump — *to help meet nutritional and metabolic requirements.*

Postoperative care

• Maintain chest tube and respiratory support *to prevent respiratory compromise.*

• Suction as needed *to remove secretions and prevent aspiration.*

• Make sure the NG tube is secure and handle with extreme caution *to avoid displacement.*

• Administer antibiotics as prescribed *to prevent infection.*

• Administer total parenteral nutrition or feedings *to maintain nutritional support.*

Teaching topics

• Explanation of the disorder and treatment plan

• Understanding proper care of the child at home, such as feeding and bathing techniques

Failure to thrive

Failure to thrive is a chronic, potentially life-threatening condition characterized by failure to maintain weight and height above the 5th percentile on age-appropriate growth charts. Most children are diagnosed before age 2. It can result from physical, emotional, or psychological causes.

CONTRIBUTING FACTORS

• May be a combination of organic and non-organic factors

Organic

• Prenatal: chromosomal abnormalities; maternal exposure to toxins, such as tobacco, alcohol, or drugs; maternal illness, such as hypertension, preeclampsia, or diabetes mellitus

• Postnatal: inadequate intake due to conditions associated with inability to suck or swallow, lack of appetite resulting from infection, or vomiting associated with GI obstruction; poor absorption of nutrients due to endocrine disorders, GI disorders (such as celiac disease), or renal failure; increased metabolic demand caused by chronic disease (such as inflammatory bowel disease) or malignancy

Nonorganic

• Poor parenting, failure to bond
• Poor feeding skills
• Family dysfunction
• Child neglect
• Difficult child
• Eating disorder

ASSESSMENT FINDINGS

• History of feeding problems
• History of a medical problem or an illness
• History of dysfunctional family or inadequate parenting
• Listlessness
• Noninteractive behavior
• Wasting
• Height, weight, and head circumference less than expected for age
• Rash or skin changes
• Hepatomegaly

DIAGNOSTIC TEST RESULTS

• Negative nitrogen balance indicates inadequate intake of protein or calories.
• Associated physiologic causes may be detected.
• Reduced creatinine-height index reflects muscle mass and estimates muscle protein depletion.

NURSING DIAGNOSES

• Delayed growth and development
• Impaired parenting
• Imbalanced nutrition: Less than body requirements

TREATMENT

• Treatment of underlying medical cause
• High-calorie diet
• Parent and child counseling

Drug therapy

• Vitamin and mineral supplements

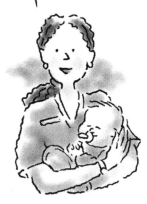

Adequate stimulation helps to prevent failure to thrive.

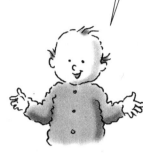

I dig visual and auditory stimulation.

INTERVENTIONS AND RATIONALES
- Weigh the child on admission *to determine baseline weight.*
- Assess growth and development using an appropriate tool, such as the Denver Developmental Screening test, *to determine the child's developmental level.*
- Properly feed and interact with the child *to promote nutrition and growth and development.*
- Establish specific times for feeding, bathing, and sleeping *to establish and maintain a structured routine.*
- Provide the child with visual and auditory stimulation *to promote normal sensory development.*
- Assess interaction of the parent with the child *to determine parent-child relationship and parenting skills.*
- Provide information on parenting skills *to assist parents with proper child care.*

Teaching topics
- Explanation of the disorder and treatment plan
- Understanding healthy parenting skills
- Normal growth and development
- Stimulation techniques
- Obtaining counseling for the parents and child, if necessary
- Understanding dietary needs

Gastroenteritis

A self-limiting disorder, gastroenteritis is characterized by diarrhea, nausea, vomiting, and acute or chronic abdominal cramping. It occurs in children of all ages, and ranks as the fifth leading cause of death in young children. Gastroenteritis can quickly become a major illness in children, especially infants and young children, because of the risk of dehydration.

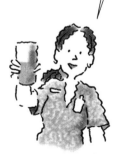

Drink that water! Increased fluid intake is crucial to combat gastroenteritis.

CAUSES
- Bacteria (responsible for acute food poisoning): *Staphylococcus aureus,* Salmonella, Shigella, *Clostridium botulinum, Eshericheria coli, Clostridium perfringens*
- Viruses: adenovirus, echovirus, coxsackievirus, rotavirus
- Food allergens
- Amoebae, especially *Entamoeba histolytica*
- Drug reactions
- Ingestion of toxins

ASSESSMENT FINDINGS
- Diarrhea
- Nausea and vomiting
- Abdominal discomfort

DIAGNOSTIC TEST RESULTS
- Stool culture identifies causative bacteria, parasite, or amoebae.
- Blood culture identifies causative organism.

NURSING DIAGNOSES
- Diarrhea
- Risk for impaired fluid volume
- Acute pain

TREATMENT
- Increased fluid intake
- I.V. fluid and electrolyte replacement
- Nutritional support

Drug therapy
- Antibiotic therapy according to the sensitivity of the causative organism
- Antidiarrheals: diphenoxylate with atropine, loperamide
- Antiemetic: prochlorperazine

INTERVENTIONS AND RATIONALES
- Early intervention with fluid and electrolyte replacement is key because of the risk of dehydration in young children.
- Administer I.V. fluids and medications.
- Encourage clear liquids and electrolyte replacement *to prevent dehydration.*
- Instruct the parents to avoid giving the child milk or milk products, *which may exacerbate the condition.*
- Monitor intake and output. Watch for signs of dehydration, such as sunken fontanels, lack of tears, and lethargy.
- Stress hand washing to the child and his family.

Teaching topics
- Explanation of the disorder and treatment plan

- Increased fluid intake
- Importance of good hand hygiene
- Recognizing signs of dehydration and seeking prompt treatment

Gastroesophageal reflux disease

GERD is the backflow of gastric or duodenal contents, or both, into the esophagus and past the lower esophageal sphincter (LES) without associated belching or vomiting. Until recently, GERD has been underdiagnosed in children. However, many infants diagnosed with GERD outgrow the disorder by age 1.

CAUSES
- Pressure within the stomach that exceeds LES pressure

ASSESSMENT FINDINGS
- Frequent or recurrent vomiting
- Regurgitation and re-swallowing
- Frequent crying and fussiness
- Choking or gagging with feeding
- Frequent or persistent cough

DIAGNOSTIC TEST RESULTS
- Barium swallow fluoroscopy indicates reflux.
- Esophageal pH probe reveals a low pH, which indicates reflux.
- Esophagoscopy shows reflux.
- Gastric emptying study shows prolonged emptying time.

NURSING DIAGNOSES
- Risk for aspiration
- Imbalanced nutrition: Less than body requirements

TREATMENT
- Positional therapy to help relieve symptoms by decreasing intra-abdominal pressure
- Low-fat, high-fiber diet
- Oxygen therapy

Drug therapy
- Histamine-2 receptor antagonists: ranitidine (Zantac), famotidine (Pepcid)

- Proton-pump inhibitor: esomeprazole (Nexium)
- Anti-gas agent: Mylicon

INTERVENTIONS AND RATIONALES
- Have the parent hold the infant for at least 30 minutes after feeding *to reduce intra-abdominal pressure.*
- Offer reassurance and emotional support to the parents *to help them cope with their child's illness.*
- Encourage the child to eat several small meals during the day *to help decrease the pressure on the LES.*

Teaching topics
- Explanation of the disorder and treatment plan
- Medication use and possible adverse effects
- Positional therapy
- Dietary modifications

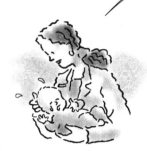

A cranky baby could be a sign of GERD. Check for crying, fussiness, gagging, coughing, and vomiting.

Intestinal obstruction

Intestinal obstruction is the partial or complete blockage of the lumen in the small or large bowel. Small-bowel obstruction is far more common and usually more serious. Complete obstruction in any part of the bowel, if untreated, can cause death within hours from shock and vascular collapse.

Intestinal obstruction can occur in three forms:

simple: blockage prevents intestinal contents from passing, with no other complications

strangulated: blood supply to part or all of the obstructed section is cut off, in addition to blockage of the lumen

close-looped: both ends of a bowel section are occluded, isolating it from the rest of the intestine.

CAUSES
Mechanical
- Adhesions and strangulated hernias (most common causes of small-bowel obstruction)

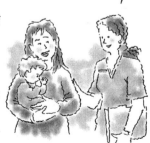

Support parents of a child with GERD. Instruct them to hold their baby for at least 30 minutes after meals to reduce intra-abdominal pressure.

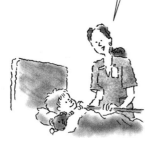

When the obstruction is high in the intestine, vomiting is marked and abdominal distention is limited. When the obstruction is low, the child has marked distention but little vomiting.

- Carcinomas (most common cause of large-bowel obstruction)
- Compression of the bowel wall due to stenosis, intussusception, volvulus of the sigmoid or cecum, tumors, or atresia
- Congenital bowel deformities
- Ingestion of foreign bodies (such as fruit pits or worms)
- Obstruction after abdominal surgery

Other
- Paralytic ileus
- Electrolyte imbalances
- Toxicity (uremia, generalized infection)
- Neurogenic abnormalities (spinal cord lesions)
- Thrombosis or embolism of mesenteric vessels

ASSESSMENT FINDINGS
Partial small-bowel obstruction
- Abdominal distention
- Colicky pain
- Constipation
- Drowsiness
- Dry oral mucous membranes and tongue
- Intense thirst
- Malaise
- Nausea
- Vomiting (the higher the obstruction, the earlier and more severe the vomiting)

Complete small-bowel obstruction
- Persistent epigastric or periumbilical pain
- Bowel contents propelled toward mouth (instead of rectum) by vigorous peristaltic waves

Partial large-bowel obstruction
- Dramatic abdominal distention
- Colicky abdominal pain; may appear suddenly, producing spasms that last less than 1 minute and recur every few minutes
- Constipation (may be only clinical effect for days)
- Continuous hypogastric pain and nausea; vomiting usually absent at first
- Leakage of liquid stools around the obstruction (common)
- Loops of large bowel becoming visible on the abdomen

Complete large-bowel obstruction
- Continuous abdominal pain
- Vomiting of fecal matter
- Localized peritonitis

DIAGNOSTIC TEST RESULTS
- X-rays confirm the diagnosis. Abdominal films show the presence and location of intestinal gas or fluid.
- With large-bowel obstruction, barium enema reveals a distended, air-filled colon or, in sigmoid volvulus, a closed loop of sigmoid with extreme distention.
- Arterial blood gas (ABG) analysis reveals metabolic alkalosis from dehydration and loss of gastric hydrochloric acid, characteristic of obstruction in the upper intestine.
- ABG analysis reveals metabolic acidosis caused by slower dehydration and loss of intestinal alkaline fluids, characteristic of lower-bowel obstruction.

NURSING DIAGNOSES
- Imbalanced nutrition: Less than body requirements
- Acute pain
- Risk for ineffective gastrointestinal perfusion
- Disturbed body image

TREATMENT
- I.V. therapy to correct fluid and electrolyte imbalances
- NG tube to decompress the bowel to relieve vomiting and distention
- Surgical resection with anastomosis, colostomy, or ileostomy
- Total parenteral nutrition for protein deficit from chronic obstruction, paralytic ileus, infection, or prolonged postoperative recovery time that requires NPO status

Drug therapy
- Analgesics (usually nonopioid to avoid reduced intestinal motility commonly caused by opioid analgesics)
- Antibiotics for peritonitis

INTERVENTIONS AND RATIONALES
- Monitor vital signs frequently. *A drop in blood pressure may indicate reduced circulating blood volume due to blood loss from*

a strangulated hernia. As much as 10 L of fluid can collect in the small bowel, drastically reducing plasma volume.

• Assess cardiovascular status *to observe for signs of shock, such as pallor, rapid pulse, and hypotension.*
• Monitor for signs and symptoms of metabolic alkalosis (changes in sensorium; slow, shallow respirations; hypertonic muscles; tetany) or acidosis (dyspnea on exertion, disorientation and, later, deep, rapid breathing, weakness, and malaise). *This allows for early detection of complications.*
• Observe for signs and symptoms of secondary infection, such as fever and chills. *Sustained temperature elevations after surgery may signal onset of pulmonary complications or wound infection.*
• Monitor intake and output carefully *to assess renal function, circulating blood volume, and possible urine retention caused by bladder compression by the distended intestine.*
• Provide oral and nasal care *to prevent mucosal breakdown.*
• Place the child in Fowler's position as much as possible *to promote pulmonary ventilation and ease respiratory distress from abdominal distention.*
• Assess GI status. Listen for bowel sounds, and watch for signs of returning peristalsis (passage of flatus and mucus through the rectum) *to promote nutritional status.*
• Arrange for an enterostomal therapist to visit the child who has had an ostomy *to provide education and information and relieve anxiety.*

Teaching topics
• Explanation of the disorder and treatment plan
• Signs and symptoms of complications
• Wound care or ostomy care, if appropriate

Lead toxicity

Lead toxicity occurs most commonly in toddlers. Lead is poorly absorbed by the body and slowly excreted, replacing calcium in the bones and increasing the permeability of central nervous system membranes.

CAUSES
• Ingestion of lead from dust, soil, paint chips, folk remedies, or use of old ceramic cookware

ASSESSMENT FINDINGS
• Abdominal pain
• Pallor
• Hyperactivity
• Constipation
• Increased intracranial pressure, cortical atrophy, behavioral changes, altered cognition and motor skills, and seizures
• Peripheral neuritis from calcium release into the blood
• Anorexia, vomiting
• Weight loss

DIAGNOSTIC TEST RESULTS
• Blood lead level (BLL) greater than 10 mcg/dl.
• Hematologic studies reveal anemia and increased erythrocyte protoporphyrin.
• Urinalysis reveals proteinuria, ketonuria, and glycosuria.
• X-rays reveal lead lines near the epiphyseal lines (areas of increased density) of long bones. The thickness of the line shows the length of time the lead ingestion has been occurring.

NURSING DIAGNOSES
• Risk for ineffective cerebral tissue perfusion
• Risk for deficient fluid volume
• Risk for poisoning
• Deficient knowledge (lead toxin)

TREATMENT
• BLL less than 10 mcg/dl: no treatment
• BLL 10 to 14 mcg/dl: repeat test in 1 month and again in 3 months if level isn't lower
• BLL 15 to 19 mcg/dl: repeat test in 1 month and again in 2 months if level isn't lower
• BLL 20 to 44 mcg/dl: repeat test in 1 week; if level remains elevated, environmental evaluation by local health department
• BLL 45 to 69 mcg/dl: repeat test in 2 days; if level confirmed, chelating agents

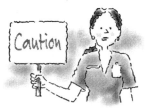

Chelating agents used to treat lead toxicity also bind with calcium, leading to decreased calcium levels. So monitor calcium carefully.

Caution

- BLL over 70 mcg/dl: hospitalization; repeat test, chelating agents
- Oral or I.V. fluid administration to lower BLL and prevent lead encephalopathy
- Low-fat diet with adequate supplies of calcium, magnesium, zinc, iron, and copper; prevents any more lead from being bound and stored in the body's fat tissues

Drug therapy
- Chelating agents: succimer (Chemet) or dimercaprol (BAL In Oil) for BLL greater than 45 mcg/dl
- Benzodiazepines (if seizures occur)

INTERVENTIONS AND RATIONALES
- Monitor calcium levels (chelating agents also bind with calcium) *to prevent tetany and seizures, which may result from hypocalcemia.*
- Monitor vital signs, intake and output, hydration status, and kidney function *to ensure that kidney function is adequate to handle the lead being excreted. If kidney function isn't adequate, EDTA may cause kidney damage.*
- Assess cardiovascular and neurologic status. *Increased levels of lead can cause severe encephalopathy with seizures and permanent neurologic damage.*
- Initiate seizure precautions, if appropriate, *to ensure patient safety.*

Teaching topics
- Explanation of the disorder and treatment plan
- Identifying sources of lead and adjusting the environment appropriately
- Stressing the importance of a well-balanced diet to ensure that the child receives adequate amounts of calcium, magnesium, zinc, iron, and copper
- Signs and symptoms of complications

Pyloric stenosis

With pyloric stenosis, also known as *infantile hypertrophic pyloric stenosis,* hyperplasia and hypertrophy of the circular muscle at the pylorus narrow the pyloric canal, thereby preventing the stomach from emptying normally. The defect is most commonly diagnosed at ages 3 to 12 weeks and occurs four times more often in males.

CAUSES
- Exact cause unknown

ASSESSMENT FINDINGS
- Olive-size bulge palpated below the right costal margin
- Poor weight gain
- Jaundice
- Symptoms of malnutrition and dehydration despite the child's apparent adequate intake of food
- Projectile emesis during or soon after feedings, preceded by reverse peristaltic waves (going left to right) but not by nausea (the child resumes eating after vomiting)
- Tetany

DIAGNOSTIC TEST RESULTS
- ABG analysis reveals metabolic alkalosis.
- Blood chemistry tests may reveal hypocalcemia, hypokalemia, and hypochloremia.
- Hematest reveals emesis containing blood.
- Ultrasound shows pyloric muscle thickness greater than 4 mm.
- Endoscopy reveals a hypertrophied sphincter.

NURSING DIAGNOSES
- Imbalanced nutrition: Less than body requirements
- Risk for imbalanced fluid volume
- Risk for infection
- Delayed growth and development

TREATMENT
- Diet: NPO status before surgery
- I.V. therapy to correct fluid and electrolyte imbalances
- Possible insertion of NG tube, kept open and elevated for gastric decompression
- Surgical intervention: pyloromyotomy performed by laparoscopy

Drug therapy
- Potassium supplements
- Calcium supplement: I.V. calcium
- Atropine sulfate for 21 days (may cause regression of pyloric hypertrophy)

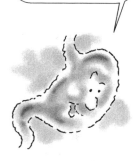

The pylorus is the outlet from the stomach to the duodenum.

INTERVENTIONS AND RATIONALES
- Weigh the child daily *to assess growth.*
- Monitor vital signs and intake and output *to assess renal function and check for signs of dehydration.*
- Assess for metabolic alkalosis and dehydration from frequent emesis *to detect early complications.*
- Assess GI and cardiovascular status *to detect early signs of compromise.*
- Provide small, frequent, thickened feedings with the head of the bed elevated; burp the child frequently (preoperatively) *to promote nutrition and prevent aspiration.*
- Position the child on his right side *to prevent the aspiration of vomitus.*

Postoperative care
- After surgery, feed the infant small amounts of oral electrolyte solution at first; then increase the amount and concentration of food until normal feeding is achieved *to meet nutritional needs and prevent vomiting.*
- Provide a pacifier *to meet nonnutritive sucking needs and maintain comfort.*
- Provide routine postoperative care *to maintain and improve the child's condition and to detect early complications. Position the child on his side so if vomiting occurs there's little chance of aspiration. Laying the child on the right side possibly aids the flow of fluid through the pyloric valve by gravity.*

Teaching topics
- Explanation of the disorder and treatment plan
- Feeding the infant, including specific formula, volume, and technique
- Signs and symptoms of complications

Salicylate toxicity

Salicylate (aspirin) is an analgesic, antipyretic, and anti-inflammatory agent that inhibits platelet aggregation. Toxicity may result from an overdose of salicylate. Symptoms begin when children ingest 150 to 200 mg of aspirin per kilogram of body weight. The peak blood level is reached within 2 to 3 hours of ingestion. The prognosis of the child with salicylate toxicity depends on the amount of salicylate ingested and how quickly treatment begins.

CAUSES
- Ingestion of salicylate beyond the recommended dosage

ASSESSMENT FINDINGS
- Nausea, vomiting
- Tinnitus
- Tachypnea and hyperpnea
- Vertigo
- Restlessness
- Lethargy, which may progress to disorientation, seizures, and coma
- High fever
- Petechiae and bleeding tendency

DIAGNOSTIC TEST RESULTS
- Ferric chloride test reveals the presence of salicylates in urine.
- ABG levels may reveal metabolic acidosis.
- Serum salicylate levels are elevated beyond therapeutic range.

NURSING DIAGNOSES
- Imbalanced nutrition: Less than body requirements
- Hyperthermia
- Risk for imbalanced fluid volume
- Risk for injury
- Ineffective breathing pattern

TREATMENT
- I.V. fluids
- Gastric lavage
- Whole-bowel irrigation with polyethylene glycol
- Hemodialysis (for serum salicylate level over 100 mg/dl)
- Hypothermia blanket
- Intubation and mechanical ventilation if respiratory failure occurs

Drug therapy
- Oral activated charcoal (Liqui-Char)
- Calcium and potassium supplements, if indicated
- Alkalinizing agent: sodium bicarbonate

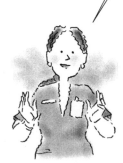

Because aspirin inhibits platelet aggregation, look for petechiae and bleeding in salicylate toxicity.

INTERVENTIONS AND RATIONALES

- Assess respiratory status *to identify respiratory failure.*
- Assess neurologic status *to recognize altered mental staus and level of consciousness and provide appropriate protective measures.*
- Administer I.V. fluids *to dilute the toxin and prevent dehydration.*
- Monitor vital signs and intake and output *to detect dehydration and early signs of compromise.*
- Assess cardiovascular and GI status *to identify signs of metabolic acidosis and GI bleeding.*
- Maintain mechanical ventilation, if required, *to ensure adequate oxygenation.*
- Ensure adequate hydration *to flush the aspirin through the kidneys.*
- Monitor urine pH; *pH over 8 aids salicylate excretion.*
- Dress the child lightly and sponge with tepid water or use a cooling blanket *to reduce high temperature.*
- Monitor body temperature every 15 to 30 minutes according to facility policy while a hypothermia blanket is in use *to evaluate its effectiveness and prevent injury.*
- Monitor ABG values *to assess acid-base balance.*
- Monitor salicylate levels *to assess the effectiveness of treatment.*

Teaching topics

- Explanation of the disorder and treatment plan
- Storing medication and taking steps to prevent aspirin overdose
- Monitoring the child's temperature and encouraging a high fluid intake

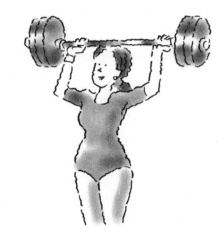

Pump up on practice questions

1. A 3-week-old infant diagnosed with pyloric stenosis is admitted to the hospital during a vomiting episode. Which action by the nurse is most appropriate?

1. Placing the infant on his back to sleep
2. Weighing the infant every 12 hours
3. Positioning the infant on his right side
4. Taking vital signs every 8 hours

Answer: 3. The nurse should position the infant on his right side to prevent aspiration. The infant should be weighed daily, not every 12 hours. Vital signs should be monitored every 4 hours, not every 8 hours.

➡ **NCLEX keys**
Client needs category: Physiological integrity
Client needs subcategory: Reduction of risk potential
Cognitive level: Application

2. A nurse teaches a mother to position an infant with a tracheoesophageal fistula with his head elevated to 30 degrees. The nurse should recognize that teaching was effective when the mother makes which statement?

1. "Positioning him with his head elevated to 30 degrees helps his breathing."
2. "Positioning him with his head elevated to 30 degrees helps with eating."
3. "Positioning him with his head elevated to 30 degrees keeps gastric juices from backing up."
4. "Positioning him with his head elevated to 30 degrees makes him comfortable."

Answer: 3. Placing the infant with his head elevated to 30 degrees helps decrease gastric reflux into the trachea. The child won't be taking food by mouth until after the fistula is surgically repaired. The infant will also breathe easier and be more comfortable with his head elevated, but they aren't the primary reasons for elevating the infant's head to 30 degrees.

➡ *NCLEX keys*
Client needs category: Physiological integrity
Client needs subcategory: Reduction of risk potential
Cognitive level: Application

3. A child with a nasogastric (NG) tube in place complains of nausea. Which action by the nurse is most appropriate?

1. Administer an antiemetic.
2. Irrigate the NG tube.
3. Notify the physician about the nausea.
4. Reposition the NG tube.

Answer: 2. The nurse should first check NG tube placement and then irrigate the tube to check for patency. If nausea continues, the NG tube may be repositioned, depending on the child's condition. If the child continues to complain of nausea after these measures, the physician should be notified and an antiemetic given as ordered.

➡ *NCLEX keys*
Client needs category: Physiological integrity
Client needs subcategory: Reduction of risk potential
Cognitive level: Application

4. The mother of a child diagnosed with celiac disease asks the nurse which foods should be eliminated from her child's diet. The nurse should advise the mother to eliminate:

1. malted milk, wheat bread, and spaghetti.
2. rice cereals, milk, and corn bread.
3. tapioca, potato bread, and peanut butter.
4. corn cereals, milk, and honey.

Answer: 1. The mother should provide her child with celiac disease with a gluten-free diet, eliminating such foods as malted milk, wheat bread, and spaghetti. Rice and corn cereals, milk, corn and potato breads, tapioca, peanut butter, and honey are all appropriate for a gluten-free diet.

➡ *NCLEX keys*
Client needs category: Physiological integrity
Client needs subcategory: Basic care and comfort
Cognitive level: Application

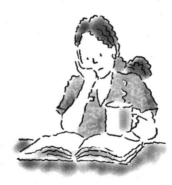

5. A nurse is caring for a toddler after surgical repair of a cleft palate. The nurse should position the child:
1. on his back.
2. on his stomach.
3. on his back with his head slightly elevated.
4. for comfort.

Answer: 2. After surgical repair of a cleft palate, the child should be positioned on his stomach to prevent pooling of secretions in the oropharynx. The child shouldn't be positioned on his back. The nurse shouldn't choose a position based on comfort.

➡ *NCLEX keys*

Client needs category: Physiological integrity
Client needs subcategory: Reduction of risk potential
Cognitive level: Application

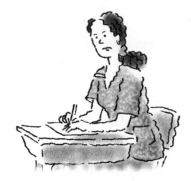

6. A nurse is caring for a child with a complete intestinal obstruction. Which is a key finding in this client?
1. Vomiting
2. Intense thirst
3. Visible peristaltic waves
4. Nausea

Answer: 3. Visible peristaltic waves propel bowel contents toward the mouth instead of the rectum. Vomiting, intense thirst, and nausea are symptoms of a small-bowel obstruction and aren't the key findings in complete intestinal obstruction.

➡ *NCLEX keys*

Client needs category: Physiological integrity
Client needs subcategory: Reduction of risk potential
Cognitive level: Comprehension

7. A nurse is caring for an infant with a cleft lip and palate. This condition places the infant at increased risk for:
1. upper respiratory infections and otitis media.
2. otitis media and diarrhea.
3. upper respiratory infections and diarrhea.
4. diarrhea and vomiting.

Answer: 1. The infant with a cleft lip and palate is at increased risk for upper respiratory infections and otitis media because the increased open space decreases natural defenses against bacteria. It doesn't increase the risk of vomiting and diarrhea.

➡ *NCLEX keys*

Client needs category: Physiological integrity
Client needs subcategory: Reduction of risk potential
Cognitive level: Application

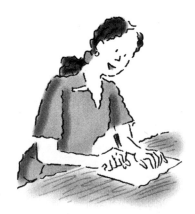

8. A nurse is caring for a toddler with salicylate toxicity. Besides salicylate levels, which values should the nurse be monitoring?
   1. Arterial blood pH
   2. Acetaminophen levels
   3. Calcium levels
   4. Phosphorus levels

Answer: 1. Salicylate toxicity results in metabolic acidosis. Monitoring arterial blood pH helps the nurse evaluate the effectiveness of treatment. Acetominophen levels should be monitored with acetominophen toxicity. Calcium and phosphorus levels can be obtained, but they aren't primarily affected by salicylate toxicity.

➡ *NCLEX keys*
Client needs category: Physiological integrity
Client needs subcategory: Reduction of risk potential
Cognitive level: Analysis

9. A 4-week-old infant is brought to the pediatrician's office. The infant has been experiencing projectile vomiting shortly after feedings. The infant most likely has:
   1. an intestinal obstruction.
   2. intussusception.
   3. a tracheoesophageal fistula.
   4. pyloric stenosis.

Answer: 4. Symptoms of pyloric stenosis generally develop between ages 4 and 6 weeks. They include a palpable bulge below the right costal margin, projectile vomiting during or shortly after feeding, resuming feeding after vomiting, poor weight gain, malnutrition, and dehydration. Intestinal obstruction presents with constipation, colicky abdominal pain, nausea, and dramatic abdominal distention. Intussusception causes sudden onset of severe abdominal pain; the infant is usually inconsolable. Tracheoesophageal fistula causes coughing, choking, and intermittent cyanosis during feeding, and abdominal distention.

➡ *NCLEX keys*
Client needs category: Physiological integrity
Client needs subcategory: Reduction of risk potential
Cognitive level: Application

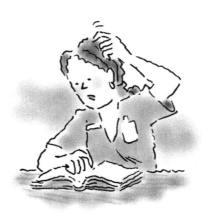

10. Which findings are common in neonates born with esophageal atresia? Select all that apply.
   1. Decreased saliva production
   2. Cyanosis
   3. Coughing
   4. Inadequate swallowing
   5. Choking
   6. Inability to cough

Answer: 2, 3, 5. Cyanosis, coughing, and choking occur when fluid from the blind pouch is aspirated into the trachea. Saliva production doesn't decrease in neonates born with esophageal atresia. The ability to swallow isn't affected by this disorder.

➡ *NCLEX keys*

Client needs category: Physiological integrity
Client needs subcategory: Physiological adaptation
Cognitive level: Analysis

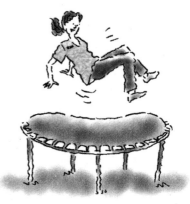

Jump for Joy! Another chapter finished. You did it!

10 | Endocrine system

Brush up on key concepts

Together with the nervous system, the endocrine system regulates and integrates the body's metabolic activities. Disorders of the endocrine system involve hyposecretion or hypersecretion of hormones, which affect the body's metabolic processes and function.

At any time, you can review the major points of this chapter by consulting the *Cheat sheet* on page 140.

Endocrine junior
Here are key points about **endocrine functioning in childhood:**
• The pituitary gland controls the release of nine different hormones and is the master gland for all age-groups.
• The adrenal cortex begins secreting glucocorticoids and mineralocorticoids early in embryonic life.
• The thyroid gland, many times larger in children than in adults, is functional at age 2 weeks. It's thought to play a role in immune function.

Ch..ch..changes
The pituitary is stimulated at puberty to produce androgen steroids responsible for **secondary sex characteristics.**

Female secondary sexual development during puberty involves increase in the size of the ovaries, uterus, vagina, labia, and breasts. The first visible sign of sexual maturity is the appearance of breast buds. Body hair appears in the pubic area and under the arms and menarche begins. The ovaries, present at birth, remain inactive until puberty.

Male secondary sexual development consists of genital growth and the appearance of pubic and body hair.

A place to integrate
The endocrine system meets the nervous system at the **hypothalamus.** The hypothalamus, the main integrative center for the endocrine and autonomic nervous systems, controls the function of endocrine organs by neural and hormonal pathways.

Neural pathways connect the hypothalamus to the posterior pituitary, or neurohypophysis. Neural stimulation to the posterior pituitary provokes the secretion of hormones (chemical transmitters released from specialized cells into the bloodstream). Hormones are then carried to specialized organ-receptor cells that respond to them.

Negative feedback
In addition to hormonal and neural controls, a **negative feedback system** regulates the endocrine system. The mechanism of feedback may be either simple or complex:
• **Simple feedback** occurs when the level of one substance regulates secretion of a hormone. For example, low serum calcium levels stimulate parathyroid hormone secretion; high serum calcium levels inhibit it.
• **Complex feedback** occurs through an axis established between the hypothalamus, pituitary gland, and target organ. For example, secretion of the hypothalamic corticotropin-releasing hormone stimulates release of pituitary corticotropin which, in turn, stimulates cortisol secretion by the adrenal gland (the target organ). A rise in serum cortisol levels inhibits corticotropin secretion by decreasing corticotropin-releasing hormone.

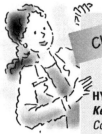

Endocrine refresher

HYPOTHYROIDISM

Key signs and symptoms
Congenital hypothyroidism
- Poor feeding
- Low temperature
- Hoarse crying
- Prolonged jaundice

Acquired hypothyroidism
- Lethargy, decreased energy
- Cold intolerance
- Heat intolerance
- Weight loss

Untreated hypothyroidism in older children
- Bone and muscle dystrophy
- Cognitive impairment
- Stunted growth (cretinism)

Key test results
- Radioimmunoassay confirms hypothyroidism with low triiodothyronine and thyroxine levels.

Key treatments
- Oral thyroid hormone: levothyroxine (Synthroid)

Key interventions
- During early management of infantile hypothyroidism, monitor blood pressure and pulse rate and report hypertension and tachycardia immediately (normal infant heart rate is approximately 120 beats/minute).
- Check rectal temperature every 2 to 4 hours. Keep the infant warm and his skin moist.
- If the infant's tongue is unusually large, position him on his side and observe him frequently.

TYPE 1 DIABETES MELLITUS

Key signs and symptoms
- Polydipsia
- Polyphagia
- Polyuria
- Weight loss and hunger

Key test results
- Two fasting plasma glucose levels (no caloric intake for at least 8 hours) are greater than or equal to 126 mg/dl.
- Glycosylated hemoglobin level is greater than 7%.
- Plasma glucose value in the 2-hour sample of the oral glucose tolerance test is greater than or equal to 200 mg/dl. This test should be performed after a loading dose of 75 g of anhydrous glucose.
- A random plasma glucose value (obtained without regard to the time of the child's last food intake) greater than or equal to 200 mg/dl accompanied by symptoms of diabetes indicates diabetes mellitus.

Key treatments
- Exercise
- Insulin replacement
- Strict diet planned to meet nutritional needs, control blood glucose levels, and reach and maintain appropriate body weight

Key interventions
- Monitor vital signs and intake and output.
- Use age-appropriate teaching materials when teaching about diabetes and the therapeutic regimen.

Keep abreast of diagnostic tests

Here are some important tests used to diagnose endocrine disorders, along with common nursing interventions associated with each test.

Function studies

An **endocrine function study** focuses on measuring the level or effect of a hormone such as the effect of insulin on blood glucose levels.

Sophisticated techniques of hormone measurement have improved diagnosis of endocrine disorders. For example, the human growth hormone stimulation test measures human growth hormone levels after I.V. administration of arginine, an amino acid that, under normal circumstances, stimulates human growth hormone. This test is used to diagnose growth hormone deficiency.

Nursing actions
- Explain the test to the child and his parents.
- Check with the laboratory and consult facility protocol to determine specific actions before the test (nothing-by-mouth for blood glucose test).

Minute measurements
A **radioimmunoassay** is used to measure minute quantities of hormones.

Nursing actions
- Explain the test to the child and his parents.

Polish up on client care

Two major pediatric endocrine disorders are hypothyroidism and type 1 diabetes mellitus.

Hypothyroidism

Hypothyroidism occurs when the body doesn't produce enough thyroid gland hormones, the hormones necessary for normal growth and development. (See *Thyroid gland hormones.*)

Two types of hypothyroidism exist. Congenital hypothyroidism is present at birth. Acquired hypothyroidism is commonly due to thyroiditis, an inflammation of the thyroid gland that results in injury or damage to thyroid tissue. Hypothyroidism is two times more common in girls than in boys.

Early diagnosis and treatment offer the best hope. Infants treated before age 3 months usually grow and develop normally. Children who remain untreated beyond age 3 months and children with acquired hypothyroidism who remain untreated beyond age 2 suffer irreversible cognitive impairment. Skeletal abnormalities may also occur; however, these may be reversible with treatment.

CAUSES
- Antithyroid drugs taken during pregnancy (in infants)
- Chromosomal abnormalities
- Chronic autoimmune thyroiditis (in children older than age 2)
- Defective embryonic development that causes congenital absence or underdevelopment of the thyroid gland (most common cause in infants)
- Inherited enzymatic defect in the synthesis of thyroxine (T_4) caused by an autosomal recessive gene (in infants)
- Irradiation of the thyroid gland

CONTRIBUTING FACTORS
- Prolonged gestation
- High birth weight

ASSESSMENT FINDINGS
General findings
- Delayed dentition
- Enlarged tongue
- Hypotonia
- Legs shorter in relation to trunk size
- Cognitive impairment (develops as the disorder progresses)
- Short stature with the persistence of infant proportions
- Short, thick neck; goiter
- Brittle nails

Congenital hypothyroidism
- Delayed stools at birth
- Prolonged jaundice
- Poor feeding
- Low temperature
- Decreased activity level
- Hoarse crying
- Galactorrhea
- Large fontanels
- Umbilical hernia

Acquired hypothyroidism
- Dry, scaly skin
- Lethargy, decreased energy
- Sleep disturbance
- Cold intolerance
- Constipation
- Heat intolerance
- Weight loss
- Sexual pseudoprecocity

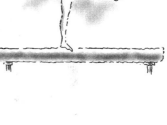

Balance is better. Too many hormones or not enough hormones can cause an endocrine disorder.

Thyroid gland hormones

- The thyroid gland secretes the iodinated hormones thyroxine and triiodothyronine.
- Thyroid hormones, necessary for normal growth and development, act on many tissues to increase metabolic activity and protein synthesis.
- Deficiency of thyroid hormone causes varying degrees of hypothyroidism, from a mild, clinically insignificant form to life-threatening myxedema coma.

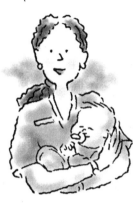

Timing is everything. If hypothyroidism is treated before the child is age 3 months, the prognosis is excellent — left untreated, it leads to cognitive impairment and skeletal abnormalities.

Key test for detecting hypothyroidism: Radioimmunoassay results show low T_3 and T_4 hormone levels.

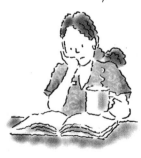

Untreated hypothyroidism in older children
- Bone and muscle dystrophy
- Cognitive impairment
- Stunted growth (cretinism)

DIAGNOSTIC TEST RESULTS
- Electrocardiogram shows bradycardia and flat or inverted T waves in untreated infants.
- Hip, knee, and thigh X-rays reveal absence of the femoral or tibial epiphyseal line and delayed skeletal development that's markedly inappropriate for the child's chronological age.
- In myxedema coma, laboratory tests may also show low serum sodium levels, decreased pH, and increased partial pressure of arterial carbon dioxide, indicating respiratory acidosis.
- Increased gonadotropin levels accompany sexual precocity in older children and may coexist with hypothyroidism.
- Serum cholesterol, alkaline phosphatase, and triglyceride levels are elevated.
- Normocytic normochromic anemia is present.
- Radioimmunoassay confirms hypothyroidism with low triiodothyronine (T_3) and T_4 levels.
- Thyroid scan and ^{131}I uptake tests show decreased uptake levels and confirm the absence of thyroid tissue in athyroid children.
- Thyroid-stimulating hormone (TSH) level is decreased when hypothyroidism results from hypothalamic or pituitary insufficiency.
- TSH level is increased when hypothyroidism results from thyroid insufficiency.

NURSING DIAGNOSES
- Delayed growth and development
- Interrupted family processes
- Deficient knowledge (treatment regimen)
- Imbalanced nutrition: Less than body requirements
- Activity intolerance
- Risk for imbalanced body temperature

TREATMENT
- Routine monitoring of T_4 and TSH levels
- Periodic evaluation of growth to ensure thyroid replacement is adequate
- Surgery to remove massive goiter (rare)

Drug therapy
- Oral thyroid hormone: levothyroxine (Synthroid)

INTERVENTIONS AND RATIONALES
- During early management of infantile hypothyroidism, monitor blood pressure and pulse rate; report hypertension and tachycardia immediately (normal infant heart rate is approximately 120 beats/minute). *These signs of hyperthyroidism indicate that the dose of thyroid replacement medication is too high.*
- Check rectal temperature every 2 to 4 hours. Keep the infant warm and his skin moist *to promote normothermia and reduce metabolic demands.*
- If the infant's tongue is unusually large, position him on his side and observe him frequently *to prevent airway obstruction.*
- Provide parents with support, referrals, and counseling as necessary *to help parents cope with the possibility of caring for a physically and cognitively impaired child.*
- Adolescent girls require future-oriented counseling that stresses the importance of adequate thyroid replacement during pregnancy. *Ideally, women should have excellent control before conception.*

Teaching topics
- Explanation of the disorder and treatment plan
- Medication use and possible adverse effects
- Recognizing signs of overdose of supplemental thyroid hormone (rapid pulse rate, irritability, insomnia, fever, sweating, weight loss)
- Understanding that the child requires lifelong treatment with thyroid supplements
- Complying with the treatment regimen to prevent further mental impairment
- Adopting a positive but realistic attitude and focusing on the child's strengths rather than his weaknesses
- Providing stimulating activities to help the child reach maximum potential (referring

parents to appropriate community resources for support)
• Preventing infantile hypothyroidism (emphasize the importance of adequate nutrition during pregnancy, including iodine-rich foods and the use of iodized salt or, in cases of sodium restriction, iodine supplements)

Type 1 diabetes mellitus

Type 1 diabetes mellitus (formerly referred to as juvenile diabetes or insulin-dependent diabetes) is a chronic metabolic disease characterized by absolute insulin insufficiency. Children with this type of diabetes must inject insulin to process carbohydrates, fat, and protein. Type 1 diabetes is most commonly diagnosed during childhood or adolescence but can occur at any time from infancy to about age 30. (See *Understanding type 1 diabetes,* page 144.)

CAUSES
• Genetic predisposition
• Viral infection
• Autoimmune response
• Congenital absence of pancreas or islet cells
• Pancreatic damage secondary to another disorder, such as cystic fibrosis or pancreatitis
• Chromosomal disorders such as Down syndrome

ASSESSMENT FINDINGS
• Polydipsia
• Polyphagia
• Polyuria
• Weight loss and hunger

Hyperglycemia
• Abdominal cramping
• Dry, flushed skin
• Fatigue
• Fruity breath odor
• Headache
• Mental status changes
• Nausea
• Thin appearance and possible malnourishment

• Vomiting
• Weakness

Hypoglycemia in conjunction with diabetes
• Behavior changes (belligerence, confusion, slurred speech)
• Diaphoresis
• Palpitations
• Tachycardia
• Tremors

DIAGNOSTIC TEST RESULTS
• Two fasting plasma glucose levels (no caloric intake for at least 8 hours) are greater than or equal to 126 mg/dl.
• Glycosylated hemoglobin level is greater than 7%.
• Plasma glucose value in the 2-hour sample of the oral glucose tolerance test is greater than or equal to 200 mg/dl. This test should be performed after a loading dose of 75 g of anhydrous glucose.
• A random plasma glucose value (obtained without regard to the time of the child's last food intake) greater than or equal to 200 mg/dl that's accompanied by symptoms of diabetes indicates diabetes mellitus.

NURSING DIAGNOSES
• Disturbed body image
• Risk for imbalanced nutrition: Less than body requirements
• Risk for imbalanced fluid volume
• Deficient knowledge (treatment regimen)

TREATMENT
• Exercise
• Strict diet planned to meet nutritional needs, control blood glucose levels, and reach and maintain appropriate body weight

Drug therapy
• Insulin replacement

INTERVENTIONS AND RATIONALES
• Monitor vital signs and fluid intake and output *to detect signs of hyperglycemia or hypoglycemia.*
• Monitor blood glucose levels and electrolytes *to detect early signs of electrolyte imbalance.*

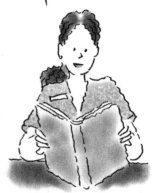

> Remember that regular study habits do more good than cramming. Plan a realistic, regular schedule and stick to it.

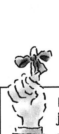

Memory jogger

Think "tri-poly" (sounds like Tripoli) to remember the key assessment findings in type 1 diabetes mellitus:

polydipsia

polyphagia

polyuria.

Understanding type 1 diabetes

Here are important points for understanding how type 1 diabetes develops.

THE KEY PLAYERS
- The endocrine part of the pancreas produces glucagon from the alpha cells and insulin from the beta cells.
- Glucagon, the hormone of the fasting state, releases stored glucose to raise the blood glucose level.
- Insulin, the hormone of the nourished state, facilitates glucose transport, promotes glucose storage, stimulates protein synthesis, and enhances free fatty acid uptake and storage.

WHAT HAPPENS
Absolute or relative insulin deficiency causes diabetes mellitus. Here's what happens:
- Pancreatic beta cells are destroyed, no insulin is produced, and the cells can't utilize glucose.
- Excess glucose in the blood spills into the urine.
- The increased level of blood glucose can act as an osmotic diuretic, resulting in dehydration, hypotension, and renal shutdown.
- The body attempts to compensate for lost energy by breaking down fatty acids to form ketones with resulting metabolic acidosis.

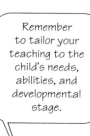

Remember to tailor your teaching to the child's needs, abilities, and developmental stage.

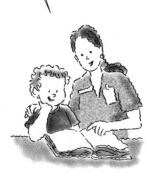

- Observe neurologic status *to detect signs of hyperglycemia or hypoglycemia.*
- Evaluate the child's or adolescent's understanding of type 1 diabetes and his attitude about the need to manage it *to help plan teaching.*
- Use age-appropriate teaching materials when teaching about diabetes and the therapeutic regimen *to increase the child or adolescent's knowledge of his condition and instill confidence in his ability to manage it.*
- Provide an opportunity for the child or adolescent to interact with peers who have experienced diabetes *to decrease his feelings of isolation and being different from others.*

Hyperglycemia
- Administer regular insulin for fast action *to promote euglycemic state and prevent complications.*
- Administer I.V. fluids without dextrose *to flush out acetone and maintain hydration.*
- Monitor electrolyte and arterial blood gas levels *to detect imbalances or acidosis.*
- Monitor blood glucose level *to detect early changes and prevent complications such as diabetic ketoacidosis.*

Hypoglycemia
- Give a fast-acting carbohydrate, such as honey, orange juice, or sugar cubes, followed later by a protein source *to increase glucose levels thereby preventing complications of hypoglycemia.*
- If the child is stuporous or unconscious, administer glucagon (subcutaneously, I.V., or I.M.) or dextrose 50% I.V. *to prevent complications of hypoglycemia.*

Teaching topics
- Explanation of the disorder and treatment plan
- Medication use and possible adverse effects
- Dietary adjustments
- Complying with the prescribed treatment program (see *Teaching about insulin administration*)
- Monitoring blood glucose levels
- Understanding the importance of good hygiene
- Preventing, recognizing, and treating hypoglycemia and hyperglycemia
- Understanding the effect of blood glucose control on long-term health
- Managing diabetes during a minor illness, such as a cold, the flu, or an upset stomach
- Providing the child or adolescent with written materials that cover the teaching topics
- Providing the child and his family with information about the Juvenile Diabetes Foundation

Management moments

Teaching about insulin administration

Teaching about insulin administration is an important part of care management for the child with type 1 diabetes and his parents. Here are some important elements to teach the child and his parents about insulin administration:
• When giving both types of insulin, draw up clear insulin first to prevent contamination.
• To prevent air bubbles, don't shake the vial; intermediate forms are suspensions and should be gently rotated.
• Rotate injection sites to prevent lipodystrophy.
• Make sure the child eats when the insulin peaks, such as midafternoon and bedtime.
• Insulin requirements may be altered with illness, stress, growth, food intake, and exercise; blood glucose measurements are the best way to determine insulin adjustments.

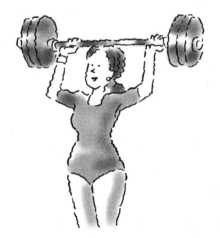

Pump up on practice questions

1. A nurse is teaching the mother of a child diagnosed with type 1 diabetes. The mother asks why her child must inject insulin and can't take pills as her uncle does. Which reply is most appropriate?
   1. "Because a child's pancreas is less developed than an adult's, antidiabetic pills aren't recommended for children."
   2. "Pills only affect fat and protein metabolism, not sugar."
   3. "The only way to replace insulin is by injection."
   4. "Your child may be able to take pills when he's older."

Answer: 3. In type 1 diabetes, the pancreas doesn't produce insulin, so the child must receive insulin replacement by injection. Oral antidiabetic agents stimulate the pancreas to produce more insulin and are only effective in treating type 2 diabetes. Because the pancreas in the child with type 1 diabetes doesn't produce insulin, the child will never be a candidate for oral antidiabetic agents.

➡ *NCLEX keys*
Client needs category: Physiological integrity
Client needs subcategory: Pharmacological and parenteral therapies
Cognitive level: Application

2. A nurse is teaching the mother of a child how to recognize the signs and symptoms of hypoglycemia. Which signs and symptoms should the nurse discuss?
   1. Behavioral changes, increased heart rate, sweating, and tremors
   2. Nausea, fruity breath odor, headache, and fatigue
   3. Polydipsia, polyuria, polyphagia, and weight loss
   4. Enlarged tongue, hypotonia, easy weight gain, and cool skin temperature

Answer: 1. The nurse should instruct the mother of a child with diabetes to recognize such signs and symptoms of hypoglycemia as behavioral changes, increased heart rate, sweating, and tremors. Nausea, fruity breath odor, headache, and fatigue are present with hyperglycemia. Polydipsia, polyuria, polyphagia, and weight loss are classic signs of diabetes. Enlarged tongue, hypotonia, easy weight gain, and cool skin temperature are associated with hypothyroidism.

➡ *NCLEX keys*

Client needs category: Physiological integrity
Client needs subcategory: Reduction of risk potential
Cognitive level: Comprehension

3. A nurse is assessing a child who might have diabetes. Which laboratory value helps confirm a diagnosis of type 1 diabetes?
1. A fasting plasma glucose level of 110 mg/dl obtained once
2. A fasting plasma glucose level of 126 mg/dl obtained at two different times
3. A random plasma glucose level of 180 mg/dl obtained once
4. A 2-hour glucose tolerance test of 140 mg/dl obtained at two different times

Answer: 2. According to the American Diabetes Association, diabetes occurs when any of the following conditions exist: symptoms of diabetes plus a random plasma glucose level greater than or equal to 200 mg/dl, two fasting plasma glucose levels greater than or equal to 126 mg/dl, or a 2-hour oral glucose tolerance test greater than or equal to 200 mg/dl.

➡ *NCLEX keys*

Client needs category: Health promotion and maintenance
Client needs subcategory: None
Cognitive level: Application

4. A nurse is caring for a child with type 1 diabetes. The nurse enters the child's room and finds him diaphoretic and unresponsive. The nurse should anticipate which of the following emergency interventions?
1. Administering honey followed by a protein source
2. Administering orange juice followed by a protein source
3. Administering dextrose 50% I.V.
4. Administering insulin

Answer: 3. The child is unconscious and experiencing a hypoglycemic reaction; therefore, the nurse should be prepared to administer 50% dextrose I.V. The child experiencing a hypoglycemic episode who's conscious should be given a fast-acting carbohydrate, such as honey, orange juice or sugar cubes, followed by a protein source. Insulin administration would further worsen the child's condition.

➡ *NCLEX keys*

Client needs category: Physiological integrity
Client needs subcategory: Pharmacological and parenteral therapies
Cognitive level: Application

5. A nurse is teaching the parents of a child with diabetes. Which agent should the nurse teach the parents to administer if their child suffers a severe hypoglycemic reaction?
1. I.V. dextrose
2. Subcutaneous insulin administration
3. Subcutaneous glucagon administration
4. Oral fast-acting carbohydrate administration

Answer: 3. The nurse should instruct the parents of a child with diabetes about proper administration of subcutaneous glucagon if their child suffers a severe hypoglycemic episode. Administering insulin subcutaneously would further worsen the child's condition. I.V. dextrose is reserved for health care professionals specially trained in I.V. drug administration. Oral administration of fast-acting carbohydrates is reserved for the conscious child who isn't suffering from a severe hypoglycemic reaction.

➡ *NCLEX keys*

Client needs category: Physiological integrity
Client needs subcategory: Reduction of risk potential
Cognitive level: Application

6. A nurse is teaching an adolescent with diabetes about situations that can alter insulin requirements. Which situation should be emphasized?
1. Illness, stress, growth, food intake, and exercise
2. Water intake, illness, stress, and exercise
3. Exposure to ultraviolet light, illness, stress, and exercise
4. Sodium intake, exercise, stress, and illness

Answer: 1. Illness, stress, growth, food intake, and exercise can alter insulin requirements. Water intake, ultraviolet light exposure, and sodium intake don't alter insulin requirements.

➡ NCLEX keys
Client needs category: Physiological integrity
Client needs subcategory: Reduction of risk potential
Cognitive level: Application

7. The nurse is teaching an adolescent with diabetes about his disease. Which statement by the adolescent indicates that teaching was effective?
1. "If I want to eat ice cream, I'll just give myself more insulin."
2. "I'm so busy, I'm glad I can still skip meals if I need to."
3. "I will remember to take my regular dose of insulin even if I'm sick."
4. "I will monitor my blood glucose level to determine how much insulin I need."

Answer: 4. Diabetic teaching is effective when the adolescent verbalizes the importance of monitoring his blood glucose level to determine his insulin needs. Teaching should stress the importance of maintaining a diabetic diet and not skipping meals. It should also address the need for adjusting insulin doses during times of illness.

➡ NCLEX keys
Client needs category: Physiological integrity
Client needs subcategory: Reduction of risk potential
Cognitive level: Analysis

8. A 10-year-old boy with type 1 diabetes comes to the pediatrician's office. Which technique best ensures responsible insulin administration?
1. The child observes his parents as they administer his injections.
2. The child learns to administer his insulin with supervision.
3. The child manages his insulin administration independently.
4. The child learns to draw up his own insulin and his parents inject it.

Answer: 2. School-age children should be encouraged to administer their own insulin with adult supervision to ensure correct procedure is followed and the correct dosage is administered. Having the child observe the parents or drawing up his insulin and not injecting it doesn't allow the child to take sufficient responsibility for his care. Allowing the child to administer his insulin without adult supervision gives him too much responsibility.

➡ NCLEX keys
Client needs category: Physiological integrity
Client needs subcategory: Reduction of risk potential
Cognitive level: Application

9. A 9-year-old boy with type 1 diabetes takes a mixture of regular and NPH insulin. He's scheduled to go on a camping trip and his mother asks the nurse whether it's safe for him to participate in this activity. What's the most appropriate response?
1. "He needs to understand the physical limitations placed on a client with diabetes."
2. "He should have a light snack before doing any hiking."
3. "He shouldn't go on this trip because it's potentially dangerous."
4. "Have him increase his morning NPH insulin to compensate for higher metabolism while hiking."

Answer: 2. A light meal before rigorous exercise gives the child adequate blood glucose levels during the peak action of his morning NPH insulin. Restricting the child's physical activity discourages a normal lifestyle. The child's diagnosis alone shouldn't be used to evaluate the danger of the trip. Increasing the child's insulin would increase the likelihood of a hypoglycemic reaction.

➡ *NCLEX keys*

Client needs category: Physiological integrity
Client needs subcategory: Reduction of risk potential
Cognitive level: Application

10. A nurse administers oral thyroid hormone to an infant with hypothyroidism. For which signs of overdose should the nurse observe the infant?

1. Tachycardia, fever, irritability, and sweating
2. Bradycardia, cool skin temperature, and dry scaly skin
3. Bradycardia, fever, hypotension, and irritability
4. Tachycardia, cool skin temperature, and irritability

Answer: 1. The infant experiencing an overdose of thyroid replacement hormone exhibits tachycardia, fever, irritability, and sweating. Bradycardia, cool skin temperature, and dry scaly skin are signs of hypothyroidism.

➡ *NCLEX keys*

Client needs category: Physiological integrity
Client needs subcategory: Pharmacological and parenteral therapies
Cognitive level: Application

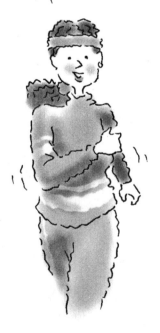

Treat yourself right while studying for the exam. Don't skip meals, miss sleep, or neglect exercise. Stay healthy and, in the long run, you'll stay ahead.

Brush up on key concepts

The genitourinary (GU) system includes the genitalia and urinary structures. This chapter focuses on the kidneys, ureters, and bladder, which are involved in renal and urinary function. The chapter also discusses two sexually transmitted diseases (STDs) that affect children.

You can review the major points of this chapter by consulting the *Cheat sheet* on pages 150 and 151.

High turnover
Water, which is controlled by the GU system, is the body's primary fluid. An infant has a much greater percentage of total body water in extracellular fluid (42% to 45%) than an adult does (20%). Because of the increased percentage of water in a child's extracellular fluid, a child's **water turnover rate** is two to three times greater than an adult's. Every day, 50% of an infant's extracellular fluid is exchanged, compared with only 20% of an adult's; a child is therefore more susceptible than an adult to dehydration.

Sweating it out
A neonate also has a greater ratio of body-surface area to body weight than an adult; this ratio results in greater **fluid loss through the skin.**

Less efficient during stress
A child's kidneys attain the adult number of **nephrons** (about a million in each kidney) shortly after birth. The nephrons, which form urine, continue to mature throughout early childhood.

An infant's renal system can maintain a healthy fluid and electrolyte status. However, it doesn't function as efficiently as an adult's during periods of stress. For example, if a child doesn't receive enough fluid to meet his needs, his kidneys can't adequately concentrate urine to prevent dehydration. Conversely, if a child receives too much fluid, he may be unable to dilute urine appropriately to get rid of the increased volume.

Concentration change
An infant's kidneys don't concentrate urine at an adult level (average **specific gravity** is less than 1.010 for an infant, compared with 1.010 to 1.030 for an adult).

Although the number of daily voidings decreases with increasing age (because of increased urine concentration), the total amount of urine produced daily may not vary significantly.

An infant usually voids 5 to 10 ml/hour, a 10-year-old child usually voids 10 to 25 ml/hour, and an adult usually voids 35 ml/hour.

Short path to the bladder
A child also has a short urethra; therefore, organisms can be easily transmitted into the bladder, increasing the risk of bladder infection.

Keep abreast of diagnostic tests

Here are the most important tests used to diagnose GU disorders, along with common nursing interventions associated with each test.

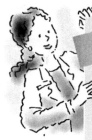

Cheat sheet

Genitourinary refresher

CHLAMYDIA

Key signs and symptoms
With conjunctivitis
- Fiery red conjunctivae with a thick pus
- Edematous eyelids

With pneumonia
- Nasal congestion
- Sharp cough that gradually worsens
- Failure to gain weight
- Tachypnea
- Crackles

Key test results
- Tissue cell cultures from infected sites reveal *Chlamydia trachomatis.*

Key treatments
- Irrigation of eyes with sterile saline solution to clear copious discharge
- Chest physiotherapy to mobilize secretions in a child with pneumonia
- Erythromycin
- Humidified oxygen to ease labored breathing and prevent hypoxemia in a child with pneumonia

Key interventions
- Check the neonate of an infected mother for signs of chlamydial infection.
- Administer medication as prescribed and monitor its effectiveness.
- Auscultate breath sounds and monitor oxygenation.
- Monitor for continued infection.

HYPOSPADIAS

Key signs and symptoms
- Altered angle of urination
- Meatus terminating at some point along lateral fusion line, ranging from the perineum to the distal penile shaft

Key test results
- Examination confirms aberrant placement of the opening.

Key treatments
- Avoiding circumcision (the foreskin may be needed later for surgical repair)

- Tubularized incised plate procedure (for distal and midshaft hypospadias); most commonly used repair for primary tubularization of the urethral plate
- Urethroplasty (surgical procedure in which the urethra is extended into a normal position with a meatus at the top of the penis); may initially be performed to restore normal urinary function
- Orthoplasty when the child is age 12 to 18 months, to release the adherent chordee (fibrous band that causes the penis to curve downward); if extensive repair is needed, delay until age 4
- Indwelling urinary catheter or suprapubic urinary catheter (postoperatively)
- Analgesics: meperidine (Demerol), acetaminophen (Tylenol) for postoperative pain relief
- Antispasmodic agent: propantheline prescribed postoperatively to treat bladder spasms

Key interventions
- Perform diligent perineal care.
- Provide emotional support to parents. Provide accurate information and answer questions thoroughly.

Postoperative care
- After the procedure, apply a pressure dressing.
- Check the tip of the penis frequently.
- Leave the dressing in place for several days.
- Avoid pressure on the child's catheter, and avoid kinking of the catheter.

NEPHRITIS

Key signs and symptoms
- Anorexia
- Burning during urination
- Flank pain
- Urinary frequency
- Shaking chills
- Temperature of 102° F (38.9° C) or higher
- Urinary urgency

Uh-oh! My renal system doesn't function as well as an adult's when it undergoes stress.

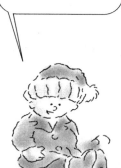

Genitourinary refresher (continued)

NEPHRITIS (CONTINUED)
Key test results
• Pyuria is present (with pyclonephritis). Urine sediment reveals the presence of leukocytes singly, in clumps, and in casts and, possibly, a few red blood cells.
• Urine culture identifies specific bacteria.

Key treatments
• Antibiotics: targeted to specific infecting organism

Key interventions
• Encourage fluid intake to achieve urine output of more than 2 L/day. However, discourage intake greater than 3 L/day.

NEPHROBLASTOMA
Key signs and symptoms
• Nontender mass, usually midline near the liver, that's commonly detected by the parent while bathing or dressing the child
• Associated congenital anomalies, such as microcephaly, mental retardation, genitourinary tract problems

Key test results
• Computed tomography scan or sonography reveals tumor, lymph node involvement, and metastasis.

Key treatments
• Nephrectomy to remove affected kidney and evaluate remaining kidney; may be preceded by chemotherapy to shrink the tumor if it has extended to the vena cava or if there's bilateral involvement
• Radiation therapy (after surgery)
• Chemotherapy (after surgery): dactinomycin (Cosmegen), doxorubicin (Doxil), vincristine

Key interventions
• Monitor vital signs and intake and output.

• Don't palpate the abdomen, and prevent others from doing so.
• Prepare the child and family members for a nephrectomy.
After nephrectomy
• Monitor urine output and report output less than 30 ml/hour.
• Assist with turning, coughing, and deep breathing.
• Encourage early ambulation.
• Provide pain medications as necessary and evaluate their effect.
• Monitor postoperative dressings for signs of bleeding.
• Provide wound care as directed.

URINARY TRACT INFECTION
Key signs and symptoms
• Frequent urges to void with pain or burning on urination
• Lethargy
• Low-grade fever
• Urine that's cloudy and foul-smelling

Key test results
• Clean catch urine culture yields large amounts of bacteria.
• Urine culture identifies specific bacteria.

Key treatments
• Increased fluid intake
• Antibiotics: gentamicin (Garamycin), cefotaxime (Claforan)

Key interventions
• Monitor intake and output.
• Assess toileting habits for proper front-to-back wiping and proper hand washing.
• Encourage increased intake of fluids.
• Assist the child when necessary to ensure that the perineal area is clean after elimination.

Blood analysis
Blood tests are used to analyze serum levels of chemical substances, such as uric acid, creatinine, and blood urea nitrogen.

Nursing actions
• Explain the procedure to the parents and child.
• Allow the child to hold a comfort object, such as a stuffed animal or blanket, to help diminish his anxiety.

Urine tests #1 and #2
Urinalysis is analysis of a urine specimen to determine characteristics, such as:
• presence of red blood cells (RBCs)
• presence of white blood cells
• presence of casts or bacteria
• specific gravity and pH
• physical properties, such as clarity, color, and odor.

    Urine culture and sensitivity identifies the type of bacteria present in the urine. Results of this test help direct antibiotic therapy.

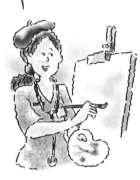

Picture this. Several tests help visualize the renal system: KUB radiography, excretory urography, and voiding cystourethrography.

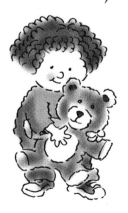

Holding a comfort object such as a stuffed animal may help decrease my anxiety.

Nursing actions
- Explain the procedure to the parents and child.
- Before specimen collection, explain the importance of cleaning the meatal area thoroughly.
- Explain that the culture specimen should be caught midstream, in a sterile container, preferably at the first voiding of the day.
- A urine specimen for culture for an infant should be obtained using a sterile straight catheter.

Urine test #3
A 24-hour urine specimen involves collecting urine over 24 hours to assess urine output or to measure the excretion of certain substances into urine over a 24-hour period.

Nursing actions
- Explain the procedure to the parents and child.
- Begin a 24-hour specimen collection after discarding the first voiding. Specimens typically necessitate special handling or preservatives and should be kept on ice or in the refrigerator until they're ready to be sent to the laboratory.
- When obtaining a urine specimen from a catheterized child, remember to avoid taking the specimen from the collection bag; instead, aspirate a specimen through the collection port in the catheter, with a sterile syringe.

Kidney pictures
Kidney-ureter-bladder (KUB) radiography is an X-ray used to assess the size, shape, position, and possible areas of calcification of the renal organs.

Nursing actions
- Explain the procedure to the parents and child.
- Tell the child that the X-ray only takes a few minutes and remind him to hold still.
- Shield the genitals of a male child to prevent irradiation of the testes.

Crisscrossing the belly
Computed tomography (CT) scan of the abdomen is an X-ray that obtains cross-sectional pictures of abdominal structures.

Nursing actions
- Explain the procedure to the parents and child.
- Complete paperwork required by the facility, including an informed consent if contrast dye is to be used.
- Tell the parents and child that he may be asked to drink barium sulfate 60 to 90 minutes before the test.
- Tell the parents and child that the CT scan should take about 30 minutes and that he'll need to remain still for the test.
- After the test, encourage the child to drink plenty of fluids for 24 to 48 hours.

I.V. action
Excretory urography is an X-ray that aids in checking renal pelvic structures (kidneys, ureters, and bladder). Contrast media is injected into the vein, allowing visualization of the collecting system and ureters.

Nursing actions
- Explain the procedure to the parents and child.
- Check the child's history for allergies.
- Tell the parents and child that the procedure may take up to 1 hour to complete and that the child will need to remain still after the dye is injected.
- Inform the child that a compression device may be placed on the abdomen to keep the contrast dye in the kidneys. The child may feel some pressure.
- Maintain the child on nothing-by-mouth status for 8 hours before the test.
- Make sure that written, informed consent has been obtained.
- Increase hydration after the procedure.

While the water is running
A voiding cystourethrogram is an X-ray that views the bladder and related structures during urination.

Nursing actions
- Explain the procedure to the child and parents.
- Check the child's history for allergies.
- Monitor the child's intake and output.
- Make sure that written, informed consent has been obtained.

• Tell the child that a small catheter will be placed in the bladder and that contrast dye will be injected through it.
• Inform the child that he'll be asked to urinate after the catheter is removed and that X-rays will be taken at the same time.
• After the procedure, encourage the child to drink lots of fluids to reduce burning on urination and to flush out residual dye.

Polish up on client care

Common pediatric GU disorders include chlamydia, hypospadias, nephritis, nephroblastoma (Wilms' tumor), and urinary tract infections (UTIs).

Chlamydia

Chlamydial infection is one of the most common STDs in the United States. In infants, the infecting organism is passed from the infected mother to the fetus during passage through the birth canal.

Chlamydia is the most common cause of ophthalmia neonatorum (eye infection at birth or during the first month) and a major cause of pneumonia in infants in the first 3 months of life. With antibiotic therapy, the prognosis is good.

CAUSES
• *Chlamydia trachomatis* exposure

ASSESSMENT FINDINGS
With conjunctivitis (occur within first 10 days of life)
• Fiery red conjunctivae with a thick puslike discharge
• Edematous eyelids

With pneumonia (occur within 3 to 6 weeks of birth)
• Nasal congestion
• Sharp cough that gradually worsens
• Failure to gain weight
• Tachypnea
• Crackles

DIAGNOSTIC TEST RESULTS
• Tissue cell cultures from infected sites reveal *C. trachomatis*.
• Blood studies show elevated levels of immunoglobulin (Ig) G and IgM antibodies.

NURSING DIAGNOSES
• Ineffective airway clearance
• Interrupted family processes
• Acute pain

TREATMENT
• Irrigation of eyes with sterile saline solution to clear copious discharge
• Humidified oxygen to ease labored breathing and prevent hypoxemia in a child with pneumonia
• Chest physiotherapy to mobilize secretions in a child with pneumonia

Drug therapy
• Erythromycin

INTERVENTIONS AND RATIONALES
• Check the neonate of an infected mother for signs of chlamydial infection *to identify infection early and initiate treatment.*
• Obtain appropriate specimens for diagnostic testing *to aid in diagnosis of infection.*
• Administer medication as prescribed and monitor its effectiveness *to improve the infant's condition.*
• Provide eye care for the neonate *to prevent complications.*
• Monitor for continued infection *to evaluate treatment.*
• Auscultate breath sounds and monitor oxygenation *to determine oxygen status and respiratory function.*
• Suction as needed *to provide airway clearance.*
• Assess for signs and symptoms of pain (increased respirations, tachycardia, increased or inconsolable crying, and frequent awakening from sleep).

Teaching topics
• Explanation of the disorder and treatment plan
• Medication use and possible adverse effects
• Completing the entire course of drug therapy

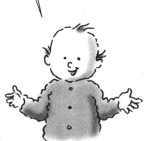

Children born of mothers who have chlamydial infection may contract conjunctivitis or pneumonia during passage through the birth canal.

- Eye care
- Signs and symptoms of complications or continued infection
- Information on safe sex practices and prevention of STDs

Hypospadias

Hypospadias is a congenital anomaly of the penis. In this condition, the urethral opening may be anywhere along the ventral side of the penis. The condition shortens the distance to the bladder, offering easier access for bacteria.

CAUSES
- Genetic factors (most likely)
- Idiopathic

ASSESSMENT FINDINGS
- Altered angle of urination
- Meatus terminating at some point along lateral fusion line, ranging from the perineum to the distal penile shaft
- Marked downward curvature of the penis

DIAGNOSTIC TEST RESULTS
- Examination confirms aberrant placement of the opening.

NURSING DIAGNOSES
- Disturbed body image
- Deficient knowledge (disease process and treatment regimen)
- Anxiety

TREATMENT
- Avoiding circumcision (the foreskin may be needed later for surgical repair)

Surgery
- Tubularized incised plate procedure (for distal and midshaft hypospadias); most commonly used repair for primary tubularization of the uretheral plate
- Urethroplasty (procedure in which the urethra is extended into a normal position with a meatus at the tip of the penis); may initially be performed to restore normal urinary function

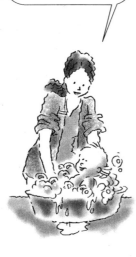

The key intervention in hypospadias is scrupulous cleaning to deter bacteria.

- Orthoplasty when the child is age 12 to 18 months, to release the adherent chordee (fibrous band that causes the penis to curve downward); if extensive repair is needed, delay until age 4
- Indwelling urinary catheter or suprapubic urinary catheter (postoperatively)

Drug therapy
- Analgesics: meperidine (Demerol), acetaminophen (Tylenol) for postoperative pain relief
- Antispasmodic agent: propantheline prescribed postoperatively to treat bladder spasms

INTERVENTIONS AND RATIONALES
- Monitor urine output *to ensure that the infant maintains a normal urine output of 5 to 10 ml/hr.*
- Perform diligent perineal care *to prevent bacteria invasion and infection.*
- Provide emotional support to the parents. Provide accurate information and answer questions thoroughly. Encourage verbalization of feelings. *Encouraging open discussion may help ease the parents' anxiety.*

Postoperative care
- After the procedure, apply a pressure dressing *to reduce bleeding and tissue swelling.*
- Check the tip of the penis frequently *to make sure that it's pink and viable.*
- Leave the dressing in place for several days *to encourage healing of the grafted skin flap.*
- Avoid pressure on the child's catheter *to prevent trauma to the incision site* and avoid kinking of the catheter *to ensure urine flow.*
- Encourage early ambulation *to prevent complications of immobility.*

Teaching topics
- Explanation of the disorder and treatment plan
- Wound care
- Hygiene of uncircumcised penis
- Understanding signs and symptoms of complications
- Follow-up care

Nephritis

Nephritis is a sudden inflammation that primarily affects the interstitial area and the renal pelvis or, less commonly, the renal tubules. Types of nephritis include acute tubulointerstitial nephritis (TIN), pyelonephritis, and glomerulonephritis. One of the most common renal diseases, nephritis is more common in females, probably because of a shorter urethra and the proximity of the urinary meatus to the vagina and the rectum.

With treatment and continued follow-up care, the prognosis is good and extensive permanent damage is rare.

CAUSES
• Bacterial infection of the kidneys (the most common cause); infecting bacteria usually are normal intestinal and fecal flora that grow readily in urine (the most common causative organism is *Escherichia coli,* but *Proteus, Pseudomonas, Staphylococcus aureus,* and *Enterococcus faecalis* [formerly *Streptococcus faecalis*] may also cause such infections)
• Hematogenic infection (as in septicemia or endocarditis)
• Lymphatic infection
• Transplant rejection
• Ureter obstruction
• Allergy or toxic response to a drug (TIN)

ASSESSMENT FINDINGS
• Anorexia
• Burning during urination
• Dysuria
• Flank pain
• Urinary frequency
• General fatigue
• Hematuria (usually microscopic but may be gross)
• Nocturia
• Rash (TIN)
• Shaking chills
• Temperature of 102° F (38.9° C) or higher
• Urinary urgency
• Urine that's cloudy and has an ammonia-like or fishy odor

DIAGNOSTIC TEST RESULTS
• Excretory urography may show asymmetrical or enlarged kidneys.

• Pyuria is present (with pyelonephritis). Urine sediment reveals the presence of leukocytes singly, in clumps, and in casts and, possibly, a few RBCs.
• Urine culture identifies specific bacteria.
• Urine specific gravity and osmolality are low, resulting from a temporarily decreased ability to concentrate urine.
• Urine pH is slightly alkaline.
• Blood chemistry reveals elevated potassium level (TIN).
• KUB radiography may reveal calculi, tumors, or cysts in the kidneys and the urinary tract.
• Kidney biopsy confirms the extent of kidney damage.

NURSING DIAGNOSES
• Impaired urinary elimination
• Hyperthermia
• Fatigue
• Deficient knowledge (disease process; treatment regimen)
• Acute pain

TREATMENT
• Follow-up treatment for antibiotic therapy: reculturing urine 1 week after drug therapy stops and periodically for 1 year after to detect residual or recurring infection
• Dialysis if acute renal failure occurs
• Surgery to relieve obstruction or correct the anomaly responsible for obstruction or vesicoureteral reflux
• Discontinuation of causative drug (TIN)

Drug therapy
• Antibiotics: targeted to specific infecting organism
• Corticosteroid: prednisone (Deltasone) (TIN)
• Antipyretic: acetaminophen (Tylenol)

INTERVENTIONS AND RATIONALES
• Monitor vital signs *to detect fever and hypertension.*
• Monitor intake and output and laboratory studies *to evaluate kidney function.*
• Assess renal status *to determine baseline renal function and detect changes from baseline.*
• Administer antipyretics *to reduce fever.*

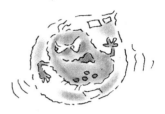

Antibiotic therapy for nephritis targets the specific infecting organism.

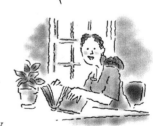

How to survive the big exam? Set goals, have an organized plan of action, and maintain a strong belief in yourself. Stick with it when the going gets tough.

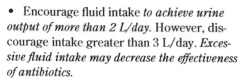

It ain't over till the pill bottle is empty. Emphasize the need to complete the prescribed antibiotic therapy, even after symptoms subside.

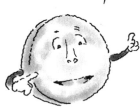

- Encourage fluid intake *to achieve urine output of more than 2 L/day.* However, discourage intake greater than 3 L/day. *Excessive fluid intake may decrease the effectiveness of antibiotics.*
- Provide a diet that contains adequate calcium (500 mg for children up to age 3, 800 mg for school-age children, and 1,300 mg for adolescents), moderately restricts sodium intake and protein, and avoids high doses of vitamin C. *These measures help to prevent renal calculi formation.*

Teaching topics
- Explanation of the disorder and treatment plan
- Medication use and possible adverse effects
- Completing prescribed antibiotic therapy, even after symptoms subside
- Understanding long-term follow-up care for high-risk children

Nephroblastoma

Key assessment finding in nephroblastoma: a nontender mass in the midline area.

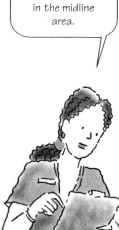

Nephroblastoma, also known as *Wilms' tumor,* is an embryonal cancer of the kidney. It's the most common childhood abdominal malignancy. The average age at diagnosis is 2 to 4 years. The prognosis is excellent if metastasis hasn't occurred.

Nephroblastoma is measured in five stages:
- In stage I, the tumor is limited to the kidney.
- In stage II, the tumor extends beyond the kidney but can be completely excised.
- In stage III, the tumor spreads but is confined to the abdomen and lymph nodes.
- In stage IV, the tumor metastasizes to the lung, liver, bone, brain, or lymph nodes outside the abdomenopelvic region.
- In stage V, bilateral renal involvement occurs.

CAUSES
- Genetic predisposition

ASSESSMENT FINDINGS
- Abdominal pain
- Fever
- Constipation

- Hematuria
- Hypertension
- Nontender mass, usually midline near the liver, that's commonly detected by the parent while bathing or dressing the child
- Associated congenital anomalies, such as microcephaly, mental retardation, and GU tract problems

DIAGNOSTIC TEST RESULTS
- CT scan or sonography reveals tumor, lymph node involvement, and metastasis.
- Abdominal ultrasonography identifies a renal mass and possible renal vein or inferior vena cava thrombosis.
- Serum blood studies show anemia.
- Histologic studies at time of nephreotomy confirm diagnosis.

NURSING DIAGNOSES
- Fear
- Chronic pain
- Anxiety

TREATMENT
- Nephrectomy to remove affected kidney and evaluate remaining kidney; may be preceded by chemotherapy to shrink the tumor if it has extended to the vena cava or if there's bilateral involvement
- Radiation therapy (after surgery): for stages III and IV

Drug therapy
- Analgesics (postoperatively)
- Chemotherapy (after surgery): dactinomycin (Cosmegen), doxorubicin (Doxil), vincristine

INTERVENTIONS AND RATIONALES
- Monitor vital signs and intake and output *to determine fluid volume status.*
- Don't palpate the abdomen, and prevent others from doing so; *palpating the abdomen may cause tumor rupture.*
- Prepare the child and family members for a nephrectomy. *Surgery must be performed quickly after diagnosis to prevent metastasis.*
- After surgery, provide routine care for a nephrectomy client:
  – monitor urine output and report output less than 30 ml/hour

– assist with turning, coughing, and deep breathing
– encourage early ambulation
– provide pain medications as necessary and evaluate their effect
– monitor postoperative dressings for signs of bleeding
– provide wound care as directed.

These measures help to prevent postoperative complications, such as pneumonia, wound infection, and kidney failure.

• Evaluate for adverse effects to chemotherapy and radiation therapy *to provide appropriate interventions.*

Teaching topics

• Explanation of the disorder and treatment plan
• Medication use and possible adverse effects
• Providing adequate nutrition and hydration
• Dealing with adverse reactions to chemotherapy
• Signs and symptoms of metastasis or recurrence
• Signs and symptoms of kidney failure
• Follow-up care
• Contacting support groups

Urinary tract infection

A UTI is a microbial invasion of the kidneys, ureters, bladder, or urethra.

The risk of UTIs varies depending on the child's age and the presence of obstructive uropathy or voiding dysfunction. In the neonatal period, UTIs occur most commonly in males, possibly because of the higher incidence of congenital abnormalities in male neonates. By age 4 months, UTIs are much more common in girls than in boys. The increased incidence in girls continues throughout childhood.

After infancy, nearly all UTIs occur when bacteria enter the urethra and ascend the urinary tract. Females are especially at risk for infection because the female urethra is much shorter than the male urethra. The female urethra is more subject to direct contamination because of its proximity to the anal opening. *Escherichia coli* causes approximately 75% to 90% of all UTIs in females.

When evaluating an infant for a UTI, a lumbar puncture may first be performed to rule out meningitis. Urine specimens for culture should be obtained by sterile straight catheterization.

CAUSES

• Incomplete bladder emptying
• Frequent bubble baths
• Poor hygiene
• Reflux

ASSESSMENT FINDINGS

• Abdominal pain
• Flank tenderness
• Enuresis
• Frequent urges to void with pain or burning on urination
• Hematuria
• Lethargy
• Low-grade fever
• Poor feeding patterns
• Urine that's cloudy and foul-smelling

DIAGNOSTIC TEST RESULTS

• Clean-catch urine culture yields large amounts of bacteria.
• Urine culture identifies specific bacteria.
• Urine pH is increased.

NURSING DIAGNOSES

• Impaired urinary elimination
• Acute pain
• Hyperthermia

TREATMENT

• Increased fluid intake

Drug therapy

• Antibiotics: gentamicin (Garamycin), cefotaxime (Claforan)
• Analgesic: acetaminophen (Tylenol)

INTERVENTIONS AND RATIONALES

• Monitor intake and output *to determine if fluid replacement therapy is adequate.*
• Monitor vital signs to detect fever and increased stress on kidneys as evidenced by elevated blood pressure *to identify complications.*
• Assess toileting habits for proper front-to-back wiping and proper hand washing *to prevent recurrent infection.*

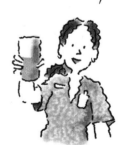

Encourage the client with a UTI to drink fluids. They improve hydration and promote kidney function.

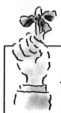

Memory jogger

To remember the clinical findings associated with urinary tract infection, think, "The urinary tract is **FULL** of infection." Look for:

Frequent urges to void

Urine that is foul-smelling and cloudy

Low-grade fever

Lethargy.

• Encourage increased intake of fluids *to keep the child hydrated and promote kidney function.*
• Assist the child when necessary to ensure that the perineal area is clean after elimination. *Cleaning the perineal area by wiping from the area of least contamination (urinary meatus) to the area of greatest contamination (anus) helps prevent UTIs.*

Teaching topics

• Explanation of the disorder and treatment plan
• Medication use and possible adverse effects
• Avoiding bubble baths
• Encouraging the child to use the toilet every 2 hours
• Performing toilet hygiene; including wiping from front to back

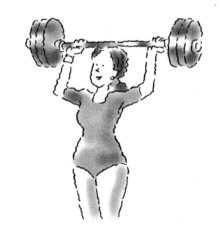

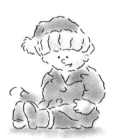

Keep your cool. There's only one more pediatric chapter to go!

Pump up on practice questions

1. A school-age child is diagnosed with acute glomerulonephritis (nephritis). Which nursing action takes priority when caring for this child?
  1. Monitoring blood pressure every 4 hours
  2. Checking urine specific gravity every 8 hours
  3. Offering the child fluids every hour
  4. Providing the child with a regular diet and snacks

Answer: 1. Hypertension is a major complication that can occur during the acute phase of glomerulonephritis; therefore, blood pressure should be monitored at least once every 4 hours. Specific gravity may also be monitored, but it doesn't take priority over blood pressure monitoring. Fluids may be limited and a low-sodium diet initiated if the child is hypertensive.

➡ **NCLEX keys**
Client needs category: Physiological integrity
Client needs subcategory: Reduction of risk potential
Cognitive level: Application

2. A nurse is assessing a young female child who may have a urinary tract infection (UTI). A female child is more susceptible to UTIs than a male because she has:
  1. no pubic hair.
  2. a shorter urethra.
  3. a smaller bladder.
  4. smaller kidneys.

Answer: 2. The female child is more susceptible to UTIs than the male because the female has a shorter urethra, making it easier for organisms to be transmitted into the bladder. The absence of pubic hair is normal in young children; pubic hair growth signals the onset of puberty. A small child voids more frequently because of a small bladder, but this doesn't make the child prone to UTI. The infant's smaller, immature kidneys cause a low glomerular filtration rate but don't make the infant prone to UTI.

➡ **NCLEX keys**
Client needs category: Health promotion and maintenance
Client needs subcategory: None
Cognitive level: Application

3. An infant is admitted to the pediatric unit for surgical repair of hypospadias. The infant's urine output is 7 ml/hr. Which nursing action is most appropriate?
  1. Notify the physician immediately.
  2. Prepare to administer I.V. fluids.
  3. Offer the infant formula every hour.
  4. Continue to monitor urine output.

Answer: 4. The normal urine output for an infant is 5 to 10 ml/hour. The urine output of this infant falls within the normal range;

therefore, the nurse should continue to monitor urine output. It isn't necessary to notify the physician, administer I.V. fluids, or increase the infant's intake.

➡ NCLEX keys

Client needs category: Physiological integrity
Client needs subcategory: Reduction of risk potential
Cognitive level: Application

4.   A nurse must obtain a urine specimen for culture from an infant. The nurse can best obtain a specimen by:
1.   inserting a sterile straight catheter for specimen.
2.   placing the infant on a pediatric bedpan.
3.   inserting an indwelling urinary catheter.
4.   wringing out a cloth diaper after the infant voids.

Answer: 1. A sterile straight catheterization is quick and the most accurate way to obtain a sterile urine specimen from an infant. Placing the infant on a pediatric bedpan, inserting an indwelling urinary catheter, or wringing out a urine-filled cloth diaper aren't appropriate methods of collecting urine specimens for culture in infants.

➡ NCLEX keys

Client needs category: Safe and effective care environment
Client needs subcategory: Safety and infection control
Cognitive level: Application

5.   A nurse is creating a teaching plan for a school-age child with a urinary tract infection (UTI). Which factor should the nurse assess first?
1.   Dietary intake
2.   Toileting habits
3.   Calcium intake
4.   Activity level

Answer: 2. The nurse should assess toileting habits before creating a teaching plan for the school-age child with a UTI. Based on her findings, the nurse should instruct the child in proper front-to-back wiping, hand washing, and toilet use every 2 hours. It isn't necessary to ask about the child's dietary intake, calcium intake, or activity level at this time.

➡ NCLEX keys

Client needs category: Physiological integrity
Client needs subcategory: Reduction of risk potential
Cognitive level: Application

6.   A child is admitted to the pediatric unit with a temperature of 102.5° F (39.2° C), shaking chills, and flank pain. From these assessment findings, the nurse should most likely suspect:
1.   urinary tract infection (UTI).
2.   pyelonephritis.
3.   nephroblastoma.
4.   urolithiasis.

Answer: 2. With pyelonephritis, the child exhibits such assessment findings as temperature of 102° F (38.9° C) or higher, shaking chills, flank pain, urgency, frequency, and burning during urination. The child experiencing a UTI may exhibit low-grade fever, dysuria, frequency, urgency, lethargy, and urine that's cloudy and foul-smelling. The child with a nephroblastoma typically presents with a nontender mass, usually midline near the liver; abdominal pain; hypertension; hematuria; and constipation. The child with urolithiasis presents with colicky flank pain, nausea, vomiting, hematuria, and dysuria.

➡ NCLEX keys

Client needs category: Physiological integrity
Client needs subcategory: Reduction of risk potential
Cognitive level: Analysis

7.   A preschooler is scheduled to have a Wilms' tumor removed. Identify the area of the urinary system where a Wilms' tumor is located.

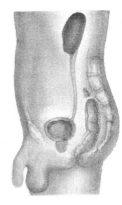

Answer: Wilms' tumor, also known as a *nephroblastoma*, is a tumor located on the kidney. It's most common in children ages 2 to 4.

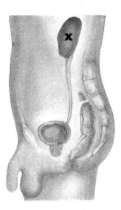

➡ **NCLEX keys**

Client needs category: Physiological integrity
Client needs subcategory: Physiological adaptation
Cognitive level: Application

8. A toddler is admitted to the pediatric unit with a diagnosis of nephroblastoma. When providing routine care for this toddler, the nurse should avoid:
   1. palpating the toddler's abdomen.
   2. positioning the toddler on the side.
   3. bathing the toddler.
   4. loosening the toddler's clothing.

Answer: 1. The nurse shouldn't palpate the toddler's abdomen and should prevent others from doing so because it may disseminate cancer cells to other sites. The toddler may be carefully positioned on his side. The toddler may be bathed but must be handled carefully. The toddler's clothes should be loosened around the abdomen.

➡ **NCLEX keys**

Client needs category: Physiological integrity
Client needs subcategory: Reduction of risk potential
Cognitive level: Application

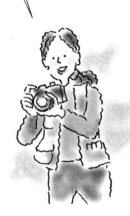

I know you think I'm goofing off, but taking a break and having some fun is also part of preparing for the exam.

9. A parent reports finding a mass in her child's abdomen. After the diagnosis of nephroblastoma is confirmed, the nurse should prepare the child and family for:
   1. immediate chemotherapy.
   2. immediate radiation therapy.
   3. nephrectomy.
   4. discharge to home with hospice care.

Answer: 3. The nurse should prepare the child and family for a nephrectomy, which is usually performed within 24 to 48 hours of diagnosis. Chemotherapy and radiation therapy are typically used as follow-up treatment once the nephrectomy is completed. The prognosis is excellent if there's no metastasis, and the tumor usually remains encapsulated for a long time.

➡ **NCLEX keys**

Client needs category: Physiological integrity
Client needs subcategory: Reduction of risk potential
Cognitive level: Knowledge

10. The nurse is doing discharge teaching with the parents of a neonate with hypospadias. Which statement by the parents indicates a need for further teaching?
   1. "We'll use disposable diapers."
   2. "We'll position him on his back to sleep."
   3. "We'll make sure we bathe him in an infant bathtub."
   4. "We'll have him circumcised by the pediatrician."

Answer: 4. The parents should be instructed to avoid having the neonate circumcised because the foreskin may be needed for surgical repair. The parents would be permitted to use disposable diapers for their neonate. The parents should be instructed to place the neonate on his back to sleep to decrease the risk of sudden infant death syndrome. It's acceptable for the parents to bathe the neonate in an infant bathtub.

➡ **NCLEX keys**

Client needs category: Physiological integrity
Client needs subcategory: Reduction of risk potential
Cognitive level: Application

12 Integumentary system

Brush up on key concepts

The skin, the primary component of the integumentary system, forms a protective barrier between internal structures and the external environment. Tough and resilient, the skin is virtually impermeable to aqueous solutions, bacteria, or toxic compounds.

At any time, you can review the major points of this chapter by consulting the *Cheat sheet* on pages 162 and 163.

Immature at birth

Like most body systems, the integumentary system isn't mature at birth. Therefore, it provides a less effective barrier to physical elements or microorganisms during birth and infancy than during childhood. This factor helps to explain why infants and young children are more prone to infection.

Untouched

The **skin** of infants and young children appears smoother than that of adults. A child's skin has less terminal hair and hasn't been subjected to long-term exposure to environmental elements.

I'm chilly

Infants have poorly developed **subcutaneous fat,** predisposing them to hypothermia. Eccrine sweat glands don't begin to function until the first month of life, which also inhibits the infant's ability to control body temperature.

Adolescent woes

With the onset of adolescence, **apocrine** glands enlarge and become active. This activity leads to axillary sweating and characteristic body odor. The sebaceous glands begin to produce sebum in response to hormone activity, which predisposes the adolescent to acne. Along with the skin glands becoming active, coarse terminal hair grows in the axillae and pubic areas of both sexes and on the faces of males.

Here's the skinny

Skin performs many vital functions. These functions include:
- protecting against trauma
- regulating body temperature
- serving as an organ of excretion and sensation
- synthesizing vitamin D in the presence of ultraviolet light.

Wearing layers

Skin has three primary layers:

✌ The **epidermis** (the outermost layer) produces keratin as its primary function. It contains two sublayers: the stratum corneum, an outer, horny layer of keratin that protects the body against harmful environmental substances and restricts water loss, and the cellular stratum, where keratin cells are synthesized. It also contains melanocytes, which produce the melanin that gives skin its color, and Langerhans cells, which are involved in various immunologic reactions.

✌ The **dermis** (the middle layer) contains collagen, which strengthens the skin to prevent it from tearing, and elastin to give it resilience.

✌ The **subcutaneous tissue** (the innermost layer) consists mainly of fat (containing mostly triglycerides), which provides heat, insulation, shock absorption, and a reserve of calories.

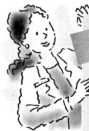

Integumentary refresher

ACNE VULGARIS

Key signs and symptoms

• Closed comedo, or whitehead (acne plug not protruding from the follicle and covered by the epidermis)
• Open comedo, or blackhead (acne plug protruding and not covered by the epidermis)
• Inflammation and characteristic acne pustules, papules or, in severe forms, acne cysts or abscesses (caused by rupture or leakage of an enlarged plug into the dermis)

Key treatments

• Phototherapy with blue and red light
• Oral retinoid: isotretinoin (Accutane) limited to those with nodulocystic or recalcitrant acne who don't respond to conventional therapy; contraindicated during pregnancy
• Systemic therapy: usually tetracycline to decrease bacterial growth; alternatively, erythromycin (tetracycline contraindicated during pregnancy and childhood because it discolors developing teeth)
• Topical medications: benzoyl peroxide (Benzac), clindamycin (Cleocin), or erythromycin (Benzamycin) antibacterial agents, alone or in combination with external retinoids such as tretinoin (Accutane, Retin-A), or a keratolytic

Key interventions

• Try to identify predisposing factors.
• Instruct the adolescent receiving tretinoin to apply it at least 30 minutes after washing the face and at least 1 hour before bedtime. Warn against using it around the eyes or lips. After treatments, the skin should look pink and dry.
• Advise the adolescent to avoid exposure to sunlight or to use a sunblock. If the prescribed regimen includes tretinoin and benzoyl peroxide, tell the adolescent to use one preparation in the morning and the other at night.
• Instruct the adolescent to take tetracycline on an empty stomach and not to take it with antacids or milk.
• Tell the adolescent who's taking isotretinoin to avoid vitamin A supplements. Also discuss how to deal with the dry skin and mucous membranes that usually occur during treatment. Warn the female adolescent about the severe risk of teratogenesis. Monitor liver function and lipid levels.
• Offer emotional support.

BURNS

Key signs and symptoms

Partial-thickness
• Dry, painful skin with edema
• Sunburn appearance
Deep, partial-thickness
• Moist, weeping blisters with edema
• Extreme pain
Full-thickness
• Avascular site without blanching or pain
• Dry, pale, leathery skin

Key test results

• The Lund and Browder chart, a body surface area chart that's corrected for age to determine the extent of injury, estimates extent of the burn.

Key treatments

• I.V. fluids to prevent and treat shock; urine output at 1 to 2 ml/kg
• Protective isolation, depending on burn severity

Key interventions

• Stop the burning in an emergency situation.
• Maintain a patent airway in the immediate postburn phase.
• Monitor vital signs, intake, and output.
• Prevent heat loss.

CONTACT DERMATITIS (DIAPER RASH)

Key signs and symptoms

• Characteristic bright red, maculopapular rash in the diaper area

Key treatments

• Cleaning affected area with mild soap and water
• Leaving affected area open to air
• Zinc oxide or vitamin A ointment

Key interventions

• Keep the diaper area clean and dry.

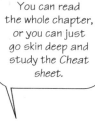

You can read the whole chapter, or you can just go skin deep and study the Cheat sheet.

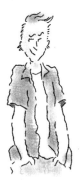

Integumentary refresher *(continued)*

HEAD LICE
Key signs and symptoms
• Pruritus of the scalp
• Presence of lice eggs, which look like white flecks, firmly attached near the base of hair shafts.

Key treatments
• Pyrethrins (RID) or permethrin (Elimite) shampoos or lindane in resistant cases

Key interventions
• Carefully follow the manufacturer's directions when applying medicated shampoo.

IMPETIGO
Key signs and symptoms
• Red, macular rash progressing to a papular and vesicular rash, which oozes and forms a moist, honey-colored crust

Key treatments
• Washing area with soap and water

Key interventions
• Apply antibiotic ointment.
• Wash the area three times daily with soap and water.

RASHES
Key signs and symptoms
• Papular rash: raised solid lesions with color changes in circumscribed areas
• Pustular rash: vesicles and bullae that fill with purulent exudate
• Vesicular rash: small, raised, circumscribed lesions filled with clear fluid

Key test results
• Aspirate from lesions may reveal cause.
• Patch test may identify cause.

Key treatments
• Antibacterial (bacitracin, neomycin [Cortisporin]), antifungal (clotrimazole [Lotrimin], ketaconazole [Nizoral]), or antiviral agent (acyclovir [Zovirax], penciclovir [Denavir]) if infection is cause
• Antihistamine (diphenhydramine [Benadryl]) if the rash is from an allergy

Key interventions
• Maintain contact precautions.
• Keep draining lesions covered.

SCABIES
Key signs and symptoms
• Minute, linear black burrows between fingers and toes and in palms, axillae, and groin

Key test results
• Drop of mineral oil placed over the burrow, followed by superficial scraping and examination of expressed material under a microscope may reveal ova or mite feces.

Key treatments
• Topical application of permethrin 8% cream (Elimite)

Key interventions
• Apply medication as prescribed.
• Teach the child and parents to apply permethrin from the neck down covering the entire body, wait 15 minutes before dressing, and avoid bathing for 8 to 12 hours.

Thinner, more sensitive
A child's skin differs from an adult's in two important ways:
• The child has thinner and more sensitive skin than the adult.
• Irritation in the neonate's skin can result from the sensitivity of the neonate's skin or clogged pores.

Keep abreast of diagnostic tests

Here are the most important tests used to diagnose skin disorders, along with common nursing interventions associated with each test.

Slide show
In **diascopy,** a lesion is covered with a glass slide or piece of clear plastic and pressure is applied. The area is observed to identify purpura (the lesion remains red) or erythema (the lesion blanches).

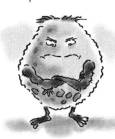

Because a child's skin is thinner and more sensitive than an adult's, it's more prone to infection.

Nursing actions
- Explain the procedure to the child and parents.

Light up and down

Sidelighting shows minor elevations or depressions in lesions; it also helps determine the configuration and degree of eruption.

Subdued lighting, another test, highlights the difference between normal skin and circumscribed lesions that are hypopigmented or hyperpigmented.

Nursing actions
- Explain the procedure to the child and parents.

Spotlight on disease

Microscopic immunofluorescence identifies immunoglobulins and elastic tissue in detecting skin manifestations of immunologically mediated disease.

Nursing actions
- Explain the procedure to the child and parents.

Organism info

Gram stains and exudate cultures help identify organisms responsible for underlying infections.

Nursing actions
- Explain the procedure to the child and parents.
- Obtain cultures as directed by institutional policy.

Patching it together

Patch tests identify contact sensitivity (usually with dermatitis).

Nursing actions
- Explain the procedure to the child and parents.
- Tell the child that the skin area tested will be evaluated 24 to 48 hours after the patch is applied.

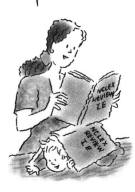

Important nursing actions following skin biopsy include preventing infection, injury, and irritation.

Tissue test

A **skin biopsy** is used to determine the histology of cells. It can be used to diagnose or confirm a disorder.

Nursing actions
Before the procedure
- Explain the procedure to the child and parents.
- Make sure that written, informed consent has been obtained.
After the procedure
- Tell the parents that the child should avoid wool or rough clothing.
- Prevent secondary infections by cutting the child's nails and applying mittens and elbow restraints.
- Suggest the child wear light, loose, nonirritating clothing.

Polish up on client care

Major pediatric skin disorders include acne vulgaris, burns, contact dermatitis (diaper rash), head lice, impetigo, rashes, and scabies.

Acne vulgaris

An inflammatory disease of the sebaceous follicles, acne vulgaris primarily affects adolescents, although lesions can appear as early as age 8. Although acne is more common and more severe in boys, it usually occurs in girls at an earlier age and tends to last longer, sometimes into adulthood. The prognosis is good with treatment.

CAUSES
- Androgen-stimulated sebum production
- Follicular occlusion
- *Propionibacterium acnes,* a normal skin flora

CONTRIBUTING FACTORS
- Androgen stimulation
- Certain drugs, including corticosteroids, corticotropin, androgens, iodides, bromides,

trimethadione (Tridione), phenytoin (Dilantin), isoniazid, lithium (Eskalith), and halothane; cobalt irradiation; or total parenteral nutrition
- Cosmetics
- Exposure to heavy oils, greases, or tars
- Heredity
- Hormonal contraceptives (many females experience acne flare-ups during their first few menses after starting or discontinuing hormonal contraceptives)
- Trauma or rubbing from tight clothing
- Unfavorable climate
- Deficient personal hygiene

ASSESSMENT FINDINGS
- Closed comedo, or whitehead (acne plug not protruding from the follicle and covered by the epidermis)
- Open comedo, or blackhead (acne plug protruding and not covered by the epidermis)
- Inflammation and characteristic acne pustules, papules or, in severe forms, acne cysts or abscesses (caused by rupture or leakage of an enlarged plug into the dermis)
- Acne scars from chronic, recurring lesions

DIAGNOSTIC TEST RESULTS
- Diagnostic testing isn't necessary. The appearance of characteristic acne lesions, especially in an adolescent client, confirms the presence of acne vulgaris.

NURSING DIAGNOSES
- Impaired skin integrity
- Disturbed body image
- Risk for infection

TREATMENT
- Phototherapy with blue and red light
- Exfoliation (mechanical or chemical)

Drug therapy
- Intralesional corticosteroid injection
- Oral retinoid: isotretinoin (Accutane) — limited to those with nodulocystic or recalcitrant acne who don't respond to conventional therapy; contraindicated during pregnancy
- Systemic therapy: usually tetracycline to decrease bacterial growth; alternatively, erythromycin (tetracycline contraindicated

during pregnancy and childhood because it discolors developing teeth)
- Topical medications: benzoyl peroxide (Benzac), clindamycin (Cleocin), or erythromycin (Benzamycin) antibacterial agents; alone or in combination with external retinoids such as tretinoin (Accutane, Retin-A), or a keratolytic
- Antiandrogenic agents: estrogens or spironolactone (Aldactazide)

INTERVENTIONS AND RATIONALES
- Review the adolescent's drug history *because some medications, such as hormonal contraceptives, may cause acne flare-ups.*
- Try to identify predisposing factors *to determine those that can be eliminated or modified.*
- Explain the causes of acne to the adolescent and family. Provide written instructions regarding treatment *to provide education.*
- Instruct the adolescent receiving tretinoin to apply it at least 30 minutes after washing the face and at least 1 hour before bedtime. Warn against using it around the eyes or lips *to prevent damage.* After treatments, the skin should look pink and dry. *If it appears red or starts to peel, the preparation may have to be weakened or applied less often.*
- Advise the adolescent to avoid exposure to sunlight or to use a sunscreen *to prevent a photosensitivity reaction.* If the prescribed regimen includes tretinoin and benzoyl peroxide, tell the adolescent to use one preparation in the morning and the other at night *to avoid skin irritation.*
- Instruct the adolescent to take tetracycline on an empty stomach and not to take it with antacids or milk *because it interacts with their metallic ions and is then poorly absorbed.*
- Tell the adolescent who's taking isotretinoin to avoid vitamin A supplements, *which can worsen adverse effects.* Also discuss how to deal with the dry skin and mucous membranes that usually occur during treatment. Warn the female adolescent about the severe risk of teratogenesis. Monitor liver function and lipid levels *to avoid toxicity.*
- Inform the adolescent that acne takes a long time to clear — possibly even years for complete resolution. Encourage continued local skin care even after acne clears. Explain

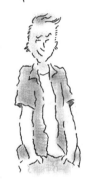

In other words, ZITS!

the adverse effects of all drugs *to promote compliance.*

• Offer emotional support *to help the adolescent cope with the effects of his skin condition.*

• Advise the female adolescent that taking oral antibiotics with hormonal contraceptives may make the contraceptive ineffective.

Teaching topics

• Explanation of the disorder and treatment plan

• Medication use and possible adverse effects

• Avoiding prolonged exposure to sunlight

• Identifying and eliminating predisposing factors, such as cosmetic use and emotional stress

Burns

A burn is tissue damage caused by heat, chemicals, electricity, sunlight, or nuclear radiation. Most pediatric burns occur to children younger than age 5. Overall, burns are the third leading cause of accidental death in children (after motor vehicle accidents and drowning). Burns are classified based on the depth of skin and tissue damage: superficial partial-thickness (first-degree), deep, partial-thickness (second-degree) or full-thickness (third-degree).

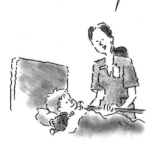

Remember that the Rule of Nines, generally used to determine the extent of a burn, is inaccurate for children. Use the Lund and Browder chart instead.

CAUSES

• Thermal burn: residential fire, motor vehicle accident, playing with matches, improperly stored gasoline, space heater, household accident (such as a child climbing on top of a stove or grabbing a hot iron), excessive exposure to sunlight (sunburn)

• Chemical burn: contact, ingestion, inhalation, or injection of acids, alkalis, or resicants

• Electrical burn: contact with faulty electrical wiring or high-voltage power line, chewing on electric cord

ASSESSMENT FINDINGS
Partial-thickness (first-degree)

• Dry, painful skin with edema

• Sunburn appearance

• Damage limited to the epidermis

Deep, partial-thickness (second-degree)

• Moist, weeping blisters with edema

• Extreme pain

• Damage to the epidermis and part of the dermis

Full-thickness (third-degree)

• Avascular without blanching or pain

• Dry, pale, leathery skin

• Fluid shift from intravascular to interstitial compartments

• Damage to the epidermis and dermis

• Hypovolemia and symptoms of shock from fluid shift, including renal function

• Infection due to altered skin integrity

Fourth-degree burn

• Damage through deeply charred subcutaneous tissue to muscle and bone

DIAGNOSTIC TEST RESULTS

• The Lund and Browder chart, a body surface area chart that's corrected for age to determine the extent of injury, estimates extent of the burn. (The Rule of Nines is inaccurate for children because the head can account for 13% to 19% of body surface area; the legs account for 10% to 16%, depending on the child's age and size.)

NURSING DIAGNOSES

• Deficient fluid volume

• Ineffective airway clearance

• Risk for infection

• Acute pain

• Interrupted family processes

• Disturbed body image

TREATMENT

• Oxygen therapy (may require intubation)

• I.V. fluids to prevent and treat shock; urine output at 1 to 2 ml/kg

• Protective isolation, depending on burn severity

• Total parenteral nutrition

• Debridement

• Escharotomy

• Diet: adequate nutritional support to avoid negative nitrogen balance and prevent overfeeding

• Skin grafting

• Physical and occupational therapy

Drug therapy
- Analgesics: morphine (Arinza), meperidine (Demerol)
- Topical antibiotics: silver sulfadiazine (Silvadene), mafenide acetate (Sulfamylon) to limit infection at the site

INTERVENTIONS AND RATIONALES
- Stop the burning in an emergency situation *to prevent further injury.*
- Maintain a patent airway in the immediate postburn phase; *inhalation of smoke may cause airway edema.*
- Monitor vital signs, intake, and output *to assess for signs of complications.*
- Assess cardiovascular, renal, respiratory, and neurologic status *to assess for signs of shock.*
- Administer I.V. fluids according to recommended rates based on extent of burn damage *to maintain fluid balance.*
- Administer I.V. analgesics *to relieve pain;* don't administer I.M. injections.
- Assist with debridement *to promote healing.*
- Elevate the burned body part *to promote venous drainage and decrease edema.*
- Spread a thin layer of topical medication, such as mafenide acetate, over the burn *to prevent infection.*
- Prevent heat loss *to reduce metabolic demands.*
- Explain treatments, pain management, and the need for the child's active participation in the treatment and offer the child choices, where appropriate, *to help the child feel less afraid and anxious.*
- Encourage family and friends to participate in the child's care when appropriate *to create a loving and supportive atmosphere.*
- Allow the child to participate in everyday activities, such as playing and school activities, *to normalize his situation.*
- Give the child the opportunity to maintain the developmental tasks already achieved, such as eating in a high chair, not using diapers if the child has been toilet-trained, and allowing self-feeding if the child is able, *to prevent regression.*

- Promote a comfortable and loving atmosphere for the child. *This encourages him to talk and act out feelings of depression and hostility and express anxieties.*

Teaching topics
- Explanation of the disorder and treatment plan
- Medication use and possible adverse effects
- Using coping strategies to deal with long-term care
- Understanding burn prevention

Contact dermatitis

Contact dermatitis, also known as *diaper rash,* is a local skin reaction in the areas normally covered by a diaper.

CAUSES
- Irritation caused by acidic urine and fecal enzymes
- Moist, warm environment contained by a plastic diaper lining
- Clothing dyes or the soaps used to wash diapers
- Body soaps, bubble baths, tight clothes, and wool or rough clothing

ASSESSMENT FINDINGS
- Characteristic bright red, maculopapular rash in the diaper area
- Irritability because the rash is painful and warm

DIAGNOSTIC TEST RESULTS
- Diagnostic testing isn't necessary. Diagnosis is based on inspection.

NURSING DIAGNOSES
- Acute pain
- Impaired skin integrity
- Risk for infection

TREATMENT
- Cleaning the affected area with mild soap and water
- Leaving the affected area open to air

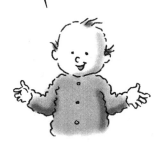

Because contact dermatitis is commonly caused by a moist, warm environment, it makes sense that an important intervention is keeping the area clean, dry, and open to the air.

Drug therapy
• Zinc oxide or vitamin A ointment to help the skin heal
• Antibiotics based on infecting organism if secondary infection occurs: levofloxacin (Levaquin)

INTERVENTIONS AND RATIONALES
• Keep the diaper area clean and dry *to maintain skin integrity.*
• Change the diaper immediately after the child voids or defecates *to prevent skin breakdown.*
• Wash the area with mild soap and water *to promote healing.*
• Keep the area open to the air without plastic bed linings, if possible, *to promote circulation and comfort.*
• Avoid using commercially prepared diaper wipes on broken skin; *the chemicals and alcohol in commercially prepared wipes may be irritating.*

Teaching topics
• Explanation of the disorder and treatment plan
• Medication use and possible adverse effects
• Preventing diaper rash

Head lice

Head lice (pediculosis capitis) are a contagious infestation of lice eggs that are firmly attached near the base of hair shafts. The cause of this disorder isn't related to the hygiene of a child or family members; however, head lice are easily transmitted among children and family members.

CAUSES
• Exposure to lice by sharing clothing, hats, or combs or close physical contact with peers

ASSESSMENT FINDINGS
• Pruritus of the scalp
• Presence of lice eggs, which look like white flecks, firmly attached near the base of hair shafts

DIAGNOSTIC TEST RESULTS
• Diagnostic testing isn't necessary.

NURSING DIAGNOSES
• Disturbed body image
• Impaired skin integrity
• Social isolation

TREATMENT
• Removal of lice and eggs using fine-toothed comb

Drug therapy
• Pyrethrins (RID) or permethrin (Elimite) shampoos; lindane in resistant cases
• Preventive drug therapy for other family members and classmates

INTERVENTIONS AND RATIONALES
• Carefully follow the manufacturer's directions when applying medicated shampoo to avoid neurotoxicity.
• Repeat treatment in 7 to 12 days *to ensure that all the eggs have been killed.*

Teaching topics
• Explanation of disorder and treatment plan
• Medication use and possible adverse effects
• Washing bed linens, hats, combs, brushes, and anything else that came in contact with the hair to prevent reinfestation
• Assessing for reinfestation
• Refraining from exchanging combs, brushes, headgear, or clothing with other children

Impetigo

Impetigo is a highly contagious superficial infection of the skin, marked by patches of tiny blisters that erupt. It's common in children ages 2 to 5. Infection is spread by direct contact; incubation period is 2 to 10 days after contact.

CAUSE
• Staphylococci

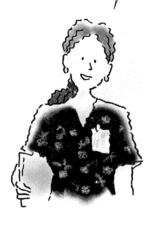

When applying insecticidal treatments, carefully follow the manufacturer's directions to avoid neurotoxicity.

ASSESSMENT FINDINGS

- Red, macular rash that progresses to a papular and vesicular rash, which oozes and forms a moist, honey-colored crust
- Commonly seen on the face and extremities but may spread to other parts of the body by scratching
- Pruritus

DIAGNOSTIC TEST RESULTS

- Diagnostic testing isn't necessary. Diagnosis is based on inspection of skin.

NURSING DIAGNOSES

- Impaired skin integrity
- Risk for infection
- Bathing or hygiene self-care deficit

TREATMENT

- Washing area with soap and water

Drug therapy

- Topical antibiotic ointment
- Systemic antibiotics (in severe cases)

INTERVENTIONS AND RATIONALES

- Apply antibiotic ointment *to eradicate the infection.*
- Wash the area three times daily with soap and water *to promote skin healing.*
- Cover the child's hands, if necessary, *to prevent secondary infection;* cut the child's nails.
- Cover the lesions *to prevent their spread.*

Teaching topics

- Explanation of the disorder and treatment plan
- Medication use and possible adverse effects
- Preventing recurrence

Rashes

A rash is a temporary skin eruption. Three types of rashes — papular, pustular, and vesicular — are described below.

A *papular rash* may erupt anywhere on the body in various configurations and may be acute or chronic. Papular rashes characterize many cutaneous disorders; they may also result from allergy or infectious, neoplastic, or systemic disorders. Common causes of papular rashes in children are infectious diseases, such as molluscum and scarlet fever; scabies; insect bites; allergies or drug reactions; and miliaria.

A *pustular rash* is made up of crops of pustules that fill with purulent exudate. These lesions vary greatly in size and shape and can be generalized or localized to the hair follicles or sweat glands. Pustules appear in skin and systemic disorders, with use of certain drugs, and with exposure to skin irritants. Disorders that produce pustular rash in children include erythema toxicum neonatorum and impetigo. Pustules typify the inflammatory lesions of acne vulgaris, common in adolescents.

A *vesicular rash* is a scattered or linear distribution of vesicles. A vesicular rash may be mild or severe and temporary or permanent. It may result from infection, inflammation, or allergic reactions. Vesicular rashes in children are caused by staphylococcal infections, varicella, hand-foot-mouth disease, and miliaria.

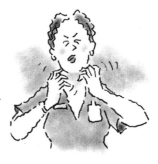

Insidious infectious itch! Impetigo rash may be spread to other parts of the body by scratching.

CAUSES

- Allergic reactions
- Environmental causes
- Viral, fungal, or bacterial infestations

ASSESSMENT FINDINGS

- Papular rash: raised solid lesions with color changes in circumscribed areas
- Pustular rash: vesicles and bullae that fill with purulent exudate
- Vesicular rash: small, raised, circumscribed lesions filled with clear fluid

DIAGNOSTIC TEST RESULTS

- Aspirate from lesions may reveal cause.
- Patch test may identify cause.

NURSING DIAGNOSES

- Impaired skin integrity
- Risk for infection
- Disturbed body image

TREATMENT

- Antibacterial (bacitracin, neomycin [Cortisporin]), antifungal (clotrimazole [Lotrimin], ketaconazole [Nizoral]) or antiviral agent (acyclovir [Zovirax], penciclovir [Denavir]) if infection is cause

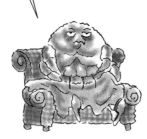

I like to make myself at home. Scabies mites can live their entire lives in human skin, causing chronic infection.

• Antihistamine (diphenhydramine [Benadryl]) if the rash is from an allergy and to decrease pruritis

INTERVENTIONS AND RATIONALES
• Keep the area cool. *Heat aggravates most skin rashes and increases pruritus; coolness decreases pruritus.*
• Keep the affected area clean and pat it dry *to promote healing.*
• Don't apply powder or cornstarch *because these agents encourage bacterial growth.*
• Maintain contact precautions *to prevent the spread of infection.*
• Keep draining lesions covered *to prevent transmission.*

Teaching topics
• Explanation of the disorder and treatment plan
• Medication use and possible adverse effects
• Understanding sanitary techniques
• Avoiding sharing combs or hats
• Avoiding scratching
• Avoiding puncturing vesicles or pustules with needles or hands

Scabies

Scabies is a parasitic skin disorder that causes severe itching. Scabies develops when microscopic itch mites enter a child's skin and provoke a sensitivity reaction. Mites can live their entire lives inside human skin, causing chronic infection. The female mite burrows into the skin to lay her eggs, from which larvae emerge to copulate and then reburrow under the skin. Scabies is transmitted through the skin or through sexual contact.

CAUSES
• Female mite that burrows into the skin and deposits eggs in areas that are thin and moist

ASSESSMENT FINDINGS
• Minute, linear black burrows between fingers and toes and in palms, axillae, and groin
• Severe itching

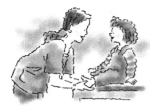

Severe itching marks scabies infestation. Linear black mite burrows may be visible between the fingers and toes or on the palms, axillae, and groin.

DIAGNOSTIC TEST RESULTS
• Drop of mineral oil placed over the burrow, followed by superficial scraping and examination of expressed material under a microscope may reveal ova or mite feces.

NURSING DIAGNOSES
• Disturbed body image
• Impaired skin integrity
• Social isolation

TREATMENT
• Treatment for all members of the family (as well as close contacts of the child)

Drug therapy
• Topical application of permethrin (Elimite) 8% cream

INTERVENTIONS AND RATIONALES
• Apply medication as prescribed *to promote healing.*
• Wash the area thoroughly with soap and water *to promote healing.*
• Teach the child and parents to apply permethrin from the neck down covering the entire body, wait 15 minutes before dressing, and avoid bathing for 8 to 12 hours *to ensure effectiveness of therapy.*
• Explain to the child and parents that if skin irritation or an allergic reaction develops, they should notify the physician immediately, stop using the cream, and wash it off thoroughly *to avoid risk of an anaphylactic reaction.*

Teaching topics
• Explanation of the disorder and treatment plan
• Medication use and possible adverse effects
• Understanding that pruritus may persist for several weeks after treatment
• Practicing proper hygiene measures
• Changing bed linens, towels, and clothing after bathing and lotion application
• Understanding the need to treat family members and close contacts because the parasite is transmitted by close personal contact and through clothes and linens
• Understanding that the length of time between infestation and physical symptoms may be 30 to 60 days

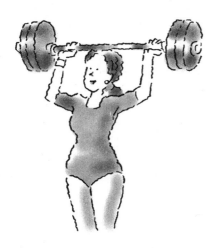

Pump up on practice questions

1. The clothes of a 16-year-old girl catch fire while she's lighting the grill for a family picnic. The girl's mother, a nurse, tells her to drop and roll to extinguish the flames. Which action should the nurse take next?

1. Move her daughter away from the grill.
2. Remove her daughter's clothing.
3. Use the garden hose to wet her daughter down.
4. Call the fire department.

Answer: 3. In emergency burn care, the priority is to stop the burning. The client shouldn't be moved because flames may intensify. Once the fire is extinguished, the client's clothes should be removed to prevent further injury. Emergency medical personnel should be summoned after the flames are extinguished.

➡ NCLEX keys

Client needs category: Physiological integrity
Client needs subcategory: Reduction of risk potential
Cognitive level: Application

2. A child has full-thickness burns of the hands, face, and chest. Which nursing diagnosis takes priority?

1. *Ineffective airway clearance related to edema*
2. *Disturbed body image related to physical appearance*
3. *Impaired urinary elimination related to fluid loss*
4. *Infection related to epidermal disruption*

Answer: 1. Initially, when a client is admitted to the hospital for burns, the primary focus is on assessing and managing an effective airway. Body image disturbance, impaired urinary elimination, and infection are all integral parts of burn management but aren't the first priority.

➡ NCLEX keys

Client needs category: Physiological integrity
Client needs subcategory: Physiological adaptation
Cognitive level: Analysis

3. A nurse is caring for a child with deep, partial-thickness and full-thickness burns. Which analgesic would most effectively manage the client's severe pain?

1. Acetaminophen administered by suppository
2. Meperidine administered I.M.
3. Codeine administered by mouth
4. Morphine administered I.V.

Answer: 4. A client with severe burns requires strong analgesia. The most effective method of administering analgesics is the I.V. route. Deep partial-thickness burns are commonly too painful to be relieved by acetaminophen. I.M. medication may not be absorbed when the client is physiologically unstable. Codeine may not provide sufficient analgesia, and oral administration usually isn't the best route for severe burn victims.

➡ NCLEX keys

Client needs category: Physiological integrity
Client needs subcategory: Pharmacological and parenteral therapies
Cognitive level: Application

To keep up your motivation for studying, remember the big picture. Conquering the exam is one of the keys to fulfilling life goals you have chosen for yourself.

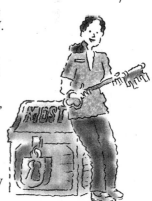

4. A 14-month-old infant is in a private room for treatment of burns. Which intervention can best meet the child's developmental needs?

1. Ask the mother to room with the child.
2. Have nursing personnel visit the child regularly throughout the day.
3. Set the television to the child's favorite cartoon shows.
4. Attach a brightly colored balloon to the child's crib.

Answer: 1. The mother can best provide for the child's developmental needs by being present all of the time. At this age, the child is most susceptible to separation anxiety. A child of this age is likely to be apprehensive toward unfamiliar adults, so regular visits by nursing personnel wouldn't help. Television is a poor substitute for human contact. A balloon is dangerous for a child this age.

➠ NCLEX keys

Client needs category: Health promotion and maintenance
Client needs subcategory: None
Cognitive level: Application

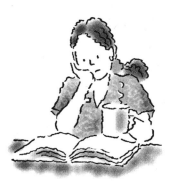

5. A 13-year-old adolescent has received third-degree burns over 20% of his body. When performing an assessment 72 hours after the burn, which finding should the nurse expect?

1. Increasing urine output
2. Severe peripheral edema
3. Respiratory distress
4. Absent bowel sounds

Answer: 1. During the resuscitative-emergent phase of a burn, fluid shifts back into the interstitial space resulting in the onset of diuresis. Edema resolves during the emergent phase, when fluid shifts back to the intravascular space. Respiratory rate increases during the first hours as a result of edema. When edema resolves, respirations return to normal. Absent bowel sounds occur in the initial stage.

➠ NCLEX keys

Client needs category: Physiological integrity
Client needs subcategory: Physiological adaptation
Cognitive level: Analysis

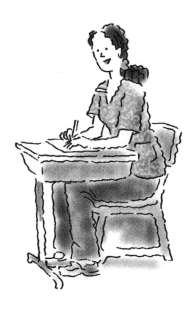

6. A child comes into the emergency department with a rash that's raised and has color changes in circumscribed areas. What type of rash should the nurse document?

1. Macular rash
2. Papular rash
3. Petechial rash
4. Vesicular rash

Answer: 2. A papular rash contains raised solid lesions with color changes in circumscribed areas. A macular rash is flat with color changes in circumscribed areas. Petechiae are pinpoint purple or red spots on the skin caused by minute hemorrhages. A vesicular rash contains small, raised circumscribed lesions filled with clear fluid.

➡ NCLEX keys
Client needs category: Physiological integrity
Client needs subcategory: Reduction of risk potential
Cognitive level: Comprehension

7. The nurse is developing a teaching plan for the mother of a neonate. The nurse should instruct the mother to prevent diaper rash by:
   1. using disposable diapers so she doesn't have to change the infant often.
   2. bathing the infant in a tub with bubble bath.
   3. not washing the infant with soap.
   4. keeping the infant's diaper area clean and dry.

Answer: 4. The mother should be instructed to keep the infant's diaper area clean and dry; to change the diaper immediately after the infant voids or defecates; to avoid bubble bath; and to wash the diaper area with mild soap and water with every diaper change.

➡ NCLEX keys
Client needs category: Health promotion and maintenance
Client needs subcategory: None
Cognitive level: Application

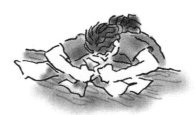

8. A mother calls the pediatrician's office because there's an outbreak of scabies at her child's day-care center. The nurse should instruct the mother to check her child for which findings associated with scabies infestation?
   1. Pruritic papules, pustules, and linear burrows of the fingers and toe webs
   2. Oval white dots adhered to the hair shafts
   3. Diffuse pruritic wheals

   4. Pain, erythema, and edema at the site of the bite

Answer: 1. The mother should be instructed to check her child for pruritic papules, vesicles, and linear burrows. Oval flecks on the hair shaft indicate head lice. Diffuse pruritic wheals can indicate an allergic reaction. The specific site of the bite reveals no trace of the insect bite.

➡ NCLEX keys
Client needs category: Health promotion and maintenance
Client needs subcategory: None
Cognitive level: Application

9. A 16-month-old infant is being treated with permethrin (Elimite) for scabies. The infant's mother is concerned that the drug hasn't been effective because her child continues to scratch. Which response by the nurse is most appropriate?
   1. Stop treatment because the drug isn't safe for children younger than age 2.
   2. Tell the mother that pruritus can be present for weeks after treatment.
   3. Apply the drug every day until the rash disappears.
   4. Tell the mother that pruritus is common in children younger than age 5 treated with permethrin.

Answer: 2. Pruritus may be present for weeks in the child treated with permethrin for scabies. The drug is safe for use in infants as young as age 2 months. Treatment with permethrin can safely be repeated in 2 weeks. Pruritus is caused by secondary reactions of mites.

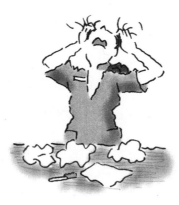

➡ NCLEX keys

Client needs category: Physiological integrity
Client needs subcategory: Pharmacological
and parenteral therapies
Cognitive level: Application

10. A child is diagnosed with head lice and
the mother asks how she should get the nits
out of her child's hair. The nurse should tell
the mother that:
1. the treatment should be repeated in
7 to 12 days.
2. combing the hair after shampooing
is necessary.
3. treatment should be repeated every
day for 7 days.
4. all children that had contact with
the child should be prophylactically
treated.

Answer: 1. Treatment should be repeated in
7 to 12 days to ensure that all of the eggs have
been killed. Combing the hair thoroughly
isn't necessary to remove lice eggs. People
exposed should be observed for infestation
before being treated.

➡ NCLEX keys

Client needs category: Physiological integrity
Client needs subcategory: Reduction of risk
potential
Cognitive level: Application

I'm just itching to
answer more practice
questions. In addition
to the questions that
follow, don't forget to
pump up on practice
questions available for
free on the Web site.

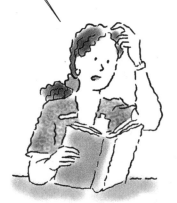

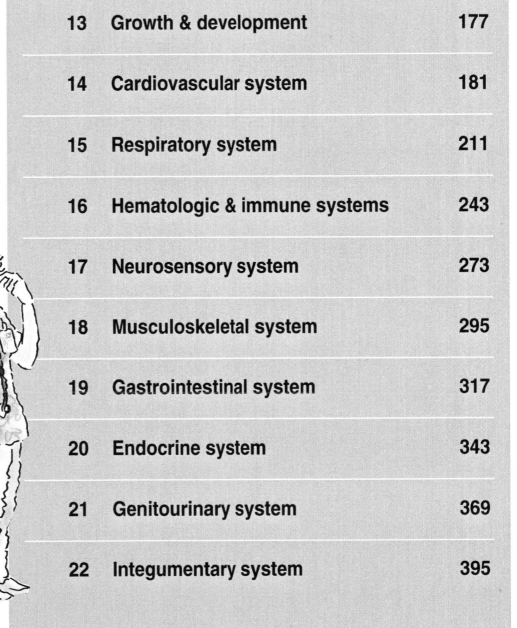

Part III   Questions & answers

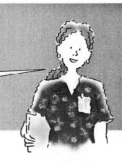

Here's a short but important chapter that covers growth and development of children. Enjoy!

Chapter 13
Growth & development

1. A mother tells a nurse that her 22-month-old child says "no" to everything. When scolded, the toddler becomes angry and starts crying loudly but then immediately wants to be held. What is the best interpretation of this behavior?
   1. The toddler isn't effectively coping with the stress.
   2. The toddler's need for affection isn't being met.
   3. This is normal behavior for a 2-year-old child.
   4. This behavior suggests the need for counseling.

2. The mother of a 12-month-old infant expresses concern about the effect of frequent thumb sucking on her child's teeth. After the nurse teaches her about this matter, which response by the mother indicates that the teaching has been effective?
   1. "Thumb sucking should be discouraged at 12 months."
   2. "I'll give the baby a pacifier instead."
   3. "Sucking is important to the baby."
   4. "I'll wrap the thumb in a bandage."

3. An adolescent client has just had surgery and has a dressing on the abdomen. Which question should the nurse expect the client to ask initially?
   1. "Did the surgery go OK?"
   2. "Will I have a large scar?"
   3. "What complications can I expect?"
   4. "When can I return to school?"

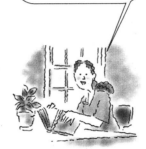

Question 1 wants you to read the rest, but go with the best.

1. 3. Toddlers are confronted with the conflict of achieving autonomy yet relinquishing the much-enjoyed dependence on—and affection of—others. As a result, their negativism is a necessary part of their growth and development. Nothing about this behavior indicates that the child is under stress, isn't receiving sufficient affection, or requires counseling.
CN: Health promotion and maintenance; CNS: None; CL: Analysis

2. 3. Sucking is the infant's chief pleasure. However, thumb sucking can cause malocclusion if it persists after age 4. Many fetuses begin sucking their fingers in utero and, as infants, refuse a pacifier as a substitute. A young child is likely to chew on a bandage, which could lead to airway obstruction.
CN: Health promotion and maintenance; CNS: None; CL: Analysis

3. 2. Adolescents are deeply concerned about their body image and how they appear to others. An adolescent wouldn't ask how the surgery went or what complications to expect, although an adult probably would. Although an adolescent may be curious as to when he can return to school, it probably wouldn't be his primary concern.
CN: Health promotion and maintenance; CNS: None; CL: Application

CN: Client needs category   CNS: Client needs subcategory   CL: Cognitive level

4. For an 8-month-old infant, the nurse should plan to provide which toy to promote the child's cognitive development?
   1. Blocks to stack
   2. Jack-in-the-box
   3. Small rubber ball
   4. Play gym strung across the crib

5. A 14-month-old is admitted to the pediatric unit with a diagnosis of croup. Which characteristics would the nurse expect the toddler to demonstrate if he's developing normally? Select all that apply:
   1. Strong hand grasp
   2. Tendency to hold one object while looking for another
   3. Recognition of familiar voices (smiles in recognition)
   4. Presence of Moro reflex
   5. Weight that's triple his birth weight
   6. Closed anterior fontanel

6. Which comment by a 7-year-old boy to his friend best typifies his developmental stage?
   1. "Girls are so yucky."
   2. "My mommy and I are always together."
   3. "I can't decide if I like Amy or Heather better."
   4. "I can turn into Batman when I come out of my closet."

7. A nurse should expect a 3-year-old child to be able to perform which action?
   1. Ride a tricycle
   2. Tie shoelaces
   3. Roller skate
   4. Jump rope

You had better treat me with "kid" gloves.

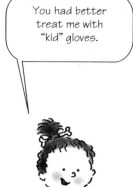

4. 2. According to Piaget's theory of cognitive development, an 8-month-old child will look for an object after it disappears from sight to develop the cognitive skill of object permanence. Stacking blocks and small balls are inappropriate because infants frequently put their fingers or objects into their mouth. Anything strung across an infant's crib is a safety hazard, especially to a child who may use it to pull to a standing position.
CN: Health promotion and maintenance; CNS: None; CL: Application

5. 1, 2, 3, 5. A strong hand grasp is demonstrated within the first month of life. Holding one object while looking for another is accomplished by the 20th week. Within the first year of life, the toddler masters smiling at familiar faces and voices, the toddler's birth weight triples, and the Moro reflex disappears. The anterior fontanel closes at approximately age 18 months.
CN: Health promotion and maintenance; CNS: None; CL: Application

6. 1. During the school-age years, the most important social interactions typically are those with peers. Peer-to-peer interactions lead to the formation of intimate friendships between same-sex children. Friendships with opposite-sex children are uncommon. At this age, children socialize more frequently with friends than with parents. Interest in peers of the opposite sex generally doesn't begin until ages 10 to 12. Magical thinking and fantasy play are more characteristic during the preschool years.
CN: Health promotion and maintenance; CNS: None; CL: Application

7. 1. At age 3, gross motor development and refinement in hand-eye coordination enable a child to ride a tricycle. The fine motor skills required to tie shoelaces and the gross motor skills required for roller-skating and jumping rope develop around age 5.
CN: Health promotion and maintenance; CNS: None; CL: Application

CN: Client needs category   CNS: Client needs subcategory   CL: Cognitive level

8. A 6-month-old infant is admitted to the pediatric unit for a 2-week course of antibiotics. His parents can visit only on weekends. Which action indicates that the nurse understands the infant's emotional needs?

1. The nurse places the infant in a four-bed unit.
2. The nurse places the infant in a room away from other children.
3. The nurse assigns the infant to a different nurse each day.
4. The nurse assigns the infant to the same nurse as often as possible.

9. A term neonate weighs 7½ lb (3 kg) at birth. When he's 1 year old, approximately how much should he weigh?

1. 16 lb (7.3 kg)
2. 22 lb (10 kg)
3. 28 lb (12.7 kg)
4. 32 lb (14.5 kg)

10. Which behavior by a preschool child indicates that the child is in the appropriate stage of growth and development?

1. He cries in protest when his mother leaves.
2. He asks for a bandage after having blood drawn.
3. He's upset about having a scar after surgery.
4. He wants to know why his friends don't visit.

11. A nurse observes parents playing with their 10-month-old daughter. Which behavior indicates that the infant is developing object permanence?

1. She looks for the toy that her parents hid under the blanket.
2. She returns the play blocks to the same spot on the table.
3. She recognizes that a ball of clay is the same object even when it's flattened out.
4. She bangs two cubes in her hands and throws them to the floor.

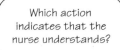

Which action indicates that the nurse understands?

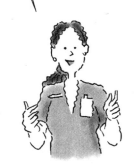

8. 4. Building a sense of trust is crucial with an infant at this stage of growth and development. Consistent caregivers will promote a sense of trust. Placing him in a four-bed unit isn't the best choice because a 6-month-old child doesn't play with other children. Placing him in a room away from other children would isolate him from others, which is neither necessary nor helpful.

CN: Health promotion and maintenance; CNS: None; CL: Application

9. 2. A term neonate who weighs 7½ lb at birth should triple his birth weight by age 1 year; therefore, he should weigh approximately 22 to 23 pounds. A weight of 16 pounds is roughly a doubling of birth weight, which should occur by 6 months. A weight of 28 or 32 pounds indicates a gain that exceeds three times the birth weight.

CN: Health promotion and maintenance; CNS: None; CL: Analysis

10. 2. A preschooler typically asks for a bandage after having blood drawn because he has poorly defined body boundaries and believes he will lose all of his blood from the hole the needle has made. A toddler cries in protest when the parent leaves. An adolescent might be upset about a surgical scar because he's concerned about body image. A school-age child might ask why his friends don't visit because peers become important by that age.

CN: Heath promotion and maintenance; CNS: None; CL: Analysis

11. 1. Object permanence is exhibited by the infant looking for objects that have been hidden from sight. Returning the blocks to the same spot on the table is imitative behavior. Recognizing that a ball of clay is the same object even when flattened out is an example of the theory of conservation, which occurs in early-school-age children. Banging two cubes in her hands and throwing them to the floor is normal behavior for a 10-month old but doesn't indicate object permanence.

CN: Health promotion and maintenance; CNS: None; CL: Application

12. A nurse is teaching the parents of a 6-month-old infant about age-specific growth and development. Which statement is true regarding infant development? Select all that apply:

1. A 6-month-old infant has trouble holding objects.
2. A 6-month-old infant can usually roll from prone to supine and supine to prone positions.
3. A teething ring is appropriate for a 6-month-old infant.
4. Head lag is commonly noted in infants at age 6 months.
5. Lack of visual coordination usually resolves by age 6 months.

12. 2, 3, 5. Gross motor skills of the 6-month-old infant include rolling from front to back and back to front. Teething usually begins around age 6 months and, therefore, a teething ring is appropriate. Visual coordination is usually resolved by age 6 months. At age 6 months, fine motor skills include purposeful grasps. The 6-month-old infant should have good head control and should no longer display head lag when pulled up to a sitting position.

CN: Health promotion and maintenance; CNS: None; CL: Application

13. A nurse is conducting a physical examination on an infant. Identify the anatomical landmark she should use to measure chest circumference.

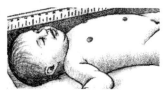

13. Chest circumference is most accurately measured by placing the measuring tape

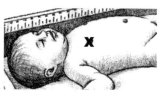

around the infant's chest with the tape covering the nipples. If measured above or below the nipples, a false measurement is obtained.

CN: Health promotion and maintenance; CNS: None; CL: Application

14. The nurse is examining the breasts of an adolescent girl. She classifies her sexual maturity as Tanner stage 3. Which graphic depicts this stage?

1.

2.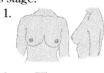

3.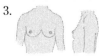

4.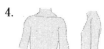

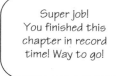

Super job! You finished this chapter in record time! Way to go!

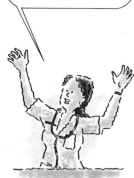

14. 2. In Tanner stage 3, the entire breast enlarges and the nipple doesn't protrude. Option 1 shows Tanner stage 5: an adult breast has developed, the nipple protrudes, and the areola no longer appears separate from the breast. Option 3 shows Tanner stage 4: the breast enlarges and the nipple and papilla protrude and appear as a secondary mound. Option 4 shows Tanner stage 2: breast buds appear and the areola is slightly widened and appears as a small mound.

CN: Physiological integrity; CNS: Reduction of risk potential; CL: Application

CN: Client needs category   CNS: Client needs subcategory   CL: Cognitive level

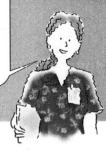

You've reached our test on cardiovascular disorders in children. Before taking this comprehensive test, why not bolster yourself with a heart-healthy snack of celery and low-fat cream cheese? Yum!

Chapter 14
Cardiovascular system

1. A nurse is performing a cardiac assessment on a 2-year-old. The first heart sound (S₁) can best be heard at which location?
1. Third or fourth intercostal space
2. The apex with the stethoscope bell
3. Second intercostal space, midclavicular line
4. Fifth intercostal space, left midclavicular line

2. The nurse auscultates the first heart sound, interpreting this sound as occurring:
1. late in diastole.
2. early in diastole.
3. with closure of the mitral and tricuspid valves.
4. with closure of the aortic and pulmonic valves.

3. A nurse is performing a cardiac assessment on a child. Which characteristic would indicate a diagnosis of a grade 1 heart murmur?
1. The murmur is equal to the heart sounds.
2. The murmur is softer than the heart sounds.
3. The murmur can be heard with the naked ear.
4. The murmur is associated with a precordial thrill.

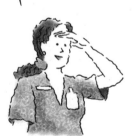

You might have a lot of questions ahead of you, but I know you can do it!

1. 4. The S₁ can best be heard at the fifth intercostal space, left midclavicular line. The fourth heart sound can be heard at the third or fourth intercostal space. The third heart sound is heard with the stethoscope bell at the apex of the heart. The second heart sound is heard at the second intercostal space.
CN: Health promotion and maintenance; CNS: None; CL: Application

2. 3. The S₁ occurs during systole with closure of the mitral and tricuspid valves. The fourth heart sound is heard late in diastole and may be a normal finding in children. The third heart sound is heard early in diastole. The second heart sound occurs during diastole with closure of the aortic and pulmonic valves.
CN: Health promotion and maintenance; CNS: None; CL: Analysis

3. 2. A grade 1 heart murmur is commonly difficult to hear and softer than the heart sounds. A grade 2 murmur is usually equal to the heart sounds. A grade 6 murmur can be heard with the naked ear or with the stethoscope off the chest. A grade 4 murmur is associated with a precordial thrill. A thrill is a palpable manifestation associated with a loud murmur.
CN: Health promotion and maintenance; CNS: None; CL: Analysis

CN: Client needs category   CNS: Client needs subcategory   CL: Cognitive level

4. A graduate nurse has started working in a pediatric intensive care unit. She's measuring the client's cardiac output. To understand cardiac output, the nurse must know that stroke volume is the:

1. volume of blood returning to the heart.
2. ability of the cardiac muscle to act as an efficient pump.
3. resistance the ventricles pump against when ejecting blood.
4. amount of blood ejected by the heart in any one contraction.

5. A child is diagnosed with cardiogenic shock. Which condition would the nurse expect to occur with this child?

1. Decreased cardiac output
2. A reduction in circulating blood volume
3. Overwhelming sepsis and circulating bacterial toxins
4. Inflow or outflow obstruction of the main bloodstream

6. Which sign is considered a late sign of shock in children?

1. Tachycardia
2. Hypotension
3. Delayed capillary refill
4. Pale, cool, mottled skin

7. Which factor indicating a cardiac defect might be found when assessing a 1-month-old?

1. Weight gain
2. Hyperactivity
3. Poor nutritional intake
4. Pink mucous membranes

8. A 2-year-old child is showing signs of shock. A 10-ml/kg bolus of normal saline solution is ordered. The child weighs 20 kg. How many milliliters should be administered?

1. 20 ml
2. 100 ml
3. 200 ml
4. 2,000 ml

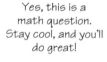

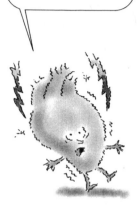

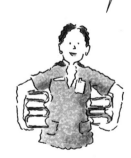

4. 4. Stroke volume is the amount of blood ejected by the heart in any one contraction. It's influenced by preload, afterload, and contractility. Preload is the amount of blood returning to the heart. Contractility is the ability of the cardiac muscle to act as an efficient pump. Afterload is the resistance the ventricles pump against when ejecting blood.

CN: Physiological integrity; CNS: Physiological adaptation; CL: Application

5. 1. *Cardiogenic shock* occurs when cardiac output is decreased and tissue oxygen needs aren't adequately met. *Hypovolemic shock* is a reduction in circulating blood volume. *Septic shock* is overwhelming sepsis and circulating bacterial toxins. *Obstructive shock* is an inflow or outflow obstruction of the main bloodstream.

CN: Physiological integrity; CNS: Physiological adaptation; CL: Application

6. 2. Hypotension is considered a late sign of shock in children. This represents a decompensated state and impending cardiopulmonary arrest. Tachycardia; delayed capillary refill; and pale, cool, mottled skin are earlier indicators of shock that may show compensation.

CN: Physiological integrity; CNS: Physiological adaptation; CL: Analysis

7. 3. Infants and children with heart defects tend to have poor nutritional intake and weight loss, indicating poor cardiac output, heart failure, or hypoxemia. The child appears lethargic or tired because of the heart failure or hypoxia. Pink, moist mucous membranes are normal.

CN: Health promotion and maintenance; CNS: None; CL: Analysis

8. 3. The correct formula for this calculation is 10 ml/kg × 20 kg. The correct answer is 200 ml. The other options are incorrect.

CN: Physiological integrity; CNS: Pharmacological and parenteral therapies; CL: Analysis

CN: Client needs category   CNS: Client needs subcategory   CL: Cognitive level

9. Which of the following arrhythmias is <u>commonly</u> found in neonates and infants?
1. Atrial fibrillation
2. Bradyarrhythmias
3. Premature atrial contractions
4. Premature ventricular contractions

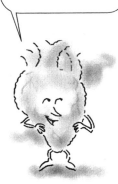

Pick an arrhythmia, any correct arrhythmia.

9. 3. Premature atrial contractions are common in fetuses, neonates, and children. They occur from increased automaticity of an atrial cell anywhere except the sinoatrial node. Atrial fibrillation is an uncommon arrhythmia in children occurring from a disorganized state of electrical activity in the atria. Bradyarrhythmias are usually congenital, surgically acquired, or caused by infection. Premature ventricular contractions are more common in adolescents.
CN: Physiological integrity; CNS: Physiological adaptation; CL: Analysis

10. A nurse is reviewing the waveforms of an electrocardiogram of an infant with a nursing student. The nurse will tell the student that which waveform indicates ventricular depolarization and contraction?
1. P wave
2. PR interval
3. QRS complex
4. T wave

10. 3. The QRS complex reflects ventricular depolarization and contraction. The P wave represents atrial depolarization and contraction. The PR interval represents the time it takes an impulse to trace from the atrioventricular node to the bundle of His. The T wave represents repolarization of the ventricles.
CN: Physiological integrity; CNS: Reduction of risk potential; CL: Application

11. Which evaluation of cardiovascular status is noninvasive?
1. Transthoracic echocardiogram
2. Cardiac enzyme levels
3. Cardiac catheterization
4. Transesophageal pacing

11. 1. A transthoracic echocardiogram is a noninvasive procedure to visualize the anatomy of the heart. Blood testing determines cardiac enzyme levels. Cardiac catheterization involves passing a catheter into the chambers of the heart for direct visualization of the heart and great vessels. Transesophageal pacing requires a probe to be placed in the esophagus for high-frequency ultrasound.
CN: Physiological integrity; CNS: Reduction of risk potential; CL: Analysis

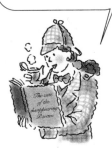

I think I detect the correct statement.

12. Which statement about using an echocardiogram to evaluate cardiac function in a child is the <u>most</u> correct?
1. The child must be sedated in order to get an accurate result.
2. It uses sound waves to measure and evaluate cardiac structures and function.
3. The transthoracic method of echocardiogram is an invasive procedure.
4. It is the most definitive method of evaluating cardiac function.

12. 2. Echocardiograms use sound waves to measure and evaluate cardiac structures and function. The transthoracic method is not an invasive procedure; however, the transesophageal method is considered invasive. The child does not have to be sedated, but lying quietly is preferred. While an echocardiogram gives the physician a good idea of cardiac function, a cardiac catheterization is the definitive method for a complete and accurate picture.
CN: Physiological integrity; CNS: Reduction of risk potential; CL: Application

13. Before a cardiac catheterization, which intervention is <u>most appropriate</u> for a child and his parents?
1. Supplying a map of the hospital
2. Limiting visitors to parents only
3. Offering a guided tour of the hospital and catheterization laboratory
4. Explaining that the child can't eat or drink for 1 to 2 days postoperatively

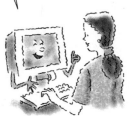

What can you do to ease the family's fears?

14. The nurse is teaching the parents of a child who is scheduled for a cardiac catheterization. Which statement by the nurse is the most accurate regarding cardiac catheterization?
1. It's a noninvasive procedure.
2. General anesthesia is required.
3. It uses high-frequency sound waves to produce an image of the heart in motion.
4. It provides visualization of the heart and great vessels with radiopaque dye.

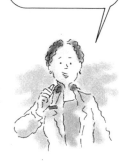

You've already answered 15 questions! See how time flies when you're taking a test?

15. Which nursing intervention is <u>most appropriate</u> when caring for a child in the immediate postcatheterization phase?
1. Elevate the head of the bed 45 degrees.
2. Encourage the child to remain flat.
3. Assess vital signs every 2 to 4 hours.
4. Replace a bloody groin dressing with a new dressing.

16. Which home care instruction is included for a child postcatheterization?
1. The child should drink fluids and eat a regular diet.
2. The child may participate in sports once home.
3. The child can routinely bathe after returning home.
4. The child may return to school the next day.

13. 3. A guided tour will help minimize fears and allay anxieties for the child and parents. It gives the opportunity for questions and teaching. A map of the hospital is helpful, but a tour provides the family with more information. Visitors should include all significant others and siblings as part of the preoperative teaching. The child will be able to start clear liquids and advance as tolerated after the procedure is completed and the child is fully awake.
CN: Physiological integrity; CNS: Physiological adaptation; CL: Analysis

14. 4. Cardiac catheterization provides visualization of the heart and great vessels. It's an invasive procedure in which a thin catheter is passed into the chambers of the heart through a peripheral vein or artery. General anesthesia may be used for more complex catheterizations or procedures that place the child at greater risk. High-frequency sound waves describe ultrasound and echocardiography. Conscious sedation is usually given before cardiac catheterization.
CN: Physiological integrity; CNS: Reduction of risk potential; CL: Application

15. 2. During recovery, the child should remain flat in bed, keeping the punctured leg straight for the prescribed time. The child should avoid raising the head, sitting, straining the abdomen, or coughing. Vital signs are taken every 15 minutes until the child is awake and stable, then every half hour, then hourly as ordered. If bleeding occurs at the insertion site, the nurse should mark the margins with a pen and monitor for changes.
CN: Physiological integrity; CNS: Physiological adaptation; CL: Analysis

16. 1. A regular diet and increased fluids are encouraged postcatheterization. Increased fluids may flush the injected dyes out of the system. Normal activities may be resumed, but strenuous physical activities or sports should be avoided for about 3 days. Prolonged bathing can be resumed in 3 days. A sponge bath is encouraged until then. The child may return to school 3 days after discharge.
CN: Physiological integrity; CNS: Physiological adaptation; CL: Analysis

CN: Client needs category   CNS: Client needs subcategory   CL: Cognitive level

17. A 2-year-old child is being monitored after cardiac surgery. Which sign represents a decrease in cardiac output?
1. Hypertension
2. Increased urine output
3. Weak peripheral pulses
4. Capillary refill less than 2 seconds

18. A 3-year-old child is experiencing distress after having cardiac surgery. Which sign indicates cardiac tamponade?
1. Hypertension
2. Muffled heart sounds
3. Widened pulse pressures
4. Increased chest tube drainage

19. A nurse is monitoring fluid and electrolyte balance in a child after cardiac surgery requiring cardiopulmonary bypass. Which finding is expected?
1. Increased urine output
2. Increased sodium level
3. Decreased sodium level
4. Increased potassium level

20. A nurse is teaching wound care to parents after cardiac surgery. Which statement is <u>most appropriate</u>?
1. Lotions and powders are acceptable.
2. Your child can take a complete bath tomorrow.
3. Tingling, itching, and numbness are normal sensations at the wound site.
4. If the sterile adhesive strips over the incision fall off, call the physician.

21. Parents ask a nurse about their 8-year-old son's activity level after cardiac surgery. Which response would be best?
1. There are no exercise limitations.
2. The child may resume school in 3 days.
3. Encourage a balance of rest and exercise.
4. Climbing and contact sports are restricted for 1 week.

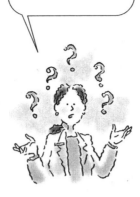

All of these signs may appear, but only one indicates cardiac tamponade. Which one?

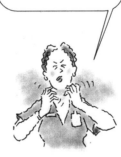

I'm itching to get question 20 correct.

17. 3. Signs of decreased cardiac output include weak peripheral pulses, hypotension, low urine output, delayed capillary refill, and cool extremities.
CN: Physiological integrity; CNS: Physiological adaptation; CL: Analysis

18. 2. Symptoms of cardiac tamponade include muffled heart sounds, hypotension, a narrowing pulse pressure, and sudden cessation of chest tube drainage. Cardiac tamponade occurs when a large volume of fluid interferes with ventricular filling and pumping and collects in the pericardial sac, decreasing cardiac output.
CN: Physiological integrity; CNS: Physiological adaptation; CL: Analysis

19. 2. In response to surgery and cardiopulmonary bypass, the body secretes aldosterone and antidiuretic hormone. This in turn increases sodium levels, decreases potassium levels, increases water retention, and decreases urine output.
CN: Physiological integrity; CNS: Physiological adaptation; CL: Analysis

20. 3. As the area heals, tingling, itching, and numbness are normal sensations and will eventually go away. Lotions and powders should be avoided during the first 2 weeks after surgery. A complete bath should be delayed for the first week, although sponge baths are allowed. Adhesive strips may loosen or fall off on their own. This is a common and normal occurrence.
CN: Physiological integrity; CNS: Physiological adaptation; CL: Analysis

21. 3. Activity should be increased gradually each day, allowing for a sensible balance of rest and exercise. School and large crowds should be avoided for at least 2 weeks to prevent exposure to people with active infections. Sports and contact activities should be restricted for about 6 weeks, giving the sternum enough time to heal.
CN: Physiological integrity; CNS: Physiological adaptation; CL: Analysis

22. Which home care instruction is <u>most appropriate</u> for a child after cardiac surgery?
1. Don't stop giving the child the prescribed drugs until the physician says so.
2. Maintain a sodium-restricted diet.
3. Routine dental care can be resumed.
4. Immunizations are delayed indefinitely.

23. A 4-year-old client with a chest tube is placed on water seal. Which statement is correct?
1. The water level rises with inhalation.
2. Bubbling is seen in the suction chamber.
3. Bubbling is seen in the water seal chamber.
4. Water seal is obtained by clamping the tube.

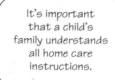
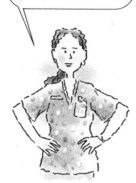

It's important that a child's family understands all home care instructions.

24. Which intervention is <u>most appropriate</u> when a chest tube falls out or becomes dislodged?
1. Place a dry gauze dressing over the insertion site.
2. Place a petroleum gauze dressing over the insertion site.
3. Wipe the tube with alcohol and reinsert it.
4. Call the physician immediately.

25. When assessing a child with heart failure, which findings should the nurse expect to find?
1. Bradycardia
2. Decreased respiratory rate
3. Gallop murmur
4. Strong, bounding pulses

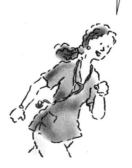

Question 25 is a milestone. Way to go!

22. 1. Drugs, such as digoxin and furosemide, shouldn't be stopped abruptly. There are no diet restrictions, and the child may resume his regular diet. Routine dental care is usually delayed 6 months after surgery. Immunizations are delayed at least 6 weeks after surgery.
CN: Physiological integrity; CNS: Reduction of risk potential; CL: Analysis

23. 1. The water seal chamber is functioning appropriately when the water level rises in the chamber with inhalation and falls with expiration. This shows that negative pressure required in the lung is being maintained. Bubbling in the suction chamber should be seen only when suction is being used. Bubbling in the water seal chamber generally indicates the presence of an air leak. The chest tube should never be clamped; a tension pneumothorax may occur. Water seal is activated when the suction is disconnected.
CN: Physiological integrity; CNS: Reduction of risk potential; CL: Application

24. 2. Petroleum gauze should be placed over the site immediately to prevent a pneumothorax. The physician should be notified after this step. A dry gauze dressing will allow air to enter pleural space, leading to a pneumothorax. The tube is reinserted only by a physician using a sterile thoracotomy tray.
CN: Physiological integrity; CNS: Reduction of risk potential; CL: Application

25. 3. When the heart stretches beyond efficiency, an extra heart sound or S_3 gallop murmur may be audible. This is related to excessive preload and ventricular dilation. Tachycardia occurs as a compensatory mechanism to the decrease in cardiac output. It also attempts to increase the force and rate of myocardial contraction and increase oxygen consumption of the heart. The respiratory rate increases, not decreases, in an attempt to increase oxygenation. Pulses are usually weak and thready.
CN: Physiological integrity; CNS: Physiological adaptation; CL: Analysis

CN: Client needs category   CNS: Client needs subcategory   CL: Cognitive level

26. An emergency room nurse is caring for a pediatric client in heart failure. Which symptom is consistent with a diagnosis of left-sided heart failure?
1. Weight gain
2. Peripheral edema
3. Neck vein distention
4. Tachypnea and dyspnea

27. Which intervention is <u>most appropriate</u> when caring for an infant with heart failure?
1. Limit fluid intake.
2. Avoid using infant seats.
3. Cluster nursing activities.
4. Place the infant prone or supine.

28. Which diet plan is recommended for an infant with heart failure?
1. Restrict fluids.
2. Weigh once a week.
3. Use low-sodium formula.
4. Increase caloric content per ounce.

29. A boy with patent ductus arteriosus was delivered 6 hours earlier and is being held by his mother. As the nurse enters the room to assess the neonate's vital signs, the mother says, "The physician says that my baby has a heart murmur. Does that mean he has a bad heart?" Which response by the nurse would be the most appropriate?
1. "He'll need more tests to determine his heart condition."
2. "He'll require oxygen therapy at home for a while."
3. "He'll be fine. Don't worry about him."
4. "The murmur is caused by the natural opening, which can take a day or two to close. It's a normal part of your baby's transition."

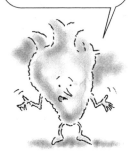

Do you know what happens when my left side isn't working properly?

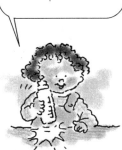

What's the diet plan?

26. 4. Respiratory symptoms, such as tachypnea and dyspnea, are seen as a result of pulmonary congestion. Peripheral edema, jugular vein distention, and weight gain are seen with systemic venous congestion or right-sided heart failure. Fluid accumulates in the interstitial spaces because of blood pooling in the venous circulation.
CN: Physiological integrity; CNS: Physiological adaptation; CL: Application

27. 3. Energy expenditures need to be limited to reduce metabolic and oxygen needs. Nursing care should be clustered, followed by long periods of undisturbed rest. Fluid may be restricted in older children, but infants' nutritional requirements depend on fluid needs. Infants should be placed in the semi-Fowler or upright position. Infant seats help maintain an upright position. This facilitates lung expansion, provides less restrictive movement of the diaphragm, relieves pressure from abdominal organs, and decreases pulmonary congestion.
CN: Physiological integrity; CNS: Physiological adaptation; CL: Analysis

28. 4. Formulas with increased caloric content are given to meet the greater caloric requirements from the overworked heart and labored breathing. Fluid restriction and low-sodium formulas aren't recommended. An infant's nutritional needs depend on fluid. Daily weights at the same time of the day on the same scale before feedings are recommended to follow trends in nutritional stability and diuresis. Low-sodium formulas may cause hyponatremia.
CN: Physiological integrity; CNS: Basic care and comfort; CL: Application

29. 4. Although the nurse may want to tell the client not to worry, the most appropriate response would be to explain the neonate's present condition, to relieve the mother and to acknowledge an awareness of the condition. A neonate's vascular system changes with birth; certain factors help to reverse the flow of blood through the ductus and ultimately favor its closure. This closure typically begins within the first 24 hours after birth and ends within a few days after birth. The other responses don't adequately address the mother's question.
CN: Health promotion and maintenance; CNS: None; CL: Analysis

30. A teenage client with heart failure is prescribed digoxin (Lanoxin) and asks the nurse, "What's the drug supposed to do?" The nurse teaches the teenager based on the understanding that this drug belongs to which classification?
1. Angiotensin-converting enzyme (ACE) inhibitor
2. Cardiac glycoside
3. Diuretic
4. Vasodilator

31. Which assessment finding would lead the nurse to suspect a child has a digoxin level greater than 2 ng/ml?
1. Weight gain
2. Tachycardia
3. Nausea and vomiting
4. Seizures

32. An 11-month-old infant with heart failure weighs 10 kg. Digoxin is prescribed as 10 mcg/kg/day in divided doses every 12 hours. How much is given per dose?
1. 10 mcg
2. 50 mcg
3. 100 mcg
4. 500 mcg

33. A client with heart failure is given captopril (Capoten), an angiotensin-converting enzyme (ACE) inhibitor. Which action occurs with this type of drug?
1. Vasoconstriction
2. Increased sodium excretion
3. Decreased sodium excretion
4. Increased vascular resistance

34. The parents of a newborn child have just been told that he has a heart defect known as *patent ductus arteriosus*. Which statement made by the parents indicates that teaching has been effective?
1. "Heart failure is uncommon in this defect."
2. "The ductus normally closes completely by age 6 weeks."
3. "An open ductus arteriosus causes decreased blood flow to the lungs."
4. "It represents a cyanotic defect with decreased pulmonary blood flow."

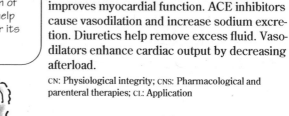
Knowing the classification of a drug can help you remember its actions.

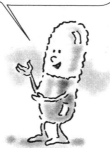

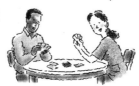
I don't think this ace will inhibit me.

30. 2. Digoxin is a cardiac glycoside. It decreases the workload of the heart and improves myocardial function. ACE inhibitors cause vasodilation and increase sodium excretion. Diuretics help remove excess fluid. Vasodilators enhance cardiac output by decreasing afterload.
CN: Physiological integrity; CNS: Pharmacological and parenteral therapies; CL: Application

31. 3. Digoxin toxicity in infants and children may present with nausea, vomiting, anorexia, or a slow, irregular apical heart rate. Weight gain, tachycardia, or seizures wouldn't be seen in digoxin toxicity.
CN: Physiological integrity; CNS: Pharmacological and parenteral therapies; CL: Analysis

32. 2. 10 kg × 10 mcg/kg/day = 100 mcg/day divided by 2 doses = 50 mcg/dose.
CN: Physiological integrity; CNS: Pharmacological and parenteral therapies; CL: Analysis

33. 2. ACE inhibitors block the conversion of angiotensin I to angiotensin II in the kidney. This causes decreased aldosterone, vasodilation, and increased sodium excretion. As a vasodilator, it also acts to reduce vascular resistance by the manipulation of afterload.
CN: Physiological integrity; CNS: Pharmacological and parenteral therapies; CL: Application

34. 2. At birth, oxygenated blood normally causes the ductus to constrict, and the vessel closes completely by age 6 weeks. This defect is considered an acyanotic defect with increased pulmonary blood flow. The open ductus arteriosus can cause an excessive blood flow to the lungs because of the high pressure in the aorta. Heart failure is common in premature infants with a patent ductus arteriosus.
CN: Physiological integrity; CNS: Physiological adaptation; CL: Analysis

CN: Client needs category   CNS: Client needs subcategory   CL: Cognitive level

35. Which intervention or drug is recommended initially for preterm neonates to close a patent ductus arteriosus?
1. Indomethacin
2. Prostaglandin E_1
3. Surgical ligation
4. Cardiac catheterization

36. A nurse is caring for a client with patent ductus arteriosus. Which assessment finding is consistent with this diagnosis?
1. Weak peripheral pulses
2. Machinelike murmur
3. Narrowed pulse pressure
4. Right ventricular hypertrophy

37. During observation of a child who has undergone cardiac catheterization, the nurse notes significant bleeding from the percutaneous femoral catheterization site. Which action should be taken <u>first</u>?
1. Apply direct, continuous pressure.
2. Assess the pulse and blood pressure.
3. Seek the assistance of another nurse.
4. Check the pulses in the affected leg.

38. Which finding is expected during an assessment of a child with an acyanotic heart defect?
1. Overweight
2. Bradycardia
3. Hepatomegaly
4. Decreased respiratory rate

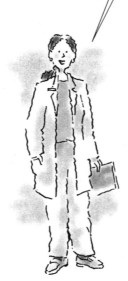

Question 36 asks which finding you *expect*, not necessarily one that may or may not occur.

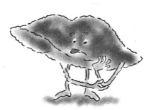

How did I get into a chapter on cardiovascular disorders?

35. 1. Preterm neonates with good renal function may receive oral indomethacin, a prostaglandin inhibitor, to encourage ductal closure. If this isn't effective, surgery is suggested. Prostaglandin E_1 will ensure patency of a patent ductus arteriosus for infants dependent on an open ductus arteriosus. Surgical ligation and a cardiac catheterization procedure may also be performed in infants and children.
CN: Physiological integrity; CNS: Physiological adaptation; CL: Analysis

36. 2. The continuous, turbulent flow of blood from the aorta through the patent ductus arteriosus to the pulmonary artery produces a machinelike murmur. There's a widened pulse pressure and bounding peripheral pulses from the runoff of blood from the aorta to the pulmonary artery. Left ventricular hypertrophy created from the left to right shunting of blood can be seen on X-ray.
CN: Physiological integrity; CNS: Physiological adaptation; CL: Analysis

37. 1. Bleeding from a major vessel must be stopped immediately to prevent massive hemorrhage. Vital signs would be taken after bleeding control measures are instituted. Calling for help is important, but pressure on the site must be applied and maintained while help is found. Pulses would be checked after bleeding is controlled.
CN: Physiological integrity; CNS: Reduction of risk potential; CL: Application

38. 3. Hepatomegaly may result from blood backing up into the liver due to the difficulty of entering the right side of the heart. The increase in blood flow to the lungs may cause tachycardia (not bradycardia) and increased respiratory rates to compensate. Poor growth and development, not excess weight gain, may be seen because of the increased energy required for breathing.
CN: Physiological integrity; CNS: Physiological adaptation; CL: Analysis

39. Eisenmenger's complex consists of pulmonary vascular resistance exceeding systemic pressure. This can occur in which cardiac anomaly when untreated?
1. Aortic stenosis
2. Atrial septal defect
3. Pulmonary stenosis
4. Ventricular septal defect

40. Which sign may be seen in a child with ventricular septal defect?
1. Cyanosis of the nailbeds
2. Above-average height on growth chart
3. Above-average weight gain on growth chart
4. Pink nailbeds with capillary refill less than 2 seconds

41. When caring for a child diagnosed with a ventricular septal defect, which description would the nurse incorporate when teaching the parents about this condition?
1. It is a narrowing of the aortic arch.
2. It is a failure of a septum to develop completely between the atria.
3. It is a narrowing of the values at the entrance of the pulmonary artery.
4. It is a failure of a septum to develop completely between the ventricles.

42. Which curative surgical intervention is recommended for a child with ventricular septal defect?
1. Surgery with pulmonary artery banding
2. Defect repair through cardiac catheterization
3. Surgery with purse-string suture or Dacron patch repair
4. Surgery when severe pulmonary hypertension is noted

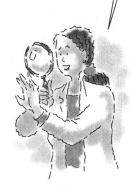

You can see this sign without a magnifying glass!

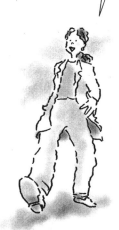

Question 42 already? Wow! You're making great strides!

39. 4. In moderate to large untreated ventricular septal defects, the constant excess flow will increase pulmonary vascular resistance. As time progresses, pressures in the right ventricle and left ventricle may change, causing higher pressures on the right side. A right-to-left shunt results, and pulmonary hypertension occurs.
CN: Physiological integrity; CNS: Physiological adaptation; CL: Analysis

40. 1. Cyanotic nailbeds can be seen when pulmonary resistance increases and causes the left to right shunt to reverse and shunt right to left. This shift leads to signs of heart failure and cyanosis. Children with the defect usually present with symptoms of heart failure, poor growth and development, and failure to thrive.
CN: Physiological integrity; CNS: Physiological adaptation; CL: Analysis

41. 4. Failure of a septum to develop between the ventricles results in a left-to-right shunt, which is noted as a ventricular septal defect. The narrowing of the aortic arch describes coarctation of the aorta. Narrowing of the valves at the pulmonary artery describes pulmonic stenosis. When the septum fails to develop between the atria, it's considered an atrial septal defect.
CN: Physiological integrity; CNS: Physiological adaptation; CL: Application

42. 3. Surgery is recommended for children ages 1 to 4. A median sternotomy incision is placed with the heart on cardiopulmonary bypass. For small defects, a stitch closure is performed. For larger defects, a patch is sewn. Surgery with pulmonary artery banding is only a palliative procedure for children too small or too ill but in heart failure. Cardiac catheterization repairs have been performed for selective cases but aren't approved for general care. Severe pulmonary hypertension would lead to an inoperable condition. If repaired, the excess blood flow to the lungs by patching the defect may be fatal.
CN: Physiological integrity; CNS: Physiological adaptation; CL: Application

CN: Client needs category   CNS: Client needs subcategory   CL: Cognitive level

43. A child with a ventricular septal defect repair is receiving dopamine (Intropin) postoperatively. The nurse should teach the child's parents that this medication is <u>most</u> likely to be given for which action?
1. To decrease heart rate
2. To decrease urine output
3. To increase cardiac output
4. To decrease cardiac contractility

44. A child returns to his room after a cardiac catheterization. Which statement regarding mobility would be appropriate for the nurse to teach the child and his parents?
1. The child may sit in a chair with the affected extremity immobilized.
2. The child will be maintained on bed rest with no further activity restrictions.
3. The child will be maintained on bed rest with the affected extremity immobilized.
4. The child may get out of bed to go to the bathroom, if necessary.

45. A client with Down syndrome (trisomy 21) comes to the pediatric clinic for a well visit. Which cardiac anomaly would this child be at risk for considering his health history?
1. Atrial septal defect
2. Pulmonic stenosis
3. Ventricular septal defect
4. Endocardial cushion defect

46. Which finding would concern the nurse who's caring for an infant after a right femoral cardiac catheterization?
1. Weak right dorsalis pedis pulse
2. Elevated temperature
3. Decreased urine output
4. Slightly bloody drainage around catheterization site dressing

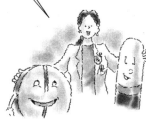

You know more about drugs than you realize!

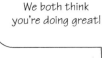

We both think you're doing great!

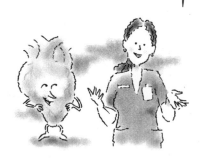

43. 3. Dopamine stimulates beta$_1$- and beta$_2$-adrenergic receptors. It's a selective cardiac stimulant that will increase cardiac output, heart rate, and cardiac contractility. Urine output increases in response to dilation of the blood vessels to the mesentery and kidneys.
CN: Physiological integrity; CNS: Pharmacological and parenteral therapies; CL: Application

44. 3. The child should be maintained on bed rest with the affected extremity immobilized after cardiac catheterization to prevent hemorrhage. Allowing the child to sit in a chair with the affected extremity immobilized, to move the affected extremity while on bed rest, or to have bathroom privileges places him at risk for hemorrhage.
CN: Physiological integrity; CNS: Reduction of risk potential; CL: Application

45. 4. Endocardial cushion defects are seen most in children with Down syndrome. Atrial septal defects account for about 10% of all cardiac anomalies. Pulmonic stenosis is responsible for about 8% of all cardiac anomalies. Ventricular septal defects are the most common cardiac anomaly.
CN: Health promotion and maintenance; CNS: None; CL: Application

46. 1. The pulse below the catheterization site should be strong and equal to the unaffected extremity. A weakened pulse may indicate vessel obstruction or perfusion problems. Elevated temperature and decreased urine output are relatively normal findings after catheterization and may be the result of decreased oral fluids. A small amount of bloody drainage is normal; however, the site must be assessed frequently for increased bleeding.
CN: Physiological integrity; CNS: Reduction of risk potential; CL: Application

47. Which cardiac anomaly produces a left-to-right shunt?
1. Atrial septal defect
2. Pulmonic stenosis
3. Tetralogy of Fallot
4. Total anomalous pulmonary venous return

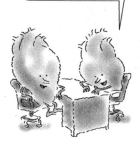

My shunt is left to right. How about yours?

48. A child with an atrial septal defect repair is entering postoperative day 3. Which intervention would be most appropriate?
1. Give the child nothing by mouth.
2. Maintain strict bed rest.
3. Take vital signs every 8 hours.
4. Administer an analgesic as needed.

49. A 3-year-old child is on postoperative day 5 for an atrial septal defect repair. Which nursing diagnosis would be most appropriate?
1. *Activity intolerance*
2. *Chronic pain*
3. *Social isolation*
4. *Risk for imbalanced fluid volume*

50. A 6-month-old infant with uncorrected tetralogy of Fallot suddenly becomes increasingly cyanotic and diaphoretic, with weak peripheral pulses and an increased respiratory rate. What should the nurse do immediately?
1. Administer oxygen.
2. Administer morphine sulfate.
3. Place the infant in a knee-chest position.
4. Place the infant in Fowler's position.

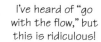

I've heard of "go with the flow," but this is ridiculous!

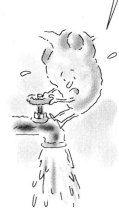

51. A client is diagnosed with coarctation of the aorta. Which finding should the nurse expect during an assessment?
1. Normal blood pressure
2. Increased blood pressure in the upper extremities
3. Decreased blood pressure in the upper extremities
4. Decreased or absent pulses in the upper extremities

47. 1. Atrial septal defects shunt from left to right because pressures are greater on the left side of the heart. Pulmonic stenosis, tetralogy of Fallot, and total anomalous pulmonary venous return will show a right-to-left shunting of blood.
CN: Health promotion and maintenance; CNS: None; CL: Analysis

48. 4. Pain management is always a priority and should be given on an as-needed basis. By day 3, the child should be advancing to a regular diet. Activity should include activity as able in the step-down unit, with coughing and deep breathing exercises. Vital signs should be performed routinely every 2 to 4 hours.
CN: Physiological integrity; CNS: Physiological adaptation; CL: Application

49. 4. Diuretics may still be used as needed at this point. By day 5, the child's activity level will be normal and there will be little to no pain. The child isn't isolated from anyone and can usually attend the playroom on day 3 or 4.
CN: Physiological integrity; CNS: Physiological adaptation; CL: Analysis

50. 3. The knee-chest position reduces the workload of the heart by increasing the blood return to the heart and keeping the blood flow more centralized. Oxygen should be administered quickly but only after placing the infant in the knee-chest position. Morphine should be administered after repositioning and oxygen administration are completed. Fowler's position wouldn't improve the situation.
CN: Safe, effective care environment; CNS: Management of care; CL: Application

51. 2. As blood is pumped from the left ventricle to the aorta, some blood flows to the head and upper extremities while the rest meets obstruction and jets through the constricted area. Pressures and pulses are greater in the upper extremities. Decreased or absent pulses are found in the lower extremities.
CN: Physiological integrity; CNS: Physiological adaptation; CL: Analysis

CN: Client needs category   CNS: Client needs subcategory   CL: Cognitive level

52. A child with coarctation of the aorta experiences a postsurgical recoarctation. Which treatment should the nurse expect the physician to recommend?
1. Bypass graft repair
2. Patch aortoplasty
3. Balloon angioplasty
4. Left subclavian flap angioplasty

53. Which factor is a necessary part of assessment for a child with a possible cardiac anomaly?
1. Skin turgor
2. Temperature
3. Pupil size and reaction to light
4. Blood pressure in four extremities

54. Which intervention is recommended postoperatively for a client with coarctation of the aorta repair?
1. Give a vasoconstrictor.
2. Maintain hypothermia.
3. Maintain a normal to low blood pressure.
4. Give a bolus of I.V. fluids.

55. Which assessment is expected when assessing a child with tetralogy of Fallot?
1. Machinelike murmur
2. Eisenmenger's complex
3. Increasing cyanosis with crying or activity
4. Higher pressures in the upper extremities than with the lower extremities

56. A child with tetralogy of Fallot has clubbing of the fingers and toes. Which condition is most likely to be causing this clubbing?
1. Polycythemia
2. Chronic hypoxia
3. Pansystolic murmur
4. Abnormal growth and development

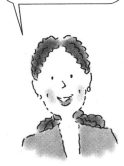

Hint: Cardiac anomalies can be extreme.

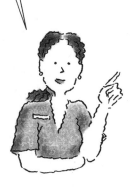

When it comes to assessment, practice makes perfect!

52. 3. Balloon angioplasty is the treatment of choice for postsurgical recoarctations. Bypass graft repair, patch angioplasty, and left subclavian flap angioplasty are surgical options to treat the original coarctation.
CN: Physiological integrity; CNS: Physiological adaptation; CL: Analysis

53. 4. Measuring blood pressure in all four extremities is necessary to document hypertension and the blood pressure gradient between the upper and lower extremities. Temperature, skin turgor, and pupillary assessment are also important, but are not as specific for cardiac assessment as the blood pressure.
CN: Physiological integrity; CNS: Physiological adaptation; CL: Application

54. 3. Blood pressure is tightly managed and kept low so there's no excessive pressure on the fresh suture lines. Vasoconstrictors would be contraindicated. Normothermia is maintained, and diuretics may be given to decrease fluid volume.
CN: Physiological integrity; CNS: Physiological adaptation; CL: Analysis

55. 3. A child with tetralogy of Fallot will be mildly cyanotic at rest and have increasing cyanosis with crying, activity, or straining, as with a bowel movement. A machinelike murmur is a characteristic of patent ductus arteriosus. Eisenmenger's complex is a complication of pulmonary pressure exceeding systemic pressure. Higher pressures in the upper extremities are characteristic of coarctation of the aorta.
CN: Physiological integrity; CNS: Physiological adaptation; CL: Application

56. 2. Chronic hypoxia longer than 6 months causes clubbing of the fingers and toes when untreated. Hypoxia varies with the degree of pulmonic stenosis. Polycythemia is an increased number of red blood cells as a result of the chronic hypoxemia. A pansystolic murmur is heard at the middle to lower left sternal border but has no impact on clubbing. Growth and development may appear normal.
CN: Physiological integrity; CNS: Physiological adaptation; CL: Analysis

57. A child with tetralogy of Fallot may assume which position of comfort during exercise?
1. Prone
2. Semi-Fowler's
3. Side-lying
4. Squat

58. A nurse is describing tetralogy of Fallot to a child's parents. Which statement by the parents demonstrates that the teaching has been effective?
1. "The condition is commonly referred to as 'blue tets.'"
2. "A child with this condition experiences hypercyanotic, or 'tet,' spells."
3. "A child with this condition experiences frequent respiratory infections."
4. "A child with this condition experiences decreased or absent pulses in the lower extremities."

59. A child diagnosed with tetralogy of Fallot has been ordered to undergo testing. Which test would indicate the direction and amount of shunting in this child?
1. Chest radiography
2. Echocardiography
3. Electrocardiography (ECG)
4. Cardiac catheterization

60. A nurse is teaching parents about tricuspid atresia. Which statement indicates that the parents understand this disorder?
1. "There's a narrowing at the aortic outflow tract."
2. "The pulmonary veins don't return to the left atrium."
3. "There's a narrowing at the entrance of the pulmonary artery."
4. "There's no communication between the right atrium and right ventricle."

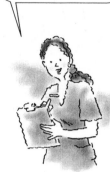

I'll bet you already know the answer!

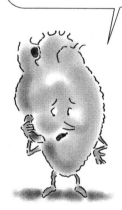

Hello? Is anybody there? I must have a bad connection.

57. 4. A child may squat or assume a knee-chest position to reduce venous blood flow from the lower extremities and to increase systemic vascular resistance, which diverts more blood flow into the pulmonary artery. Prone, semi-Fowler's, and side-lying positions won't produce this effect.
CN: Physiological integrity; CNS: Physiological adaptation; CL: Analysis

58. 2. Hypercyanotic, or "tet," spells may occur as a result of increasing obstruction of right ventricular outflow, resulting in decreased pulmonary blood flow and increased right-to-left shunting. Infants with mild obstruction to blood flow have little or no right-to-left shunting and appear pink, or "pink tets." Frequent respiratory infections are seen in defects with increased pulmonary blood flow, such as a patent ductus arteriosus. Decreased or absent pulses in the lower extremities is a sign of Coarctation of the aorta.
CN: Physiological integrity; CNS: Physiological adaptation; CL: Analysis

59. 4. Cardiac catheterization provides specific information about the direction and amount of shunting, coronary anatomy, and each portion of the heart defect. Chest radiographs will show right ventricular hypertrophy pushing the heart apex upward, resulting in a boot-shaped silhouette. Echocardiogram scans define such defects as large ventricular septal defects, pulmonic stenosis, and malposition of the aorta. ECG shows right ventricular hypertrophy with tall R waves.
CN: Physiological integrity; CNS: Reduction of risk potential; CL: Application

60. 4. Tricuspid atresia is failure of the tricuspid valve to develop, leaving no communication between the right atrium and right ventricle. Narrowing at the aortic outflow tract is aortic stenosis. Total anomalous pulmonary venous return is a defect in which the pulmonary veins don't return to the left atrium but abnormally return to the right side of the heart. The narrowing at the entrance of the pulmonary artery represents pulmonic stenosis.
CN: Physiological integrity; CNS: Physiological adaptation; CL: Analysis

CN: Client needs category   CNS: Client needs subcategory   CL: Cognitive level

61. Which characteristic can be noted during the assessment of a child with tricuspid atresia?
1. Cyanosis
2. Machinelike murmur
3. Decreased respiratory rate
4. Capillary refill more than 2 seconds

62. A child with tricuspid atresia develops polycythemia. Which statement is the most accurate concerning this manifestation?
1. The red blood cell count is normal.
2. There is an increased ability for the oxygen to carry blood.
3. There is little to no effect on the blood clotting system.
4. The viscosity of the blood is unchanged.

63. A child has been diagnosed with tricuspid atresia. Which operation should a nurse expect the physician to recommend?
1. Blalock-Taussig operation
2. Fontan procedure
3. Jatene procedure
4. Patch closure

64. Which guideline should the nurse follow when administering digoxin (Lanoxin) to an infant?
1. Mix the digoxin with the infant's food.
2. Double the subsequent dose if a dose is missed.
3. Give the digoxin with antacids when possible.
4. Withhold the dose if the apical pulse rate is less than 90 beats/minute.

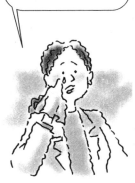

Tricuspid atresia always makes me blue.

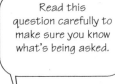

Read this question carefully to make sure you know what's being asked.

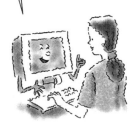

61. 1. Cyanosis is the most consistent clinical sign of tricuspid atresia. Tachypnea and dyspnea are commonly present because of the decreased pulmonary blood flow and right-to-left shunting. Tricuspid atresia doesn't have a characteristic murmur. A machinelike murmur is characteristic of a patent ductus arteriosus. Decreased oxygenation would increase capillary refill time.
CN: Physiological integrity; CNS: Physiological adaptation; CL: Analysis

62. 2. Polycythemia is an increased number of red blood cells, thereby increasing the ability of the blood to carry oxygen to the cells. Due to this clinical manifestation, the viscosity of the blood increases, and there is not as much room for clotting factors. This leaves the child at risk for blood clotting disorders.
CN: Physiological integrity; CNS: Physiological adaptation; CL: Application

63. 2. The Fontan procedure is used to correct tricuspid atresia. It separates the systemic and pulmonary circulations by closing septal defects and previous shunts and connecting the systemic venous structures with the pulmonary arteries. The Blalock-Taussig operation is used to palliate children with tricuspid atresia. The Jatene procedure is used to correct a mixed defect such as transposition of the great arteries. Patch closures are used for defects such as a ventricular or atrial septal defect.
CN: Physiological integrity; CNS: Physiological adaptation; CL: Application

64. 4. Digoxin is used to decrease heart rate; however, the apical pulse must be carefully monitored to detect a severe reduction. Administering digoxin to an infant with a heart rate of less than 90 beats/minute could further reduce the rate and compromise cardiac output. Mixing digoxin with food may interfere with accurate dosing. Double-dosing should never be done. Antacids may decrease drug absorption.
CN: Physiological integrity; CNS: Pharmacological and parenteral therapies; CL: Application

65. What part of the assessment of a child who has undergone complete repair of total anomalous pulmonary venous connection would lead the nurse to suspect that the complication of pulmonary venous obstruction has occurred?
1. Decreased work of breathing
2. Decreasing respiratory rate
3. Decreasing oxygenation saturation levels
4. Increasing urine output

66. Which finding is <u>common</u> during an assessment of a child with a total anomalous pulmonary venous return defect?
1. Hypertension
2. Frequent respiratory infections
3. Normal growth and development
4. Above-average weight gain on the growth chart

67. Which complication may result <u>after</u> the repair of total anomalous pulmonary venous return?
1. Hypotension
2. Pulmonary hypertension
3. Ventricular arrhythmias
4. Pulmonary vein dilatation

68. An infant has recently been diagnosed with tricuspid atresia and the parents have been told that their child will need a series of three, staged surgeries. Which statement indicates that the parents have an understanding of the procedures?
1. "My child will have this dusky color for the rest of his life."
2. "These procedures will make my child have a normal heart."
3. "Once fixed, my baby will not have to take any more medicine."
4. "My baby will be just like all of the other children once the surgeries are all done."

69. Which finding commonly occurs during an assessment of a child with truncus arteriosus?
1. Weak, thready pulses
2. Narrowed pulse pressure
3. Pink and moist mucous membranes
4. Harsh systolic regurgitant murmur

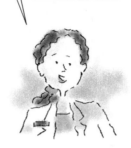

You're halfway there. Fantastic!

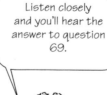

Listen closely and you'll hear the answer to question 69.

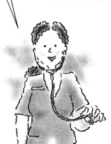

65. 3. A child who has pulmonary venous obstruction will exhibit signs of increasing respiratory distress, such as increased respiratory rate, dyspnea, and shortness of breath. Oxygen saturation levels will decrease. Urine output will decrease as the heart fails.
CN: Physiological integrity; CNS: Physiological adaptation; CL: Application

66. 2. Children with total anomalous pulmonary venous return defects are prone to repeated respiratory infections due to increased pulmonary blood flow. Hypertension usually occurs with coarctation of the aorta, an acyanotic defect with obstructive flow. Poor feeding and failure to thrive are also signs. Infants look thin and malnourished.
CN: Physiological integrity; CNS: Physiological adaptation; CL: Application

67. 2. Pulmonary hypertension, atrial arrhythmias, and pulmonary vein obstruction are complications that may result postoperatively. The left atrium is small and sensitive to fluid volume loading. An increase in the pressure in the right atrium is required to ensure left atrial filling.
CN: Physiological integrity; CNS: Physiological adaptation; CL: Analysis

68. 1. The child will be dusky, particularly around mucus membranes and nail beds, for the rest of its life as a result of chronic hypoxemia. The surgeries do not make the child have a "normal" heart, as they do not fix the original defect. The child will more than likely be on medications for the rest of its life, and the child will more than likely be smaller in stature than other children.
CN: Physiological integrity; CNS: Physiological adaptation; CL: Analysis

69. 4. As a result of the ventricular septal defect, a harsh systolic regurgitant murmur is heard along the left sternal border and is usually accompanied by a thrill. Increasing pulmonary blood flow causes bounding pulses and a widened pulse pressure. Systemic and pulmonary blood mixing leads to mild or moderate cyanosis, so mucous membranes may appear dull or gray.
CN: Physiological integrity; CNS: Physiological adaptation; CL: Analysis

CN: Client needs category   CNS: Client needs subcategory   CL: Cognitive level

70. Treatment for truncus arteriosus includes digoxin and diuretics. Which technique would be best for giving these drugs to an infant?
1. Usc a mcasuring spoon.
2. Use a graduated dropper.
3. Mix the drug with baby food.
4. Mix the drug in a bottle with juice or milk.

71. Which change would the nurse expect after administering oxygen to an infant with uncorrected tetralogy of Fallot?
1. Disappearance of the murmur
2. No evidence of cyanosis
3. Improvement of finger clubbing
4. Less agitation

72. Which statement about transposition of the great arteries is correct?
1. Electrocardiography will always show arrhythmias.
2. Diagnosis can be made in utero.
3. Chest X-ray can show an accurate view of the defect.
4. Heart failure isn't a related complication.

73. A nurse is assessing a child with transposition of the great arteries. Which associated defect should the nurse expect to see in this client?
1. Mitral atresia
2. Atrial septal defect
3. Patent foramen ovale
4. Hypoplasia of the left ventricle

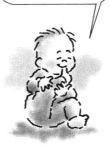

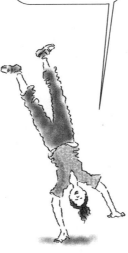

70. 2. Using a dropper allows the exact dosage to be given. A measuring spoon isn't as exact as a dropper. Mixing drugs with juice, milk, or food may cause a problem if the child doesn't completely finish the meal because then how much the child received isn't definite. In addition, this may prevent the child from drinking or eating for fear of tasting the drug.
CN: Physiological integrity; CNS: Pharmacological and parenteral therapies; CL: Application

71. 4. Supplemental oxygen will help the infant breathe more easily and feel less anxious or agitated. Disappearance of the murmur, no evidence of cyanosis, and improvement of finger clubbing would not occur as a result of supplemental oxygen administration.
CN: Physiological integrity; CNS: Physiological adaptation; CL: Application

72. 2. Echocardiography done by a fetal cardiologist can diagnose transposition of the great arteries in utero. The other defects associated with this defect include a patent foramen ovale and a ventricular septal defect that contribute to developing heart failure. Electrocardiography may or may not reveal arrhythmias. Chest X-ray can show cardiomegaly and pulmonary vascular markings only. Echocardiography or cardiac catheterization may be required preoperatively to show the coronary artery anatomy before surgical repair.
CN: Physiological integrity; CNS: Physiological adaptation; CL: Analysis

73. 3. A patent foramen ovale, patent ductus arteriosus, and ventricular septal defect are associated defects related to transposition of the great arteries. A patent foramen ovale is the most common and is necessary to provide adequate mixing of blood between the two circulations. An atrial septal defect is common in association with total anomalous pulmonary venous return. Hypoplasia of the left ventricle and mitral atresia are two defects associated with hypoplastic left heart syndrome.
CN: Physiological integrity; CNS: Physiological adaptation; CL: Analysis

74. Administration of which drug would be the <u>most important</u> in treating transposition of the great arteries?
1. Digoxin
2. Diuretics
3. Antibiotics
4. Prostaglandin E₁

75. Which surgical procedure is recommended for repair of transposition of the great arteries?
1. Jatene procedure
2. Fontan procedure
3. Balloon atrial septostomy
4. Blalock-Taussig operation

76. Which statement best describes a characteristic of valvular pulmonic stenosis?
1. The valve is normal.
2. The right ventricle is hypoplastic.
3. Left ventricular hypertrophy develops.
4. Divisions between the cusps are fused.

77. During the assessment of a child with pulmonic stenosis, which finding is <u>most common</u>?
1. Hyperactivity
2. Normal respiratory rate
3. Systolic ejection murmur
4. Capillary refill more than 2 seconds

78. Which finding is seen during cardiac catheterization of a child with pulmonic stenosis?
1. Right-to-left shunting
2. Left-to-right shunting
3. Decreased pressure in the right side of the heart
4. Increased oxygenation in the left side of the heart

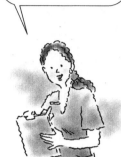

It's most important that you read each question carefully.

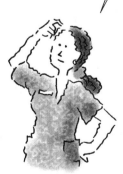
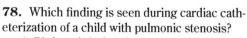

All of these conditions may occur, but which occurs most commonly?

74. 4. Prostaglandin E₁ is necessary to maintain patency of the patent ductus arteriosus and improve systemic arterial flow in children with inadequate intracardiac mixing. Digoxin and diuretics will treat heart failure when present. Antibiotics are given in the immediate preoperative phase.
CN: Physiological integrity; CNS: Pharmacological and parenteral therapies; CL: Application

75. 1. The Jatene procedure involves transposing the great arteries and mobilizing and reimplanting the coronary arteries. The Fontan procedure is recommended for repair of tricuspid atresia. Balloon atrial septostomy is a palliative procedure used during cardiac catheterization for those children without a coexisting lesion. The Blalock-Taussig operation is used to palliate tricuspid atresia and pulmonic atresia.
CN: Physiological integrity; CNS: Physiological adaptation; CL: Application

76. 4. Blood flow through the valve is restricted by fusion of the divisions between the cusps. The valve may be normal or malformed. Right ventricular hypertrophy develops due to resistance to blood flow.
CN: Physiological integrity; CNS: Physiological adaptation; CL: Analysis

77. 3. A systolic ejection murmur, which may be accompanied by a thrill, can be heard at the upper left sternal border. The decrease in pulmonary blood flow causes fatigue and dyspnea. Systemic cyanosis may result from right ventricular failure that increases the capillary refill time.
CN: Physiological integrity; CNS: Physiological adaptation; CL: Analysis

78. 1. Right-to-left shunting develops through a patent foramen ovale, an atrial septal defect, or a ventricular septal defect due to right ventricular failure and an increase in pressure in the right side of the heart. Decreased oxygenation in the left side of the heart is noted because of the right-to-left shunt and decreased pulmonary blood flow.
CN: Physiological integrity; CNS: Physiological adaptation; CL: Analysis

CN: Client needs category   CNS: Client needs subcategory   CL: Cognitive level

79. A nurse is caring for a 16-year-old client with aortic stenosis. Which finding is associated with aortic stenosis when the child is active?
1. Chest pain
2. Right ventricular failure
3. Increased cardiac output
4. Loud systolic regurgitant murmur with a thrill

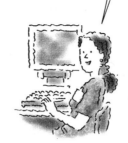

Keep going! You're doing great!

79. 1. Children with aortic stenosis may develop chest pain similar to angina when they're active. They're also at risk for tachycardia, syncope, hypotension, left ventricular failure, dyspnea, fatigue, and palpitations. Poor left ventricular ejection leads to a decreased cardiac output. Loud systolic regurgitant murmurs are heard with ventricular septal defects.
CN: Physiological integrity; CNS: Physiological adaptation; CL: Application

80. A nurse is teaching the parents of a child with congenital aortic stenosis. Which statement should the nurse include in her teaching about this disorder?
1. It can result from rheumatic fever (infection with group A streptococci).
2. It accounts for 25% of all congenital defects.
3. It causes an increase in cardiac output.
4. It's classified as an acyanotic defect with increased pulmonary blood flow.

80. 1. Aortic stenosis can result from rheumatic fever, which can damage the aortic valve in the first 8 weeks of pregnancy. It accounts for about 5% of all congenital defects. It causes a decrease in cardiac output. Aortic stenosis is classified as an acyanotic defect with obstructed flow from the ventricles.
CN: Physiological integrity; CNS: Physiological adaptation; CL: Analysis

81. Which instruction would be most appropriate for a child with aortic stenosis?
1. Restrict exercise.
2. Avoid prostaglandin E_1.
3. Avoid digoxin and diuretics.
4. Allow the child to exercise freely.

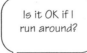

Is it OK if I run around?

81. 1. Exercise should be restricted because of low cardiac output and left ventricular failure. Strenuous activity has been reported to result in sudden death from the development of myocardial ischemia. Prostaglandin E_1 is recommended to maintain the patency of the ductus arteriosus in the neonate with critical aortic stenosis. This allows for improved systemic blood flow. Digoxin and diuretics may be required for the critically ill infant experiencing heart failure as a result of severe aortic stenosis.
CN: Physiological integrity; CNS: Physiological adaptation; CL: Application

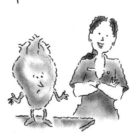

82. The nurse is planning care for a 9-year-old male child with heart failure. Which nursing diagnosis should receive priority?
1. *Risk for decreased cardiac tissue perfusion related to sympathetic response to heart failure*
2. *Imbalanced nutrition: Less than body requirement related to rapid tiring while feeding*
3. *Anxiety (parent) related to unknown nature of child's illness*
4. *Decreased cardiac output related to cardiac defect*

82. 4. The primary nursing diagnosis for a child with heart failure is *Decreased cardiac output related to cardiac defect*. The most common cause of heart failure in children is congenital heart defects. Some defects result from the blood being pumped from the left side of the heart to the right side of the heart. The heart can't manage the extra volume, resulting in the pulmonary system becoming overloaded. *Risk for decreased cardiac tissue perfusion, Imbalanced nutrition,* and *Anxiety* don't take priority over decreased cardiac output.
CN: Physiological integrity; CNS: Physiological adaptation; CL: Application

83. Which nursing diagnosis is the most appropriate when caring for an infant with hypoplastic left heart syndrome?
　1. *Death anxiety*
　2. *Delayed growth and development*
　3. *Deficient diversional activity*
　4. *Risk for activity intolerance*

83. 1. Without intervention, death usually occurs within the first few days of life as a result of progressive hypoxia, acidosis, and shock as the ductus closes and systemic perfusion diminishes. If the parents choose cardiac transplantation, the child may die waiting for a donor heart. For those who choose surgery, the child may not survive the three stages of the surgery. The other three choices don't apply to this type of defect because of the low survival rates.
CN: Physiological integrity; CNS: Physiological adaptation; CL: Analysis

84. A child receives prednisone after undergoing a heart transplant. What is the desired effect of this medication?
　1. Stimulate appetite.
　2. Suppress immune response.
　3. Improve wound healing.
　4. Prevent fluid retention.

84. 2. The goal of prednisone for this client is to suppress the immune system, thereby preventing organ rejection. Prednisone is often used in combination with other immunosuppressant medications in order to prevent rejection. While corticosteroids do stimulate appetites, that is not the desired effect for this child. Prednisone and other corticosteroids cause decreased ability of wounds to heal; fluid retention is one of the side effects.
CN: Physiological integrity; CNS: Pharmacological and parenteral therapies; CL: Application

85. Which adverse reaction to prednisone would a nurse expect to observe in a child who has received a heart transplant?
　1. Weight loss
　2. Hyperpyrexia
　3. Anorexia
　4. Poor wound healing

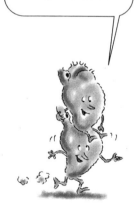

Hey, I'm just along for the ride.

85. 4. Common adverse reactions to prednisone include poor wound healing, weight gain, delayed temperature response, increased appetite, delayed sexual maturation, growth impairment, and a cushingoid appearance. The school-age child who has received prednisone is usually overweight and has a moon-shaped face.
CN: Physiological integrity; CNS: Pharmacological and parenteral therapies; CL: Application

86. A child is given 0.5 mg/kg/day of prednisone divided into two doses. The child weighs 10 kg. How much is given in each dose?
　1. 2.5 mg
　2. 5 mg
　3. 10 mg
　4. 1.5 mg

86. 1. The child should receive 2.5 mg/dose. Use the following equations:
$$0.5 \text{ mg/kg} \times 10 \text{ kg} = 5 \text{ mg};$$
$$5 \text{ mg/2 doses} = 2.5 \text{ mg/dose}$$
CN: Physiological integrity; CNS: Pharmacological and parenteral therapies; CL: Analysis

87. A 3-year-old client has a high red blood cell count and polycythemia. In planning care, the nurse would anticipate which goal to help prevent clot formation?
　1. The child won't have signs of dehydration.
　2. The child won't have signs of dyspnea.
　3. The child will be pain free.
　4. The child will attain the 40th percentile of weight for his age.

87. 1. When dehydration occurs, blood is thicker and more prone to clotting. Dyspnea would be a sign of hypoxia. Pain and weight gain would not be indicators of blood clot formation.
CN: Physiological integrity; CNS: Reduction of risk potential; CL: Application

CN: Client needs category　CNS: Client needs subcategory　CL: Cognitive level

88. Which statement about bacterial/infective endocarditis is the <u>most</u> accurate?
1. Bacteria invading only tissues of the heart
2. Infection of the valves and inner lining of the heart
3. Inappropriate fusion of the endocardial cushions in fetal life
4. Caused by alterations in cardiac preload, afterload, contractility, or heart rate

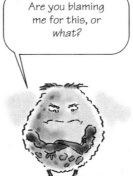

Are you blaming me for this, or what?

88. 2. Bacterial or infective endocarditis is an infection of the valves and inner lining of the heart. It's usually caused by the bacteria *Streptococcus viridans* and commonly affects children with acquired or congenital anomalies of the heart or great vessels. Bacteria may grow into adjacent tissues and may break off and embolize elsewhere, such as the spleen, kidney, lung, skin, and central nervous system. Endocardial cushion defects represent inappropriate fusion of the endocardial cushions in fetal life. Alterations in preload, afterload, contractility, or heart rate refer to heart failure.
CN: Physiological integrity; CNS: Physiological adaptation; CL: Application

89. A child with suspected bacterial endocarditis arrives at the emergency department. Which finding is expected during assessment?
1. Weight gain
2. Bradycardia
3. Low-grade fever
4. Increased hemoglobin level

89. 3. Symptoms may include a low-grade intermittent fever, decrease in hemoglobin level, tachycardia, anorexia, weight loss, and decreased activity level. Bacteremia leads to these signs of an infection.
CN: Physiological integrity; CNS: Physiological adaptation; CL: Application

90. Which factor may lead to bacterial endocarditis in a child with underlying heart disease?
1. History of a cold for 3 days
2. Dental work pretreated with antibiotics
3. Peripheral I.V. catheter in place for 1 day
4. Indwelling urinary catheter for 2 days leading to a urinary tract infection

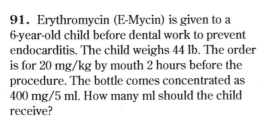

Wow! You finished question 90! The rest should be a snap!

90. 4. Bacterial organisms can enter the bloodstream from any site of infection such as a urinary tract infection. Gram-negative bacilli are common causative agents. Colds are usually viral, not bacterial. Dental work is a common portal of entry if not pretreated with antibiotics. A peripheral I.V. catheter is an entry site, but only if signs and symptoms of infection are present. Long-term indwelling catheters pose a higher risk for infection.
CN: Physiological integrity; CNS: Physiological adaptation; CL: Analysis

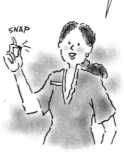

SNAP

91. Erythromycin (E-Mycin) is given to a 6-year-old child before dental work to prevent endocarditis. The child weighs 44 lb. The order is for 20 mg/kg by mouth 2 hours before the procedure. The bottle comes concentrated as 400 mg/5 ml. How many ml should the child receive?
1. 2.5 ml
2. 5 ml
3. 5.5 ml
4. 10 ml

91. 2. The child should receive 5 ml. Use the following equations:
Convert pounds to kilograms:
44 lb/2.2 kg = 20 kg
Then, determine how many mg to give:
20 mg/kg × 20 kg = 400 mg
Next, determine how many ml to give:
400 mg/400 mg × 5 ml = 5 ml
(desired/have × amount on hand = amount to administer)
CN: Physiological integrity; CNS: Pharmacological and parenteral therapies; CL: Analysis

92. What would be the <u>most</u> common adverse reaction a nurse might observe after administering enteric-coated erythromycin (Ery-tab)?

1. Weight gain
2. Constipation
3. Increased appetite
4. Nausea and vomiting

93. A child is hospitalized with bacterial endocarditis. Which nursing diagnosis is <u>most appropriate</u>?

1. *Constipation*
2. *Excess fluid volume*
3. *Deficient diversional activity*
4. *Imbalanced nutrition: More than body requirements*

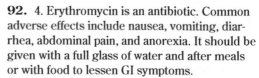
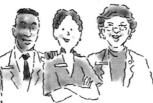

Nursing diagnoses: Share the knowledge!

94. When assessing a child with suspected Kawasaki disease, which symptom is common?

1. Low-grade fever
2. "Strawberry" tongue
3. Pink, moist mucous membranes
4. Bilateral conjunctival infection with yellow exudate

95. A nurse is teaching the parents of a child with Kawasaki disease. Which statement should the nurse include in her teaching about this disorder?

1. It mostly occurs in the summer and fall.
2. Diagnosis can be made with laboratory testing.
3. It's an acute systemic vasculitis of unknown cause.
4. It manifests in two different stages: acute and subacute.

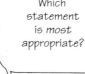

Which statement is most appropriate?

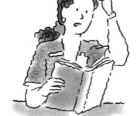

92. 4. Erythromycin is an antibiotic. Common adverse effects include nausea, vomiting, diarrhea, abdominal pain, and anorexia. It should be given with a full glass of water and after meals or with food to lessen GI symptoms.
CN: Physiological integrity; CNS: Pharmacological and parenteral therapies; CL: Application

93. 3. Treatment for bacterial endocarditis requires long-term hospitalization or home care for I.V. antibiotics. Children may be bored and depressed, needing age-appropriate activities. *Excess fluid volume, Constipation,* and *Imbalanced nutrition: More than body requirements* may be possible nursing diagnoses related to the adverse reactions of antibiotics, such as GI upset.
CN: Physiological integrity; CNS: Physiological adaptation; CL: Analysis

94. 2. Inflammation of the pharynx and oral mucosa develops, causing red, cracked lips and a "strawberry" tongue in which the normal coating of the tongue sloughs off. A high fever of 5 or more days unresponsive to antibiotics and antipyretics is also part of the diagnostic criteria. The eyes are generally dry without exudation.
CN: Physiological integrity; CNS: Physiological adaptation; CL: Application

95. 3. Kawasaki disease can best be described as an acute systemic vasculitis of unknown cause. Most cases are geographic and seasonal, with most occurring in the late winter and early spring. Diagnosis is based on clinical findings of five of the six diagnostic criteria and associated laboratory results. There's no specific laboratory test for diagnosis. There are three stages: acute, subacute, and convalescent.
CN: Physiological integrity; CNS: Physiological adaptation; CL: Application

CN: Client needs category   CNS: Client needs subcategory   CL: Cognitive level

96. Which characteristic indicates that a child with Kawasaki disease has entered the <u>subacute</u> phase?
1. Polymorphous rash
2. Normal blood values
3. Cervical lymphadenopathy
4. Desquamation of the hands and feet

97. A nurse is caring for a child with Kawasaki disease. Which symptom should concern the nurse the most?
1. Mild diarrhea
2. Pain in the joints
3. Abdominal pain with vomiting
4. Increased erythrocyte sedimentation rate (ESR)

98. A child is undergoing testing to rule out a diagnosis of Kawasaki disease. Which test result may lead to this diagnosis?
1. Hematuria
2. Elevated leukocyte count
3. Normal or decreased platelet count
4. Decreased erythrocyte sedimentation rate

99. Therapy for Kawasaki disease includes I.V. gamma globulin, prescribed at 400 mg/kg/day for 4 days. The child weighs 10 kg. How much is given per dose?
1. 200 mg
2. 400 mg
3. 2,000 mg
4. 4,000 mg

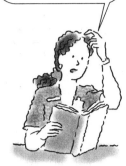

What happens during the subacute phase of this disease?

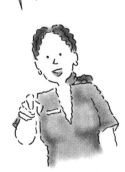

Here's another dosing question. You can do it!

96. 4. The subacute phase shows characteristic desquamation of the hands and feet. Blood values return to normal at the end of the convalescent phase. Cervical lymphadenopathy and a polymorphous rash can be seen in the acute phase due to the onset of inflammation and fever.
CN: Physiological integrity; CNS: Physiological adaptation; CL: Analysis

97. 3. The most serious complication of this disease is cardiac involvement. Abdominal pain, vomiting, and restlessness are the main symptoms of an acute myocardial infarction in children. Mild diarrhea can be treated with oral fluids. Pain in the joints is an expected sign of arthritis that usually occurs in the subacute phase. An increased ESR is a reflection of the inflammatory process and may be seen for 2 to 4 weeks after the onset of symptoms.
CN: Physiological integrity; CNS: Physiological adaptation; CL: Analysis

98. 2. Inflammation of the small vessels, along with pancarditis, leads to an elevated leukocyte count, increased platelet count, and proteinuria or sterile pyuria. The capillaries, venules, and arterioles are affected first, then the medium-sized muscular arteries. These laboratory results contribute to the clinical presentation and diagnosis of Kawasaki disease.
CN: Physiological integrity; CNS: Physiological adaptation; CL: Analysis

99. 4. The child should receive 4,000 mg. Use the following equation:
400 mg/kg × 10 kg = 4,000 mg or 4 g
CN: Physiological integrity; CNS: Pharmacological and parenteral therapies; CL: Analysis

100. A child is receiving 8 g of I.V. gamma globulin for treatment of Kawasaki disease. The child weighs 20 kg. The order is for 8 g of gamma globulin over 12 hours. The concentration is 8 g in 300 ml of normal saline. How many milliliters per hour will this child receive?
1. 12 ml/hour
2. 25 ml/hour
3. 50 ml/hour
4. 40 ml/hour

101. A child is prescribed aspirin as part of the therapy for Kawasaki disease. The order is for 80 mg/kg/day orally in four divided doses until the child is afebrile. The child weighs 15 kg. How much is given in one dose?
1. 60 mg
2. 300 mg
3. 320 mg
4. 1,200 mg

102. A nurse is giving discharge instructions to the parents of a child with Kawasaki disease. Which statement by the parents shows an understanding of the treatment plan?
1. "A regular diet can be resumed at home."
2. "Black, tarry stools are considered normal."
3. "My child should use a soft-bristled toothbrush."
4. "My child can return to playing football next week."

103. A nurse is preparing the family of a client with Kawasaki disease for discharge. Which instruction is most appropriate?
1. Stop the aspirin when you return home.
2. Immunizations can be given in 2 weeks.
3. The child may return to school in 1 week.
4. Frequent echocardiography will be needed.

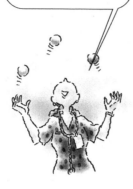

The numbers just keep coming!

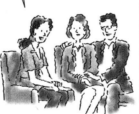

Listen for feedback to find out if your instructions were understood.

100. 2. The child should receive 25 ml/hour. Use the following equation:
300 ml/12 hours = 25 ml/hour
CN: Physiological integrity; CNS: Pharmacological and parenteral therapies; CL: Analysis

101. 2. The child should receive 300 mg in one dose. Use the following equation:
First, determine how many mg should be given in one day:
80 mg/kg × 15 kg = 1,200 mg
Then, determine how many mg should be given in one dose:
1,200 mg/4 doses = 300 mg/dose
CN: Physiological integrity; CNS: Pharmacological and parenteral therapies; CL: Analysis

102. 3. Because of the anticoagulant effects of aspirin therapy, a soft-bristled toothbrush will prevent bleeding of the gums. A low-cholesterol diet should be followed until coronary artery involvement resolves. Black, tarry stools are abnormal and are signs of bleeding that should be reported to the physician immediately. Contact sports should be avoided because of the cardiac involvement and excessive bruising that may occur as a result of aspirin therapy.
CN: Physiological integrity; CNS: Physiological adaptation; CL: Analysis

103. 4. Because of the risk of coronary artery involvement and possible aneurysm development, repeat echocardiography and electrocardiography will be required the first few weeks and at 6 months. Aspirin therapy may be continued for 2 weeks after the onset of symptoms. If signs of coronary artery involvement are present, aspirin therapy may be continued indefinitely. Live-virus vaccines should be avoided for 6 to 11 months after gamma globulin therapy because of an increased risk of a cross-sensitivity reaction to the antibodies found in the dose given. Returning to school should be avoided until cleared by the physician.
CN: Physiological integrity; CNS: Physiological adaptation; CL: Analysis

CN: Client needs category   CNS: Client needs subcategory   CL: Cognitive level

104. A nurse is teaching the parents of a child with <u>acute</u> rheumatic fever about the disorder. Which statement would be the most accurate concerning this condition?
1. A progressive inflammation of the small vessels
2. A mucocutaneous lymph node syndrome
3. A serious infection of the endocardial surface of the heart
4. A sequela of group A beta-hemolytic streptococcal infections

105. Which assessment finding is expected in a child with acute rheumatic fever?
1. Leukocytosis
2. Normal electrocardiogram
3. High fever for 5 or more days
4. Normal erythrocyte sedimentation rate

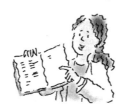

Read carefully. Question 104 asks about acute rheumatic fever, not chronic.

106. Which criteria is required to establish a diagnosis of acute rheumatic fever?
1. Laboratory tests
2. Fever and four Jones criteria
3. Positive blood cultures for *Staphylococcus* organisms
4. Use of Jones criteria and presence of a streptococcal infection

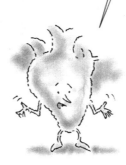

I was just trying to "keep up with the Jones."

107. Which diagnostic criteria is considered major for Jones criteria for acute rheumatic fever?
1. Carditis
2. Prolonged PR interval
3. Low-grade fever
4. Previous heart disease

108. A nurse is caring for a child with acute rheumatic fever. Which symptom would indicate Sydenham's chorea, a major manifestation of acute rheumatic fever?
1. Cardiomegaly
2. Regurgitant murmur
3. Pericardial friction rubs
4. Involuntary muscle movements

104. 4. Acute rheumatic fever is a multisystem disorder caused by group A beta-hemolytic streptococcal infections. It may involve the heart, joints, central nervous system, and skin. Kawasaki disease is also known as a mucocutaneous lymph node syndrome characterized by a progressive inflammation of the small vessels. Endocarditis describes a serious infection of the endocardial surface of the heart.
CN: Health promotion and maintenance; CNS: None; CL: Application

105. 1. Leukocytosis can be seen as an immune response triggered by colonization of the pharynx with group A streptococci. The electrocardiogram will show a prolonged PR interval as a result of carditis. The inflammatory response will cause an elevated erythrocyte sedimentation rate. A low-grade fever is a minor manifestation. A high fever of 5 or more days may represent Kawasaki disease.
CN: Physiological integrity; CNS: Physiological adaptation; CL: Application

106. 4. Two major or one major and two minor manifestations from Jones criteria and the presence of a streptococcal infection justify the diagnosis of rheumatic fever. There's no single laboratory test for diagnosis. Fever and four diagnostic criteria are required to diagnose Kawasaki disease. Blood cultures would be positive for *Streptococcus*, not *Staphylococcus*, organisms.
CN: Physiological integrity; CNS: Physiological adaptation; CL: Analysis

107. 1. Carditis is a major diagnostic criteria of acute rheumatic fever. It's the only manifestation that can lead to death or long-term sequelae. Prolonged PR interval, low-grade fever, and previous heart disease are considered minor diagnostic criteria for Jones criteria.
CN: Physiological integrity; CNS: Physiological adaptation; CL: Application

108. 4. Sydenham's chorea is an involvement of the central nervous system by the rheumatic process. This is seen as muscular incoordination; purposeless, involuntary movements; and emotional lability. A regurgitant murmur, cardiomegaly, and a pericardial friction rub are clinical signs of rheumatic carditis.
CN: Physiological integrity; CNS: Physiological adaptation; CL: Application

109. Criteria for rheumatic fever are being discussed with parents. A nurse realizes that the parents understand chorea when they make which statement?
1. "My child may not be able to walk."
2. "Long movies may help for relaxation."
3. "My child might have difficulty in school."
4. "Many activities and visitors are recommended."

110. A 3-year-old child has a positive culture for *Streptococcus* organisms. Which intervention is <u>most appropriate</u>?
1. Give aspirin.
2. Give antibiotics.
3. Give corticosteroids.
4. Encourage fluid intake.

111. A nurse is preparing a child for discharge after being diagnosed with rheumatic fever without carditis. What instructions should the nurse give the parents?
1. Give aspirin for signs of chorea.
2. Give penicillin for 1 month total.
3. Only give penicillin for dental work.
4. It isn't necessary to give penicillin before dental procedures.

112. Which nursing diagnosis is <u>most appropriate</u> for a child with rheumatic fever?
1. *Imbalanced nutrition: More than body requirements*
2. *Risk for injury*
3. *Delayed growth and development*
4. *Impaired gas exchange*

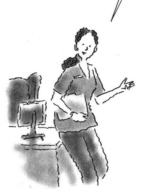

Question 110 is asking for the most appropriate intervention.

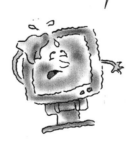

Don't sweat it! You're almost there.

109. 3. Chorea may last 1 to 6 months. Central nervous system involvement contributes to a shortened attention span, so children might have difficulty learning in school. A quiet environment is required for treatment. Muscle incoordination may cause the child to be more clumsy than usual when walking.
CN: Physiological integrity; CNS: Physiological adaptation; CL: Analysis

110. 2. Infection caused by *Streptococcus* organisms is treated with antibiotics, mainly penicillin. Antipyretics, such as acetaminophen, may be given for fever. Aspirin isn't recommended. Corticosteroids have no implication. Fluid intake is encouraged to prevent dehydration from decreased oral intake due to the sore throat or to replace fluids lost because of possible diarrhea from the antibiotics.
CN: Physiological integrity; CNS: Physiological adaptation; CL: Analysis

111. 4. Children who might benefit from prophylactic penicillin include those with unrepaired congenital heart defects, heart defects repaired with synthetic material, or prior infective endocarditis, and some children with heart transplants. Prophylactic antibiotic therapy isn't otherwise recommended.
CN: Physiological integrity; CNS: Pharmacological and parenteral therapies; CL: Application

112. 2. Because of symptoms of chorea, safety measures should be taken to prevent falls or injury. There may be *Imbalanced nutrition: Less than body requirements* due to a sore throat and dysphagia. Growth and development usually aren't delayed. *Impaired gas exchange* usually isn't an issue unless the condition worsens with carditis and heart failure is present.
CN: Physiological integrity; CNS: Physiological adaptation; CL: Analysis

CN: Client needs category   CNS: Client needs subcategory   CL: Cognitive level

113. The nurse is teaching the parents of a child with sinus bradycardia. Which statement about the condition is the most correct?
1. "It is a heart rate less than normal for age."
2. "It is a heart rate greater than normal for age."
3. "It is a variation of the normal cardiac rhythm."
4. "It is an increase in sinus node impulse formation."

114. In which condition or group is sinus bradycardia a <u>normal</u> finding?
1. Hypoxia
2. Hypothermia
3. Growth-delayed adolescent
4. Physically conditioned adolescent

115. Treatment for a child with sinus bradycardia includes atropine 0.02 mg/kg/dose. If the child weighs 20 kg, how much is given per dose?
1. 0.02 mg
2. 0.04 mg
3. 0.2 mg
4. 0.4 mg

116. Atropine, an anticholinergic agent, is being administered to a child with sinus bradycardia. Which statement is the most accurate about the administration of this medication?
1. It increases heart rate.
2. It raises blood pressure.
3. It dilates bronchial tubes.
4. It decreases heart rate.

117. A nurse has given atropine to treat sinus bradycardia in an 11-month-old infant. Which <u>adverse reaction</u> may be noted?
1. Lethargy
2. Diarrhea
3. No tears when crying
4. Increased urine output

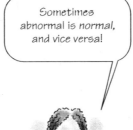

Sometimes abnormal is normal, and vice versa!

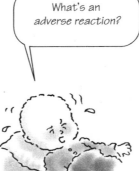

What's an adverse reaction?

113. 1. Sinus bradycardia can best be described as a heart rate less than normal for age. Sinus tachycardia refers to a heart rate greater than normal for age or an increase in sinus node impulse formation. A sinus arrhythmia is a variation of the normal cardiac rhythm.
CN: Physiological integrity; CNS: Physiological adaptation; CL: Application

114. 4. A physically conditioned adolescent might have a lower than normal heart rate; this is of no significance. Hypoxia and hypothermia are pathologic states in which a slow heart rate may produce a compromised hemodynamic state. Growth-delayed adolescents won't have bradycardia as a normal finding.
CN: Physiological integrity; CNS: Physiological adaptation; CL: Analysis

115. 4. The child should receive 0.4 mg. Use the following equation:
$$0.02 \text{ mg/kg} \times 20 \text{ kg} = 0.4 \text{ mg}$$
CN: Physiological integrity; CNS: Pharmacological and parenteral therapies; CL: Analysis

116. 1. Atropine blocks vagal impulses to the myocardium and stimulates the cardio-inhibitory center in the medulla, thereby increasing heart rate and cardiac output. Atropine is not given to directly increase blood pressure or dilate the bronchial tubes.
CN: Physiological integrity; CNS: Pharmacological and parenteral therapies; CL: Application

117. 3. Atropine dries up secretions and also lessens the response of ciliary and iris sphincter muscles in the eye, causing mydriasis. It usually causes paradoxical excitement in children. Constipation and urinary retention can be seen due to a decrease in smooth-muscle contractions of the GI and genitourinary tracts.
CN: Physiological integrity; CNS: Pharmacological and parenteral therapies; CL: Application

118. Which condition could cause sinus tachycardia?
1. Fever
2. Hypothermia
3. Hypothyroidism
4. Hypoxia

119. Which arrhythmia commonly seen in children involves heart rate changes related to respirations?
1. Sinus arrhythmia
2. Sinus block
3. Sinus bradycardia
4. Sinus tachycardia

120. Which condition may lead to sinus arrest or sinus pause in a child?
1. Hypokalemia
2. Hyperthermia
3. Valsalva's maneuver
4. Decreased intracranial pressure

121. Which statement is the most correct regarding the use of amiodarone (Cordarone)?
1. It is used to treat atrial dysrhythmias.
2. It is used to treat ventricular dysrhythmias.
3. It is used to treat both atrial and ventricular dysrhythmias.
4. It is used to treat heart failure.

118. 1. Sinus tachycardia is commonly seen in children with a fever. It's usually a result of a noncardiac cause. Hypothermia, hypothyroidism, and hypoxia will result in sinus bradycardia.
CN: Physiological integrity; CNS: Physiological adaptation; CL: Analysis

119. 1. In sinus arrhythmia, heart rate increases with inhalation and decreases with exhalation in response to changes in intrathoracic pressure during respiration. Sinus arrhythmia is a common occurrence in childhood and adolescence. Sinus block, sinus bradycardia, and sinus tachycardia are respiration-independent arrhythmias.
CN: Physiological integrity; CNS: Physiological adaptation; CL: Analysis

120. 3. Sinus arrest may occur in children when vagal tone is increased such as during Valsalva's maneuver in vomiting, gagging, or straining during a bowel movement. This represents a failure of the sinoatrial node to generate an impulse. A straight line or pause occurs, indicating the absence of electrical activity. After the pause, another impulse will be generated and a cardiac complex will appear. Hyperkalemia, hypothermia, and increased intracranial pressure are pathologic conditions that may also produce sinus arrest.
CN: Physiological integrity; CNS: Physiological adaptation; CL: Analysis

121. 3. Amiodarone is used to treat both atrial and ventricular dysrhythmias. It is not used in the treatment of heart failure.
CN: Physiological integrity; CNS: Pharmacological and parenteral therapies; CL: Application

CN: Client needs category   CNS: Client needs subcategory   CL: Cognitive level

122. To which classification does isoproterenol belong?
   1. Adrenergic agonist
   2. Anticholinergic
   3. Beta-adrenergic blocker
   4. Vasopressor

123. Which finding may be seen in a 1-year-old child with supraventricular tachycardia?
   1. Heart rate of 100 beats/minute
   2. Heart rate of 180 beats/minute
   3. Heart rate less than 80 beats/minute
   4. Heart rate more than 240 beats/minute

In question 124, the word *first* is your clue to the right answer.

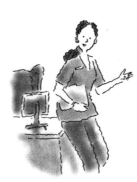

124. A 2-year-old child is experiencing supraventricular tachycardia. Which intervention should be attempted first?
   1. Administration of digoxin
   2. Administration of verapamil
   3. Synchronized cardioversion
   4. Immersion of the child's hands in cold water

125. A 2-month-old infant arrives in the emergency department with a heart rate of 180 beats/minute and a temperature of 103.1° F (39.5° C) rectally. Which intervention is most appropriate?
   1. Give acetaminophen (Tylenol).
   2. Encourage fluid intake.
   3. Apply carotid massage.
   4. Place the infant's hands in cold water.

122. 3. Isoproterenol acts as a beta-adrenergic blocker to reduce peripheral resistance and increase the force of cardiac contraction without producing vasoconstriction. It also acts as a bronchodilator, relaxing bronchial smooth muscle and creating peripheral vasodilation.
CN: Physiological integrity; CNS: Pharmacological and parenteral therapies; CL: Analysis

123. 4. Supraventricular tachycardia may be related to increased automaticity of an atrial cell other than the sinoatrial node, or as a reentry mechanism. The rhythm is regular and can occur at rates of 240 beats/minute or more. A heart rate of 100 beats/minute is a normal finding for a 1-year-old child. A heart rate around 180 beats/minute may represent sinus tachycardia. A heart rate of less than 80 beats/minute can be characterized as sinus bradycardia.
CN: Physiological integrity; CNS: Physiological adaptation; CL: Analysis

124. 4. Vagal maneuvers such as immersion of the hands in cold water are commonly tried first as a mechanism to decrease the heart rate. Other vagal maneuvers include breath-holding, carotid massage, gagging, and placing the head lower than the rest of the body. Synchronized cardioversion may be required if vagal maneuvers and drugs are ineffective. If a child has low cardiac output, cardioversion may be used instead of drugs. Verapamil isn't recommended. Digoxin is one of the most common drugs given to help decrease heart rate by increasing myocardial contractility and automaticity and reducing excitability.
CN: Physiological integrity; CNS: Reduction of risk potential; CL: Application

125. 1. Acetaminophen should be given first to decrease the temperature. A heart rate of 180 beats/minute is normal in an infant with a fever. A tepid sponge bath may be given to help decrease the temperature and calm the infant. Carotid massage is an attempt to decrease the heart rate as a vagal maneuver. This won't work in this infant because the source of the increased heart rate is fever. Fluid intake is encouraged after the acetaminophen is given to help replace insensible fluid losses.
CN: Physiological integrity; CNS: Physiological adaptation; CL: Application

126. A critically ill 4-year-old is in the pediatric intensive care unit. Telemetry monitoring reveals junctional tachycardia. Identify where this arrhythmia originates.

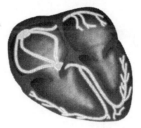

127. An infant who weighs 8 kg is to receive ampicillin 25 mg/kg I.V. every 6 hours. How many milligrams should the nurse administer per dose? Record your answer using a whole number.

_____ milligrams

128. The nurse is caring for an infant with a heart defect that involves increased pulmonary blood flow. Which illustration shows a congenital heart disorder with increased pulmonary blood flow?

1.

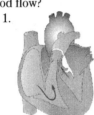

2.

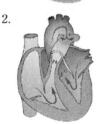

3.

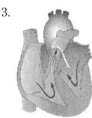

4.

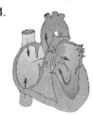

126. In junctional tachycardia, the atrioventricular node rapidly fires.
CN: Physiological integrity;
CNS: Physiological adaptation;
CL: Analysis

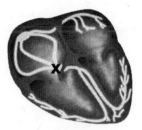

127. 200. The nurse should calculate the correct dose using the following equation: 25 mg/kg × 8 kg = 200 mg.
CN: Physiological integrity; CNS: Pharmacological and parenteral therapies; CL: Application

128. 2. In patent ductus arteriosus, an accessory fetal structure that connects the pulmonary artery to the aorta fails to close at birth. This allows blood to shunt from the aorta to the pulmonary artery. Option 1 depicts aortic stenosis (narrowed aortic valve) and option 3 shows pulmonic stenosis (narrowed pulmonic valve); both are obstruction to blood flow disorders. Option 4 shows tricuspid atresia (failure of the tricuspid valve to develop), a decreased pulmonary blood flow disorder.
CN: Physiological integrity; CNS: Physiological adaptation; CL: Analysis

CN: Client needs category   CNS: Client needs subcategory   CL: Cognitive level

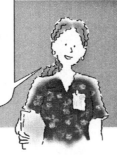

Chapter 15
Respiratory system

1. Following the death of an infant from sudden infant death syndrome (SIDS), which response by a nurse to the grieving parents is most appropriate?

1. "You didn't cause your infant's death."
2. "An autopsy will confirm the cause of your infant's death."
3. "Don't worry, you'll have more children."
4. "Be sure to place your next infant on his back to sleep."

2. Which child has an increased risk of sudden infant death syndrome (SIDS)?

1. A neonate born at 32 weeks' gestation weighing 4 lb (1.8 kg)
2. A 2-year-old with a broken arm
3. An infant hospitalized with a temperature of 103.4° F (39.7° C)
4. A first-born child

3. A 6-week-old infant is brought to the emergency department not breathing; a preliminary finding of sudden infant death syndrome (SIDS) is made to the parents. Which intervention should the nurse take <u>initially</u>?

1. Call their spiritual advisor.
2. Explain the etiology of SIDS.
3. Allow them to see their infant.
4. Collect the infant's belongings and give them to the parents.

Cool! You made it to chapter 15. Keep up the good work!

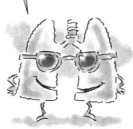

Careful. This question is asking you to prioritize.

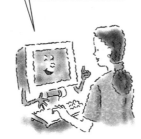

1. 1. The nurse can best support grieving parents by correcting the common falsehood that they could have prevented the infant's death. While an autopsy may need to be performed, it isn't a supportive response to grieving parents. Telling the parents that they will have more children minimizes the death of this infant and belittles the parent's feelings of grief. Instructing the parents to position future infants on their back suggests that the parents could have prevented this child's death.

CN: Psychosocial integrity; CNS: None; CL: Analysis

2. 1. Premature infants, especially those with low birth weight, have an increased risk for SIDS. Infants with apnea, central nervous system disorders, or respiratory disorders have a higher risk of SIDS. Peak age for SIDS is 2 to 4 months. Hospitalization for fever is insignificant. There's an increased risk of SIDS in subsequent siblings of two or more SIDS victims.

CN: Physiological integrity; CNS: Reduction of risk potential; CL: Analysis

3. 3. The parents need time with their infant to assist with the grieving process. Calling their pastor and collecting the infant's belongings are also important steps in the plan of care but aren't priorities. The parents will be too upset to understand an explanation of SIDS at this time.

CN: Psychosocial integrity; CNS: None; CL: Application

4. The family of an infant that died from sudden infant death syndrome (SIDS) asks the nurse what risk factors could have predisposed their child to SIDS. Which response would be the <u>most</u> accurate?
　　1. Breast feeding the infant
　　2. Gestational age of 42 weeks
　　3. Immunizations
　　4. Low birth weight

5. An infant is brought to the emergency department (ED) and pronounced dead with the preliminary finding of sudden infant death syndrome (SIDS). Which question to the parents is appropriate?
　　1. Did you hear the infant cry out?
　　2. Was the infant's head buried in a blanket?
　　3. Were any of the siblings jealous of the new baby?
　　4. How did the infant look when you found him?

6. Which diagnostic test should be included in the care plan for children with an increased risk of sudden infant death syndrome (SIDS)?
　　1. Pulmonary function tests at regular intervals
　　2. Home apnea monitor
　　3. Pulse oximetry while sleeping
　　4. Chest X-ray at age 1 month

7. Which reaction is usually exhibited by the family of an infant who has died from sudden infant death syndrome (SIDS)?
　　1. Feelings of blame or guilt
　　2. Acceptance of the diagnosis
　　3. Requests for the infant's belongings
　　4. Questions regarding the etiology of the diagnosis

8. The parents of an infant who just died from sudden infant death syndrome (SIDS) are angry at God and refuse to see any member of the clergy. Which nursing diagnosis is most appropriate?
　　1. *Ineffective coping*
　　2. *Spiritual distress*
　　3. *Complicated grieving*
　　4. *Chronic sorrow*

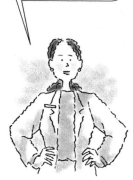

It's important to be sensitive to a family's feelings when they've lost a child to SIDS.

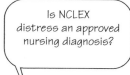

Is NCLEX distress an approved nursing diagnosis?

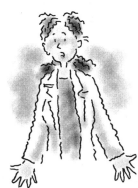

4. 4. Prematurity, low birth weight, maternal smoking, and multiple births are important risk factors associated with SIDS. Breast feeding and a gestational age of 42 weeks aren't significant. Immunizations have been disproved to be associated with the disorder.
CN: Physiological integrity; CNS: Reduction of risk potential; CL: Application

5. 4. Only factual questions should be asked during the initial history in the ED. The other questions imply blame, guilt, or neglect.
CN: Physiological integrity; CNS: Physiological adaptation; CL: Application

6. 2. A home apnea monitor is recommended for infants with an increased risk for SIDS. Diagnostic tests, such as pulmonary function tests, pulse oximetry, and chest X-rays can't diagnose the risk of surviving or dying from SIDS.
CN: Physiological integrity; CNS: Reduction of risk potential; CL: Application

7. 1. During the first few moments, the parents often are in shock and have overwhelming feelings of blame or guilt. Acceptance of the diagnosis and questions regarding the etiology may not occur until the parents have had time to see the child. The infant's belongings are usually packaged for the family to take home but some parents may see this as a painful reminder.
CN: Psychosocial integrity; CNS: None; CL: Application

8. 2. The defining characteristics of *Spiritual distress* include anger and refusing to interact with spiritual leaders. While anger is part of the grieving process, there's no indication that the parents aren't coping effectively or are experiencing *Complicated grieving*. Since *Chronic sorrow*, as the name implies, occurs over a period of time and may be cyclical, this isn't an appropriate nursing diagnosis since the death has just occurred.
CN: Psychosocial integrity; CNS: None; CL: Analysis

CN: Client needs category   CNS: Client needs subcategory   CL: Cognitive level

9. Which plan is most appropriate for a nurse scheduling a home visit to parents who lost an infant to sudden infant death syndrome (SIDS)?
  1. One visit in 2 weeks
  2. No visit is necessary
  3. As soon after death as possible
  4. One visit with parents only, no siblings

10. About 1 week after the death of an infant from sudden infant death syndrome (SIDS), which behavior should a nurse expect to observe in a parent?
  1. Disorganized thinking
  2. Feelings of guilt
  3. Repressed thoughts
  4. Structured thinking

11. Which position is recommended for placing an infant to sleep?
  1. Prone position
  2. Supine position
  3. Side-lying position
  4. With head of bed elevated 30 degrees

12. Which activity should be recommended for <u>long-term</u> support of parents with an infant who has died of sudden infant death syndrome (SIDS)?
  1. Attending support groups
  2. Attending church regularly
  3. Attending counseling sessions
  4. Discussing feelings with family and friends

Make sure you understand the grieving process necessary for SIDS parents.

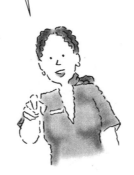

9. 3. When parents return home, a visit is necessary as soon after the death as possible. The nurse should assess what the parents have been told, what they think happened, and how they've explained this to the other siblings. Not all of these issues will be resolved in one visit. The number of visits and plan for intervention must be flexible. The needs of the siblings must always be considered.
CN: Psychosocial integrity; CNS: None; CL: Application

10. 4. About 1 week after the death, the parent of the infant would most likely be in the turmoil phase. In the turmoil phase, structured thinking is common. Almost immediately, at the time of death, parents may have repressed thoughts and feelings of guilt or blame. Within a day or two, the parents enter the impact phase of crisis. This consists of disorganized thoughts in which they can't deal with the crisis in concrete terms.
CN: Psychosocial integrity; CNS: None; CL: Application

11. 2. The American Academy of Pediatrics endorses placing infants face-up in their cribs as a way to reduce sudden infant death syndrome (SIDS). Placing infants on their stomach is thought to make an attack of apnea harder to fight off but how exactly the sleeping position predisposes a child to SIDS is still unclear. The side-lying position promotes gastric emptying. Raising the head of the bed 30 degrees is recommended for infants with gastroesophageal reflux.
CN: Health promotion and maintenance; CNS: None; CL: Application

12. 1. The best support will come from parents who have had the same experience. Attending church and discussing feelings with family and friends can offer support but they may not understand the experience. Counseling sessions are usually a short-term support.
CN: Psychosocial integrity; CNS: None; CL: Application

13. Which intervention is best to help a 2-year-old child adapt to hospitalization?
1. Allow the child to have favorite toys.
2. Allow the child to play with equipment used on him.
3. Explain procedures in simple terms.
4. Ask one or both parents to stay with the child.

14. A 2-year-old child comes to the emergency department with inspiratory stridor and a barking cough. A preliminary diagnosis of croup has been made. Which action should be an <u>initial</u> intervention?
1. Administer I.V. antibiotics.
2. Provide oxygen by facemask.
3. Establish and maintain the airway.
4. Ask the mother to go to the waiting room.

15. Which action is the best intervention for parents to take if their child is experiencing an episode of "midnight croup," or acute spasmodic laryngitis?
1. Give warm liquids.
2. Raise the heat on the thermostat.
3. Provide humidified air with cool mist.
4. Take the child into the bathroom with a warm running shower.

16. Which sign is <u>most characteristic</u> of a child with croup?
1. Barking cough
2. Fever
3. High heart rate
4. Respiratory distress

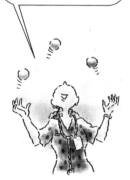

Congratulations! You've finished the first 15 questions! Good job!

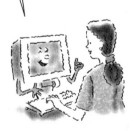

This question is asking for the symptom most commonly associated with croup.

13. 4. The most important factor in helping a child cope with new and strange surroundings is to have the security of the parents being present. This is the hallmark of family-centered care. Placing the child's favorite toys in the room provides distraction and allows the child to have something of his own with him but may *not* alleviate fears. Allowing the child to play with the equipment may pose a safety hazard and isn't appropriate. Explaining procedures in simple terms is important but a 2-year-old has limited understanding.
CN: Psychosocial integrity; CNS: None; CL: Application

14. 3. The initial priority is to establish and maintain the airway. Edema and accumulation of secretions may contribute to airway obstruction. Antibiotics aren't indicated for viral illnesses. Oxygen should be administered by tent as soon as possible to decrease the child's distress. Allowing the child to stay with the mother reduces anxiety and distress.
CN: Physiological integrity; CNS: Physiological adaptation; CL: Application

15. 3. High humidity with cool mist provides the most relief. Raising the heat on the thermostat will result in dry, warm air, which may cause secretions to adhere to the airway wall. A warm, running shower provides a mist that may be helpful to moisten and decrease the viscosity of airway secretions and may also decrease laryngeal spasm, but cool liquids would be best for the child. If unable to take liquid, the child needs to be in the emergency department.
CN: Physiological integrity; CNS: Physiological adaptation; CL: Application

16. 1. A resonant cough described as "barking" is the most characteristic sign of croup. The child may present with a low-grade or high fever depending on whether the etiologic agent is viral or bacterial. While the child with croup may have a rapid heart rate, it isn't a characteristic sign of croup. The child may have varying degrees of respiratory distress related to swelling or obstruction.
CN: Physiological integrity; CNS: Physiological adaptation; CL: Analysis

CN: Client needs category   CNS: Client needs subcategory   CL: Cognitive level

17. Which sign should alert a nurse that an 18-month-old child with croup is experiencing increased respiratory distress?
1. A barking cough
2. Intercostal retractions
3. Clubbing of the fingers
4. Increased anterior-posterior chest diameter

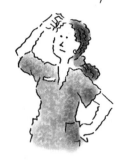

I know what's important, but what's the *most* important?

18. Which intervention is the <u>most important</u> goal for a child with ineffective airway clearance?
1. Reducing the child's anxiety
2. Maintaining a patent airway
3. Providing adequate oral fluids
4. Administering medications as ordered

19. A 19-month-old child with croup is crying as a nurse tries to auscultate breath sounds. Which intervention by the nurse would be most appropriate?
1. Ignore the crying and listen to breaths sounds as best as possible.
2. Tell the parents that they are upsetting the child and to wait outside the room.
3. Tell the child, in a loud and firm voice, that he must sit still and cooperate.
4. Hand the stethoscope to the child to examine before auscultating his lungs.

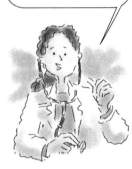

It's important to gain the child's trust.

20. Which precaution is recommended when caring for children with respiratory infections such as croup?
1. Enforce hand washing.
2. Place the child in isolation.
3. Teach children to use tissues.
4. Keep siblings in the same room.

21. What is the <u>best</u> time to administer a nebulizer treatment to a child with croup?
1. During naptime
2. During playtime
3. After the child eats
4. After the parents leave

17. 2. Intercostal retractions occur as the child's breathing becomes more labored and the use of other muscles is necessary to draw air into the lungs. A barking cough occurs in a child with croup and itself isn't a sign that the condition is worsening. Clubbing of the fingers and a change in chest diameter occur with chronic respiratory conditions.
CN: Physiological integrity; CNS: Physiological adaptation; CL: Analysis

18. 2. The most important goal is to maintain a patent airway. Reducing anxiety and administering medications will follow after the airway is secure. The child shouldn't be allowed to eat or drink anything to prevent the risk of aspiration.
CN: Physiological integrity; CNS: Physiological adaptation; CL: Application

19. 4. Developmentally, children at this age are curious. Therefore, encouraging the child to play with the stethoscope will distract him and help gain trust so that the nurse will be able to auscultate the lungs. Ignoring the child's crying may only get him more upset and won't help the nurse gain his trust. The nurse should use the parents to help quiet and comfort the child. Asking the parents to leave may only upset the child more. The nurse should speak to the child in a soft, comforting tone of voice.
CN: Health promotion and maintenance; CNS: None; CL: Analysis

20. 1. Hand washing helps prevent the spread of infections. Ill children should be placed in separate bedrooms if possible but don't need to be isolated. Teaching children to use tissues properly is important, but the key is disposal and hand washing after use.
CN: Health promotion and maintenance; CNS: None; CL: Application

21. 1. The nurse should administer nebulizer treatments at prescribed intervals. During naptime allows for as little disruption as possible. Administering treatment during playtime will disrupt the child's daily pattern. A child should be given a treatment before eating so the airway will be open and the work of eating will be decreased. Parents are usually helpful when administering treatments. The child can sit on the parents' lap to help decrease anxiety or fear.
CN: Physiological integrity; CNS: Pharmacological and parenteral therapies; CL: Application

22. During the recovery stages of croup, a nurse should explain which intervention to parents?
1. Limiting oral fluid intake
2. Recognizing signs of respiratory distress
3. Providing three nutritious meals per day
4. Allowing the child to go to the playground

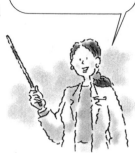

Adequate parent teaching is essential for managing a child with croup.

23. Which instruction should a nurse give the parents of a 2-year-old child who wakes in the night with a barking cough?
1. Provide humidified air for the child to breath.
2. Call for an ambulance immediately.
3. Place the child in a warm, dry room.
4. Begin rescue breathing at once.

24. The nurse is assessing a child recently brought to the emergency department. Which observations would cause the nurse to suspect epiglottitis?
1. Decreased secretions
2. Drooling
3. Low-grade fever
4. Spontaneous cough

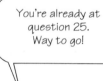

You're already at question 25. Way to go!

25. Which strategy is the best plan of care for a child with acute epiglottitis?
1. Encourage oral fluids for hydration.
2. Maintain the client in semi-Fowler's position.
3. Administer I.V. antibiotic therapy.
4. Maintain respiratory isolation for 48 hours.

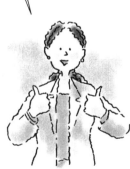

22. 2. Although most children recover without complications, the parents should be able to recognize signs and symptoms of respiratory distress and know how to access emergency services. Oral fluids should be encouraged because fluids help to thin secretions. Although nutrition is important, frequent small nutritious snacks are usually more appealing than an entire meal. Children should have optimal rest and engage in quiet play. A comfortable environment free from noxious stimuli lessens respiratory distress.
CN: Physiological integrity; CNS: Physiological adaptation; CL: Application

23. 1. Humidified air reduces laryngeal irritation and spasm and helps liquefy secretions. The child doesn't need emergency care at this time; however, if the child develops respiratory distress, the parents should be instructed to call emergency medical services and not to drive the child to the hospital themselves. The child shouldn't be placed in a warm, dry room as cool, humidified air is used to reduce laryngospasm. The child doesn't require rescue breathing at the time. Rescue breathing is necessary if the child stops breathing.
CN: Physiological integrity; CNS: Reduction of risk potential; CL: Application

24. 2. Drooling of saliva is common due to the pain of swallowing, excessive secretions, and sore throat. The child usually has a high fever and the absence of a spontaneous cough. The classic picture is the child in a tripod position with mouth open and tongue protruding.
CN: Physiological integrity; CNS: Physiological adaptation; CL: Application

25. 3. The etiologic agent for epiglottitis is usually bacterial; therefore, the treatment consists of I.V. antibiotic therapy. The client shouldn't be allowed anything by mouth during the initial phases of the infection to prevent aspiration. The client should be placed in Fowler's position or any position that provides the most comfort and security. Respiratory isolation isn't required.
CN: Physiological integrity; CNS: Physiological adaptation; CL: Application

CN: Client needs category   CNS: Client needs subcategory   CL: Cognitive level

26. A 2-year-old child is found on the floor next to his toy chest. After first determining unresponsiveness and calling for help, which step should be taken <u>next?</u>
1. Start mouth-to-mouth resuscitation.
2. Begin chest compressions.
3. Check for a pulse.
4. Open the airway.

27. A 10-month-old infant is found in respiratory arrest and cardiopulmonary resuscitation is started. Which site is best to check for a pulse?
1. Brachial
2. Carotid
3. Femoral
4. Radial

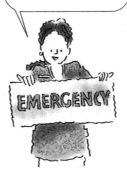

It's important to prioritize in an emergency situation.

28. When giving rescue breathing to an infant under age 1, what is the <u>ratio</u> of breaths per second?
1. 1 breath every 2 to 3 seconds
2. 1 breath every 3 to 5 seconds
3. 1 breath every 4 to 6 seconds
4. 1 breath every 5 to 7 seconds

29. When performing chest compressions on a 2-year-old child, which depth is correct?
1. ½″ to 1″ (1 to 2.5 cm)
2. 1″ to 1½″ (2.5 to 3.5 cm)
3. 1½″ to 2″ (3.5 to 5 cm)
4. 2″ to 2½″ (5 to 6.5 cm)

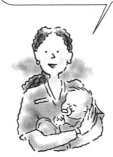

The procedure for rescue breathing for infants is different from that for adults.

30. A nurse rescuer knows that chest compressions must be coordinated with ventilations. Which ratio should the nurse rescuer use for a 3-year-old child?
1. 15 compressions to 1 ventilation
2. 15 compressions to 2 ventilations
3. 30 compressions to 1 ventilation
4. 30 compressions to 2 ventilations

26. 4. The airway should be opened by using the chin thrust and breathlessness should be determined at the start of cardiopulmonary resuscitation. The sequence of airway, breathing, and circulation needs to be followed.
CN: Physiological integrity; CNS: Physiological adaptation; CL: Application

27. 1. Palpation of the brachial artery is recommended. The short, chubby neck of infants makes rapid location of the carotid artery difficult. After age 1, the carotid would be used. The femoral pulse, often palpated in a hospital setting, may be difficult to assess because of the infant's position, fat folds, and clothing. The radial pulse isn't a good indicator of central artery perfusion.
CN: Physiological integrity; CNS: Physiological adaptation; CL: Application

28. 2. Rescue breathing should be performed once every 3 to 5 seconds until spontaneous breathing resumes. This provides approximately 20 breaths/minute. One breath every 2 to 3 seconds may cause gastric distention. One breath every 5 to 6 seconds is recommended for adults.
CN: Physiological integrity; CNS: Physiological adaptation; CL: Application

29. 2. The chest compressions should equal approximately one-third to one-half the total depth of the chest. This corresponds to about 1 to 1½″ in a child age 1 to 8, ½″ to 1″ for an infant younger than age 1, and 1½″ to 2″ for an adult.
CN: Physiological integrity; CNS: Physiological adaptation; CL: Application

30. 4. A single health care provider rescuer should use a ratio of 30 chest compressions to 2 ventilations for children ages 1 year to the onset of adolescence. Ratios of 15:1, 15:2, and 30:1 won't provide optimal compression and ventilation.
CN: Physiological integrity; CNS: Physiological adaptation; CL: Application

31. A 10-month-old child is found choking and soon becomes unconscious. Which intervention should a nurse attempt <u>first</u> after opening the airway?
1. Look inside the child's mouth for a foreign object.
2. Give five back blows and five chest thrusts.
3. Attempt a blind finger sweep.
4. Attempt rescue breathing.

32. Using which part of the hands is appropriate when performing chest compressions on a child between ages 1 and 8?
1. Heels of both hands
2. Heel of one hand
3. Index and middle fingers
4. Thumbs of both hands

33. A 3-year-old child is brought to the emergency department not breathing, cyanotic, and lethargic. The mother states that she thinks he swallowed a penny. Which intervention should the nurse take <u>first</u>?
1. Give 100% oxygen.
2. Administer five back blows.
3. Attempt a blind finger sweep.
4. Administer abdominal thrusts.

34. Which statement by the parent of a 4-year-old boy who just had a tonsillectomy indicates that a nurse's discharge instruction has been successful?
1. "I will keep him flat on his back in bed."
2. "I will sit him in bed at a 45-degree angle."
3. "I will place him on his stomach with his head to the side."
4. "I will place him on his back with his head on a pillow."

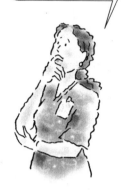

I am going to feel like a real heel if I get this answer wrong.

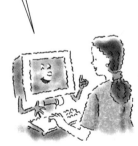

Again, you're being asked to prioritize.

31. 1. After the airway is open, the nurse should check for a foreign object and remove it with a finger sweep if it can be seen. After this step, rescue breathing should be attempted. If ventilation is unsuccessful, the nurse should then give five back blows and five chest thrusts in an attempt to dislodge the object. Blind finger sweeps should never be performed because this may push the object further back into the airway.
CN: Physiological integrity; CNS: Physiological adaptation; CL: Application

32. 2. The heel of one hand is recommended for performing chest compressions on children between ages 1 and 8. Two hands are used for adult cardiopulmonary resuscitation. Chest thrusts administered with the middle and third fingers, and in some cases the thumbs of each hand, are used on infants younger than age 1.
CN: Physiological integrity; CNS: Physiological adaptation; CL: Application

33. 4. A child between ages 1 and 8 should receive abdominal thrusts to help dislodge the object. Administering 100% oxygen won't help if the airway is occluded. Infants younger than age 1 should receive back blows before chest thrusts. Blind finger sweeps should never be performed because this could push the object further back into the airway.
CN: Physiological integrity; CNS: Physiological adaptation; CL: Application

34. 3. Laying the child on his stomach with the head turned to the side allows blood and other secretions to drain from the mouth and pharynx, reducing the risk of aspiration. Placing the child flat on his back, on his back with a pillow, or at a 45-degree angle doesn't promote drainage and increases the likelihood of aspiration.
CN: Physiological integrity; CNS: Reduction of risk potential; CL: Application

35. A 7-month-old child is diagnosed with otitis media; the physician orders amoxicillin 40 mg/kg/day to be administered three times per day. The child weighs 9 kg. How much amoxicillin should the child receive per dose?
1. 120 mg
2. 180 mg
3. 200 mg
4. 360 mg

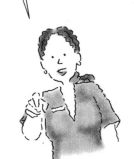

Make sure you understand this formula. You'll use it again later in this chapter.

35. 1. The child should receive 120 mg per dose. Here are the calculations: 40 mg × 9 kg = 360 mg/day; 360 mg/3 doses = 120 mg/dose.
CN: Physiological integrity; CNS: Pharmacological and parenteral therapies; CL: Application

36. Children with chronic otitis media commonly require surgery for a myringotomy and ear tube placement. Which management strategy explains the purpose of the ear tubes?
1. To administer antibiotics
2. To flush the middle ear
3. To increase pressure
4. To drain fluid

36. 4. Ear tubes allow normal fluid to drain (not flush) from the middle ear. They also allow ventilation. The purpose isn't to administer medication. The tubes also allow pressure to equalize in the middle ear.
CN: Physiological integrity; CNS: Physiological adaptation; CL: Application

37. A nurse is discharging a 10-month-old client with eardrops. Which information should she give the parent about how to administer the drops?
1. Pull the earlobe upward.
2. Pull the earlobe up and back.
3. Pull the earlobe down and back.
4. Pull the earlobe down and forward.

37. 3. For infants, the parent should be told to gently pull the earlobe down and back to visualize the external auditory canal. For children over age 3 and for adults, the earlobe is gently pulled slightly up and back.
CN: Physiological integrity; CNS: Pharmacological and parenteral therapies; CL: Application

38. A child is diagnosed with right chronic otitis media. After the child returns from surgery for myringotomy and placement of ear tubes, which intervention is appropriate?
1. Apply gauze dressings.
2. Position the child on the left side.
3. Position the child on the right side.
4. Apply warm compresses to both ears.

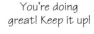

You're doing great! Keep it up!

38. 3. The child should be positioned on the right side to facilitate drainage. Gauze dressings aren't necessary after surgery. Some physicians may prefer a loose cotton wick. The left side isn't an area of concern for drainage. Warm compresses may help to facilitate drainage only when used on the affected ear.
CN: Physiological integrity; CNS: Physiological adaptation; CL: Application

39. To reduce the risk of an infant developing otitis media, a nurse should instruct the parents to:
1. treat all cold symptoms with antibiotics.
2. place the infant in an upright position when feeding from a bottle.
3. avoid washing the ears to keep them dry.
4. swab the outer ear with a cotton-tipped swab.

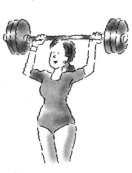

39. 2. The risk of otitis media can be reduced by bottle feeding an infant in the upright position. Formula that pools in the nasopharynx is a good medium for bacterial growth which can move through the shortened, horizontal eustachian tube of the infant. Administering antibiotics with cold symptoms won't reduce the risk of otitis media since colds are due to viral causes. Washing the ears, getting them wet or swabbing the outer ear doesn't contribute to otitis media.
CN: Health promotion and maintenance; CNS: None; CL: Application

40. The nurse is assessing with an otoscope a child suspected of acute otitis media. Which assessment would be indicative of this condition?
  1. Pearl-gray tympanic membrane
  2. Bright red, bulging tympanic membrane
  3. Dull gray membrane with fluid behind the eardrum
  4. Bright red or yellow, bulging or retracted, tympanic membrane

41. A nurse is teaching the parents of a 1-year-old infant with otitis media. Which statement regarding predisposing factors for otitis media would be the <u>most</u> accurate for the nurse to make?
  1. The cartilage lining is overdeveloped.
  2. When infants sit up, it favors the pooling of fluid.
  3. Humoral defense mechanisms decrease the risk of infection.
  4. Eustachian tubes are short, wide, and straight and lie in a horizontal plane.

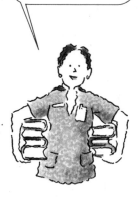

Question 41 is asking about a proximate cause of otitis media.

42. Which complication is most commonly related to acute otitis media?
  1. Eardrum perforation
  2. Hearing loss
  3. Meningitis
  4. Tympanosclerosis

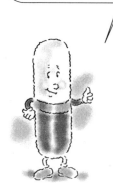

It's important that I stay the course.

43. Which statement by the parent of a child with otitis media indicates an understanding of a nurse's discharge instruction on the use of antibiotics?
  1. "I will give my child the full course of antibiotics."
  2. "I will stop the antibiotics when my child no longer has ear pain."
  3. "I will give the antibiotics whenever my child has ear pain."
  4. "I will put antibiotics in the affected ear."

40. 4. With acute otitis media, the tympanic membrane may present as bright red or yellow, bulging or retracted. A pearl-gray tympanic membrane is a normal finding. Dull gray membrane fluid is consistent with subacute or chronic otitis media.
CN: Physiological integrity; CNS: Physiological adaptation; CL: Application

41. 4. In an infant or child, the eustachian tubes are short, wide, and straight, and lie in a horizontal plane, allowing them to be more easily blocked by conditions such as large adenoids and infections. Until the eustachian tubes change in size and angle, children are more susceptible to otitis media. Cartilage lining is underdeveloped, making the tubes more distensible and more likely to open inappropriately. The usual lying-down position of infants favors the pooling of fluid such as formula in the pharyngeal cavity. Immature humoral defense mechanisms increase the risk of infection.
CN: Physiological integrity; CNS: Physiological adaptation; CL: Analysis

42. 1. Eardrum perforation is the most common complication as the exudate accumulates and pressure increases. Hearing loss in most cases is conductive in nature and mild in severity but is less common than eardrum perforation. Hearing tests aren't usually performed during episodes of otitis media. Tympanosclerosis and meningitis are possible but uncommon when adequate antibiotic therapy is implemented.
CN: Physiological integrity; CNS: Physiological adaptation; CL: Application

43. 1. Antibiotics should be given for the full prescribed course of therapy regardless of whether the child has symptoms. Antibiotics are taken at prescribed intervals and not for episodes of ear pain. Oral antibiotics are used to treat otitis media.
CN: Physiological integrity; CNS: Pharmacological and parental therapies; CL: Application

CN: Client needs category   CNS: Client needs subcategory   CL: Cognitive level

44. A 2-year-old child is diagnosed with epiglottitis. Ampicillin is ordered 50 mg/kg/day in 6 divided doses. The client weighs 12 kg. How much ampicillin is given per dose?
1. 50 mg
2. 100 mg
3. 200 mg
4. 300 mg

45. A 3-year-old child is receiving ampicillin for acute epiglottitis. Which of the following would lead the nurse to suspect an adverse effect to ampicillin?
1. Constipation
2. Generalized rash
3. Increased appetite
4. Low-grade temperature

46. A 3-year-old child is given a preliminary diagnosis of acute epiglottitis. Which nursing intervention is appropriate?
1. Obtain a throat culture immediately.
2. Place the child in a side-lying position.
3. Don't attempt to visualize the epiglottis.
4. Use a tongue blade to look inside the throat.

47. An infant is brought to the clinic for her 6-month vaccines. The nurse tells the mother that administration of which vaccine is an appropriate step for prevention of epiglottitis?
1. Diphtheria vaccine
2. *Haemophilus influenzae* type B (Hib) vaccine
3. Measles vaccine
4. Oral poliovirus vaccine (OPV)

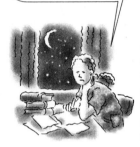

What did I tell you? Here's that formula again!

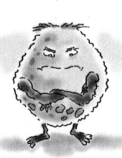

Vaccines. Who needs them?

44. 2. The child should receive 100 mg per dose. Here are the calculations:
50 mg × 12 kg = 600 mg/day;
600 mg/6 doses = 100 mg/dose.
CN: Physiological integrity; CNS: Pharmacological and parenteral therapies; CL: Application

45. 2. Some clients may develop an erythematous or maculopapular rash after 3 to 14 days of therapy; however, this complication doesn't necessitate discontinuing the drug. Nausea, vomiting, epigastric pain, and diarrhea are adverse effects that may necessitate discontinuation of the drug.
CN: Physiological integrity; CNS: Pharmacological and parenteral therapies; CL: Application

46. 3. The nurse shouldn't attempt to visualize the epiglottis. The use of tongue blades or throat culture swabs may cause the epiglottis to spasm and totally occlude the airway. Throat inspection should be attempted only when immediate intubation or tracheostomy can be performed in the event of further or complete obstruction. The child should always remain in the position that provides the most comfort and security and ease of breathing.
CN: Physiological integrity; CNS: Physiological adaptation; CL: Application

47. 2. Epiglottitis is caused by the bacterial agent *H. influenzae*. The American Academy of Pediatrics recommends that, beginning at age 2 months, children receive the Hib conjugate vaccine. A decline in the incidence of epiglottitis has been seen as a result of this vaccination regimen. The OPV, measles, mumps, and rubella vaccine, and diphtheria vaccine are preventive for those diseases.
CN: Health promotion and maintenance; CNS: None; CL: Application

48. Which sign in a 3-year-old child with acute epiglottitis indicates that the client's respiratory distress is <u>increasing</u>?
1. Progressive barking cough
2. Increasing irritability
3. Increasing heart rate
4. Productive cough

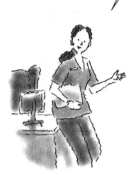

This question is asking about an increase—not just a presence—of symptoms.

49. While examining a child with acute epiglottitis, a nurse should have which item available?
1. Cool mist tent
2. Intubation equipment
3. Tongue blades
4. Viral culture medium

50. A 2-year-old child is brought to the emergency department in respiratory distress. The child is drooling, sitting upright and leaning forward with chin thrust out, mouth open, and tongue protruding. Which nursing intervention is most appropriate?
1. Check the child's gag reflex with a tongue blade.
2. Allow the child to cry to keep the lungs expanded.
3. Check the airway for a foreign body obstruction.
4. Support the child in an upright position on the parent's lap.

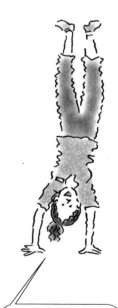

Congratulations! You've finished more than 50 questions! Keep up the good work!

51. What is the best position for a nurse to place a 3-year-old child with right lower lobe pneumonia?
1. On the right side
2. On the left side
3. Supine
4. Prone

48. 3. Increasing heart rate is an early sign of hypoxia. A progressive barking cough is characteristic of spasmodic croup. A child in respiratory distress will be irritable and restless. As distress increases, the child will become lethargic related to the work of breathing and impending respiratory failure. A productive cough shows that secretions are moving and the child can effectively clear them.
CN: Physiological integrity; CNS: Physiological adaptation; CL: Application

49. 2. Emergency intubation equipment should be at the bedside to secure the airway if examination precipitates further or complete obstruction. Viral culture medium and cool mist tents are recommended for the diagnosis and treatment of croup. Tongue blades are contraindicated and may cause the epiglottis to spasm.
CN: Physiological integrity; CNS: Physiological adaptation; CL: Application

50. 4. The classic signs of epiglottitis are drooling, sitting upright, and leaning forward with chin thrust out, mouth open, and tongue protruding. The child with epiglottitis should be kept in an upright position to ease the work of breathing and to avoid aspiration of secretions and obstruction of the airway by the swollen epiglottis. Placing the child on the lap of a parent may help reduce the child's anxiety. The gag reflex of a child with epiglottitis should never be checked unless emergency personnel and equipment are immediately available to perform a tracheotomy if the airway should become obstructed by the swollen epiglottis. Likewise, crying and inspecting the airway for a foreign body may also cause entrapment of the epiglottis and obstruction of the airway.
CN: Physiological integrity; CNS: Reduction of risk potential; CL: Application

51. 2. The child with right lower lobe pneumonia should be placed on his left side. This places the unaffected left lung in a position so that gravity will promote blood flow to the healthy lung tissue, improving gas exchange. Placing the child on the right side, his back, or his stomach doesn't promote circulation to the unaffected lung.
CN: Physiological integrity; CNS: Physiological adaptation; CL: Application

CN: Client needs category   CNS: Client needs subcategory   CL: Cognitive level

52. The arterial blood gas analysis of a child with asthma shows a pH of 7.30, P_{CO_2} of 56 mm Hg, and HCO_3^- of 25 mEq/L. The nurse determines that the child has which condition?

   1. Metabolic acidosis
   2. Metabolic alkalosis
   3. Respiratory acidosis
   4. Respiratory alkalosis

53. Which neonate is at high risk for developing bronchopulmonary dysplasia?

   1. A neonate born at 38 weeks' gestation receiving 1 to 4 L oxygen during feedings
   2. A premature neonate born at 36 weeks' gestation receiving supplemental oxygen
   3. A premature neonate born at 28 weeks' gestation on a high-pressure ventilator
   4. A neonate born at 42 weeks' gestation who requires treatments for respiratory syncytial virus

54. Which nursing diagnosis is the priority for an infant with bronchopulmonary dysplasia?

   1. *Imbalanced nutrition: Less than body requirements*
   2. *Effective breast-feeding*
   3. *Impaired gas exchange*
   4. *Risk for imbalanced fluid volume*

55. Which management strategy is recommended when caring for an infant with bronchopulmonary dysplasia?

   1. Provide frequent playful stimuli.
   2. Decrease oxygen during feedings.
   3. Place the infant on a set schedule.
   4. Place the infant in an open crib.

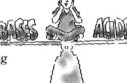

I think I sense an acid-base disturbance coming on.

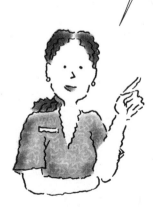

Which management strategy is recommended in question 55?

52. 3. Respiratory acidosis is an acid-base disturbance characterized by excess CO_2 in the blood, indicated by a P_{CO_2} greater than 45 mm Hg. The pH level is usually below the normal range of 7.36 to 7.45. The HCO_3^- level is normal in the acute stage and elevated in the chronic stage.

CN: Physiological integrity; CNS: Physiological adaptation; CL: Analysis

53. 3. Premature neonates with low birth weight on high-pressure ventilators are at highest risk for developing bronchopulmonary dysplasia. Supplemental oxygen, respiratory treatments, and 1 to 4 L oxygen for feedings are *not* high risk factors for bronchopulmonary dysplasia.

CN: Physiological integrity; CNS: Reduction of risk potential; CL: Application

54. 3. The infant will have *Impaired gas exchange* related to retention of carbon dioxide and borderline oxygenation secondary to fibrosis of the lungs. Although the infant may require increased caloric intake and may have excess fluid volume, *Imbalanced nutrition: Less than body requirements, Effective breast-feeding,* and *Risk for imbalanced fluid volume* aren't priority nursing diagnoses.

CN: Physiological integrity; CNS: Physiological adaptation; CL: Analysis

55. 3. Timing care activities with rest periods to avoid fatigue and to decrease respiratory effort is essential. Early stimulation activities are recommended but the infant will have limited tolerance for them because of the illness. Oxygen is usually increased during feedings to help decrease respiratory and energy requirements. Thermoregulation is important because both hypothermia and hyperthermia will increase oxygen consumption and may increase oxygen requirements. These infants are usually maintained on warmer beds or inside Isolettes.

CN: Safe, effective care environment; CNS: Management of care; CL: Application

56. The nurse is planning care for a child admitted to the pediatric unit with bronchopulmonary dysplasia. Which symptom is the nurse most likely to assess?
1. Minimal work of breathing
2. Tachypnea and dyspnea
3. Easily consolable
4. Hypotension

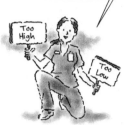

Be sure not to confuse the prefixes hyper and hypo!

57. Which intervention is <u>most appropriate</u> for helping parents to cope with a child <u>newly diagnosed</u> with bronchopulmonary dysplasia?
1. Teach cardiopulmonary resuscitation.
2. Refer them to support groups.
3. Help parents identify necessary lifestyle changes.
4. Evaluate and assess parents' stress and anxiety levels.

58. The nursing care plan for an infant with bronchopulmonary dysplasia includes the nursing diagnosis of *Impaired gas exchange.* Which nursing action would be most appropriate for a nurse to include?
1. Provide chest physiotherapy.
2. Provide enteral feedings.
3. Provide appropriate age-related activities.
4. Promote bonding between parent and child.

59. Theophylline is ordered for a 1-year-old client with bronchopulmonary dysplasia. The recommended dosage is 24 mg/kg/day. The client weighs 10 kg. How much is given per dose when administered 4 times per day?
1. 60 mg/dose
2. 80 mg/dose
3. 120 mg/dose
4. 240 mg/dose

Here's that formula again!

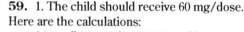

60. Infants with bronchopulmonary dysplasia require frequent, prolonged rest periods. Which sign indicates overstimulation?
1. Increased alertness
2. Good eye contact
3. Cyanosis
4. Lethargy

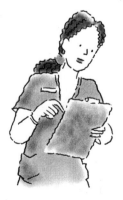

56. 2. Tachypnea, dyspnea, and wheezing are intermittently or chronically present secondary to airway obstruction and increased airway resistance. These infants usually show increased work of breathing and increased use of accessory muscles. They're frequently described as irritable and difficult to comfort. Pulmonary hypertension is a common finding resulting from fibrosis and chronic hypoxia.
CN: Physiological integrity; CNS: Physiological adaptation; CL: Application

57. 4. The emotional impact of bronchopulmonary dysplasia is clearly a crisis situation. The parents are experiencing grief and sorrow over the loss of a "healthy" child. The other strategies are more appropriate for long-term intervention.
CN: Psychosocial integrity; CNS: None; CL: Application

58. 1. All these activities are appropriate to include in the care of a child with bronchopulmonary dysplasia; however, providing chest physiotherapy addresses the nursing diagnosis of *Impaired gas exchange.*
CN: Physiological integrity; CNS: Basic care and comfort; CL: Analysis

59. 1. The child should receive 60 mg/dose. Here are the calculations:
24 mg/kg × 10 kg = 240 mg/day;
240 mg/4 doses = 60 mg/dose.
CN: Physiological integrity; CNS: Pharmacological and parenteral therapies; CL: Application

60. 3. Signs of overstimulation in an immature child include cyanosis, avoidance of eye contact, vomiting, diaphoresis, or falling asleep. The child may also become irritable and show signs of respiratory distress.
CN: Physiological integrity; CNS: Basic care and comfort; CL: Analysis

CN: Client needs category   CNS: Client needs subcategory   CL: Cognitive level

61. Which outcome should be anticipated of parental care of a child with bronchopulmonary dysplasia?
1. Reports increased levels of stress
2. Makes safe decisions with professional assistance only
3. Participates in routine, but not complex, caretaking activities
4. Verbalizes the causes, risks, therapy options, and nursing care

62. Bronchopulmonary dysplasia can be classified into four categories. Which characteristic is noted during the early or <u>first</u> stage of the disease?
1. Interstitial fibrosis
2. Signs of emphysema
3. Hyperexpansion on chest X-ray
4. Resemblance to respiratory distress syndrome

63. Bronchopulmonary dysplasia can cause increased fluid in the lungs due to disruption of the alveolar-capillary membrane, and the client may begin receiving furosemide (Lasix). Which adverse effect is possible?
1. Hypercalcemia
2. Hyperkalemia
3. Hypernatremia
4. Irregular heart rhythm

64. A pediatric client is to receive furosemide (Lasix) 4 mg/kg/day in one daily dose. The client weighs 20 kg. How many milligrams should be administered in each dose?
1. 20
2. 40
3. 80
4. 160

65. A 2-year-old child with bronchopulmonary dysplasia is placed on furosemide (Lasix) once per day. The parents are being educated on foods that are rich in potassium. Which food should the nurse recommend?
1. Apples
2. Oranges
3. Peaches
4. Raisins

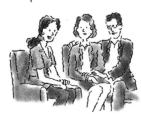

Encourage parents to verbalize their understanding of their infant's disorder.

We're raising awareness about our potassium content.

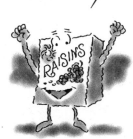

61. 4. The parents should understand the causes, risks, and care of their infant by the time of discharge. Having the parents verbalize this information is the only way to assess their understanding. The parents should report decreased levels of stress, be capable of making decisions independently, and participate in routine and complex care.
CN: Physiological integrity; CNS: Basic care and comfort; CL: Analysis

62. 4. Stage I can be characterized by early interstitial changes and resembles respiratory distress syndrome. Stage IV shows interstitial fibrosis and hyperexpansion on chest X-ray. Stage III shows signs of the beginning of chronic disease with interstitial edema, signs of emphysema, and pulmonary hypertension.
CN: Physiological integrity; CNS: Physiological adaptation; CL: Analysis

63. 4. An irregular heart rhythm and muscle cramps are adverse effects related to hypokalemia and hypocalcemia and not hypercalcemia or hyperkalemia. Diuretics cause volume depletion by inhibiting reabsorption of sodium and chloride. Hypocalcemia is related to the urinary excretion of calcium. Hypokalemia can occur with excessive fluid loss or as part of contraction alkalosis.
CN: Physiological integrity; CNS: Pharmacological and parenteral therapies; CL: Application

64. 3. The child should receive 80 mg per dose. Here are the calculations:
$$4 \text{ mg/kg} \times 20 \text{ kg} = 80 \text{ mg}.$$
CN: Physiological integrity; CNS: Pharmacological and parenteral therapies; CL: Application

65. 4. Raisins, dates, figs, and prunes are among the highest potassium-rich foods. They average 17 to 20 mEq of potassium. Apples, oranges, and peaches have very low amounts of potassium. They average 3 to 4 mEq.
CN: Physiological integrity; CNS: Pharmacological and parenteral therapies; CL: Application

66. Which reason necessitates tracheostomy tube placement in long-term care of infants with bronchopulmonary dysplasia?
1. Increased risk of tracheomalacia
2. Inability to wean from the ventilator
3. Need to allow for gastrostomy tube feedings
4. Increased signs of respiratory distress

67. A 1-year-old infant with bronchopulmonary dysplasia has just received a tracheostomy. Which intervention is <u>appropriate</u>?
1. Keep extra tracheostomy tubes at the bedside.
2. Secure ties at the side of the neck for easy access.
3. Change the tracheostomy tube 2 weeks after surgery.
4. Secure the tracheostomy ties tightly to prevent dislodgment of the tube.

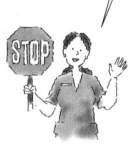

Ask yourself what you would need if the worst occurred.

68. An 11-month-old infant with bronchopulmonary dysplasia and a tracheostomy experiences a decline in oxygen saturation from 97% to 88%. He appears anxious and his heart rate is 180 beats/minute. Which intervention is most appropriate?
1. Change the tracheostomy tube.
2. Suction the tracheostomy tube.
3. Obtain an arterial blood gas (ABG) level.
4. Increase the oxygen flow rate.

69. Which intervention is appropriate when suctioning a tracheostomy tube?
1. Hypoventilate the child before suctioning.
2. Repeat the suctioning process for two intervals.
3. Insert the catheter 1 to 2 cm below the tracheostomy tube.
4. Inject a small amount of normal saline solution into the tube before suctioning.

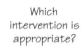

Which intervention is appropriate?

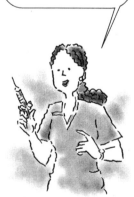

66. 2. Tracheostomy may be required after a child has been ventilator dependent for 6 to 8 weeks and is unable to wean from the ventilator. This will allow for oral feedings and reduce the risks of tracheomalacia and bronchomalacia.
CN: Physiological integrity; CNS: Physiological adaptation; CL: Analysis

67. 1. Extra tracheostomy tubes should be kept at the bedside in case of an emergency, including one size smaller in case the appropriate size doesn't fit due to edema or lack of a tract formation. Ties are usually placed at the back of the neck. The ties should be placed securely but allow the width of a little finger for room to prevent excessive pressure or skin breakdown. The first tracheostomy tube change is usually performed by the physician after 7 days.
CN: Physiological integrity; CNS: Reduction of risk potential; CL: Application

68. 2. Tracheostomy tubes, particularly in small children, require frequent suctioning to remove mucus plugs and excessive secretions. The tracheostomy tube can be changed if suctioning is unsuccessful. Obtaining an ABG level may be beneficial if oxygen saturation remains low and the child appears to be in respiratory distress. Increasing the oxygen flow rate will only help if the airway is patent.
CN: Physiological integrity; CNS: Reduction of risk potential; CL: Analysis

69. 4. Injecting a small amount (1–2 drops) of normal saline solution helps to loosen secretions for easier aspiration. Preservative-free normal saline solution should be used. The child should be hyperventilated before and after suctioning to prevent hypoxia. The suctioning process should be repeated until the trachea is clear. If the catheter is inserted too far, it will irritate the carina and may cause blood-tinged secretions. The catheter should be inserted *0.5 cm beyond* the tracheostomy tube.
CN: Physiological integrity; CNS: Reduction of risk potential; CL: Application

CN: Client needs category   CNS: Client needs subcategory   CL: Cognitive level

70. Which characteristic distinguishes allergies from colds?
1. Skin tests can diagnose a cold.
2. Allergies are accompanied by fever.
3. Colds cause itching of the eyes and nose.
4. Allergies trigger constant and consistent bouts of sneezing.

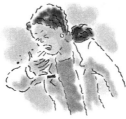

Cold or allergies? That is the (Ah-choo) question!

71. A 2-year-old with pneumonia is placed in an oxygen tent with mist. Which nursing action is a priority?
1. Change the child's bed linens and pajamas frequently.
2. Maintain a steady body temperature.
3. Avoid the use of equipment or toys that can produce sparks.
4. Keep the plastic sides of the tent tucked in.

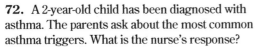

We really need to watch out for those triggers.

72. A 2-year-old child has been diagnosed with asthma. The parents ask about the most common asthma triggers. What is the nurse's response?
1. Weather
2. Peanut butter
3. The cat next door
4. One parent with asthma

73. The nurse is assessing breath sounds of a child admitted with asthma. Which breath sound is the most common in asthma?
1. Stridor
2. Rhonchi
3. Rales
4. Wheezing

70. 4. Allergies elicit consistent bouts of sneezing, are seldom accompanied by fever, and tend to cause itching of the eyes and nose. Skin testing is performed to determine the client's sensitivity to specific allergens. Colds are accompanied by fever and are characterized by sporadic sneezing.
CN: Health promotion and maintenance; CNS: None; CL: Analysis

71. 3. While all the interventions are appropriate for caring for a child in an oxygen tent with mist, sparks in the presence of oxygen can cause a fire. Therefore, all equipment and toys that may produce a spark should be avoided. Bed linens and pajamas may become damp due to the cool mist and should be changed when needed, but only after the risk of fire has been addressed. Keeping the child dry will help promote a steady body temperature which is important since shivering increases oxygen intake. The sides of the tent should be tucked in since oxygen is heavier than air, making oxygen loss greater at the bottom of the tent.
CN: Safe, effective care environment; CNS: Management of care; CL: Analysis

72. 1. Excessively cold air, wet or humid changes in weather and seasons, and air pollution are some of the most common asthma triggers. Household pets are also a trigger. Evidence suggests that asthma is partly hereditary in nature. Food allergens are rarely responsible for airway reactions in children.
CN: Physiological integrity; CNS: Physiological adaptation; CL: Application

73. 4. Asthma frequently presents with wheezing and coughing. Airway inflammation and edema increase mucus production. Other signs include dyspnea, tachycardia, and tachypnea. Stridor is heard in croup. Rhonchi and rales are not as common in asthma as wheezing.
CN: Physiological integrity; CNS: Physiological adaptation; CL: Application

74. The presence of which factor would place a child at increased risk for an asthma-related death?
1. Use of an inhaler at home
2. One admission for asthma last year
3. Prior admission to the general pediatric floor
4. Prior admission to an intensive care unit for asthma

74. 4. Asthma results in varying degrees of respiratory distress. A prior admission to an intensive care unit marks an increased severity and need of immediate therapy. Two or more hospitalizations for asthma, a recent hospitalization or emergency department visit in the past month, or three or more emergency department visits in the past year puts a child at high risk for asthma-related death. Current use of systemic steroids would also be a risk factor.
CN: Physiological integrity; CNS: Reduction of risk potential; CL: Analysis

75. Which characteristic distinguishes status asthmaticus from asthma?
1. Several attacks per month
2. Less than six attacks per year
3. Little or no response to bronchodilators
4. Constant and unrelieved by bronchodilators

This question is asking you to distinguish between varying degrees of asthma.

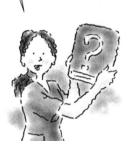

75. 4. Status asthmaticus can best be described as constant and unrelieved by bronchodilators. Moderate asthma is characterized by several attacks per month. Mild asthma is less than 6 attacks per year. Little or no response to bronchodilators would describe severe asthma.
CN: Physiological integrity; CNS: Physiological adaptation; CL: Application

76. A 2-year-old child with status asthmaticus is admitted to the pediatric unit and begins to receive continuous treatment with albuterol (Proventil), given by nebulizer. The nurse should observe for which adverse reaction?
1. Bradycardia
2. Lethargy
3. Tachycardia
4. Tachypnea

76. 3. Albuterol is a rapid-acting bronchodilator. Common adverse effects include tachycardia, nervousness, tremors, insomnia, irritability, and headache.
CN: Physiological integrity; CNS: Pharmacological and parenteral therapies; CL: Application

77. A 10-year-old child is admitted with asthma. The physician orders an aminophylline infusion. A loading dose of 6 mg/kg is ordered. The client weighs 30 kg. How much aminophylline is contained in the loading dose?
1. 60 mg
2. 90 mg
3. 120 mg
4. 180 mg

Do you know why it's called a loading dose?

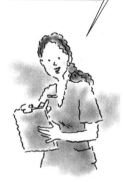

77. 4. The child should receive 180 mg per dose. Here are the calculations:
$$6 \text{ mg/kg} \times 30 \text{ kg} = 180 \text{ mg}.$$
CN: Physiological integrity; CNS: Pharmacological and parenteral therapies; CL: Application

CN: Client needs category   CNS: Client needs subcategory   CL: Cognitive level

78. A 10-year-old client with asthma has recently started receiving I.V. aminophylline. He begins to vomit and complains of his stomach hurting. Which nursing intervention is appropriate?
1. Check the theophylline level.
2. Increase the infusion rate.
3. Take no action; aminophylline can cause nausea.
4. Stop the infusion and call the physician.

79. Which finding should a nurse expect on a typical X-ray of a child with asthma?
1. Atelectasis
2. Hemothorax
3. Infiltrates
4. Pneumothoraces

80. Which intervention is most appropriate for a client with atelectasis?
1. Perform chest physiotherapy.
2. Give increased I.V. fluids.
3. Administer oxygen.
4. Obtain arterial blood gas (ABG) levels.

81. The parents of a 10-year-old child recently diagnosed with asthma ask if the child can continue to play sports. Which response is most appropriate?
1. Sports don't cause asthma attacks.
2. You should limit activities to quiet play.
3. It's okay to play some sports but swimming isn't recommended.
4. Physical activity and sports are encouraged, provided the asthma is under control.

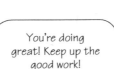

You're doing great! Keep up the good work!

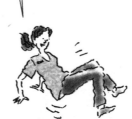

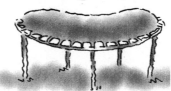

78. 1. Although nausea and GI upset are adverse effects of aminophylline, they can also represent signs of toxicity. The theophylline level should be checked to make sure the blood level is in the therapeutic range of 10 to 20 mcg/ml. The aminophylline drip may need to be decreased based on the blood level. The infusion shouldn't be stopped until a theophylline level is obtained.
CN: Physiological integrity; CNS: Pharmacological and parenteral therapies; CL: Analysis

79. 1. Hyperexpansion, atelectasis, and a flattened diaphragm are typical X-ray findings for a child with asthma. Air becomes trapped behind the narrowed airways and the residual capacity rises, leading to hyperinflation. Hypoxemia results from areas of the lung not being well perfused. A hemothorax isn't a finding related to asthma. Infiltrates and pneumothoraces are uncommon.
CN: Physiological integrity; CNS: Physiological adaptation; CL: Analysis

80. 1. Chest physiotherapy and incentive spirometry help to enhance the clearance of mucus and open the alveoli. I.V. and oral fluids are recommended to help liquefy and thin secretions. Administration of oxygen will *not* give enough pressure to open the alveoli. Obtaining ABG levels isn't necessary.
CN: Physiological integrity; CNS: Physiological adaptation; CL: Application

81. 4. Participation in sports is encouraged but should be evaluated on an individual basis provided the asthma is under control. Exercise-induced asthma is an example of the airway hyperactivity common to asthmatics. Swimming is well-tolerated related to the type of breathing and the moisture in the air. Exclusion from sports or activities may hamper peer interaction.
CN: Physiological integrity; CNS: Physiological adaptation; CL: Analysis

82. The nurse is caring for a child with asthma who is being treated with aminophylline. The child's aminophylline level is returned as normal. Which level falls within the normal range?

1. 2 to 4 mcg/ml
2. 5 to 15 mcg/ml
3. 10 to 20 mcg/ml
4. 20 to 30 mcg/ml

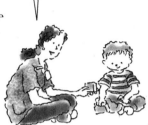

Keep this client's age in mind when answering question 83.

83. Which nursing intervention is appropriate to correct dehydration for a 2-year-old client with asthma?

1. Give warm liquids.
2. Give cold juice or ice pops.
3. Provide three meals and three snacks.
4. Give I.V. fluid boluses.

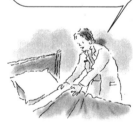

"Allergy proofing" a home can be just as important as "kid proofing" it.

84. Which intervention by the parents is appropriate to "allergy proof" the home?

1. Cover floors with carpeting.
2. Designate the basement as the play area.
3. Dust and clean the house thoroughly twice a month.
4. Use foam rubber pillows and synthetic blankets.

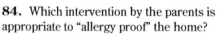

85. Which nursing diagnosis is appropriate for a client with acute asthma?

1. *Imbalanced nutrition: More than body requirements*
2. *Excess fluid volume*
3. *Activity intolerance*
4. *Constipation*

82. 3. The normal therapeutic range of aminophylline is considered to be 10 to 20 mcg/ml. Levels below 10 mcg/ml are considered to be less than therapeutic. Symptoms of toxicity such as nausea, tachycardia, and irritability can appear when levels exceed 20 mcg/ml. Levels greater than 30 mcg/ml can cause seizures and arrhythmias.

CN: Physiological integrity; CNS: Pharmacological and parenteral therapies; CL: Application

83. 1. Liquids are best tolerated if they're warm. Cold liquids may cause bronchospasm and should be avoided. Dehydration should be corrected slowly. Small, frequent meals should be provided to avoid abdominal distention that may interfere with diaphragm excursion. Overhydration may increase interstitial pulmonary fluid and exacerbate small airway obstruction.

CN: Physiological integrity; CNS: Physiological adaptation; CL: Application

84. 4. Bedding should be free from allergens with hypoallergenic covers. Unnecessary rugs should be removed and floors should be bare and mopped a few times a week to reduce dust. Basements or cellars should be avoided to lessen the child's exposure to molds and mildew. Dusting and cleaning should occur daily or at least weekly.

CN: Physiological integrity; CNS: Physiological adaptation; CL: Application

85. 3. Ineffective oxygen supply and demand may lead to activity intolerance. The nurse should promote rest and encourage developmentally appropriate activities. Nutrition may be decreased due to respiratory distress and GI upset. Dehydration is common due to diaphoresis, insensible water loss, and hyperventilation. Medications given to treat asthma may cause nausea, vomiting, and diarrhea, *not* constipation.

CN: Physiological integrity; CNS: Physiological adaptation; CL: Analysis

CN: Client needs category   CNS: Client needs subcategory   CL: Cognitive level

86. A nurse is explaining bronchiolitis to the parents of an infant admitted with the condition. Which explanation by the nurse would be the <u>most</u> accurate?
1. Acute inflammation and obstruction of the bronchioles
2. Airway obstruction from aspiration of a solid object
3. Inflammation of the pulmonary parenchyma
4. Acute highly contagious crouplike syndrome

86. 1. Bronchiolitis is an infection of the bronchioles, causing the mucosa to become edematous, inflamed, and full of mucus. Lower airway obstruction from a solid object is a form of a foreign body aspiration. Pneumonia is characterized by inflammation of the pulmonary parenchyma. Crouplike syndromes are generally upper airway infections or obstructions.
CN: Physiological integrity; CNS: Physiological adaptation; CL: Application

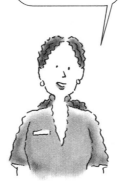

Consider the pathology of bronchiolitis when answering question 87.

87. A 2-month-old infant is brought to the emergency department and a preliminary diagnosis of bronchiolitis is given. Which symptom should a nurse expect to find on assessment?
1. Bradycardia
2. Increased appetite
3. Wheezing on auscultation
4. No signs of an upper respiratory infection

87. 3. In bronchiolitis, the bronchioles become narrowed and edematous. This can cause wheezing. These infants typically have a 2- to 3-day history of an upper respiratory infection and feeding difficulties with loss of appetite due to nasal congestion and increased work of breathing. This combination leads to respiratory distress with tachypnea and tachycardia.
CN: Physiological integrity; CNS: Physiological adaptation; CL: Application

88. In most cases, bronchiolitis is caused by a viral agent, most commonly respiratory syncytial virus (RSV). The nurse should keep in mind which statement regarding RSV infections?
1. It's more prevalent in the summer and fall months.
2. It's most likely to attack the respiratory tract mucosa.
3. It's more commonly seen in children older than age 5.
4. It's not particularly contagious.

88. 2. RSV attacks the respiratory tract mucosa. The virus is most prevalent in the winter and early spring months. Most children develop the infection between ages 2 and 6 months, and RSV generally occurs during the first 3 years of life. RSV is a highly contagious respiratory virus.
CN: Physiological integrity; CNS: Physiological adaptation; CL: Application

89. Which precaution should a nurse caring for a 2-month-old infant with respiratory syncytial virus (RSV) take to <u>prevent</u> the spread of infection?
1. Gloves only
2. Gown, gloves, and mask
3. No precautions required; the virus isn't contagious
4. Proper hand washing between clients

You better take precautions if you want to avoid the likes of me.

89. 2. RSV is highly contagious and is spread through direct contact with infectious secretions via hands, droplets, and fomites. Gowns, gloves, and masks should be worn for client care to prevent the spread of infection.
CN: Safe, effective care environment; CNS: Safety and infection control; CL: Application

90. The nurse teaches parents that the test used to diagnose respiratory syncytial virus (RSV) is:
1. Blood test
2. Nasopharyngeal washings
3. Sputum culture
4. Throat culture

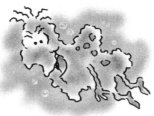

90. 2. RSV can only be diagnosed with direct aspiration of nasal secretions or nasopharyngeal washings. Positive identification is accomplished using the enzyme-linked immunosorbent assay. Blood, throat, and sputum cultures can't definitively diagnose RSV.
CN: Physiological integrity; CNS: Physiological adaptation; CL: Application

91. Which child would be at <u>increased risk</u> for a respiratory syncytial virus (RSV) infection?
1. A 2-month-old child managed at home
2. A 2-month-old child with bronchopulmonary dysplasia
3. A 3-month-old child requiring low-flow oxygen
4. A 2-year-old child

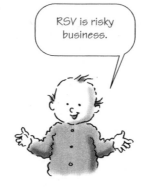

RSV is risky business.

91. 2. Infants with cardiac or pulmonary conditions are at highest risk for RSV. Because of their underlying conditions, they usually require mechanical ventilation. Many infants can be managed at home; few require hospitalization. A 3-month-old on low-flow oxygen has some risks of progression but is *not* at a high risk. A 2-year-old child has built up the immune system and can tolerate the infection without major problems.
CN: Physiological integrity; CNS: Reduction of risk potential; CL: Analysis

92. Which medication can help to prevent respiratory syncytial virus (RSV)?
1. Aminophylline
2. Bronchodilators
3. Corticosteroids
4. Respigam

92. 4. Respigam is I.V. RSV immune globulin. It can help to prevent serious lower respiratory tract infections caused by RSV. The first dose is given before RSV season, with monthly doses given throughout the season for protection. This agent is indicated for children younger than age 24 months with bronchopulmonary dysplasia or a history of prematurity. Bronchodilators, aminophylline, and corticosteroids are sometimes used for treatment.
CN: Health promotion and maintenance; CNS: None; CL: Analysis

93. Which medication is an antiviral agent used to treat bronchiolitis caused by respiratory syncytial virus (RSV)?
1. Albuterol
2. Aminophylline
3. Cromolyn sodium
4. Ribavirin (Virazole)

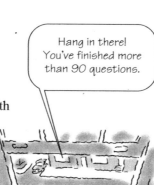

Hang in there! You've finished more than 90 questions.

93. 4. Ribavirin is an antiviral agent sometimes used to reduce the severity of bronchiolitis caused by RSV. Aminophylline and albuterol are bronchodilators and haven't been proven effective in viral bronchiolitis. Cromolyn sodium is an inhaled anti-inflammatory agent.
CN: Physiological integrity; CNS: Pharmacological and parenteral therapies; CL: Analysis

94. Which intervention is <u>most important</u> when monitoring dehydration in an infant with bronchiolitis?
1. Measurement of intake and output
2. Blood levels every 4 hours
3. Urinalysis every 8 hours
4. Weighing each diaper

94. 1. Accurate measurement of intake and output is essential to assess for dehydration. Blood levels may be obtained daily or every other day. A urinalysis every 8 hours isn't necessary. Urine specific gravities are recommended but can be obtained with diaper changes. Weighing diapers is a way of measuring output only.
CN: Physiological integrity; CNS: Physiological adaptation; CL: Application

CN: Client needs category   CNS: Client needs subcategory   CL: Cognitive level

95. Which nursing diagnosis is the priority for an infant with bronchiolitis?
1. *Imbalanced nutrition: More than body requirements*
2. *Deficient diversional activity*
3. *Impaired gas exchange*
4. *Social isolation*

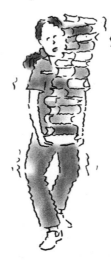

Your hard work is paying off! Keep going!

96. Which teaching point is essential for parents caring for a child with bronchiolitis at home?
1. Place the child in a prone position for comfort.
2. Use warm mist to replace insensible fluid loss.
3. Recognize signs of increasing respiratory distress.
4. Engage the child in many activities to prevent developmental delay.

97. The nurse is teaching the parents of a child with pneumonia about the condition. Which description is correct?
1. Inflammation of the large airways
2. Severe infection of the bronchioles
3. Inflammation of the pulmonary parenchyma
4. Acute viral infection with maximum effect at the bronchiolar level

98. Which organism is the <u>most common</u> causative agent for bacterial pneumonia?
1. Mycoplasma
2. Parainfluenza virus
3. Pneumococci
4. Respiratory syncytial virus (RSV)

95. 3. Infants with bronchiolitis will have impaired gas exchange related to bronchiolar obstruction, atelectasis, and hyperinflation. Nutrition may be seen as less than body requirements. If respiratory distress is present, these infants should have nothing by mouth and fluids given I.V. only. *Deficient diversional activity* and *Social isolation* usually aren't priorities. These infants are too uncomfortable to respond to social stimuli and need quiet, soothing activities that minimize energy.
CN: Physiological integrity; CNS: Physiological adaptation; CL: Analysis

96. 3. It's essential for parents to be able to recognize signs of increasing respiratory distress and know how to count the respiratory rate. The child should be positioned with the head of the bed elevated for comfort and to facilitate removal of secretions. Use of cool mist may help to replace insensible fluid loss. Quiet play activities are required only as the child's energy level permits. These infants show clinical improvement in 3 to 4 days; therefore, developmental delay isn't an issue.
CN: Physiological integrity; CNS: Physiological adaptation; CL: Analysis

97. 3. Pneumonia is an inflammation of the pulmonary parenchyma. Bronchitis is inflammation of the large airways. Bronchiolitis is a severe infection of the bronchioles. Bronchiolitis and respiratory syncytial virus are terms for an acute viral infection with maximum effect at the bronchiolar level.
CN: Physiological integrity; CNS: Physiological adaptation; CL: Application

98. 3. Pneumococcal pneumonia is the most common causative agent, accounting for about 90% of bacterial pneumonia. Mycoplasma is a causative agent for primary atypical pneumonia. Parainfluenza virus and RSV account for viral pneumonia.
CN: Physiological integrity; CNS: Physiological adaptation; CL: Application

99. The nurse is caring for an 8-year-old child admitted with pneumonia. Based on the child's age, which type of pneumonia would the nurse suspect?

1. Enteric bacilli
2. Mycoplasma pneumonia
3. Staphylococcal pneumonia
4. Streptococcal pneumonia

100. The nurse knows to monitor a child with a diagnosis of pertussis for the development of which sign or symptom?

1. Barking cough
2. Whooping cough
3. Abrupt high fever
4. Inspiratory stridor

101. Which test is the definitive means of diagnosing tuberculosis (TB)?

1. Chest X-ray
2. Sputum sample
3. Tuberculin test
4. Urine culture

102. The nurse is assessing a child who has been admitted to the emergency department with a diagnosis of tuberculosis. Which symptom would the nurse expect to observe?

1. Chills
2. Hyperactivity
3. Lymphadenitis
4. Weight gain

103. Which adverse effect can be <u>expected</u> by the parents of a 2-year-old child who has been started on rifampin (Rifadin) after testing positive for tuberculosis?

1. Hyperactivity
2. Orange body secretions
3. Decreased bilirubin levels
4. Decreased levels of liver enzymes

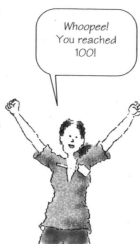

Whoopee! You reached 100!

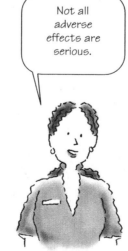

Not all adverse effects are serious.

99. 2. Mycoplasma pneumonia is a primary atypical pneumonia seen in children between ages 5 and 12. Enteric bacilli, staphylococcal pneumonia, and streptococcal pneumonia are mostly seen in children in the 3 month to 5 year age-group.

CN: Physiological integrity; CNS: Physiological adaptation; CL: Application

100. 2. Pertussis is characterized by consistent short, rapid coughs followed by a sudden inspiration with a high-pitched whooping sound. A barking cough and inspiratory stridor are noted with croup. Pertussis is usually accompanied by a low-grade fever.

CN: Physiological integrity; CNS: Physiological adaptation; CL: Application

101. 2. A sputum culture is the definitive test. X-rays usually appear normal in children with TB. The tuberculin test isn't necessarily the most reliable test for TB in children. Stool cultures and gastric washings will show positive results on acid-fast smears but aren't specific for *Mycobacterium tuberculosis*. Sputum samples are difficult to obtain from children, so gastric washings commonly replace them.

CN: Physiological integrity; CNS: Physiological adaptation; CL: Analysis

102. 3. Children are usually asymptomatic and typically don't manifest the usual pulmonary symptoms, but lymphadenitis is more likely in infants and children than in adults. Weight loss, anorexia, night sweats, fatigue, and malaise are general responses to the disease.

CN: Physiological integrity; CNS: Physiological adaptation; CL: Application

103. 2. Rifampin and its metabolites will turn urine, feces, sputum, tears, and sweat an orange color. This isn't a serious adverse effect. Rifampin may also cause GI upset, headache, drowsiness, dizziness, visual disturbances, and fever. Liver enzyme and bilirubin levels increase because of hepatic metabolism of the drug. Parents should be taught the signs and symptoms of hepatitis and hyperbilirubinemia such as jaundice of the sclera or skin.

CN: Physiological integrity; CNS: Pharmacological and parenteral therapies; CL: Application

CN: Client needs category   CNS: Client needs subcategory   CL: Cognitive level

104. Children younger than age 3 are prone to aspirating foreign bodies. Which action is recommended to prevent aspiration?
1. Cut hot dogs in half.
2. Limit popcorn and peanuts.
3. Cut grapes into small pieces.
4. Limit hard candy to special occasions.

105. A child is admitted with a possible tracheal foreign body. Which findings would <u>most</u> likely indicate a foreign body in the trachea?
1. Cough, dyspnea, and drooling
2. Cough, stridor, and changes in phonation
3. Expiratory wheeze and inspiratory stridor
4. Cough, asymmetrical breath sounds, and wheeze

106. Which activity is recommended to prevent foreign body aspiration during meals?
1. Insist that children are seated.
2. Give children toys to play with.
3. Allow children to watch television.
4. Allow children to eat in a separate room.

107. The nurse is preparing a child for testing for a foreign body aspiration. The nurse explains to the child's parents that the best diagnostic tool for diagnosis of foreign body aspiration is:
1. Bronchoscopy
2. Chest X-ray
3. Fluoroscopy
4. Lateral neck X-ray

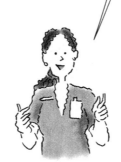

The next four questions address foreign body aspiration.

104. 3. Grapes, hotdogs, and sausage should be cut into many small pieces. Hard candy, raisins, popcorn, and peanuts should be avoided for children age 4 and younger.
CN: Physiological integrity; CNS: Reduction of risk potential; CL: Application

105. 3. Expiratory and inspiratory noise indicates that the foreign body is in the trachea. Cough, dyspnea, drooling, and gagging indicate supraglottic obstruction. A cough with stridor and changes in phonation would occur if the foreign body were in the larynx. Asymmetrical breath sounds indicate that the object may be located in the bronchi.
CN: Physiological integrity; CNS: Physiological adaptation; CL: Application

106. 1. Children should remain seated while eating. The risk of aspiration increases if the child is running, jumping, or talking with food in their mouth. Television and toys are a dangerous distraction to toddlers and young children and should be avoided. Children need constant supervision and should be monitored while eating snacks and meals.
CN: Safe, effective care environment; CNS: Safety and infection control; CL: Application

107. 1. Bronchoscopy can give a definitive diagnosis of the presence of foreign bodies and is also the best choice for removal of the object with direct visualization. Chest X-ray and lateral neck X-ray may also be used but findings vary. Some films may appear normal or show changes such as inflammation related to the presence of the foreign body. Fluoroscopy is valuable in detecting and localizing foreign bodies in the bronchi.
CN: Physiological integrity; CNS: Physiological adaptation; CL: Application

108. Which intervention is <u>most</u> appropriate for a child with cystic fibrosis who is having difficulty clearing secretions?
   1. Perform chest physiotherapy four times per day.
   2. Administer pancreatic enzymes with meals.
   3. Provide oxygen by nasal cannula at all times.
   4. Provide a high-calorie, high-protein diet at each meal.

109. Which statement by the parent of a 16-month-old child with cystic fibrosis should alert a nurse to investigate further?
   1. "My child is not walking yet."
   2. "My child is saying a few words and short phrases."
   3. "My child doesn't interact with other 16-month-olds."
   4. "My child cries when I leave the room."

110. A nurse is performing an assessment on a newborn with a possible diagnosis of cystic fibrosis. Which of the following is an early sign of the disease?
   1. Constipation
   2. Decreased appetite
   3. Hyperalbuminemia
   4. Meconium ileus

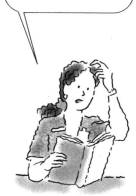

Which of these options would be most likely?

108. 1. Chest physiotherapy should be performed to mobilize secretions so they can be more easily cleared. Pancreatic enzymes should be administered with meals to aid in digestion. Administering oxygen may improve oxygenation but won't help clear secretions. A high-calorie, high-protein diet is important for normal growth and development, but won't aid in clearing secretions.
CN: Physiological integrity; CNS: Reduction of risk potential; CL: Application

109. 1. A toddler should be walking by 15 months. At 10 months, an infant holds on to furniture while walking, walks with support at 11 months, and takes his first steps at 12 months. By 12 months, a child can say a few words, with more words and short phrases being added each month. A child at 16 months engages in solitary play and has little interaction with other children. Separation anxiety is common in toddlers.
CN: Psychosocial integrity; CNS: None; CL: Analysis

110. 4. Meconium ileus is commonly a presenting sign of cystic fibrosis. Thick, mucilaginous meconium blocks the lumen of the small intestine, causing intestinal obstruction, abdominal distention, and vomiting. Large-volume, loose, frequent, foul-smelling stools are common. These infants may have an increased appetite related to poor absorption from the intestine. The undigested food is excreted, increasing the bulk of feces. Hypoalbuminemia is a common result from the decreased absorption of protein.
CN: Physiological integrity; CNS: Physiological adaptation; CL: Application

CN: Client needs category   CNS: Client needs subcategory   CL: Cognitive level

111. Which intervention would be most appropriate for a nurse to perform when the parents of a child with cystic fibrosis tell her they are having difficulty coping?
1. Tell the parents they shouldn't expect to have a normal family life.
2. Refer the parents to a cystic fibrosis support group.
3. Show the parents how to perform chest physiotherapy at home.
4. Tell the parents that with good medical care their child can live into adulthood.

112. A toddler with suspected cystic fibrosis is admitted for testing. The nurse explains that the diagnostic criteria for chloride levels is:
1. Below 20 mEq/L
2. Below 40 mEq/L
3. 40 to 60 mEq/L
4. Above 60 mEq/L

113. The parents ask which diet is recommended for their child, who has cystic fibrosis. What is the nurse's response?
1. Fat-restricted
2. High-calorie
3. Low-protein
4. Sodium-restricted

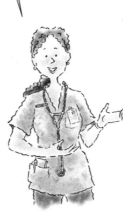

In light of the pathology of cystic fibrosis, which is the only diet that makes sense?

114. Which statement concerning pancreatic enzymes for a cystic fibrosis client is correct?
1. Capsules may not be opened.
2. Microcapsules can be crushed.
3. Encourage eating throughout the day.
4. Administer enzymes at each meal and with snacks.

111. 2. Support groups can provide the parents with the support they need to cope with their child's condition as well as provide them with accurate information on the disorder. The family shouldn't be discouraged from having as normal a life as possible. Showing the parents how to perform chest physiotherapy is an important intervention, but won't help them cope with their child's condition. With good medical care, children with cystic fibrosis can live into adulthood, but telling the parent this doesn't promote the coping skills the parents need.
CN: Physiological integrity; CNS: None; CL: Application

112. 4. A chloride concentration greater than 60 mEq/L is diagnostic of cystic fibrosis. Normal sweat chloride content is less than 40 mEq/L, with the average being 18 mEq/L. Levels between 40 and 60 mEq/L are highly suggestive of cystic fibrosis.
CN: Physiological integrity; CNS: Physiological adaptation; CL: Application

113. 2. A well-balanced high-calorie, high-protein diet is recommended for a child with cystic fibrosis due to the impaired intestinal absorption. Fat restriction isn't required because digestion and absorption of fat in the intestine are impaired. The child usually increases enzyme intake when high-fat foods are eaten. Low-sodium foods can lead to hyponatremia; therefore, high-sodium foods are recommended, especially during hot weather or when the child has a fever.
CN: Physiological integrity; CNS: Basic care and comfort; CL: Application

114. 4. Enzymes are administered with each feeding, meal, and snack to optimize absorption of the nutrients consumed. Regular capsules may be opened and the contents mixed with a small amount of applesauce or other nonalkaline food. Microcapsules can't be crushed due to the enteric coating. Eating throughout the day should be discouraged. Three meals and two or three snacks per day are recommended.
CN: Physiological integrity; CNS: Physiological adaptation; CL: Application

115. A nurse should include which information on nutrition when teaching the family of a child with cystic fibrosis?

1. Provide a high-calorie, high-protein diet.
2. Place the child on a daily 1,200 ml fluid restriction.
3. Restrict daily intake of sodium to 1.5 g/day.
4. Provide adequate amounts of fat-soluble vitamins.

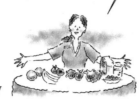

Teach the family about proper nutrition.

115. 1. To promote growth and development, the child should eat a high-calorie, high-protein diet. The child with cystic fibrosis should also be encouraged to consume higher than usual amounts of fluids and sodium. The child should be given water-soluble forms of fat-soluble vitamins.

CN: Physiological integrity; CNS: Basic care and comfort; CL: Application

116. A nurse is caring for a client with cystic fibrosis. Ranitidine (Zantac) 4 mg/kg/day every 12 hours is ordered. The child weighs 20 kg. How many milligrams are given per dose?

1. 16
2. 20
3. 40
4. 80

116. 3. The child should receive 40 mg per dose. Here are the calculations:

$20 \text{ kg} \times 4 \text{ mg/kg} = 80 \text{ mg};$
$24 \text{ hr}/12 \text{ hr} = 2 \text{ doses};$
$80 \text{ mg}/2 \text{ doses} = 40 \text{ mg}.$

CN: Physiological integrity; CNS: Pharmacological and parenteral therapies; CL: Application

117. Which intervention is appropriate for care of the child with cystic fibrosis?

1. Decrease exercise and limit physical activity.
2. Administer cough suppressants and antihistamines.
3. Administer chest physiotherapy two to four times per day.
4. Administer bronchodilator or nebulizer treatments after chest physiotherapy.

117. 3. Chest physiotherapy is recommended two to four times per day to help loosen and move secretions to facilitate expectoration. Exercise and physical activity is recommended to stimulate mucus secretion and to establish a good habitual breathing pattern. Cough suppressants and antihistamines are contraindicated. The goal is for the child to be able to cough and expectorate mucus secretions. Bronchodilator or nebulizer treatments are given before chest physiotherapy to help open the bronchi for easier expectoration.

CN: Safe, effective care environment; CNS: Management of care; CL: Application

118. Which statement is appropriate for a nurse to address to the parents of a child with cystic fibrosis who are planning to have a second child?

1. Genetic counseling is recommended.
2. There's a 50% chance the child will be normal.
3. There's a 50% chance of the child being affected.
4. There's a 25% chance the child will only be a carrier.

118. 1. Genetic counseling should be recommended. Cystic fibrosis is an autosomal-recessive disease. Therefore, there's a 25% chance of the child having the disease, a 25% chance of the child being normal, and a 50% chance of the child being a carrier.

CN: Health promotion and maintenance; CNS: None; CL: Application

CN: Client needs category   CNS: Client needs subcategory   CL: Cognitive level

119. Parents ask the nurse about the cause of their child's cystic fibrosis. Which statement best describes this autosomal-recessive disorder?
1. The genetic disorder is carried on the X chromosome.
2. Both parents must pass the defective gene or set of genes.
3. Only one defective gene or set of genes is passed by one parent.
4. The child has an extra chromosome, resulting in an XXY karyotype.

120. When a nurse enters the room to give an antibiotic elixir to a 3-year-old child, the child says the medication is "yucky" and refuses to take it. Which response by the nurse is best?
1. "Do you want to take the medicine with vanilla ice cream or chocolate ice cream?"
2. "If you don't take the medicine I will tell your mother."
3. "The doctor says you must take the medicine."
4. "You need to take this medicine to get better."

121. Ceftazidime (Fortaz) has been ordered for a client with cystic fibrosis. The order states to give 40 mg/kg every 8 hours. The child is 2 years old and weighs 38.5 lb. How many milligrams of the ceftazidime is given in one dose?
1. 116
2. 233
3. 260
4. 466

122. A child with cystic fibrosis is placed on an oral antibiotic to be given in four equally divided doses per day for 14 days. Which time schedule is most appropriate?
1. 8 a.m., 12 p.m., 4 p.m., 8 p.m.
2. 8 a.m., 2 p.m., 8 p.m., 2 a.m.
3. 9 a.m., 1 p.m., 5 p.m., 9 p.m.
4. 10 a.m., 2 p.m., 6 p.m., 10 p.m.

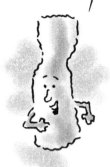

They just keep passing me along.

119. 2. In recessive disorders such as cystic fibrosis, both parents must pass the defective gene or set of genes to the child. Sex-linked genetic disorders are carried on the X chromosome. Dominant disorders are characterized by only one defective gene or set of genes passed by one parent. A child with an XXY karyotype would have Klinefelter's syndrome.

CN: Health promotion and maintenance; CNS: None; CL: Application

120. 1. Offering the child a choice of how he wants to take the medication provides the child with some control. Threatening to tell the child's mother won't help and erodes any trust between the child and nurse. Telling the child that the doctor says he must take the medication also isn't helpful. At age 3, trying to reason with the child about why he needs to take the medication won't work because his thinking is still concrete.

CN: Psychosocial integrity; CNS: None; CL: Analysis

121. 2. The child should receive 233 mg per dose. Here are the calculations: 38.5 lb/2.2 kg = 17.5 kg (1 lb equals 2.2 kg); 40 mg/kg × 17.5 kg = 700 mg; 24 hours/8 hours = 3 doses; 700 mg/3 doses = 233 mg.

CN: Physiological integrity; CNS: Pharmacological and parenteral therapies; CL: Application

122. 2. The doses should be given routinely every 6 hours. This helps maintain a therapeutic blood level of the antibiotic. The other answers have doses only every 4 hours during the day and then no doses for 12 hours at night.

CN: Physiological integrity; CNS: Pharmacological and parenteral therapies; CL: Analysis

123. Which complication of cystic fibrosis may eventually lead to death?
1. Rectal prolapse
2. Pulmonary obstruction
3. Gastroesophageal reflux
4. Reproductive system obstruction

124. Which method is best for evaluation of a 6-year-old child with cystic fibrosis who has been placed on an aerosol inhaler?
1. Ask if the parents have any questions.
2. Ask if the child can explain the procedure.
3. Ask the parents if they understand the usage.
4. Ask the client to perform a return demonstration.

125. Which intervention is appropriate for a 2-year-old client with chest trauma who has a left lower chest tube in place?
1. Stripping or milking the tubing
2. Requiring routine dressing changes
3. Clamping the chest tube during transport
4. Inspecting tubing for kinks or obstructions

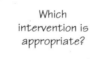

Which intervention is appropriate?

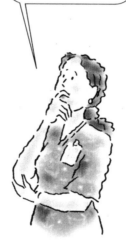

123. 2. Pulmonary obstruction related to thickened mucus secretions can lead to a progressive pulmonary disturbance and secondary infections that can lead to death. Rectal prolapse is managed with enzyme replacement therapy and manipulation of the rectum back into place. Gastroesophageal reflux can be managed with medications and proper reflux precautions. Obstruction of the reproductive system can lead to infertility due to increased mucus blocking sperm entry in the female or blockage of the vas deferens in the male.
CN: Physiological integrity; CNS: Physiological adaptation; CL: Analysis

124. 4. A return demonstration is the best evaluation. It will show if the client can repeat the steps shown and appropriately use the inhaler. The parents should understand how the inhaler should be used and ask questions, but the child must be able to correctly demonstrate usage first. The child may have difficulty explaining the procedure at age 6.
CN: Physiological integrity; CNS: Pharmacological and parenteral therapies; CL: Application

125. 4. Tubing should be inspected for kinks or obstructions so that drainage can flow freely. Manipulation of the tubing should be avoided. The pressure created from stripping can damage the pleural space or mediastinum. There's no need for routine dressing changes if the dressing isn't soiled and there's no evidence of infection. Inspect and palpate around the dressing routinely. The chest tube should never be clamped because it may lead to a tension pneumothorax. Waterseal will protect the client during transit.
CN: Physiological integrity; CNS: Physiological adaptation; CL: Application

CN: Client needs category   CNS: Client needs subcategory   CL: Cognitive level

126. A toddler in respiratory distress is admitted to the pediatric intensive care unit. When he refuses to keep his oxygen face mask on, his mother tries to help. Which action by a nurse is most appropriate?

1. Giving the child his favorite toy to play with
2. Having the mother read the child's favorite book to him
3. Administering a strong sedative so the child will sleep
4. Telling the child that the face mask will help him breathe better

127. A 12-year-old boy is discharged from the hospital after an acute asthma attack with a prescription for budesonide (Pulmicort Turbuhaler). Which signs and symptoms should the nurse instruct him and his parents to report to the physician immediately?

1. Diarrhea
2. Bradycardia
3. Weight loss
4. Oral candidiasis

128. A 6-year-old with a history of asthma is being evaluated by an allergist who orders skin testing to be done at the next visit. Which action by a nurse will help ensure accurate skin testing results?

1. Making sure the child doesn't have a runny nose
2. Making sure the child hasn't received antihistamines in the past 7 days
3. Using the child's posterior legs for testing
4. Limiting testing to environmental allergens

129. Which sign should alert a nurse to a potentially life-threatening complication in a child who received an allergy shot 30 minutes earlier?

1. Urinary output less than 30 ml/hour
2. Heart rate of 58 beats per minute
3. Blood pressure of 82/48 mm Hg
4. Rash

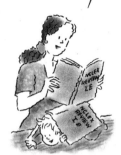

I know this is one of your favorite books.

Moving along nicely! Keep it up!

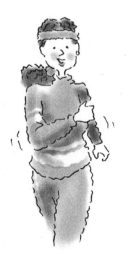

126. 2. Having the mother read the child's favorite book will ease his anxiety and provide comfort to the child. Although giving the child a favorite toy is also appropriate, the child needs his mother's comfort because the face mask is frightening. Sedation is contraindicated because it can mask signs of respiratory distress. A toddler is too young to understand that something will make him feel better.

CN: Safe, effective care environment; CNS: Management of care; CL: Application

127. 4. One of the adverse reactions to budesonide is oral candidiasis and parents should be instructed to monitor the child's mouth for this. Diarrhea, bradycardia, and weight loss are not adverse reactions to this corticosteroid.

CN: Physiological integrity; CNS: Pharmacological and parenteral therapies; CL: Analysis

128. 2. Antihistamines may alter results of skin testing and should be withheld at least 1 week before testing. A runny nose won't alter test results. The forearm and upper back are the best sites for allergy testing. Testing only for environmental allergens precludes diagnosis of allergies to other substances.

CN: Physiological integrity; CNS: Pharmacological and parenteral therapies; CL: Application

129. 3. Anaphylaxis can cause hypotension and tachycardia (not bradycardia). Urinary urgency and incontinence, not anuria, may also be reported. A rash may signal an allergic reaction, but not a severe one such as anaphylaxis.

CN: Physiological integrity; CNS: Physiological adaptation; CL: Analysis

130. The nurse is caring for a 17-year-old female client with cystic fibrosis who has been admitted to the hospital to receive I.V. antibiotic and respiratory treatment for exacerbation of a lung infection. The client has many questions about her future and the consequences of the disease. Which statements about the course of cystic fibrosis are true? Select all that apply:

1. Breast development is frequently delayed.
2. The client is at risk for developing diabetes.
3. Pregnancy and childbearing aren't affected.
4. Normal sexual relationships can be expected.
5. Only males carry the gene for the disease.
6. By age 20, the client should be able to decrease the frequency of respiratory treatment.

131. A nurse is preparing to administer the first dose of tobramycin (Nebcin) to an adolescent with cystic fibrosis. The order is for 3 mg/kg I.V. daily in three divided doses. The client weighs 110 lb. How many milligrams should the nurse administer per dose? Record your answer using a whole number.

_____ milligrams

132. A parent is planning to enroll her 9-month-old infant in a daycare facility. She asks the nurse what to look for as indicators that the daycare facility is adhering to good infection control measures. How should the nurse reply? Select all that apply:

1. The facility keeps boxes of gloves in the director's office.
2. Diapers are discarded into covered receptacles.
3. Toys are kept on the floor for the children to share.
4. Disposable papers are used on the diaper-changing surfaces.
5. Facilities for hand hygiene are located in every classroom.
6. Soiled clothing and cloth diapers are sent home in labeled paper bags.

130. 1, 2, 4. Cystic fibrosis delays growth and the onset of puberty. Children with cystic fibrosis tend to be smaller than average size and develop secondary sex characteristics later in life. In addition, clients with cystic fibrosis are at risk for developing diabetes mellitus because the pancreatic duct becomes obstructed as pancreatic tissues are destroyed. Clients with cystis fibrosis can expect to have normal sexual relationships, but fertility becomes difficult because thick secretions obstruct the cervix and block sperm entry. Both men and women carry the gene for cystic fibrosis. Pulmonary disease commonly progresses as the client ages, requiring additional respiratory treatment, not less.

CN: Physiological integrity; CNS: Physiological adaptation; CL: Analysis

131. 50. To perform this dosage calculation, the nurse should first convert the client's weight to kilograms using this formula: 1 kg/ 2.2 lb = X kg/110 lb; 2.2X = 110; X = 50 kg. Then, she should calculate the client's daily dose using this formula: 50 kg × 3 mg/kg = 150 mg. Finally, the nurse should calculate the divided dose: 150 mg ÷ 3 doses = 50 mg/dose.

CN: Physiological integrity; CNS: Pharmacological and parenteral therapies; CL: Application

132. 2, 4, 5. A parent can assess infection control measures by appraising steps taken by the facility to prevent the spread of potential diseases. Placing diapers in covered receptacles, covering the diaper-changing surfaces with disposable papers, and ensuring that there are hand sanitizers and sinks available for personnel to wash their hands after activities are all indicators that infection control measures are being followed. Gloves should be readily available to personnel and, therefore, should be kept in every room, not in an office. Typically, toys are shared by numerous children; however, this contributes to the spread of germs and infections. All soiled clothing and cloth diapers should be placed in a sealed plastic bag prior to being sent home.

CN: Safe, effective care environment; CNS: Safety and infection control; CL: Application

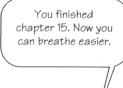

You finished chapter 15. Now you can breathe easier.

CN: Client needs category   CNS: Client needs subcategory   CL: Cognitive level

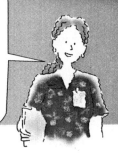

This chapter covers sickle cell disease, varicella, Rocky Mountain spotted fever, leukemia, and many other blood and immune system disorders in kids. It's a whopper of a chapter on a critically important area. If you're ready, let's begin!

Chapter 16
Hematologic & immune systems

1. A child comes to the emergency department feeling feverish and lethargic. Which assessment finding suggests Reye's syndrome?
   1. Fever, profoundly impaired consciousness, and hepatomegaly
   2. Fever, splenomegaly, and hyperactive reflexes
   3. Afebrile, intractable vomiting, and rhinorrhea
   4. Malaise, cough, and sore throat

2. Which aspect is <u>most important</u> for successful management of the child with Reye's syndrome?
   1. Early diagnosis
   2. Initiation of antibiotics
   3. Isolation of the child
   4. Staging of the illness

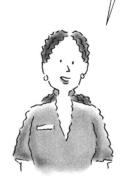

Early diagnosis is crucial to treating Reye's syndrome.

3. A child with Reye's syndrome is in stage I of the illness. Which measure can be taken to prevent further progression of the illness?
   1. Invasive monitoring
   2. Endotracheal intubation
   3. Hypertonic glucose solution
   4. Pancuronium bromide (Pavulon)

1. 1. Reye's syndrome is defined as toxic encephalopathy, characterized by fever, profoundly impaired consciousness, and disordered hepatic function. Intractable vomiting occurs during the first stage of Reye's syndrome, but rhinorrhea usually precedes the onset of the illness. Reye's syndrome doesn't affect the spleen but causes fatty degeneration of the liver. Hyperactive reflexes occur with central nervous system involvement. Malaise, cough, and sore throat are viral symptoms that commonly precede the illness.
CN: Physiological integrity; CNS: Physiological adaptation; CL: Analysis

2. 1. Early diagnosis and therapy are essential because of the rapid clinical course of the disease and its high mortality. Reye's syndrome is associated with a viral illness, and antibiotic therapy isn't crucial to preventing the initial progression of the illness. Isolation isn't necessary because the disease isn't communicable. Staging, although important to therapy, occurs after a differential diagnosis is made.
CN: Physiological integrity; CNS: Reduction of risk potential; CL: Application

3. 3. For children in stage I of Reye's syndrome, treatment is primarily supportive and directed toward restoring blood glucose levels and correcting acid-base imbalances. I.V. administration of dextrose solutions with added insulin helps to replace glycogen stores. Noninvasive monitoring is adequate to assess status at this stage. Endotracheal intubation may be necessary later. Pancuronium bromide is used as an adjunct to endotracheal intubation and wouldn't be used in this stage of Reye's syndrome.
CN: Physiological integrity; CNS: Reduction of risk potential; CL: Application

CN: Client needs category   CNS: Client needs subcategory   CL: Cognitive level

4. Which group of laboratory results, along with the clinical manifestations, <u>establishes</u> a diagnosis of Reye's syndrome?
1. Elevated liver enzymes and prolonged prothrombin and partial thromboplastin times
2. Increased serum glucose and insulin levels
3. Increased bilirubin and alkaline phosphatase levels
4. Decreased serum glucose and ammonia levels

5. In the latter stages of Reye's syndrome, which major intervention is directed toward preventing or reducing cerebral edema?
1. Noninvasive pressure monitoring
2. Paralysis and sedation
3. Liberal fluid replacement
4. Nonassisted ventilation

6. Which assessment change would indicate increased intracranial pressure (ICP) in a child acutely ill with Reye's syndrome?
1. Irritability and quick pupil response
2. Increased blood pressure and decreased heart rate
3. Decreased blood pressure and increased heart rate
4. Sluggish pupil response and decreased blood pressure

7. A client with Reye's syndrome is exhibiting increased intracranial pressure (ICP). Which nursing intervention would be the <u>most</u> appropriate for this client?
1. Position the child with the head elevated and the neck in a neutral position.
2. Maintain the child in the prone position.
3. Cluster together interventions that may be perceived as noxious.
4. Position the child in the supine position, with the child's head turned to the side.

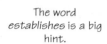

The word establishes is a big hint.

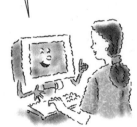

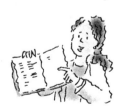

Read this question carefully.

4. 1. Reye's syndrome causes fatty degeneration of the liver, altering results of liver function studies. Decreased serum glucose levels, with reduced insulin levels, occur secondary to dehydration caused by intractable vomiting. Serum bilirubin and alkaline phosphatase usually aren't affected.

CN: Physiological integrity; CNS: Physiological adaptation; CL: Analysis

5. 2. Skeletal muscles are paralyzed with the administration of pancuronium (Pavulon). This prevents activity, especially coughing, that might increase intracranial pressure (ICP). Invasive monitoring is essential to detect increased ICP. Liberal fluid replacement may increase cerebral edema and should be strictly monitored. Tracheal intubation is performed as soon as possible to prevent hypoventilation and increased carbon dioxide levels.

CN: Physiological integrity; CNS: Reduction of risk potential; CL: Analysis

6. 2. A marked increase in ICP will trigger the pressure response; increased ICP produces an elevation in blood pressure with a reflex slowing of the heart rate. Irritability is commonly an early sign, but pupillary response becomes more sluggish in response to increased ICP.

CN: Physiological integrity; CNS: Physiological adaptation; CL: Application

7. 1. Positioning the child with the head elevated and neck in the neutral position helps decrease ICP. The prone and supine positions cause increased ICP. Interventions that may be perceived as noxious should be spaced over time because, if clustered together, they may have a cumulative effect in increasing ICP. Turning the head to the side may impede venous return from the head and increase ICP.

CN: Physiological integrity; CNS: Physiological adaptation; CL: Application

CN: Client needs category   CNS: Client needs subcategory   CL: Cognitive level

8. The goal of nursing care for a client with Reye's syndrome is to minimize intracranial pressure (ICP). Which nursing intervention helps to meet this goal?

1. Keeping the head of bed flat
2. Frequent position changes
3. Positioning to avoid neck flexion
4. Suctioning and chest physiotherapy

9. Which nursing intervention should be included in the care of an unconscious child with Reye's syndrome?

1. Keeping the arms and legs flexed
2. Placing the child on a sheepskin
3. Avoiding the use of lotions on the skin
4. Placing the client in a supine position

10. Which medication has been connected to the development of Reye's syndrome?

1. Acetaminophen (Tylenol)
2. Aspirin
3. Ibuprofen (Motrin)
4. Guaifenesin (Robitussin)

11. Parents should be told to stop acetylsalicylic acid (aspirin) administration and notify a physician if their child is exposed to which condition?

1. Stress
2. Scabies
3. Influenza
4. Environmental allergies

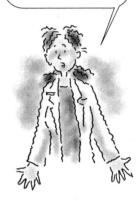

Stay calm when encountering NCLEX questions you're unsure about. That's what I do.

OK. OK. So I'm to blame.

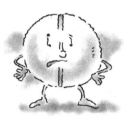

8. 3. Jugular vein compression can increase ICP by interfering with venous return. The head of the bed should be elevated to help promote venous return. Nursing procedures such as frequent positioning tend to cause overstimulation; therefore, care should be taken to avoid such procedures to prevent increased ICP. Suctioning and percussion are poorly tolerated and are contraindicated, unless concurrent respiratory problems are present.
CN: Physiological integrity; CNS: Physiological adaptation; CL: Application

9. 2. Placing the child on a sheepskin helps to prevent pressure on prominent areas of the body. Keeping extremities in a flexed position can lead to contractures. Rubbing the extremities with lotion stimulates circulation and helps prevent drying of the skin. Placing the child supine would be contraindicated because of the risk of aspiration and increasing intracranial pressure. The supine position puts undue pressure on the sacral and occipital areas.
CN: Physiological integrity; CNS: Physiological adaptation; CL: Application

10. 2. Aspirin administration is associated with the development of Reye's syndrome. Acetaminophen, ibuprofen, and guaifenesin haven't been associated with the development of Reye's syndrome. In fact, there has been a decreased incidence of Reye's syndrome with the increased use of acetaminophen and ibuprofen for management of fevers in children.
CN: Physiological integrity; CNS: Pharmacological and parenteral therapies; CL: Application

11. 3. A strong association exists between influenza and aspirin administration and the development of Reye's syndrome. There's no contraindication with the other conditions.
CN: Physiological integrity; CNS: Pharmacological and parenteral therapies; CL: Application

12. Which nursing intervention should be included in the care of a client with Reye's syndrome who's receiving pancuronium (Pavulon)?
1. Applying artificial tears as needed
2. Providing regular tactile stimulation
3. Performing active range-of-motion (ROM) exercises
4. Placing the client in a supine position

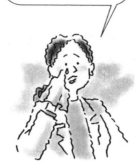

You're doing so well I'm going to cry.

13. Which goal should be achieved by performing a craniotomy on a client with Reye's syndrome?
1. Decreasing carbon dioxide levels
2. Determining the extent of brain injury
3. Reducing pressure from an edematous brain
4. Allowing continuous monitoring of intracranial pressure (ICP)

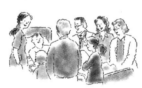

Be sensitive not only to your client's needs, but to the family's needs as well.

14. Parents of a child with Reye's syndrome need a great deal of emotional support. Which nursing intervention should be included to reduce stress and alleviate fears?
1. Not accepting aggressive behavior from the parents
2. Encouraging the parents not to overreact and to hope for the best
3. Letting the parents interpret the child's behaviors and responses
4. Explaining therapies and clarifying or reinforcing the information given

15. Which clinical manifestation should you expect to see in a client in stage V of Reye's syndrome?
1. Vomiting, lethargy, and drowsiness
2. Seizures, flaccidity, and respiratory arrest
3. Hyperventilation and coma
4. Disorientation, aggressiveness, and combativeness

12. 1. Pancuronium suppresses the corneal reflex, making the eyes prone to irritation. Artificial tears prevent drying. Tactile stimulation isn't appropriate because it may elicit a pressure response. Active ROM exercises may cause an increase in pressure. The head of the bed should be elevated slightly, with the paralyzed client in a side-lying or semiprone position to prevent aspiration and minimize intracranial pressure.
CN: Physiological integrity; CNS: Pharmacological and parenteral therapies; CL: Application

13. 3. In severe cases of cerebral edema, creating bilateral bone flaps (craniotomy) is most effective in decreasing ICP. Carbon dioxide levels can be decreased through mechanical ventilation. Most clients with Reye's syndrome recover without any resulting brain injury. Continuous monitoring of ICP is implemented through central venous pressure lines.
CN: Physiological integrity; CNS: Reduction of risk potential; CL: Analysis

14. 4. Explaining treatments and therapies will help to alleviate undue stress in the parents. An awareness of the potential for aggressive behaviors provides nurses with the understanding that helps them support the parents in their grief. Being too quick to reassure may block a parent's expression of fears. Parents may need help interpreting their child's behavior to avoid assigning erroneous meanings to the many signs their child exhibits.
CN: Psychosocial integrity; CNS: None; CL: Application

15. 2. Staging criteria were developed to help evaluate the client's progress and to evaluate the efficacy of therapies. The clinical manifestations of stage V include seizures, loss of deep tendon reflexes, flaccidity, and respiratory arrest. Vomiting, lethargy, and drowsiness occur in stage I. Hyperventilation and coma occur in stage III. Disorientation and aggressive behavior occur in stage II.
CN: Physiological integrity; CNS: Physiological adaptation; CL: Analysis

CN: Client needs category   CNS: Client needs subcategory   CL: Cognitive level

16. A nurse is administering an immunization to a 2-month-old child. Which immunity will the child form?
1. Acquired immunity
2. Active immunity
3. Natural immunity
4. Passive immunity

17. The parent of a neonate asks the nurse what is the recommended age for beginning hepatitis B immunization. Which response is the <u>most</u> accurate?
1. Birth
2. 4 months
3. 6 months
4. 1 year

18. It would be most appropriate for which infant to begin receiving the measles vaccine?
1. A 6-month-old
2. A 12-month-old
3. An 18-month-old
4. A 24-month-old

19. Which immunization should a healthy 2-month-old infant receive?
1. Measles, mumps, rubella (MMR), and inactivated polio (IPV)
2. Measles, mumps, and rubella (MMR), and varicella
3. Diphtheria, tetanus, and pertussis (DTP), and influenza nasal mist
4. DTP and IPV

20. The child who's diagnosed with thalassemia major (Cooley's anemia) typically suffers complications from the disease and from the treatment. This child is at risk for which condition?
1. Hypertrophy of the thyroid
2. Hypertrophy of the thymus
3. Polycythemia vera and thrombosis
4. Chronic hypoxia and iron overload

What's with all the shots?

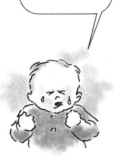

Test-taking tip: Read every question and all the options carefully before selecting your answer.

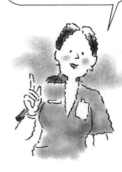

16. 2. Active immunity occurs when the individual forms immune bodies against certain diseases, either by having the disease or by the introduction of a vaccine into the individual. Acquired immunity results from exposure to the bacteria, virus, or toxins. Natural immunity is resistance to infection or toxicity. Passive immunity is a temporary immunity caused by transfusion of immune plasma proteins.
CN: Health promotion and maintenance; CNS: None; CL: Application

17. 1. According to the American Academy of Pediatrics, birth to age 2 months is the recommended time for beginning hepatitis B immunizations.
CN: Health promotion and maintenance; CNS: None; CL: Application

18. 2. According to the American Academy of Pediatrics, the first dose of the measles vaccine should be administered at age 12 to 15 months.
CN: Health promotion and maintenance; CNS: None; CL: Application

19. 4. At age 2 months, DTP and IPV are the recommended immunizations. DTP and IPV are given again at 4 months, and DTP is given again alone at 6 months. MMR is given at age 12 months. Influenza nasal mist is a weakened live vaccine which should be given to health individuals over 2 years of age.
CN: Health promotion and maintenance; CNS: None; CL: Application

20. 4. In thalassemia major, increased destruction of red blood cells (RBCs) causes anemia. RBCs also have a shortened life span. The body responds by increasing the production of RBCs, but it can't adequately produce enough mature cells to meet the body's demands. This process results in chronic hypoxia. Children with the disorder are given multiple transfusions of packed RBCs. The combination of excessive RBC destruction and multiple transfusions causes too much iron to be deposited in organs and tissues and results in damage to the involved organs. The thymus and thyroid aren't involved. Polycythemia vera refers to excessive RBC production, which can result in thrombosis.
CN: Physiological integrity; CNS: Reduction of risk potential; CL: Analysis

21. Which is the treatment of choice for severe aplastic anemia?
1. Liver transplantation
2. Exchange transfusion
3. Bone marrow transplantation
4. Administration of intravenous immunoglobulins

21. 3. Aplastic anemia refers to either a congenital or an acquired condition in which severe pancytopenia, or decrease in cellular components of the blood, occurs. Children with the condition have profound anemia, are susceptible to infections, and risk bleeding. When a good match of donor bone marrow is available, transplantation is the treatment of choice. Liver transplantation, exchange transfusion, and the administration of intravenous immunoglobulins aren't treatments for aplastic anemia.

CN: Physiological integrity; CNS: Physiological adaptation; CL: Application

22. Which type of transfusion is most likely to be given to a child with sickle cell anemia?
1. Plasma
2. Platelets
3. Whole blood
4. Packed red blood cells (RBCs)

22. 4. Packed RBCs are given to children when their hemoglobin is dangerously low. Severe anemia decreases oxygen perfusion and leads to increased sickling of cells. Packed cells are RBCs with plasma removed. If enough whole blood were given to reach the desired hemoglobin level, fluid overload could occur. Thus, the plasma is removed and packed RBCs are infused. The RBCs are needed to transport oxygen. Platelets are given to children with low platelets, not anemia.

CN: Physiological integrity; CNS: Pharmacological and parenteral therapies; CL: Analysis

23. Which direction is <u>most important</u> when administering immunizations?
1. Properly store the vaccine, and follow the recommended procedure for injection.
2. Monitor clients for approximately 1 hour after administration for adverse reactions.
3. Take the vaccine out of refrigeration 1 hour before administration.
4. Inject multiple vaccines at the same injection site.

Stop and think: Which direction would be of primary importance?

23. 1. Vaccines must be properly stored to ensure their potency. The nurse must be familiar with the manufacturer's directions for storage and reconstitution of the vaccine. Faulty refrigeration is a major cause of primary vaccine failure. It isn't necessary to monitor the clients, but the nurse should teach parents to call the physician and report any adverse effects. Taking the vaccine out of refrigeration too early can affect its potency. If more than one vaccine is to be administered, different injection sites should be used. The nurse should note which vaccine is given and at what site in case of a local reaction.

CN: Health promotion and maintenance; CNS: None; CL: Application

CN: Client needs category   CNS: Client needs subcategory   CL: Cognitive level

24. Which symptom is the most common manifestation of severe combined immunodeficiency disease (SCID)?
1. Bruising
2. Failure to thrive
3. Prolonged bleeding
4. Susceptibility to infection

24. 4. SCID is characterized by absence of both humoral and cell-mediated immunity. The most common manifestation is susceptibility to infection early in life, most often by age 3 months. SCID is characterized by chronic infection, failure to completely recover from an infection, and frequent reinfection. The history reveals no logical source for infection. Failure to thrive is a consequence of persistent illnesses. Prolonged bleeding and bruising indicate abnormalities in the clotting system.
CN: Physiological integrity; CNS: Physiological adaptation; CL: Analysis

25. A child is admitted to the hospital for an asthma exacerbation. The nursing history reveals this client was exposed to chickenpox 1 week ago. When would this client require isolation, if he were to remain hospitalized?
1. Isolation isn't required.
2. Immediate isolation is required.
3. Isolation would be required 10 days after exposure.
4. Isolation would be required 12 days after exposure.

25. 2. The incubation period for chickenpox is 2 to 3 weeks, commonly 13 to 17 days. A client is commonly isolated 1 week after exposure to avoid the risk of an earlier breakout. A person is infectious from 1 day before eruption of lesions to 6 days after the vesicles have formed crusts.
CN: Safe, effective care environment; CNS: Safety and infection control; CL: Application

Here's to you! Twenty-five questions, and you're doing great.

26. On assessment of a child's skin, the nurse notes a papular pruritic rash with some vesicles. The rash is profuse on the trunk and sparse on the distal limbs. Based on this assessment, which illness does the client have?
1. Measles
2. Mumps
3. Roseola
4. Chickenpox

26. 4. Chickenpox rash is highly pruritic. The rash begins as a macule, rapidly progresses to a papule, then becomes a vesicle. All three stages are present in varying degrees at one time. Measles begins as an erythematous maculopapular eruption on the face; the eruption gradually spreads downward. Mumps isn't associated with a skin rash. Roseola rash is nonpruritic and is described as discrete rose-pink macules, appearing first on the trunk and then spreading to the neck, face, and extremities.
CN: Health promotion and maintenance; CNS: None; CL: Analysis

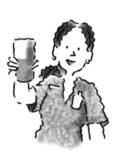

27. Which response would be appropriate to a parent inquiring about when her child with chickenpox can return to school?
1. When the child is afebrile
2. When all vesicles have dried
3. When vesicles begin to crust over
4. When lesions and vesicles are gone

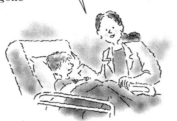

Chickenpox is highly contagious. Teach parents how to assess when it's safe to send kids back to school.

28. Which symptoms are clinical manifestations associated with roseola?
1. Apparent sickness, fever, and rash
2. Fever for 3 to 4 days, followed by rash
3. Rash, without history of fever or illness
4. Rash for 3 to 4 days, followed by high fevers

29. Which assessment finding is consistent with a roseola rash?
1. Maculopapular red spots
2. Macular and pruritic, with papules and vesicles
3. Rose-pink macules that fade on pressure
4. Red maculopapular eruption, beginning on the face

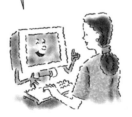

Read each question carefully, and don't do anything rash.

30. Which complication can be caused by a child with chickenpox scratching open and severely irritating the vesicles on his abdomen?
1. Myocarditis
2. Neuritis
3. Obstructive laryngitis
4. Secondary bacterial infection

27. 2. Chickenpox is contagious. It's transmitted through direct contact, droplet spread, and contact with contaminated objects. Vesicles break open; therefore, a person is potentially contagious until all vesicles have dried. It isn't necessary to wait until dried lesions have disappeared. Some vesicles may be crusted over, and new ones may have formed. Macules, papules, vesicles, and crusting are present in varying degrees at one time. A child may be free from fever but continue to have vesicles. Isolation is usually necessary only for about 1 week after the onset of the disease.
CN: Health promotion and maintenance; CNS: None; CL: Analysis

28. 2. Roseola is manifested by persistent high fever for 3 to 4 days in a child who appears well. Fever precedes the rash. When the rash appears, a precipitous drop in fever occurs and the temperature returns to normal.
CN: Health promotion and maintenance; CNS: None; CL: Analysis

29. 3. Roseola rashes are discrete, rose-pink macules or maculopapules that fade on pressure and usually last 1 to 2 days. Maculopapular red spots may indicate fifth disease. Chickenpox rash is macular, with papules and vesicles. Roseola isn't pruritic. Measles begin as a maculopapular eruption on the face.
CN: Health promotion and maintenance; CNS: None; CL: Application

30. 4. Secondary bacterial infections can occur as a complication of chickenpox. Irritation of skin lesions can lead to cellulitis or even an abscess. Myocarditis isn't considered a complication of chickenpox but has been noted as a complication of mumps. Neuritis has been associated with diphtheria. Obstructive laryngitis occurs as a complication of measles.
CN: Physiological integrity; CNS: Reduction of risk potential; CL: Application

CN: Client needs category   CNS: Client needs subcategory   CL: Cognitive level

31. Which characteristic <u>best</u> describes the cough of an infant who was admitted to the hospital with suspected pertussis?

1. Dry, hacking, more frequent on awakening
2. Loose and nonproductive
3. Occurring more frequently during the day
4. Harsh, associated with a high-pitched crowing sound

32. Which communicable disease requires isolating an infected child from pregnant women?

1. Pertussis
2. Roseola
3. Rubella
4. Scarlet fever

33. The nurse would expect the physician to order which medication as the treatment of choice for scarlet fever?

1. Acyclovir (Zovirax)
2. Amphotericin B
3. Ibuprofen (Motrin)
4. Penicillin

34. Which period of isolation is indicated for a child with scarlet fever?

1. Until the associated rash disappears
2. Until completion of antibiotic therapy
3. Until the client is fever-free for 24 hours
4. Until 24 hours after initiation of treatment

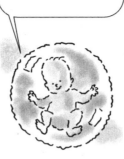

Think before you respond: Can I contract rubella?

31. 4. The cough associated with pertussis is a harsh series of short, rapid coughs, followed by a sudden inspiration and a high-pitched crowing sound. Cheeks become flushed or cyanotic, eyes bulge, and the tongue protrudes. Paroxysm may continue until a thick mucus plug is dislodged. This cough occurs most commonly at night.

CN: Physiological integrity; CNS: Physiological adaptation; CL: Analysis

32. 3. Rubella (German measles) has a teratogenic effect on the fetus. An infected child must be isolated from pregnant women. Pertussis, roseola, and scarlet fever don't have any teratogenic effects on a fetus.

CN: Safe, effective care environment; CNS: Safety and infection control; CL: Application

33. 4. The causative agent of scarlet fever is group A beta-hemolytic streptococci, which is susceptible to penicillin. Erythromycin is used for penicillin-sensitive children. Anti-inflammatory drugs, such as ibuprofen, aren't indicated for these clients. Acyclovir is used in the treatment of herpes infections. Amphotericin B is used to treat fungal infections.

CN: Physiological integrity; CNS: Pharmacological and parenteral therapies; CL: Application

34. 4. A child requires respiratory isolation until 24 hours after initiation of treatment. Rash may persist for 3 weeks. It isn't necessary to wait until the end of treatment. Fever usually breaks 24 hours after therapy has begun. It isn't necessary to maintain isolation for an additional 24 hours.

CN: Safe, effective care environment; CNS: Safety and infection control; CL: Application

35. Which instruction should be included in the teaching about care of a child with chickenpox?
  1. Administer penicillin or erythromycin as ordered.
  2. Administer local or systemic antipruritics as ordered.
  3. Offer periods of interaction with other children to provide distraction.
  4. Avoid administering varicella-zoster immune globulin to children receiving long-term salicylate therapy.

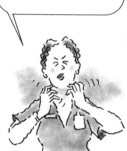

So this is what they mean by "highly pruritic."

35. 2. Chickenpox is highly pruritic. Preventing the child from scratching is necessary to prevent scarring and secondary infection caused by irritation of lesions. Penicillin and erythromycin aren't usually used in the treatment of chickenpox. Interaction with other children would be contraindicated because of the risk of communication, unless the other children previously have had chickenpox or been immunized. Varicella-zoster immune globulin *should* be administered to exposed children who are on long-term aspirin therapy because of the possible risk of Reye's syndrome.
CN: Physiological integrity; CNS: Pharmacological and parenteral therapies; CL: Application

36. A child is admitted with scarlet fever. Which causative agent does the nurse identify as a contributor to this infection?
  1. Roseola
  2. Staphylococcal parotitis
  3. Streptococcal pharyngitis
  4. Chickenpox

36. 3. The causative agent of scarlet fever is group A beta-hemolytic streptococci; therefore, scarlet fever may follow a strep throat infection. Roseola, parotitis, and chickenpox aren't strep infections and don't contribute to scarlet fever.
CN: Physiological integrity; CNS: Reduction of risk potential; CL: Analysis

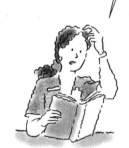

In which body fluids has HIV been isolated?

37. A mother infected with human immunodeficiency virus (HIV) inquires about the possibility of breast-feeding her newborn. Which statement would be a correct response?
  1. Breast-feeding isn't an option.
  2. Breast-feeding would be best for your baby.
  3. Breast-feeding is only an option if the mother is taking zidovudine (Retrovir).
  4. Breast-feeding is an option if milk is expressed and fed by a bottle.

37. 1. Mothers infected with HIV are unable to breast-feed because HIV has been isolated in breast milk and could be transmitted to the infant. Taking zidovudine doesn't prevent transmission. The risk of breast-feeding isn't associated with direct contact with the breast but with the possibility of HIV contained in the breast milk.
CN: Health promotion and maintenance; CNS: None; CL: Application

38. Which subjective assessment finding helps diagnose human immunodeficiency virus (HIV) infection in children?
  1. Excessive weight gain
  2. Arrhythmia
  3. Intermittent diarrhea
  4. Tolerance of feedings

38. 3. A differential diagnosis may be based on the presence of an underlying cellular immunodeficiency-related disease; symptoms include intermittent episodes of diarrhea, repeated respiratory infections, and the inability to tolerate feedings. Poor weight gain and failure to thrive are objective assessment findings that result from intolerance of feedings and frequent infections. Arrhythmia isn't associated with HIV.
CN: Physiological integrity; CNS: Physiological adaptation; CL: Analysis

CN: Client needs category   CNS: Client needs subcategory   CL: Cognitive level

39. Which approach should be included in the diagnostic workup for a 12-month-old infant who's suspected of having acquired immunodeficiency syndrome (AIDS)?
1. Sputum culture
2. Esophageal biopsy
3. Parental counseling prior to testing
4. Human immunodeficiency syndrome (HIV) enzyme-linked immunosorbent assay (ELISA)

40. Parents of a child with Kawasaki disease should be taught the importance of keeping follow-up appointments to monitor and prevent which complication?
1. Encephalitis
2. Glomerulonephritis
3. Myocardial infarction (MI)
4. Idiopathic thrombocytopenia

41. The nurse is working overnight in the emergency department when a client is admitted with sickle cell crisis. Which intervention should the nurse expect to perform?
1. Giving blood transfusions
2. Giving antibiotics
3. Increasing fluid intake and giving analgesics
4. Preparing the client for a splenectomy

42. A child comes to the emergency department suspected of being in vaso-occlusive crisis. Which assessment findings would indicate that the client is having a vaso-occlusive crisis?
1. Hypotension and thready pulse
2. Pallor and poor capillary refill
3. Anemia, jaundice, and reticulocytosis
4. Acute leg pain and hand-foot syndrome

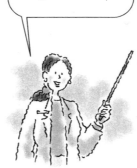

Which approach should the nurse include in the diagnostic workup?

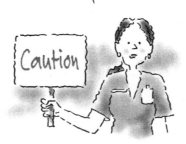

Question 42 is testing your knowledge of the four types of episodic crisis.

Caution

39. 3. AIDS and HIV are devastating diagnoses. Before testing, parents should be counseled regarding the disease, reasons for the tests, confidentiality, and benefits of early treatment. Sputum culture might help diagnose an upper respiratory infection associated with AIDS but isn't a diagnostic test for AIDS. Esophageal biopsy isn't indicated. ELISA isn't used diagnostically for children younger than 18 months because of the maternal antibodies in the child's blood.
CN: Psychosocial integrity; CNS: None; CL: Application

40. 3. In Kawasaki disease, inflammation of small and medium blood vessels can result in weakening of the vessels and aneurysm formation, especially in the heart. Blood flow through damaged vessels can cause thrombus formation and MI. Encephalitis, glomerulonephritis, and idiopathic thrombocytopenia aren't associated with Kawasaki disease.
CN: Health promotion and maintenance; CNS: None; CL: Application

41. 3. The primary therapy for sickle cell crisis is to increase fluid intake according to age and to give analgesics. Blood transfusions are only given conservatively to avoid iron overload. Antibiotics are given to clients with fever. Routine splenectomy isn't recommended. Splenectomy in clients with sickle cell anemia is controversial.
CN: Physiological integrity; CNS: Physiological adaptation; CL: Application

42. 4. Vaso-occlusive crises are the result of sickled cells obstructing the blood vessels. The major symptoms are fever, acute pain from visceral hypoxia, hand-foot syndrome, and arthralgia. A precipitous drop in blood volume is indicative of a splenic sequestration crisis and is exhibited by hypotension and a thready pulse. Aplastic crisis exhibits pallor and poor capillary refill and may result in symptoms of shock. Hyperhemolytic crisis is characterized by anemia, jaundice, and reticulocytosis and may also produce symptoms of shock.
CN: Physiological integrity; CNS: Physiological adaptation; CL: Analysis

43. Which response would be appropriate to give to a parent inquiring about a child who tests positive for <u>sickle cell trait</u>?
1. "Your child has sickle cell anemia."
2. "Your child is a carrier of the disorder but doesn't have sickle cell anemia."
3. "Your child is a carrier of the disease and will pass the disease to any offspring."
4. "Your child doesn't have the disease at present but may show evidence of the disease as he gets older."

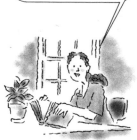

Know the difference between a positive test for sickle cell trait and a positive test for sickle cell anemia.

44. What is the primary nursing objective in caring for a child with sickle cell anemia in vaso-occlusive crisis?
1. Managing pain
2. Providing a cool environment
3. Immobilizing the affected part
4. Restricting fluids

45. The nurse avoids palpating the abdomen of a child in vaso-occlusive crisis to prevent which complication?
1. Risk of splenic rupture
2. Risk of inducing vomiting
3. Increase in abdominal pain
4. Risk of blood cell destruction

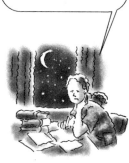

Which nursing intervention will help me keep going?

46. Which intervention is the most effective in maximizing tissue perfusion for a child in vaso-occlusive crisis?
1. Administering analgesics
2. Monitoring fluid restrictions
3. Encouraging activity as tolerated
4. Administering oxygen as prescribed

43. 2. A child with sickle cell trait is only a carrier and may never show any symptoms, except under special hypoxic conditions. A child with sickle cell trait doesn't have the disease and will never test positive for sickle cell anemia. Sickle cell anemia would be transmitted to offspring only as the result of a union between two individuals who are positive for the trait.
CN: Health promotion and maintenance; CNS: None; CL: Application

44. 1. Pain management is an important aspect in the care of a client with sickle cell anemia in vaso-occlusive crisis. The goal is to prevent sickling. This can be accomplished by promoting tissue oxygenation, hydration, and rest, which minimize energy expenditure and oxygen utilization. A cool environment can cause vasoconstriction and thus more sickling and pain. Immobilization can promote stasis and increase sickling.
CN: Physiological integrity; CNS: Basic care and comfort; CL: Analysis

45. 1. Palpating a child's abdomen in vaso-occlusive crisis should be avoided because sequestered red blood cells may precipitate splenic rupture. Abdominal pain alone wouldn't be a reason to avoid palpation. Vomiting or blood cell destruction wouldn't occur from palpation of the abdomen.
CN: Physiological integrity; CNS: Reduction of risk potential; CL: Application

46. 4. Administering oxygen is the most effective way to maximize tissue perfusion. Short-term oxygen therapy helps to prevent hypoxia, which leads to metabolic acidosis, causing sickling. Long-term oxygen therapy will depress erythropoiesis. Analgesics are used to control pain. Hydration is essential to promote hemodilution and maintain electrolyte balance. Bed rest should be promoted to reduce oxygen utilization.
CN: Physiological integrity; CNS: Reduction of risk potential; CL: Application

CN: Client needs category   CNS: Client needs subcategory   CL: Cognitive level

47. Which nursing measure is most important to decrease the postoperative complications of a client with sickle cell anemia?
1. Increasing fluids
2. Preparing the child psychologically
3. Discouraging coughing
4. Limiting the use of analgesics

47. 1. The main surgical risk of anesthesia is hypoxia; however, emotional stress, demands of wound healing, and the potential for infection can each increase the sickling phenomenon. Increased fluids are encouraged because keeping the child well-hydrated is important for hemodilution to prevent sickling. Preparing the child psychologically to decrease fear will minimize undue emotional stress. Deep coughing is encouraged to promote pulmonary hygiene and prevent respiratory tract infection. Analgesics are used to control wound pain and to prevent abdominal splinting and decreased ventilation.
CN: Physiological integrity; CNS: Reduction of risk potential; CL: Application

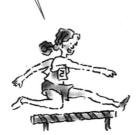

Don't let question 48 trip you up! It's asking you to prioritize.

48. Which factor should be included as a priority in teaching parents about prevention of infection in children with sickle cell anemia?
1. Providing adequate nutrition
2. Avoiding emotional stress
3. Visiting the physician when sick
4. Avoiding strenuous physical exertion

48. 1. The nurse must stress adequate nutrition. Avoiding strenuous physical exertion and emotional stress are important aspects to prevent sickling, but adequate nutrition remains a priority. Frequent medical supervision is imperative to prevention because infection is commonly a predisposing factor toward development of a crisis.
CN: Health promotion and maintenance; CNS: None; CL: Application

49. Which schedule is recommended for the immunization of normal infants and children in the first year of life?
1. Birth, 2 months, 4 months, 6 months, 12 months
2. 1 month, 3 months, 5 months, 9 months, 18 months
3. 2 months, 6 months, 9 months, 12 months, 14 months
4. 2 months, 4 months, 6 months, 12 to 15 months

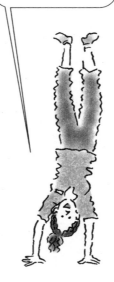

You've reached question 50! You're doing great!

49. 1. The nurse needs to be aware of the schedule for immunizations, as well as the latest recommendations for their use. According to the American Academy of Pediatrics, the recommended age for beginning primary immunizations of normal infants is at birth.
CN: Health promotion and maintenance; CNS: None; CL: Application

50. Which assessment findings would indicate vaso-occlusive crisis in a child with sickle cell anemia?
1. Painful urination
2. Pain with ambulation
3. Complaints of throat pain
4. Fever with associated rash

50. 2. Bone pain is one of the major symptoms of vaso-occlusive crisis in clients with sickle cell anemia. Hand-foot syndrome, characterized by edematous painful extremities, is usually exhibited in the refusal of the child to bear weight and ambulate. Painful urination doesn't occur, but sickle cell anemia can cause kidney abnormalities. Throat pain isn't a symptom of vaso-occlusive crisis. Fever commonly accompanies vaso-occlusive crisis but isn't associated with rash.
CN: Physiological integrity; CNS: Physiological adaptation; CL: Analysis

51. The nurse is assessing a child with sickle cell anemia. Which bone-related complications would the nurse be alert for during assessment?
   1. Arthritis
   2. Osteoporosis
   3. Osteogenic sarcoma
   4. Spontaneous fractures

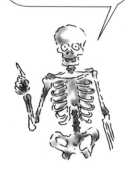

I was minding my own business when things got really complicated.

52. What is a nurse's role with the parents of a child who has been diagnosed with sickle cell anemia?
   1. Encouraging selective birth methods or abortion
   2. Referring only sickle cell–positive parents for counseling
   3. Rendering support to parents of newly diagnosed children
   4. Reinforcing the idea that transmission is unlikely in subsequent pregnancies

53. A 14-year-old girl is admitted for sickle cell crisis. Which nursing intervention would be the most important?
   1. Gathering information about the child's ability to cope with this condition
   2. Monitoring the child's temperature every 2 hours
   3. Providing adequate oxygenation, hydrations, and pain management
   4. Making sure the family is involved in every step of the child's care

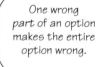

One wrong part of an option makes the entire option wrong.

54. A nurse is administering a blood transfusion to a client with sickle cell anemia. Which assessment findings would indicate that the client is having a transfusion reaction?
   1. Diaphoresis and hot flashes
   2. Urticaria, flushing, and wheezing
   3. Fever, urticaria, and red raised rash
   4. Fever, disorientation, and abdominal pain

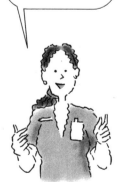

51. 2. Sickle cell anemia causes hyperplasia and congestion of the bone marrow, resulting in osteoporosis. Arthritis doesn't occur secondary to sickle cell anemia; however, a crisis can cause localized swelling over joints, resulting in arthralgia. Bones do become weakened, but spontaneous fractures don't occur as a result. Osteogenic sarcoma is bone cancer; sickle cell anemia isn't a contributing factor to bone cancer.
CN: Physiological integrity; CNS: Physiological adaptation; CL: Application

52. 3. The nurse can be instrumental in providing genetic counseling. She can give parents correct information about the disease and render support to parents of newly diagnosed children. Alternative birth methods are discussed, but parents make their own decisions. All heterozygous, or trait-positive, parents should be referred for genetic counseling. The risk of transmission in subsequent pregnancies remains the same.
CN: Health promotion and maintenance; CNS: None; CL: Application

53. 3. The most critical need of a client in sickle cell crisis is to provide adequate oxygenation, hydrations, and pain management until the crisis passes. Obtaining a temperature every 2 hours would not be the priority intervention. While assessing the client's ability to cope and involving the family in the child's care are important, they aren't the priority interventions during a sickle cell crisis.
CN: Safe, effective care environment; CNS: Management of care; CL: Analysis

54. 2. Allergic reactions may occur when the recipient reacts to allergens in the donor's blood; this reaction causes urticaria, flushing, and wheezing. A febrile reaction can occur, causing fever and urticaria, but it isn't accompanied by rash. Diaphoresis, hot flashes, disorientation, and abdominal pain aren't symptoms of a transfusion reaction.
CN: Physiological integrity; CNS: Reduction of risk potential; CL: Analysis

CN: Client needs category   CNS: Client needs subcategory   CL: Cognitive level

55. A mother brings her 5-year-old child to the clinic and asks the nurse how often a child should receive the influenza virus vaccine. Which response would be the most accurate?
   1. Annually
   2. Twice a year
   3. Never; contraindicated in children
   4. Only with the outbreak of illness

56. A 3-year-old sister of a neonate is diagnosed with pertussis. The mother has a history of having been immunized as a child. Which information should be included in teaching the mother about possible infection of her neonate?
   1. The baby will inevitably contract pertussis.
   2. Immune globulin is effective in protecting the infant.
   3. The risk to the infant depends on the mother's immune status.
   4. Erythromycin should be administered prophylactically to the infant.

57. A child has recently been admitted to the pediatric unit with laboratory values indicating an increase in hemoglobin A_2. Based on this finding, the nurse should expect to follow a care plan based on which condition?
   1. Beta-thalassemia trait
   2. Iron deficiency
   3. Lead poisoning
   4. Sickle cell anemia

58. A 4-year-old child has a petechial rash but is otherwise well. The platelet count is 20,000/ μl, and the hemoglobin level and white blood cell (WBC) count are normal. Which diagnosis is most likely?
   1. Acute lymphoblastic leukemia (ALL)
   2. Disseminated intravascular coagulation (DIC)
   3. Idiopathic thrombocytopenic purpura (ITP)
   4. Systemic lupus erythematosus (SLE)

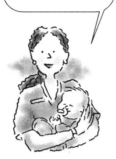

Prevention is commonly the best medicine!

55. 1. The influenza virus vaccine is usually administered annually. The vaccine isn't contraindicated in children but is targeted at clients with chronic cardiac, pulmonary, hematologic, and neurologic problems. The vaccine is given to prevent the onset of illness before an outbreak occurs.
CN: Health promotion and maintenance; CNS: None; CL: Application

56. 4. In exposed, high-risk persons such as neonates, erythromycin may be effective in preventing or lessening severity of the disease if administered during the preparoxysmal stage. Immune globulin isn't indicated because it's used as an immunization against hepatitis A. Neonates exposed to pertussis are at considerable risk for infections, regardless of the mother's immune status; however, infection isn't inevitable.
CN: Health promotion and maintenance; CNS: None; CL: Application

57. 1. The concentration of hemoglobin A_2 is increased with beta-thalassemia trait. In severe iron deficiency, hemoglobin A_2 may be decreased. The hemoglobin A_2 level is normal in lead poisoning and sickle cell anemia.
CN: Physiological integrity; CNS: Reduction of risk potential; CL: Application

58. 3. The onset of ITP typically occurs between ages 1 and 6. Clients look well, except for a petechial rash. ALL is associated with a low platelet count but an *abnormal* hemoglobin level and WBC count. DIC is secondary to a severe underlying disease. SLE is rare in a 4-year-old child.
CN: Physiological integrity; CNS: Physiological adaptation; CL: Analysis

59. Which instruction should be included in a nurse's discharge teaching for the parents of a newborn diagnosed with sickle cell anemia?
1. Stressing the importance of iron supplementation
2. Stressing the importance of monthly vitamin B$_{12}$ injections
3. Reviewing signs of abdominal pain in infants and demonstrating how to take a temperature
4. Explaining that immunizations are contraindicated

60. Which finding yields a poor prognosis for a child with leukemia?
1. Presence of a mediastinal mass
2. Late central nervous system (CNS) leukemia
3. Normal white blood cell (WBC) count at diagnosis
4. Disease presents between ages 2 and 10

61. A 1-year-old boy in the pediatrician's office for an examination is noted to be pale. He's in the 75th percentile for weight and the 25th percentile for length. His physical examination is normal, but his hematocrit is 24%. Which question would be <u>most helpful</u> in establishing a diagnosis of anemia?
1. Is the child on any medications?
2. What's the child's usual daily diet?
3. Did the child receive phototherapy for jaundice?
4. What's the pattern and appearance of bowel movements?

62. A nurse is teaching the parents of a child newly diagnosed with Hodgkin's disease. Which statement should the nurse include in her teaching?
1. Staging laparotomy is mandatory for every client.
2. Excessive weight gain can be a symptom.
3. Hodgkin's disease is rare before age 5.
4. Incidence of Hodgkin's disease peaks between ages 11 and 15.

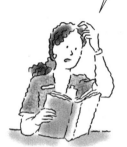

Question 60 asks about a prognosis, not a diagnosis.

59. 3. Acute splenic sequestration is a serious complication of sickle cell anemia. Early detection of splenomegaly by parents is an important aspect of client management. Parents should be able to take the temperature and identify abdominal pain. A temperature of 101.3° F to 102.2° F (38.5° C to 39° C) calls for emergency evaluation, even if the child appears well. Folic acid requirement is increased; therefore, supplementation may be indicated. Vitamin B$_{12}$ supplementation and iron supplementation aren't necessary. Parents should be encouraged to keep immunizations up to date.
CN: Health promotion and maintenance; CNS: None; CL: Application

60. 1. The presence of a mediastinal mass indicates a poor prognosis for children with leukemia. The prognosis is poorer if age at onset is younger than 2 years or older than 10 years. A WBC count of 100,000/μl or higher and early CNS leukemia also indicate a poor prognosis for a child with leukemia.
CN: Physiological integrity; CNS: Physiological adaptation; CL: Analysis

61. 2. Iron deficiency anemia is the most common nutritional deficiency in children between ages 9 months and 15 months. Anemia in a 1-year-old child is mostly nutritional in origin, and its cause will be suggested by a detailed nutritional history. None of the other selections would be helpful in diagnosing anemia.
CN: Health promotion and maintenance; CNS: None; CL: Analysis

62. 3. Hodgkin's disease is rare before age 5. Staging laparotomy is *not* recommended for clients who have obvious intra-abdominal disease by noninvasive studies. Systemic symptoms of Hodgkin's disease include fever, night sweats, malaise, weight loss, and pruritus. The peak incidence of Hodgkin's disease occurs in late adolescence and young adulthood (ages 15 to 34).
CN: Physiological integrity; CNS: Physiological adaptation; CL: Analysis

CN: Client needs category   CNS: Client needs subcategory   CL: Cognitive level

63. The nurse is caring for a child with perinatally acquired human immunodeficiency virus. At which age do children usually demonstrate symptoms of acquired immunodeficiency syndrome (AIDS)?
   1. Within the first month of life
   2. At 1 to 3 months of age
   3. At 18 to 24 months of age
   4. At 3 to 5 years of age

64. Which factors may make adolescent girls at risk for iron deficiency anemia?
   1. Menses
   2. Vegetarian diet
   3. Weight-loss diets
   4. All of the above

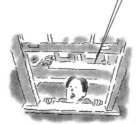

These questions are tough! Hang in there!

65. Which treatment would be most appropriate for a child diagnosed with iron deficiency anemia?
   1. Blood transfusion
   2. Oral ferrous sulfate
   3. An iron-fortified cereal
   4. Intramuscular iron dextran

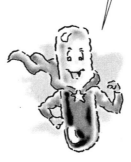

I can help with iron deficiency anemia.

66. A child is admitted to the hospital with flu-like symptoms. Diagnostic testing reveals the IgM antibody parvovirus B19 is present. The nurse interprets this finding as being indicative of which condition?
   1. Roseola
   2. Fifth disease
   3. Varicella
   4. Mumps

63. 3. The majority of children with perinatally transmitted AIDS appear normal in early infancy. Symptoms usually develop at 18 to 24 months of age.
CN: Physiological integrity; CNS: Physiological adaptation; CL: Application

64. 4. All the options make adolescent girls, who are still growing, at risk for iron deficiency anemia. That's because these girls lose blood monthly with menstrual periods, and they typically consume inadequate amounts of nutrients because of their eating patterns, which include hurried meals, vegetarian diets, and weight-loss diets.
CN: Health promotion and maintenance; CNS: None; CL: Analysis

65. 2. A prompt rise in hemoglobin level and hematocrit follows the administration of oral ferrous sulfate. Blood transfusion is rarely indicated unless a child becomes symptomatic or is further compromised by a superimposed infection. Dietary modifications are appropriate long-term measures, but they won't make enough iron available to replenish iron stores. Intramuscular dextran is reserved for situations in which compliance can't be achieved because it's expensive, painful, and no more effective than oral iron.
CN: Physiological integrity; CNS: Physiological adaptation; CL: Application

66. 2. Fifth disease is known to be caused by human parvovirus B19. Roseola is thought to be caused by the human herpes virus 6. Varicella is caused by the varicella-zoster virus. Mumps is caused by the paramyxovirus.
CN: Physiological integrity; CNS: Reduction of risk potential; CL: Application

67. A 6-year-old child has been diagnosed with Rocky Mountain spotted fever. In teaching the parents about the cause of the illness, a nurse would be correct in telling them that a bite by which animal or insect caused the illness?
1. Cat
2. Mosquito
3. Spider
4. Tick

68. An iron dextran (InFeD) injection has been ordered for an 8-month-old child with iron deficiency anemia whose parents haven't been compliant with oral supplements. What is the correct method of injection for InFeD?
1. Intradermal
2. Subcutaneous
3. Intramuscular
4. Intramuscular using the Z-track method

69. Which food is an appropriate source of dietary iron for the prevention of nutritional anemia?
1. Citrus fruits
2. Fish
3. Green vegetables
4. Milk products

70. Which instruction should a nurse provide when teaching parents the proper administration of liquid oral iron supplements?
1. Give the supplements with food.
2. Stop the medication if vomiting occurs.
3. Decrease the dose if constipation occurs.
4. Give the medicine via a dropper or through a straw.

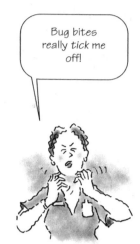

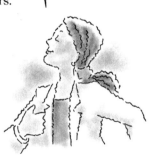

67. 4. Rocky Mountain spotted fever is caused by *Rickettsia rickettsii*, which is transmitted by the bite of a tick. Mosquito, spider, and cat bites haven't been known to transmit *R. rickettsii*.
CN: Safe, effective care environment; CNS: Safety and infection control; CL: Application

68. 4. If iron dextran is ordered, it must be injected deeply into a large muscle mass, using the Z-track method to minimize skin staining and irritation. Neither a subcutaneous nor an intradermal injection would inject the dextran into the muscle. The Z-track method is preferred over a normal intramuscular injection.
CN: Physiological integrity; CNS: Pharmacological and parenteral therapies; CL: Application

69. 3. Green vegetables are good sources of iron. Citrus foods aren't sources of iron but help with the absorption of iron. Fish isn't a good source of dietary iron. Milk is deficient in iron and should be limited in cases of nutritional anemia.
CN: Physiological integrity; CNS: Basic care and comfort; CL: Application

70. 4. Liquid iron preparations may temporarily stain the teeth; therefore, the drug should be given by dropper or through a straw. Supplements should be given between meals, when the presence of free hydrochloric acid is greatest. If vomiting occurs, supplementation shouldn't be stopped; instead, it should be administered with food. Constipation can be decreased by increasing intake of fruits and vegetables.
CN: Physiological integrity; CNS: Pharmacological and parenteral therapies; CL: Application

CN: Client needs category   CNS: Client needs subcategory   CL: Cognitive level

71. Which symptom is the primary clinical manifestation of hemophilia?
1. Petechiae
2. Prolonged bleeding
3. Decreased clotting time
4. Decreased white blood cell (WBC) count

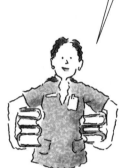

Careful! All of these answers may be accurate, but this question is asking for the most common site.

72. The nurse would be alert for signs and symptoms of internal bleeding <u>most commonly</u> at which site for a client with hemophilia?
1. Brain tissue
2. GI tract
3. Joint cavities
4. Spinal cord

73. Which measure should parents of a hemophilic child be taught to prepare them to initiate immediate treatment before blood loss is excessive?
1. Apply heat to the area.
2. Withhold factor replacement.
3. Apply pressure for at least 5 minutes.
4. Immobilize and elevate the affected area.

74. A 2-year-old child with hemophilia who sustains a joint injury is <u>best</u> treated promptly in which location?
1. Home
2. Clinic
3. Hospital unit
4. Emergency department

71. 2. The effect of hemophilia is prolonged bleeding, anywhere from or within the body. With severe deficiencies, hemorrhage can occur as a result of minor trauma. Petechiae are uncommon in persons with hemophilia because repair of small hemorrhages depends on platelet function, not on blood clotting mechanisms. Clotting time is increased in a client with hemophilia. A decrease in WBCs is *not* indicative of hemophilia.
CN: Physiological integrity; CNS: Physiological adaptation; CL: Analysis

72. 3. The joint cavities, especially the knees, ankles, and elbows, are the most common site of internal bleeding. This bleeding typically results in bone changes and crippling, disabling deformities. Intracranial hemorrhage occurs less commonly than expected because the brain tissue has a high concentration of thromboplastin. Hemorrhage along the GI tract and spinal cord can occur but are less common.
CN: Physiological integrity; CNS: Physiological adaptation; CL: Application

73. 4. Elevating the area above the level of the heart will decrease blood flow. Cold, not heat, should be applied to promote vasoconstriction. Factor replacement should *not* be delayed. Pressure should be applied to the area for at least 10 to 15 minutes to allow clot formation.
CN: Physiological integrity; CNS: Physiological adaptation; CL: Application

74. 1. Prompt treatment to prevent joint injury and other complications is best delivered in the home. After the child reaches age 2 or 3 years, parents can learn venipuncture techniques so treatment can be done at home and further injury avoided. The life of the child and family is also less disrupted. The child may be transfused on a regular basis to prevent bleeding and will be given additional doses of the missing factor when an injury occurs. By mid- to late-school age, children can learn to administer their own treatment.
CN: Physiological integrity; CNS: Reduction of risk potential; CL: Application

75. Which nursing measure is an important aid in <u>prevention</u> of the crippling effects of joint degeneration caused by hemophilia?
 1. Avoiding the use of analgesics
 2. Using aspirin for pain relief
 3. Administering replacement factor
 4. Using active range-of-motion (ROM) exercises

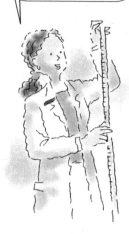

Read carefully. This question is looking for a preventive measure.

76. When comparing bleeding disorders, an increased tendency to bleed in which area differentiates von Willebrand's disease from hemophilia?
 1. Brain tissue
 2. GI tract
 3. Mucous membranes
 4. Spinal cord

77. Which nursing measure should be implemented for a client with von Willebrand's disease who's having <u>epistaxis</u>?
 1. Lying the child supine
 2. Avoiding packing of the nostrils
 3. Avoiding pressure to the nose
 4. Applying pressure to the nose

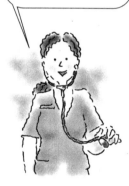

Epistaxis is a term from early in your program. Remember?

78. A nurse is teaching the parents of a child with acute lymphoblastic leukemia. The parents ask for information about what helps determine long-term survival. The nurse discusses which of the following as the three most important prognostic factors?
 1. Histologic type of disease, initial platelet count, and type of treatment
 2. Type of treatment, stage at diagnosis, and child's age at diagnosis
 3. Histologic type of disease, initial white blood cell (WBC) count, and client's age at diagnosis
 4. Progression of illness, WBC count at time of diagnosis, and client's age at diagnosis

75. 3. Prevention of bleeding is the goal and is achieved by factor replacement therapy. Active ROM exercises are contraindicated after a bleeding episode because the joint capsule can be stretched, causing bleeding. Acetaminophen should be used for pain relief because aspirin has anticoagulant effects. Analgesics should be administered before physical therapy to control pain and provide the maximum benefit.
CN: Physiological integrity; CNS: Physiological adaptation; CL: Application

76. 3. The most characteristic clinical feature of von Willebrand's disease is an increased tendency to bleed from mucous membranes, which may be seen as frequent nosebleeds or menorrhagia. In hemophilia, the joint cavities are the most common site of internal bleeding. Bleeding into the GI tract, spinal cord, and brain tissue can occur, but these are *not* the most common sites for bleeding.
CN: Physiological integrity; CNS: Physiological adaptation; CL: Application

77. 4. Applying pressure to the nose may stop bleeding because most bleeds occur in the anterior part of the nasal septum. Encourage mouth breathing at this time. The child should be instructed to sit up and lean forward to avoid aspiration of blood. Packing with tissue or cotton may be used to help stop bleeding, although care must be taken in removing packing to avoid dislodging the clot. Pressure should be maintained for at least 10 minutes to allow clotting to occur.
CN: Physiological integrity; CNS: Physiological adaptation; CL: Application

78. 3. Histologic type of leukemia is the factor whose prognostic value is considered to be of greatest significance in determining long-range outcome. Children with a normal or low WBC count appear to have a much better prognosis than those with a high WBC count. Children diagnosed between ages 2 and 10 have consistently demonstrated a better prognosis than those diagnosed before age 2 or after age 10.
CN: Physiological integrity; CNS: Physiological adaptation; CL: Analysis

CN: Client needs category CNS: Client needs subcategory CL: Cognitive level

79. Which complications are the three main consequences of leukemia?
1. Bone deformities, spherocytosis, and infection
2. Anemia, infection, and bleeding tendencies
3. Lymphocytopoiesis, growth delays, and hirsutism
4. Polycythemia, decreased clotting time, and infection

You, my friend, are doing extraordinarily well. Keep up the good work!

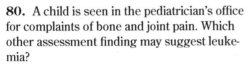

80. A child is seen in the pediatrician's office for complaints of bone and joint pain. Which other assessment finding may suggest leukemia?
1. Abdominal pain
2. Increased activity level
3. Increased appetite
4. Petechiae

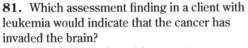

81. Which assessment finding in a client with leukemia would indicate that the cancer has invaded the brain?
1. Headache and vomiting
2. Restlessness and tachycardia
3. Hypervigilant and anxious behavior
4. Increased heart rate and decreased blood pressure

79. 2. The three main consequences of leukemia are anemia, caused by decreased erythrocyte production; infection secondary to neutropenia; and bleeding tendencies, from decreased platelet production. Bone deformities don't occur with leukemia, although bones may become painful because of the proliferation of cells in the bone marrow. Spherocytosis refers to erythrocytes taking on a spheroid shape and isn't a feature in leukemia. Lymphocytopoesis is production of lymphocytes with leukemia. Mature cells aren't produced in adequate numbers. Hirsutism and growth delay can be a result of large doses of steroids but aren't common in leukemia. Anemia, not polycythemia, occurs. Clotting times would be prolonged.
CN: Physiological integrity; CNS: Physiological adaptation; CL: Application

80. 4. The most common signs and symptoms of leukemia are a result of infiltration of the bone marrow. These include fever, pallor, fatigue, anorexia, and petechiae, along with bone and joint pain. Abdominal pain may be caused by areas of inflammation from normal flora within the GI tract or any number of other causes. Increased appetite can occur, but it usually isn't a presenting symptom.
CN: Physiological integrity; CNS: Physiological adaptation; CL: Application

81. 1. The usual effect of leukemic infiltration of the brain is increased intracranial pressure. The proliferation of cells interferes with the flow of cerebrospinal fluid in the subarachnoid space and at the base of the brain. The increased fluid pressure causes dilation of the ventricles, which creates symptoms of severe headache, vomiting, irritability, lethargy, increased blood pressure, decreased heart rate and, eventually, coma. Children with a variety of illnesses are typically hypervigilant and anxious when hospitalized.
CN: Physiological integrity; CNS: Physiological adaptation; CL: Analysis

82. A student nurse asks the nurse on the hematology unit which type of leukemia has the best prognosis. Which response would be the <u>most</u> accurate?
1. Acute lymphoblastic leukemia
2. Acute myelogenous leukemia
3. Basophilic leukemia
4. Eosinophilic leukemia

83. Which finding is the reason to perform a spinal tap on a client newly diagnosed with leukemia?
1. To rule out meningitis
2. To decrease intracranial pressure (ICP)
3. To aid in classification of the leukemia
4. To assess for central nervous system (CNS) infiltration

84. Which test is performed on a client with leukemia before initiation of therapy to evaluate the child's ability to metabolize chemotherapeutic agents?
1. Lumbar puncture
2. Liver function studies
3. Complete blood count (CBC)
4. Peripheral blood smear

85. Which statement by the nurse most accurately explains the need for a child with pauciarticular juvenile rheumatoid arthritis (JRA) to have an annual eye exam?
1. "Detached retinas are commonly associated with the disease."
2. "Painless iritis (inflammation of the iris) is commonly seen with the disease."
3. "Glaucoma is commonly seen with the disease."
4. "Strabismus is commonly seen with the disease."

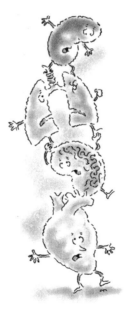

Think back to basic physiology. Which organs metabolize drugs?

82. 1. Acute lymphoblastic leukemia, which accounts for more than 80% of all childhood cases, carries the best prognosis. Acute myelogenous leukemia, with several subtypes, accounts for most of the other leukemias affecting children. Basophilic and eosinophilic leukemia are named for the specific cells involved. These are much rarer and carry a poorer prognosis.
CN: Physiological integrity; CNS: Physiological adaptation; CL: Application

83. 4. A spinal tap is performed to assess for CNS infiltration. A spinal tap can be done to rule out meningitis, but this isn't the indication for the test on a leukemic client. It wouldn't be done to decrease ICP, nor does it aid in the classification of the leukemia. Spinal taps can result in brain stem herniation in cases of increased ICP.
CN: Physiological integrity; CNS: Physiological adaptation; CL: Application

84. 2. Liver and kidney function studies are done before initiation of chemotherapy to evaluate the child's ability to metabolize the chemotherapeutic agents. A lumbar puncture is performed to assess for central nervous system infiltration. A CBC is performed to assess for anemia and white blood cell count. A peripheral blood smear is done to assess the maturity and morphology of red blood cells.
CN: Physiological integrity; CNS: Pharmacological and parenteral therapies; CL: Analysis

85. 2. Painless iritis may be found in 75% of children with pauciarticular JRA. If it's not detected and is left untreated, permanent scarring in the anterior chamber of the eye may occur, with loss of vision. Children should have annual slit lamp examinations by an ophthalmologist. Detached retinas, glaucoma, and strabismus aren't commonly associated with the disease.
CN: Health promotion and maintenance; CNS: None; CL: Application

CN: Client needs category   CNS: Client needs subcategory   CL: Cognitive level

86. Which medication would the nurse expect the physician to order most commonly for a client with leukemia as prophylaxis against *Pneumocystic carinii* pneumonia?
1. Co-trimoxazole (Bactrim)
2. Oral nystatin suspension
3. Prednisone
4. Vincristine

Here's a prescription for the drug of choice. Do you know which one it is?

86. 1. The most common cause of death from leukemia is overwhelming infection. *P. carinii* infection is lethal to a child with leukemia. As prophylaxis against *P. carinii* pneumonia, continuous low dosages of co-trimoxazole are typically prescribed. Oral nystatin suspension would be indicated for the treatment of thrush. Prednisone isn't an antibiotic and increases susceptibility to infection. Vincristine is an anti-neoplastic agent.
CN: Physiological integrity; CNS: Pharmacological and parenteral therapies; CL: Application

87. A 4-year-old child is diagnosed as having acute lymphocytic leukemia. His white blood cell (WBC) count, especially the neutrophil count, is low. Which intervention should the nurse teach the parents?
1. Protect the child from falls because of his increased risk of bleeding.
2. Protect the child from infections because his resistance to infection is decreased.
3. Provide rest periods because the oxygen-carrying capacity of the child's blood is diminished.
4. Treat constipation, which frequently accompanies a decrease in WBC.

87. 2. One of the complications of both acute lymphocytic leukemia and its treatment is a decreased WBC count, especially a decreased absolute neutrophil count. Because neutrophils are the body's first line of defense against infection, the child must be protected from infection. Bleeding is a risk factor if platelets or other coagulation factors are decreased. A decreased hemoglobin level, hematocrit, or both would reduce the oxygen-carrying capacity of the child's blood. Constipation isn't related to the WBC count.
CN: Safe, effective care environment; CNS: Safety and infection control; CL: Application

88. Which treatment measure should be implemented for a child with leukemia who has been exposed to chickenpox?
1. No treatment is indicated.
2. Acyclovir (Zovirax) should be started on exposure.
3. Varicella-zoster immune globulin (VZIG) should be given with evidence of the disease.
4. VZIG should be given within 72 hours of exposure.

Sometimes timing is everything!

88. 4. Varicella is a lethal organism to a child with leukemia. VZIG, given within 72 hours, may favorably alter the course of the disease. Giving the vaccine at the onset of symptoms wouldn't likely decrease the severity of the illness. Acyclovir may be given if the child develops the disease but not if the child has just been exposed.
CN: Health promotion and maintenance; CNS: None; CL: Analysis

89. Nausea and vomiting are common adverse effects of radiation and chemotherapy. When should a nurse administer antiemetics?
1. 30 minutes before initiation of therapy
2. With the administration of therapy
3. Immediately after nausea begins
4. When therapy is completed

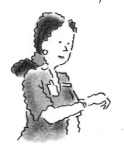

89. 1. Antiemetics are most beneficial if given before the onset of nausea and vomiting. To calculate the optimum time for administration, the first dose is given 30 minutes to 1 hour before nausea is expected, and then every 2, 4, or 6 hours for approximately 24 hours after chemotherapy. If the antiemetic was given with the medication or after the medication, it could lose its maximum effectiveness when needed.
CN: Physiological integrity; CNS: Pharmacological and parenteral therapies; CL: Application

90. A child is admitted to the pediatric unit with an unknown mass in her lower left abdomen. Which action should be the nurse's priority?
1. Obtain the history of the illness.
2. Place a "Do not palpate abdomen" sign over the child's bed.
3. Obtain a complete set of vital signs.
4. Schedule a hemoglobin and hematocrit test for early morning.

91. Which nursing measure is helpful when mouth ulcers develop as an adverse effect of chemotherapy?
1. Using lemon glycerin swabs
2. Administering milk of magnesia
3. Providing a bland, moist, soft diet
4. Frequently washing the mouth with full-strength hydrogen peroxide

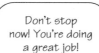

Don't stop now! You're doing a great job!

92. The parents of a child undergoing irradiation are taught about post-irradiation somnolence. Which statement, if made by the parents, indicates that the teaching has been effective?
1. "This neurologic syndrome will occur immediately."
2. "This neurologic syndrome usually occurs within 1 to 2 weeks."
3. "This neurologic syndrome usually occurs within 5 to 8 weeks."
4. "This neurologic syndrome usually occurs within 3 to 6 months."

93. Which intervention can prevent hemorrhagic cystitis caused by bladder irritation from chemotherapeutic medications?
1. Giving antacids
2. Giving antibiotics
3. Restricting fluid intake
4. Increasing fluid intake

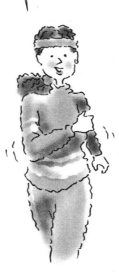

90. 2. The nurse must take measures to prevent palpation of the mass, if possible. If the mass is a malignant tumor, a do-not-palpate warning will help prevent trauma and rupture of the suspected tumor capsule. Rupture of the tumor capsule may cause seeding of cancer cells throughout the abdomen. Obtaining the history and vital signs and scheduling laboratory work are important, but not the priority.
CN: Physiological integrity; CNS: Physiological adaptation; CL: Analysis

91. 3. Oral ulcers are red, eroded, and painful. Providing a bland, moist, soft diet will make chewing and swallowing less painful. The use of lemon glycerin swabs and milk of magnesia should be avoided. Glycerin, a trihydric alcohol, absorbs water and dries the membranes. Milk of magnesia also has a drying effect because unabsorbed magnesium salts exert an osmotic pressure on tissue fluids. Many children also find the taste unpleasant. Frequent mouthwashes without alcohol are indicated. Peroxide shouldn't be used because it's irritating to tissues.
CN: Physiological integrity; CNS: Basic care and comfort; CL: Application

92. 3. Postirradiation somnolence may develop 5 to 8 weeks after CNS irradiation and may last 3 to 15 days. It's characterized by somnolence with or without fever, anorexia, nausea, and vomiting. Although the syndrome isn't thought to be clinically significant, parents should be prepared to expect such symptoms and encouraged to allow the child needed rest.
CN: Physiological integrity; CNS: Physiological adaptation; CL: Application

93. 4. Sterile hemorrhagic cystitis is an adverse effect of chemical irritation of the bladder from cyclophosphamide. It can be prevented by liberal fluid intake (at least 1½ times the recommended daily fluid requirement). Antibiotics don't aid in the prevention of sterile hemorrhagic cystitis. Restricting fluids would only increase the risk of developing cystitis. Antacids wouldn't be indicated for treatment.
CN: Physiological integrity; CNS: Reduction of risk potential; CL: Application

CN: Client needs category   CNS: Client needs subcategory   CL: Cognitive level

94. The parents of a child diagnosed with leukemia have stated that they'll give aspirin to their child for pain relief. Which statement about aspirin by the nurse would be the <u>most</u> accurate?
1. "It's contraindicated because it decreases platelet production."
2. "It's contraindicated because it promotes bleeding tendencies."
3. "It's not a strong enough analgesic."
4. "It decreases the effects of methotrexate (Trexall)."

95. Which nursing measure helps prepare the parent and child for alopecia, a common adverse effect of several chemotherapeutic agents?
1. Introducing the idea of a wig after hair loss occurs
2. Explaining that hair typically begins to regrow in 6 to 9 months
3. Stressing that hair loss during a second treatment with the same medication will be more severe
4. Explaining that, as hair thins, keeping it clean, short, and fluffy may camouflage partial baldness

96. A nurse is discussing childhood cancer with the parents of a child in an oncology unit. Which statement by the nurse would be the <u>most</u> accurate?
1. "The most common site for children's cancer is the bone marrow."
2. "All childhood cancers have a high mortality rate."
3. "Children with leukemia have a higher survival rate if they're older than 11 when diagnosed."
4. "The prognosis for children with cancer isn't affected by treatment strategies."

97. Which condition assessed by the nurse would be an early warning sign of childhood cancer?
1. Difficult in swallowing
2. Nagging cough or hoarseness
3. Slight change in bowel and bladder habits
4. Swellings, lumps, or masses anywhere on the body

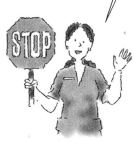

What other conditions is aspirin used for?

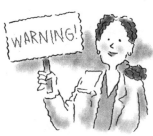

Know the early warning signs of childhood cancer.

94. 2. Aspirin would be contraindicated because it promotes bleeding. Aspirin use has also been associated with Reye's syndrome in children. For home use, acetaminophen (Tylenol) is recommended for mild to moderate pain. Aspirin enhances the effects of methotrexate and has no effect on platelet production. Nonopioid analgesia has been effective for mild to moderate pain in clients with leukemia.
CN: Physiological integrity; CNS: Pharmacological and parenteral therapies; CL: Application

95. 4. The nurse must prepare parents and children for possible hair loss. Cutting the hair short lessens the impact of seeing large quantities of hair on bed linens and clothing. Sometimes, keeping the hair short and fuller can make a wig unnecessary. Hair usually regrows in 6 months, depending on the treatment protocol. A child should be encouraged to pick out a wig similar to his own hair style and color before the hair falls out to foster adjustment to hair loss. Hair loss during a second treatment with the same medication is usually less severe.
CN: Psychosocial integrity; CNS: None; CL: Application

96. 1. Childhood cancers occur most commonly in rapidly growing tissue, especially in the bone marrow. Mortality depends on the time of diagnosis, the type of cancer, and the age at which the child was diagnosed. Children who are diagnosed between the ages of 2 and 9 consistently demonstrate a better prognosis. Treatment strategies are tailored to produce the most favorable prognosis.
CN: Physiological integrity; CNS: Physiological adaptation; CL: Application

97. 4. By being aware of early signs of childhood cancer, nurses can refer children for further evaluation. Swellings, lumps, or masses anywhere on the body are early warning signals of childhood cancer. Difficulty swallowing, cough, and hoarseness are early signs of cancer in adults. Usually there's also a marked change in bowel or bladder habits, not associated with dietary intake.
CN: Health promotion and maintenance; CNS: None; CL: Application

98. Which nursing intervention helps to decrease the adverse effects of radiation therapy on the GI tract?
1. Avoiding the use of antispasmodics
2. Encouraging fluids and a soft diet
3. Giving antiemetics when nausea or vomiting occurs
4. Avoiding mouthwashes to prevent irritation of mouth ulcers

99. Short-term steroid therapy is used in clients with leukemia to promote which reaction?
1. Increased appetite
2. Altered body image
3. Increased platelet production
4. Decreased susceptibility to infection

100. Teaching children with leukemia and their families should include potential adverse effects of treatments. Which of the following is an adverse effect of prednisone?
1. Decreased appetite
2. Increased blood glucose
3. Decreased risk of infection
4. Decreased hair growth

101. Which intervention is a priority for a hemophilic child who has fallen and badly bruised his leg?
1. Appropriate dose of aspirin and rest
2. Immobilization of the leg and a dose of ibuprofen
3. Heating pad and administration of factor VIII concentrate
4. Pressure on the site and administration of the required clotting factor

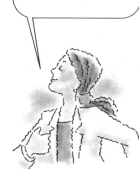

One hundred questions! You must be proud!

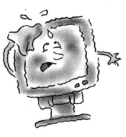

The pressure is really on to prioritize.

98. 2. Radiation therapy can cause adverse effects such as nausea and vomiting, anorexia, mucosal ulceration, and diarrhea. Antispasmodics are used to help reduce diarrhea. Encouraging fluids and a soft diet will help with anorexia. Antiemetics should be given before the onset of nausea. Frequent mouthwashes are indicated to prevent mycosis.
CN: Physiological integrity; CNS: Physiological adaptation; CL: Application

99. 1. Short-term steroid therapy produces no acute toxicities and results in two beneficial reactions: increased appetite and a sense of well-being. Physical changes, such as "moon face," a result of steroid use, can cause alterations in body image and can be extremely distressing to children. Prednisone (steroid therapy) has no effect on platelet production but may increase susceptibility to infection.
CN: Physiological integrity; CNS: Pharmacological and parenteral therapies; CL: Application

100. 2. Prednisone may cause an increase in blood glucose requiring doses of insulin, especially when other factors are involved. Increased appetite, increased risk of infection, and increased hair growth are also adverse effects of prednisone.
CN: Physiological integrity; CNS: Pharmacological and parenteral therapies; CL: Application

101. 4. With any bleeding injury in a client with hemophilia, the first line of treatment is always to replace the clotting factor. Pressure is applied along with cool compresses, and the extremity is immobilized. Aspirin isn't used because of its anticoagulant properties and the risk of Reye's syndrome in children. Immobilizing the leg and giving ibuprofen would be done after applying pressure and administering the necessary clotting factor. Heat isn't used because it increases bleeding.
CN: Safe, effective care environment; CNS: Management of care; CL: Application

CN: Client needs category   CNS: Client needs subcategory   CL: Cognitive level

102. When teaching an adolescent with iron deficiency anemia about diet choices, which menu selection would indicate that more instruction is necessary?

1. Caesar salad and pretzels
2. Cheeseburger with milkshake
3. Red beans and rice with sausage
4. Egg sandwich and snack peanuts

103. A nurse is speaking to the mother of a child with leukemia who wants to know why her child is so susceptible to infection if he has too many white blood cells (WBCs). Which response would be most accurate?

1. This is an adverse effect of the medication he has to take.
2. He hasn't been able to eat a proper diet since he's been sick.
3. Leukemia is a problem of tumors in the internal organs that prevent his ability to fight infection.
4. Leukemia causes production of too many immature WBCs, which can't fight infection very well.

104. A nurse is developing a teaching plan for parents of a toddler who was just diagnosed with sickle cell anemia. Which statement is important to emphasize in the teaching plan?

1. If they have any more children, those children will also have sickle cell anemia.
2. Knowing how to prevent vaso-occlusive crisis is an important part of the parent's role.
3. The child will have a greater tendency to bleed and should avoid contact sports.
4. Vaso-occlusive crisis will occur eventually, requiring medical care.

Good diet choices are important for clients of all ages.

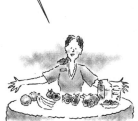

Prevention is the key to not ending up like me.

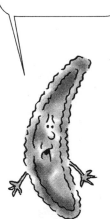

102. 1. Caesar salad and pretzels aren't foods high in iron and protein. Meats (especially organ meats), eggs, and nuts have high protein and iron.
CN: Physiological integrity; CNS: Basic care and comfort; CL: Analysis

103. 4. Leukemia is an unrestricted proliferation of immature WBCs, which don't function properly and are a poor defense against infection. Diet contributes to overall health but doesn't cause the overproduction of WBCs. There are no solid tumors in the internal organs in leukemia. Medications such as chemotherapy can diminish the immune system's effectiveness; however, they don't cause the overproduction of immature WBCs and the poor resistance to infection that the mother asked about.
CN: Physiological integrity; CNS: Physiological adaptation; CL: Application

104. 2. Prevention is the key to teaching a family of a child with sickle cell anemia. The nurse should emphasize the daily use of prescribed oral antibiotics and avoidance of dehydration, high altitudes, and cold. These interventions can dramatically reduce the incidence of crisis. The disease is autosomal recessive, so each pregnancy has a 1 in 4 chance of the child having the disease, a 1 in 4 chance of not having the disease, and a 2 in 4 chance of carrying the trait. Abnormal bleeding and the need to avoid contact sports are associated with hemophilia.
CN: Health promotion and maintenance; CNS: None; CL: Application

105. A grandmother calls the pediatric children's clinic to find out whether her 3-year-old grandson can get shingles from her. Which response would be appropriate?

1. No, shingles don't occur in small children.
2. Yes, the grandson can get shingles from her. Shingles are caused by the herpes zoster virus.
3. The grandson could develop shingles if the lesions are on exposed skin areas and are weeping.
4. No, but the grandson would be exposed to the varicella-zoster virus, which could lead to the development of chickenpox.

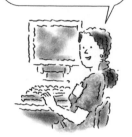

Which response would be appropriate?

105. 4. Shingles occur when a dormant varicella-zoster virus in a nerve becomes inflamed. The vesicles of shingles contain the virus and would expose others to it. The grandson couldn't develop shingles from such exposure. A herpes virus doesn't cause shingles. Shingles can occur in children, but only if they have previously had chickenpox. The impetus for the inflammation is internal, not external.

CN: Safe, effective care environment; CNS: Safety and infection control; CL: Analysis

106. A child with idiopathic thrombocytopenic purpura is admitted to the hospital with a platelet count of 20,000/mm³. He should be closely monitored for which condition?

1. Hyperactivity
2. Proteinuria
3. Hand-foot syndrome
4. Change in level of consciousness (LOC)

106. 4. When the platelet count drops to 20,000/mm³, the child is at risk for spontaneous bleeding, including intracranially. A change in LOC is an important sign of increased intracranial pressure. This child is likely to become somnolent and difficult to arouse—not hyperactive. Proteinuria is more common in glomerulonephritis. With blood in the urine, protein also increases—but this isn't the primary concern. Hand-foot syndrome occurs in a child with sickle cell disease.

CN: Physiological integrity; CNS: Reduction of risk potential; CL: Application

107. Infants must be monitored closely because they can't report changes in their condition. In a 1-month-old infant, which are the signs of increased intracranial pressure (ICP)?

1. Bulging fontanels, a high-pitched cry, vomiting
2. Frequent crying, sunken fontanel, pulse rate above 120 beats/minute
3. Blood-tinged vomitus, legs flexed to the abdomen, frequent crying
4. Falling asleep during feeding, pulse rate above 120 beats/minute when fussing, irregular arm and leg movements

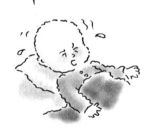

I can't tell you what's wrong, so look for the signs.

107. 1. Because fontanels haven't closed by the age of 1 month, they bulge with increasing ICP. A high-pitched cry and vomiting also signal increased ICP. Quality of the cry is an important sign in an infant. Vomiting should be distinguished from a small amount of formula regurgitation, which is normal. Frequent crying may result from various stressors, and quality of the cry should be assessed. Blood-tinged vomitus, flexed legs, and crying indicate an abdominal disorder and pain. Infants normally have irregular arm and leg movements. A pulse rate of 120 beats/minute is normal for a 1-month-old infant at rest; in fact, the pulse may increase to 200 beats/minute during stress.

CN: Physiological integrity; CNS: Reduction of risk potential; CL: Analysis

CN: Client needs category   CNS: Client needs subcategory   CL: Cognitive level

108. Discharge teaching for the family of a school-age child with idiopathic thrombocytopenia should include restriction of which activity?
1. Swimming
2. Bicycle riding
3. Computer games
4. Exposure to large crowds

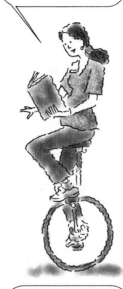

Let's see. Which activity should be restricted?

109. A 17-year-old boy with classic hemophilia (hemophilia A) is admitted to the hospital for surgery. His preoperative preparation should include which treatment?
1. Bed rest
2. Transfusion of clotting factor 8
3. I.V. analgesics given around the clock
4. Hydration at 50% above the normal fluid requirement

110. A child with hemophilia is hospitalized with bleeding into the knee. Which action should the nurse take <u>first</u>?
1. Prepare to administer a whole blood transfusion.
2. Prepare to administer a plasma transfusion
3. Perform active range-of-motion (ROM) exercise on the affected part.
4. Elevate the affected part.

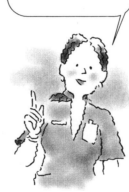

Hint! It's the first action the nurse should take.

111. Which measure is indicated for a child in sickle cell vaso-occlusive crisis?
1. Immobilizing the affected part
2. Applying warm packs to the affected part
3. Applying cool packs to the affected part
4. Performing active range-of-motion (ROM) exercises to the affected part

108. 2. When routine blood counts reveal the platelet level is 100,000/mm^3 or less, the child shouldn't engage in contact sports, bicycle or scooter riding, climbing, or other activities that could lead to injury (especially to the head). Swimming releases energy, builds muscle, and allows the child to compete without risking injury, as long as she follows normal safety precautions. Computer games don't cause physical injury. This child need not avoid large crowds because idiopathic thrombocytopenia doesn't suppress the immune system.
CN: Safe, effective care environment; CNS: Safety and infection control; CL: Application

109. 2. In classic hemophilia or hemophilia A, clotting factor 8 is deficient. This factor must be transfused before surgery and at intervals afterward to prevent bleeding during and after surgery. Analgesics would be indicated if the child experienced bleeding, especially into the joints. Hydration above the normal requirement isn't needed. Because the child wasn't admitted for bleeding, bed rest isn't necessary.
CN: Physiological integrity; CNS: Reduction of risk potential; CL: Application

110. 4. Bleeding into the joints is the most common type of bleeding episode in the more severe hemophilia forms. Elevating the affected part and applying pressure and cold are indicated. The nurse should anticipate transfusing the missing clotting factor — not whole blood or plasma, which won't stop the bleeding promptly and may pose a risk of fluid overload. Active ROM exercises are contraindicated because they may cause more bleeding, injury, and pain.
CN: Physiological integrity; CNS: Reduction of risk potential; CL: Application

111. 2. Applying warm packs promotes vasodilation and perfusion and provides pain relief and comfort. Immobilization leads to stasis, which promotes sickling. Cool packs are contraindicated because they cause vasoconstriction and may precipitate red blood cell sickling. A child in vaso-occlusive crisis experiences acute pain and limits movement of the affected part. After the acute crisis passes, the child should be encouraged to ambulate. Active ROM exercises increase pain in the affected part.
CN: Physiological integrity; CNS: Basic care and comfort; CL: Application

112. A 4-year-old child has recently been diagnosed with acute lymphocytic leukemia (ALL). What information about ALL should the nurse provide when educating the client's parents? Select all that apply:

1. Leukemia is a rare form of childhood cancer.
2. ALL affects all blood-forming organs and systems throughout the body.
3. The child shouldn't brush his teeth because of the increased risk of bleeding.
4. Adverse effects of treatment include sleepiness, alopecia, and stomatitis.
5. There's a 95% chance of remission with treatment.
6. The child shouldn't be disciplined during this difficult time.

113. A child with sickle cell anemia is being treated for a crisis. The physician orders morphine sulfate (Duramorph) 2 mg I.V. The concentration of the vial is 10 mg/1 ml of solution. How many milliliters of solution should the nurse administer? Record your answer using one decimal point.

_____ milliliters

114. A child with sickle cell anemia is being discharged after treatment for a crisis. Which instructions for avoiding future crises should the nurse provide to the client and his family? Select all that apply:

1. Avoid foods high in folic acid.
2. Drink plenty of fluids.
3. Use cold packs to relieve joint pain.
4. Report a sore throat to an adult immediately.
5. Restrict activity to quiet board games.
6. Wash hands before meals and after playing.

112. 2, 4, 5. In ALL, abnormal white blood cells proliferate, but they don't mature past the blast stage. These blast cells crowd out the healthy white blood cells, red blood cells, and platelets in the bone marrow, leading to bone marrow depression. The blast cells also infiltrate the liver, spleen, kidneys, and lymph tissue. Common adverse effects of chemotherapy and radiation include nausea, vomiting, diarrhea, sleepiness, alopecia, anemia, stomatitis, mucositis, pain, reddened skin, and increased susceptibility to infection. There's a 95% chance of obtaining remission with treatment. Leukemia is the most common form of childhood cancer. The child still needs appropriate discipline and limits. A lack of consistent parenting may lead to negative behaviors and fear.
CN: Physiological integrity; CNS: Reduction of risk potential; CL: Application

113. 0.2. The nurse should calculate the volume to be given using this equation: $2 \text{ mg}/X$ $\text{ml} = 10 \text{ mg}/1 \text{ ml}; 10X = 2; X = 0.2 \text{ ml}$.
CN: Physiological integrity; CNS: Pharmacological and parenteral therapies; CL: Application

114. 2, 4, 6. Fluids should be encouraged to prevent stasis in the bloodstream, which can lead to sickling. Sore throats, and any other cold symptoms, should be reported because they may indicate the presence of an infection, which can precipitate a crisis (red blood cells sickle and obstruct blood flow to tissues). Children with sickle cell anemia should learn appropriate measures to prevent infection, such as proper hand-washing techniques and good nutrition practices. Folic acid intake should be encouraged to help support new cell growth because new cells replace fragile, sickled cells. Warm packs should be applied to provide comfort and relieve pain; cold packs cause vasoconstriction. The child should maintain an active, normal life. When the child experiences a pain crisis, he limits his own activity according to his pain level.
CN: Physiological integrity; CNS: Reduction of risk potential; CL: Application

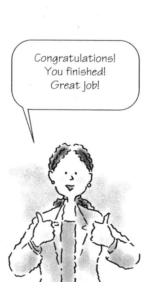

Congratulations! You finished! Great job!

CN: Client needs category   CNS: Client needs subcategory   CL: Cognitive level

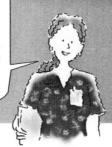

Chapter 17
Neurosensory system

1. A mother of a 3-year-old with a myelomeningocele is thinking about having another baby. A nurse should inform the woman that she should increase her intake of which acid?
1. Folic acid to 0.4 mg/day
2. Folic acid to 4 mg/day
3. Ascorbic acid to 0.4 mg/day
4. Ascorbic acid to 4 mg/day

1. 2. The American Academy of Pediatrics recommends that a woman who has had a child with a neural tube defect increase her intake of folic acid to 4 mg per day one month before becoming pregnant and continue this regimen through the first trimester. A woman who has no family history of neural tube defects should take 0.4 mg. All women of childbearing age should be encouraged to take a folic acid supplement because the majority of pregnancies in the United States are unplanned. Ascorbic acid hasn't been shown to have any effect on preventing neural tube defects.
CN: Health promotion and maintenance; CNS: None; CL: Application

2. Which nursing diagnosis is <u>most relevant</u> in the first 12 hours of life for a neonate born with a myelomeningocele?
1. *Risk for infection*
2. *Constipation*
3. *Impaired physical mobility*
4. *Delayed growth and development*

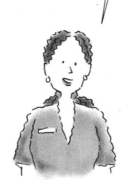

Most relevant—that's the key phrase for question 2.

2. 1. All of these diagnoses are important for a child with a myelomeningocele. However, during the first 12 hours of life, the most life-threatening event would be an infection. The other diagnoses will be addressed as the child develops.
CN: Physiological integrity; CNS: Reduction of risk potential; CL: Application

3. A neonate has been brought to the emergency room by its mother. The nurse suspects that the child may have hydrocephalus. Which observations would indicate this condition?
1. Bulging fontanel, low-pitched cry
2. Depressed fontanel, low-pitched cry
3. Bulging fontanel, eyes rotated downward
4. Depressed fontanel, eyes rotated downward

3. 3. Hydrocephalus is caused from the alteration in circulation of the cerebrospinal fluid (CSF). The amount of CSF increases, causing the fontanel to bulge. This also causes an increase in intracranial pressure. This increase in pressure causes the neonate's eyes to deviate downward (the "setting sun sign"), and the neonate's cry becomes high-pitched.
CN: Health promotion and maintenance; CNS: None; CL: Analysis

CN: Client needs category   CNS: Client needs subcategory   CL: Cognitive level

4. Which nursing action should be included in the care plan for a child following shunt insertion on the right side of the head to relieve hydrocephalus?

1. Place the child flat in bed on the right side.
2. Place the child flat in bed on the left side.
3. Place the child in a semi-Fowler's position.
4. Place the child in an upright position.

5. Which nursing action is <u>appropriate</u> when a child has a seizure?

1. Inserting a nasogastric tube to prevent emesis
2. Restraining the extremities with a pillow or blanket
3. Inserting a tongue blade to prevent injury to the tongue
4. Padding the side rails of the bed to protect the child from injury

6. A mother brings her infant to the emergency department and says he had a seizure. While a nurse is obtaining a history, the mother says she was running out of formula so she stretched the formula by adding three times the normal amount of water. Electrolytes and blood glucose levels are drawn on the infant. The nurse should expect which laboratory value?

1. Blood glucose: 120 mg/dl
2. Chloride: 104 mmol/L
3. Potassium: 4 mmol/L
4. Sodium: 125 mmol/L

7. For which symptom should a nurse assess a neonate diagnosed with bacterial meningitis?

1. Hypothermia, irritability, and poor feeding
2. Positive Babinski's reflex, mottling, and pallor
3. Headache, nuchal rigidity, and developmental delays
4. Positive Moro's embrace reflex, hyperthermia, and sunken fontanel

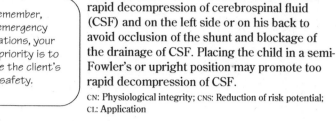

Remember, in emergency situations, your first priority is to ensure the client's safety.

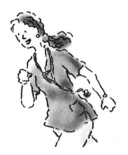

For the NCLEX, you need to be familiar with normal lab values.

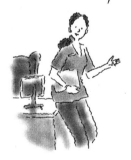

4. 2. The child should be flat in bed to avoid rapid decompression of cerebrospinal fluid (CSF) and on the left side or on his back to avoid occlusion of the shunt and blockage of the drainage of CSF. Placing the child in a semi-Fowler's or upright position may promote too rapid decompression of CSF.
CN: Physiological integrity; CNS: Reduction of risk potential; CL: Application

5. 4. A child having a seizure could fall out of bed or injure himself on anything, including the side rails of the bed. Attempts to insert anything into the child's mouth may injure the child. Attempting to restrain the child won't stop seizures. In fact, tactile stimulation may increase the seizure activity; therefore, it must be limited as much as possible.
CN: Safe, effective care environment; CNS: Safety and infection control; CL: Application

6. 4. Diluting formula in a different manner than is recommended alters the infant's electrolyte levels. Normal serum sodium for an infant is 135 to 145 mmol/L. When formula is diluted, the infant's sodium is also diluted and will decrease. Hyponatremia is one of the causes of seizures in infants. The other values are all within normal limits.
CN: Physiological integrity; CNS: Reduction of risk potential; CL: Analysis

7. 1. The clinical appearance of a neonate with meningitis is different from that of a child or an adult. Neonates may be either hypothermic or hyperthermic. The irritation to the meninges causes the neonates to be irritable and to have a decreased appetite. They may be pale and mottled with a bulging, full fontanel. Older children and adults with meningitis have headaches, nuchal rigidity, and hyperthermia as clinical manifestations. Normal neonates have positive Moro's embrace and Babinski's reflexes. Developmental delays, if present, would appear when the child was older.
CN: Physiological integrity; CNS: Physiological adaptation; CL: Application

CN: Client needs category   CNS: Client needs subcategory   CL: Cognitive level

8. Which type of behavior demonstrated by a 6-year-old should help a school nurse differentiate between attention deficit hyperactivity disorder (ADHD) and learning disability?
1. The child reverses letters and words while reading.
2. The child is easily distracted and reacts impulsively.
3. The child is always getting into fights during recess.
4. The child has a difficult time reading a chapter book.

9. Which statement by the parent of a child with cerebral palsy indicates that a nurse's teaching has been successful?
1. "My child's muscles will get stronger over time."
2. "My child's condition will get progressively worse."
3. "My child will have low intelligence."
4. "My child will need continual therapy to maintain functioning."

10. While assessing a full-term neonate, which symptom should cause the nurse to suspect a neurologic impairment?
1. A weak sucking reflex
2. A positive rooting reflex
3. A positive Babinski's reflex
4. Startle reflex in response to a loud noise

11. A mother reports that her school-age child has been reprimanded for daydreaming during class. This is a new behavior, and the child's grades are dropping. The nurse should suspect which problem?
1. The child may have a hearing problem and needs to have his hearing checked.
2. The child may have a learning disability and needs referral to the special education department.
3. The child may have attention deficit hyperactivity disorder (ADHD) and needs medication.
4. The child may be having absence seizures and needs to see his primary health care provider for evaluation.

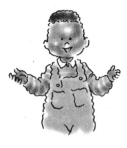

I'm trying to pay attention. Really I am.

You're through the first 10! Keep going!

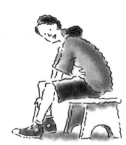

8. 2. Two of the most common characteristics of children with ADHD include inattention and impulsiveness. Children who reverse letters and words while reading have dyslexia. Although aggressiveness may be common in children with ADHD, it isn't a characteristic that will help diagnose this disorder. Six-year-old children aren't usually cognitively ready to read a chapter book.
CN: Health promotion and maintenance; CNS: None; CL: Analysis

9. 4. The child with cerebral palsy needs continual treatment and therapy to maintain or improve functioning. Without therapy, muscles will get progressively weaker and more spastic. Although some children with cerebral palsy are mentally retarded, many have normal intelligence.
CN: Health promotion and maintenance; CNS: None; CL: Analysis

10. 1. Normal neonates have a strong, vigorous sucking reflex. The rooting reflex is present at birth and disappears when the infant is between ages 3 and 4 months. A positive Babinski's reflex is present at birth and disappears by the time the infant is age 2 years. The startle reflex is present at birth and disappears when the infant is about age 4 months.
CN: Health promotion and maintenance; CNS: None; CL: Application

11. 4. Absence seizures are commonly misinterpreted as daydreaming. The child loses awareness but no alteration in motor activity is exhibited. A mild hearing problem is usually exhibited as leaning forward, talking louder, listening to louder TV and music than usual, and a repetitive "what?" from the child. There isn't enough information to indicate a learning disability. ADHD isn't characterized by episodes of quietness.
CN: Physiological integrity; CNS: Physiological adaptation; CL: Analysis

12. A 2-month-old infant is brought to the well-baby clinic for his first check-up. On initial assessment, the nurse notes the infant's head circumference is at the 95th percentile. Which action should the nurse take <u>initially</u>?
   1. Assess vital signs.
   2. Measure the head again.
   3. Assess neurologic signs.
   4. Notify the primary health care provider.

13. Which observation indicates to a nurse that the mother of a child with cerebral palsy needs further instruction?
   1. The mother gives the child assistive devices for eating.
   2. The mother fusses over the mess the child is making.
   3. The mother provides adequate time for the child to finish eating.
   4. The mother provides finger foods.

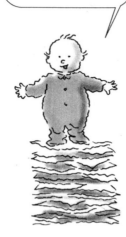

Now I should be in the 1000th percentile.

14. A 2-year-old child is admitted to the pediatric unit with the diagnosis of bacterial meningitis. Which measure would be appropriate for a nurse to perform first?
   1. Obtain a urine specimen.
   2. Draw ordered laboratory tests.
   3. Place the toddler in respiratory isolation.
   4. Explain the treatment plan to the parents.

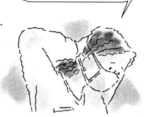

Take the necessary precautions to protect yourself and others from possible infection.

15. Which sign or symptom should a nurse expect to be present in a 12-year-old child admitted to the pediatric unit with a diagnosis of possible brain tumor?
   1. Bulging fontanel
   2. High-pitched cry
   3. Behavioral changes
   4. Change in vital signs

12. 2. Whenever there's a question about vital signs or assessment data, the first logical step would be to reassess to determine if an error had been made initially. Notifying the primary health care provider and assessing neurologic and vital signs are important and would follow the reassessment.
CN: Health promotion and maintenance; CNS: None; CL: Analysis

13. 2. Parents should encourage the child with cerebral palsy to be as independent as possible even if a mess is made while attempting to eat. Assistive devices can help the child with weak or spastic muscles eat independently. The child with cerebral palsy requires more time to bring food to the mouth and to chew and shouldn't be rushed. The parents should provide a calm and stress-free environment for eating. Providing the child with finger foods helps him eat independently.
CN: Physiological integrity; CNS: Basic care and comfort; CL: Analysis

14. 3. Nurses should take necessary precautions to protect themselves and others from possible infection from the bacterial organism causing meningitis. The affected child should immediately be placed in respiratory isolation; then the parents can be informed about the treatment plan. This should be done before laboratory tests are performed.
CN: Safe, effective care environment; CNS: Safety and infection control; CL: Application

15. 3. In a school-age child with a closed cranium, a common symptom of a brain tumor is behavior change due to the increased cranial pressure. A bulging fontanel and high-pitched cry are typical signs in an infant. A change in vital signs is a later sign of increased intracranial pressure.
CN: Physiological integrity; CNS: Physiological adaptation; CL: Application

CN: Client needs category   CNS: Client needs subcategory   CL: Cognitive level

16. A preschool-age child has just been admitted to the pediatric unit with a diagnosis of bacterial meningitis. A nurse should include which recommendation in the nursing plan?

1. Take vital signs every 4 hours.
2. Monitor temperature every 4 hours.
3. Decrease environmental stimulation.
4. Encourage the parents to hold the child.

17. A child has just returned to the pediatric unit following ventriculoperitoneal shunt placement for hydrocephalus. Which intervention should a nurse perform first?

1. Assess intake and output.
2. Place the child on the side opposite the shunt.
3. Offer fluids because the child has a dry mouth.
4. Administer pain medication by mouth as ordered.

18. An otherwise healthy 18-month-old child has a history of febrile seizures and is in the well-child clinic today. Which statement by the father would indicate to the nurse that additional teaching needs to be done?

1. "I have ibuprofen available in case it's needed."
2. "My child will outgrow these seizures by age 5."
3. "I always keep phenobarbital with me in case of a fever."
4. "The most likely time for a seizure is when the fever is rising."

19. When assessing a 5-month-old infant, which symptom should alert a nurse that the infant needs further follow-up?

1. Absent grasp reflex
2. Rolls from back to side
3. Balances head when sitting
4. Moro's embrace reflex present

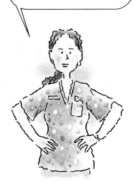

The important word in the question is first!

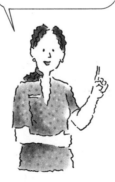

Note that for question 18, you're looking for an incorrect response from the father.

16. 3. A child with the diagnosis of meningitis is much more comfortable with decreased environmental stimuli. Noise and bright lights stimulate the child and can be irritating, causing the child to cry, in turn increasing intracranial pressure. Vital signs would be taken initially every hour and temperature monitored every two hours. Children are usually much more comfortable if allowed to lie flat because this position doesn't cause increased meningeal irritation.
CN: Physiological integrity; CNS: Physiological adaptation; CL: Application

17. 2. Following shunt placement surgery, the child should be placed on the side opposite of the surgical site to prevent pressure on the shunt valve. Intake and output will be assessed, but that isn't the priority nursing intervention. The child is usually on nothing-by-mouth status until the nasogastric tube is removed and bowel sounds return. Pain medication should be administered by an I.V. route initially postoperatively.
CN: Physiological integrity; CNS: Basic care and comfort; CL: Application

18. 3. Anticonvulsant drugs, such as phenobarbital, are administered to children with prolonged seizures or neurologic abnormalities. Ibuprofen, not phenobarbital, is given for fever. Febrile seizures usually occur after age 6 months and are unusual after age 5 years. Treatment is to decrease the temperature because seizures occur as the temperature rises.
CN: Health promotion and maintenance; CNS: None; CL: Application

19. 4. Moro's embrace reflex should be absent at 4 months. Grasp reflex begins to fade at 2 months and should be absent at 3 months. A 4-month-old infant should be able to roll from back to side and balance his head when sitting.
CN: Health promotion and maintenance; CNS: None; CL: Application

20. An adolescent is started on valproic acid (Depakene) to treat seizures. Which statement should be included when educating the adolescent?
1. This medication has no adverse effects.
2. A common adverse effect is weight gain.
3. Drowsiness and irritability commonly occur.
4. Early morning dosing is recommended to decrease insomnia.

21. Which statement about cerebral palsy is accurate?
1. Cerebral palsy is a condition that runs in families.
2. Cerebral palsy means there will be many disabilities.
3. Cerebral palsy is a condition that doesn't get worse.
4. Cerebral palsy occurs because of too much oxygen to the brain.

22. An older child has a craniotomy for removal of a brain tumor. Which statement would be appropriate for a nurse to say to the parents?
1. "Your child really had a close call."
2. "I'm sure your child will be back to normal soon."
3. "I'm so glad to hear your child doesn't have cancer."
4. "What has the physician told you about the tumor?"

23. A 6-month-old infant is being admitted with a diagnosis of bacterial meningitis. A nurse should place the infant in which room?
1. A room with a 12-month-old infant with urinary tract infection
2. A room with an 8-month-old infant with failure to thrive
3. An isolation room near the nurses' station
4. A two-bed room in the middle of the hall

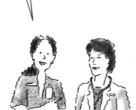

For question 22, keep in mind the difference between the nurse's and physician's roles.

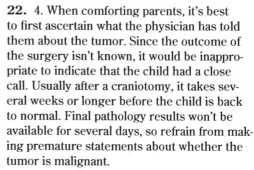

20. 2. Weight gain is a common adverse effect of valproic acid. Drowsiness and irritability are adverse effects more commonly associated with phenobarbital. Felbamate (Felbatol) more commonly causes insomnia.

CN: Physiological integrity; CNS: Pharmacological and parenteral therapies; CL: Application

21. 3. By definition, cerebral palsy is a nonprogressive neuromuscular disorder. It can be mild or quite severe and is believed to be the result of a hypoxia event during the pregnancy or the birth process.

CN: Physiological integrity; CNS: Physiological adaptation; CL: Application

22. 4. When comforting parents, it's best to first ascertain what the physician has told them about the tumor. Since the outcome of the surgery isn't known, it would be inappropriate to indicate that the child had a close call. Usually after a craniotomy, it takes several weeks or longer before the child is back to normal. Final pathology results won't be available for several days, so refrain from making premature statements about whether the tumor is malignant.

CN: Psychosocial integrity; CNS: None; CL: Application

23. 3. A child who has the diagnosis of bacterial meningitis will need to be placed in isolation near the nurses' station until that child has received I.V. antibiotics for 24 hours. The child is considered contagious. Additionally, bacterial meningitis can be quite serious; therefore, the child should be placed near the nurse's station for close monitoring and easier access in case of a crisis.

CN: Safe, effective care environment; CNS: Safety and infection control; CL: Application

CN: Client needs category   CNS: Client needs subcategory   CL: Cognitive level

24. In caring for a 9-year-old child immediately after a head injury, a nurse notes a blood pressure of 110/60, a heart rate of 78, dilated and nonreactive pupils, minimal response to pain, and slow response to name. Which symptom should cause the nurse the most concern?

1. Vital signs
2. Nonreactive pupils
3. Slow response to name
4. Minimal response to pain

25. Which assignment made by a charge nurse would be <u>appropriate</u>?

1. A registered nurse (RN) to an infant newly diagnosed with bacterial meningitis
2. A student nurse to an adolescent with cystic fibrosis and many medications
3. A licensed practical nurse (LPN) or a licensed vocational nurse (LVN) to a newly admitted child with acute leukemia, receiving blood
4. A nursing assistant to a transfer client with a head injury and frequent seizures

26. An infant has returned to the pediatric unit after repair of a myelomeningocele. A nurse notices that the infant has had no urine output in the past 2 hours. Which nursing intervention would be most appropriate?

1. Perform Credé's maneuver on the infant's bladder.
2. Catheterize the infant's bladder.
3. Ask the mother to breast-feed the infant.
4. Increase the I.V. fluid rate.

27. A 2-month-old infant who had an L4-L5 myelomeningocele repair comes to the clinic for a well-baby checkup. The mother reports that she catheterizes the infant every 2 to 3 hours. Which aspect of care should a nurse discuss with the mother?

1. Changing to a special diet
2. Scheduled immunizations
3. Normal gross motor function
4. Possibility of developing a latex allergy

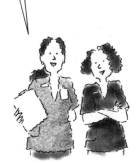

The ability to delegate responsibly is often tested on the NCLEX.

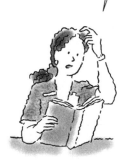

Is this mother doing the correct thing or not?

24. 2. Dilated and nonreactive pupils indicate that anoxia or ischemia of the brain has occurred. If the pupils are also fixed (don't move), then herniation of the brain stem has occurred. The vital signs are normal. Slow response to name can be normal after a head injury. Minimal response to pain is an indication of the child's level of consciousness.
CN: Physiological integrity; CNS: Physiological adaptation; CL: Application

25. 1. An RN would be appropriately assigned to care for an infant with meningitis. The RN would make frequent assessments and provide a high level of care. Student nurses may not be allowed to give medications without supervision and it may be easier for the RN or LPN to provide care to this client. In many institutions, LPNs (or LVNs) aren't allowed to monitor clients receiving blood or blood products. A transfer client with a head injury would need frequent assessments that only an RN or an LPN would be able to provide.
CN: Safe, effective care environment; CNS: Management of care; CL: Application

26. 2. Swelling around the surgical site may cause transient urinary retention and catheterization is required to empty the bladder. Credé's maneuver isn't recommended because it can cause renal rupture. Breast-feeding the infant would be inappropriate in this situation. The fluid rate wouldn't be increased because there's no indication that the infant is dehydrated.
CN: Physiological integrity; CNS: Reduction of risk potential; CL: Application

27. 4. Children who are exposed repeatedly to latex products, such as during bladder catheterizations, are at high risk for developing a latex allergy. There's no need for a special diet unless another problem indicates that it would be necessary. This infant would receive the regularly scheduled immunizations. Gross motor function will be abnormal in an infant with an L4-L5 repair.
CN: Health promotion and maintenance; CNS: None; CL: Application

28. Which intervention prevents a 17-month-old child with spastic cerebral palsy from going into a scissoring position?
1. Keep the child in leg braces 23 hours per day.
2. Let the child lay down as much as possible.
3. Try to keep the child as quiet as possible.
4. Place the child on your hip.

28. 4. To interrupt the scissoring position, flex the knees and hips. Placing the child on the hip is an easy way to stop this common spastic positioning. Wearing leg braces 23 hours per day is inappropriate and doesn't allow the child to move freely. Trying to keep the child quiet and flat are inappropriate. This child needs stimulation and movement to reach the goal of development to the fullest potential.
CN: Physiological integrity; CNS: Basic care and comfort; CL: Application

29. The mother of a child with a ventriculo-peritoneal shunt says her child has a temperature of 101.2° F (38.4° C), a blood pressure of 108/68 mm Hg, and a pulse of 100. The child is lethargic and vomited the night before. Other children in the family have had similar symptoms. Which nursing intervention is most appropriate?
1. Provide symptomatic treatment.
2. Advise the mother this is a viral infection.
3. Consult the primary health care provider.
4. Have the mother bring the child to the primary health care provider's office.

29. 4. One of the complications of a ventriculoperitoneal shunt is a shunt infection. Shunt infections can have similar symptoms as a viral infection, so it's best to have the child examined. These symptoms may be due to the same viral infection that the siblings have, but it's better to have the child examined to rule out a shunt infection because infection can progress quickly to a very serious illness.
CN: Physiological integrity; CNS: Reduction of risk potential; CL: Application

Make sure both parents understand the rationale for treatment of a sick child.

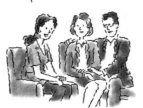

30. The mother of a 10-year-old child with attention deficit hyperactivity disorder says her husband won't allow their child to take more than 5 mg of methylphenidate (Ritalin) every morning. The child isn't doing better in school. Which recommendation should a nurse make to the mother?
1. Sneak the medication to the child anyway.
2. Put the child in charge of administering the medication.
3. Bring the child's father to the clinic to discuss the medication.
4. Have the school nurse give the child the rest of the medication.

30. 3. Bringing the father to the clinic for a teaching session about the medication should assist him in understanding why it's necessary for the child to receive the full dose. A nurse shouldn't advise dishonesty to a client or family. The father should be included in the treatment as much as possible.
CN: Physiological integrity; CNS: Pharmacological and parenteral therapies; CL: Application

31. A hospitalized child is to receive 75 mg of acetaminophen (Tylenol) for fever control. How much will the nurse administer if the acetaminophen is 40 mg per 0.4 ml?
1. 0.37 ml
2. 0.75 ml
3. 1.12 ml
4. 1.5 ml

31. 2. The nurse will administer 0.75 ml. Because 10 mg equals 0.1 ml, then 75 mg equals 0.75 ml.
CN: Physiological integrity; CNS: Pharmacological and parenteral therapies; CL: Application

CN: Client needs category   CNS: Client needs subcategory   CL: Cognitive level

32. The nurse is preparing a toddler for a lumbar puncture. For this procedure, the nurse should place the child in which position?

1. Lying prone, with the neck flexed
2. Sitting up, with the back straight
3. Lying on one side, with the back curved
4. Lying prone, with the feet higher than the head

32. 3. Lumbar puncture involves placing a needle between the lumbar vertebrae into the subarachnoid space. For this procedure, the nurse should position the client on one side, with the back curved, because curving the back maximizes the space between the lumbar vertebrae, facilitating needle insertion. Prone and seated positions don't achieve separation of the vertebrae.

CN: Physiological integrity; CNS: Reduction of risk potential; CL: Application

33. When caring for a school-age child who has had a brain tumor removed, a nurse makes the following assessment: pupils equal and reactive to light; motor strength equal; knows name, date, but not location; and complains of a headache. Which nursing intervention would be most appropriate?

1. Provide medication for the headache.
2. Immediately notify the primary health care provider.
3. Check what the child's level of consciousness (LOC) has been.
4. Call the child's parents to come and sit at the child's bedside.

33. 3. When there's an abnormality in current assessment data, it's vital to determine what the client's previous status was. Determine whether the status has changed or remained the same. Providing medication for the headache would be done after ascertaining the previous LOC. Contacting the primary health care provider and the child's parents isn't necessary before a final assessment has been made.

CN: Physiological integrity; CNS: Physiological adaptation; CL: Application

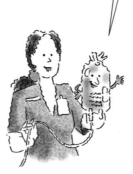

I'm happy to accommodate any drip rate that is needed.

34. Following a craniotomy on a child, I.V. fluids are ordered to run at 27 ml/hour. The tubing delivers 60 ml/hour. How many drops per minute should the nurse set the pump for?

1. 14 drops/minute
2. 27 drops/minute
3. 54 drops/minute
4. 60 drops/minute

34. 2. The pump should be set for 27 drops/minute. Tubing that delivers 60 ml per 60 minutes would deliver 1 ml/minute. To deliver 27 ml/hour, the nurse would set the pump at 27.

CN: Physiological integrity; CNS: Pharmacological and parenteral therapies; CL: Application

35. The parents of a 19-month-old child bring their toddler to the clinic for a regular checkup. When palpating the toddler's fontanels, what should the nurse expect to find?

1. Closed anterior fontanel and open posterior fontanel
2. Open anterior fontanel and closed posterior fontanel
3. Closed anterior and posterior fontanels
4. Open anterior and posterior fontanels

35. 3. By age 18 months, the anterior and posterior fontanels should be closed. The diamond-shaped anterior fontanel normally closes between ages 9 and 18 months. The triangular posterior fontanel normally closes between ages 2 and 3 months.

CN: Health promotion and maintenance; CNS: None; CL: Application

36. A 10-year-old child with a concussion is admitted to the pediatric unit. A nurse should place this child in a room with which roommate?
1. A 6-year-old child with osteomyelitis
2. An 8-year-old child with gastroenteritis
3. A 10-year-old child with rheumatic fever
4. A 12-year-old child with a fractured femur

37. A nurse notes that a 4-year-old child with cerebral palsy has a weight at the 30th percentile and a height at the 60th percentile. Which requirement should a nurse advise the family about the child?
1. He should eat fewer calories per day.
2. His height and weight are within the normal range.
3. He needs to increase his number of calories per day.
4. He is small for a 4-year-old child and will never be average.

38. After a pathogen compromises the blood-brain and blood-cerebrospinal fluid (CSF) barriers, infection will spread to the meninges for which reason?
1. The spinal fluid has a rich erythrocyte content.
2. Glucose content of the spinal fluid is relatively high.
3. There's a build-up of infectious exudate within the ventricular system.
4. CSF is devoid of the body's major defense systems.

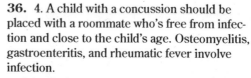

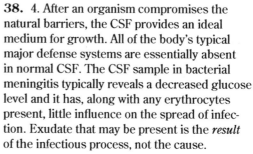
You've completed almost 40 questions. Looking good!

39. Which mechanism causes the severe headache that accompanies an increase in intracranial pressure (ICP)?
1. Cervical hyperextension
2. Stretching of the meninges
3. Cerebral ischemia related to altered circulation
4. Reflex spasm of the neck extensors to splint the neck against cervical flexion

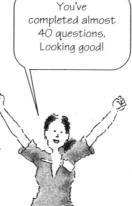

36. 4. A child with a concussion should be placed with a roommate who's free from infection and close to the child's age. Osteomyelitis, gastroenteritis, and rheumatic fever involve infection.
CN: Safe, effective care environment; CNS: Management of care; CL: Application

37. 2. The height and weight are between the 25th and 75th percentile, so the child is considered normal.
CN: Health promotion and maintenance; CNS: None; CL: Application

38. 4. After an organism compromises the natural barriers, the CSF provides an ideal medium for growth. All of the body's typical major defense systems are essentially absent in normal CSF. The CSF sample in bacterial meningitis typically reveals a decreased glucose level and it has, along with any erythrocytes present, little influence on the spread of infection. Exudate that may be present is the *result* of the infectious process, not the cause.
CN: Physiological integrity; CNS: Physiological adaptation; CL: Analysis

39. 2. The mechanism producing the headache that accompanies increased ICP may be the stretching of the meninges and pain fibers associated with blood vessels. With nuchal rigidity, cervical flexion is painful due to the stretching of the inflamed meninges, and the pain triggers a reflex spasm of the neck extensors to splint the area against further cervical flexion. It occurs in response to the pain; it doesn't cause it. Cerebral ischemia occurs because of vascular obstruction and decreased perfusion of the brain tissue.
CN: Physiological integrity; CNS: Physiological adaptation; CL: Analysis

CN: Client needs category   CNS: Client needs subcategory   CL: Cognitive level

40. While assessing the breath sounds of a child admitted with fever, seizures, and vomiting, the nurse notes petechiae on the child's back. What is the most appropriate initial action by the nurse?
  1. Cover the petechiae with dry sterile dressings.
  2. Initiate seizure precautions.
  3. Suspect that the child has been abused.
  4. Assess the child's neurologic status.

41. A nurse is assessing a 3-year-old child with suspected nuchal rigidity. Which assessment data indicates nuchal rigidity?
  1. Positive Kernig's sign
  2. Negative Brudzinski's sign
  3. Positive Homans' sign
  4. Negative Kernig's sign

42. A nurse is caring for a child with spina bifida. The child's mother asks the nurse what she did to cause the birth defect. Which statement would be the nurse's <u>best</u> response?
  1. "Older age at conception is one of the major causes of the defect."
  2. "It's a common complication of amniocentesis."
  3. "It has been linked to maternal alcohol consumption during pregnancy."
  4. "The cause is unknown and there are many environmental factors that may contribute to it."

43. A child with a diagnosis of meningococcal meningitis develops signs of sepsis and a purpuric rash over both lower extremities. The primary health care provider should be notified immediately because these signs could be indicative of which complication?
  1. A severe allergic reaction to the antibiotic regimen with impending anaphylaxis
  2. Onset of the syndrome of inappropriate antidiuretic hormone (SIADH)
  3. Fulminant (Waterhouse–Friderichsen syndrome) meningococcemia
  4. Adhesive arachnoiditis

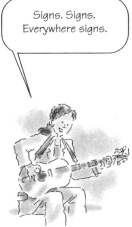

Signs. Signs. Everywhere signs.

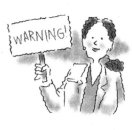

Check these signs carefully. They're critical for answering question 43.

40. 4. Since fever, seizures, vomiting, and petechiae are signs of meningitis, the nurse should promptly assess the child's neurologic status and report the findings to the physician. Petechiae are tiny purple or red spots within the dermal or submucosal layers of the skin and do not require dry sterile dressings nor are they signs of abuse. While the nurse should already have initiated seizure precautions, the finding of petechiae wouldn't be a reason to initiate seizure precautions.
CN: Physiological integrity; CNS: Physiological adaptation; CL: Analysis

41. 1. A positive Kernig's sign indicates nuchal rigidity, caused by an irritative lesion of the subarachnoid space. Brudzinski's sign is also indicative of the condition. Homans' sign indicates venous inflammation of the lower leg, not nuchal rigidity.
CN: Physiological integrity; CNS: Physiological adaptation; CL: Application

42. 4. There is no known cause of spina bifida, but scientists believe that it's linked to hereditary and environmental factors; neural tube defects, including spina bifida, have been strongly linked to low dietary intake of folic acid. Maternal age doesn't have an impact on spina bifida. An amniocentesis is performed to help diagnose spina bifida in utero but doesn't cause the disorder. Maternal alcohol intake during pregnancy has been linked to mental retardation, craniofacial defects, and cardiac abnormalities, not spina bifida.
CN: Physiological integrity; CNS: Physiological adaptation; CL: Application

43. 3. Meningococcemia is a serious complication usually associated with meningococcal infection. When onset is severe, sudden, and rapid (fulminant), it's known as Waterhouse–Friderichsen syndrome. Anaphylactic shock would need to be differentiated from septic shock. SIADH can be an acute complication, but it wouldn't be accompanied by the purpuric rash. Adhesive arachnoiditis occurs in the chronic phase of the disease and leads to obstruction of the flow of cerebrospinal fluid.
CN: Physiological integrity; CNS: Reduction of risk potential; CL: Application

44. A 1-month-old infant is admitted to the pediatric unit and diagnosed with bacterial meningitis. Which assessment findings by the nurse support the diagnosis?
  1. Hemorrhagic rash, first appearing as petechiae
  2. Photophobia
  3. Fever, change in feeding pattern, vomiting, or diarrhea
  4. Fever, lethargy, and purpura or large necrotic patches

45. To alleviate the child's pain and fear of lumbar puncture, which intervention should a nurse perform?
  1. Sedate the child with fentanyl (Sublimaze).
  2. Apply a topical anesthetic to the skin 5 to 10 minutes prepuncture.
  3. Have a parent hold the child in their lap during the tap procedure.
  4. Have the child inhale small amounts of nitrous oxide gas prepuncture.

46. Antimicrobial therapy to treat meningitis should be instituted <u>immediately after</u> which event?
  1. Admission to the nursing unit
  2. Initiation of I.V. therapy
  3. Identification of the causative organism
  4. Collection of cerebrospinal fluid (CSF) and blood for culture

47. A nurse is teaching the parents of a child diagnosed with meningitis about the child's medications. Which statement by the nurse is the most accurate with respect to the use of steroid therapy (dexamethasone) in conjunction with antimicrobial therapy?
  1. "It's the treatment of choice in aseptic meningitis."
  2. "It's used for the prevention of GI hemorrhage."
  3. "It's used for the management of problems related to blood pressure."
  4. "It's used for the prevention of deafness with *Haemophilus influenzae* meningitis."

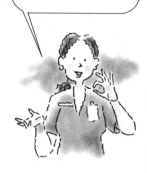

I see you've finished 44 questions. Super! Are you at least having "a little bit" of fun?

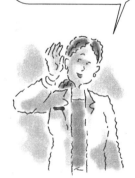

If you listen carefully, you can almost hear the answer to this question.

44. 3. Fever, change in feeding patterns, vomiting, and diarrhea are commonly observed in children with bacterial meningitis. Hemorrhagic rashes, petechiae, photophobia, fever, lethargy, and purpura are common manifestations in older children with meningitis.
CN: Physiological integrity; CNS: Physiological adaptation; CL: Application

45. 1. Sedation with fentanyl or other drugs can alleviate the pain and fear associated with a lumbar puncture. A topical anesthetic can be applied, but it should be done 1 hour before the procedure to be fully effective. Parents holding a child in their lap increases the risk of neurologic injury due to the inability to assume and maintain the proper anatomic position required for a safe lumbar puncture. Use of nitrous oxide gas isn't recommended.
CN: Physiological integrity; CNS: Basic care and comfort; CL: Application

46. 4. Antibiotics are always begun immediately after the collection of CSF and blood cultures. Admission and initiation of I.V. therapy aren't, by themselves, appropriate times to begin antimicrobial therapy. After the specific organism is identified, bacteria-specific antibiotics can be administered if the organism isn't covered by the initial choice of antibiotic therapy.
CN: Physiological integrity; CNS: Pharmacological and parenteral therapies; CL: Analysis

47. 4. Dexamethasone may play a role in the prevention of bilateral deafness in children with *H. influenzae* type b meningitis, and its use is recommended by the American Academy of Pediatrics. Treatment of aseptic meningitis is primarily symptomatic with acetaminophen for headache and muscle pain and positioning for comfort. Use of dexamethasone could complicate rather than prevent GI bleeding and problems related to blood pressure.
CN: Physiological integrity; CNS: Pharmacological and parenteral therapies; CL: Application

CN: Client needs category   CNS: Client needs subcategory   CL: Cognitive level

48. Which description is accurate about the incidence of sequelae in a client with bacterial meningitis?
1. Occur during the first 2 months of life
2. Occur in children with meningococcal meningitis
3. Primarily involve the fourth ventricle of the brain
4. Tend to affect the ocular nerves, leading to retinal damage

49. Which goal of nursing care is the most difficult to accomplish in caring for a child with meningitis?
1. Protecting self and others from possible infection
2. Avoiding actions that increase discomfort such as lifting the head
3. Keeping environmental stimuli to a minimum such as reduced light and noise
4. Maintaining I.V. infusion to administer adequate antimicrobial therapy

50. Which nursing assessment data should be given the <u>highest priority</u> for a child with clinical findings related to tubercular meningitis?
1. Onset and character of fever
2. Degree and extent of nuchal rigidity
3. Signs of increased intracranial pressure (ICP)
4. Occurrence of urine and fecal incontinence

51. The clinical manifestations of acute bacterial meningitis are dependent on which factor?
1. Age of the child
2. Length of the prodromal period
3. Time span from bacterial invasion to onset of symptoms
4. Degree of elevation of cerebrospinal fluid (CSF) glucose compared to serum glucose level

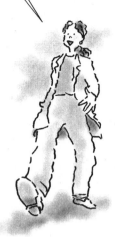

You're making great strides. Keep going.

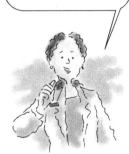

All of the choices in question 50 may be correct. So you need to prioritize.

48. 1. In infants younger than age 2 months with bacterial meningitis, communicating hydrocephalus and the effects of cerebritis on the immature brain leads to the frequent occurrence of sequelae. Sequelae are least commonly seen in children experiencing meningococcal meningitis. Meningitis primarily affects the nerves for hearing rather than vision.
CN: Physiological integrity; CNS: Physiological adaptation; CL: Application

49. 4. One of the most difficult problems in the nursing care of children with meningitis is maintaining the I.V. infusion for the length of time needed to provide adequate therapy. All of the other options are important aspects in the provision of care to the child with meningitis, but they're secondary to antimicrobial therapy.
CN: Physiological integrity; CNS: Basic care and comfort; CL: Application

50. 3. Assessment of fever and evaluation of nuchal rigidity are important aspects of care, but assessment for signs of increasing ICP should be the highest priority due to the life-threatening implications. Urinary and fecal incontinence can occur in a child who's ill from nearly any cause but don't pose a great danger to life.
CN: Physiological integrity; CNS: Reduction of risk potential; CL: Analysis

51. 1. Clinical manifestations of acute bacterial meningitis depend largely on the age of the child. Clinical manifestations aren't dependent on the prodromal or initial period of the disease nor the time from invasion of the host to the onset of the symptoms. The glucose level of the CSF is reduced, not elevated. A serum glucose level is drawn one-half hour before lumbar puncture so that the relationship between the CSF glucose and the serum glucose levels can be determined.
CN: Physiological integrity; CNS: Physiological adaptation; CL: Application

52. The mother of a child with a history of closed head injury asks the nurse why her son would begin having seizures without warning. Which response by the nurse is the <u>most</u> accurate?
1. "Clonic seizure activity is usually interpreted as falling."
2. "It's not unusual to develop seizures after a head injury because of brain trauma."
3. "Focal discharge in the brain may lead to absence seizures that go unnoticed."
4. "The epileptogenic focus in the brain needs multiple stimuli because it will discharge to cause a seizure."

53. A student nurse asks the nurse how anticonvulsant drugs work. Which statement by the nurse would be the most accurate?
1. Suppression of sodium influx through the gated pores in the cell membrane
2. Enhancement of calcium influx through the gated pores in the cell membrane
3. Potentiation of dopamine, facilitating passage across the neuronal cell membrane
4. Suppression of potassium removal from the neuronal intracellular compartment

54. During the trial period to determine the efficacy of an anticonvulsant drug, which caution should be explained to the parents?
1. Plasma levels of the drug will be monitored on a daily basis.
2. Drug dosage will be adjusted depending on the frequency of seizure activity.
3. The drug must be discontinued immediately if even the slightest problem occurs.
4. The child shouldn't participate in activities that could be hazardous if a seizure occurs.

55. Which nursing action should be included in the care plan to promote comfort in a 4-year-old child hospitalized with meningitis?
1. Avoid making noise when in the child's room.
2. Rock the child frequently.
3. Have the child's 2-year-old brother stay in the room.
4. Keep the lights on brightly so that he can see his mother.

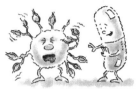

I'm sorry! I didn't mean to steal your thunder.

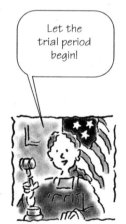

Let the trial period begin!

52. 2. Stimuli from an earlier injury may eventually elicit seizure activity, a process known as kindling. Atonic seizures, not clonic, are frequently accompanied by falling. Focal seizures are partial seizures; absence seizures are generalized seizures. Focal seizures don't lead to absence seizures. The epileptogenic focus consists of a group of hyperexcitable neurons responsible for initiating synchronous, high-frequency discharges leading to a seizure rather than needing multiple stimuli.
CN: Physiological integrity; CNS: Physiological adaptation; CL: Application

53. 1. Anticonvulsant drugs, such as phenytoin (Dilantin), suppress the influx of sodium, thereby decreasing the ability of the neurons to fire. Some anticonvulsant drugs, such as valproate sodium (Depakene) used for absence seizures, suppress the influx of calcium. The role of potassium and dopamine in the generation of seizure activity hasn't been identified.
CN: Physiological integrity; CNS: Pharmacological and parenteral therapies; CL: Application

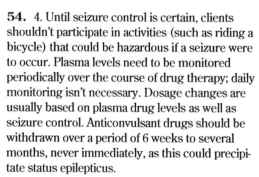

54. 4. Until seizure control is certain, clients shouldn't participate in activities (such as riding a bicycle) that could be hazardous if a seizure were to occur. Plasma levels need to be monitored periodically over the course of drug therapy; daily monitoring isn't necessary. Dosage changes are usually based on plasma drug levels as well as seizure control. Anticonvulsant drugs should be withdrawn over a period of 6 weeks to several months, never immediately, as this could precipitate status epilepticus.
CN: Physiological integrity; CNS: Pharmacological and parenteral therapies; CL: Analysis

55. 1. Meningeal irritation may cause seizures and heightens a child's sensitivity to all stimuli, including noise, lights, movement, and touch. Frequent rocking, presence of a younger sibling, and bright lights would increase stimulation.
CN: Physiological integrity; CNS: Basic care and comfort; CL: Application

CN: Client needs category   CNS: Client needs subcategory   CL: Cognitive level

56. The parents of a child with a history of seizures who has been taking phenytoin (Dilantin) ask the nurse why it's difficult to maintain therapeutic levels of this medication. Which statement by the nurse would be the <u>most</u> accurate?
1. "A drop in the plasma drug level will lead to a toxic state."
2. "The capacity to metabolize the drug becomes overwhelmed in time."
3. "Small increments in dosage lead to sharp increases in plasma drug levels."
4. "Large increases in dosage lead to more rapid stabilizing therapeutic effect."

57. Client teaching should stress which rule in relation to the differences in bioavailability of different forms of phenytoin?
1. Use the cheapest formulation the pharmacy has on hand at the time of refill.
2. Shop around to get the least expensive formulation.
3. There's no difference in one formulation from another, regardless of price.
4. Avoid switching formulations without the primary health care provider's approval.

58. To detect complications as early as possible in a child with meningitis who's receiving I.V. fluids, monitoring for which condition should be the nurse's *priority*?
1. Cerebral edema
2. Renal failure
3. Left-sided heart failure
4. Cardiogenic shock

59. Which instruction should be included in client teaching specifically related to anticonvulsant drug efficacy?
1. Wear a medical identification bracelet.
2. Maintain a seizure frequency chart.
3. Avoid potentially hazardous activities.
4. Discontinue the drug immediately if adverse effects are suspected.

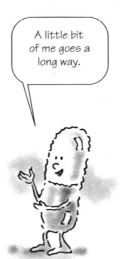

A little bit of me goes a long way.

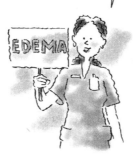

I'll give you this one...just because you've worked so hard.

EDEMA

56. 3. Within the therapeutic range for phenytoin, small increments in dosage produce sharp increases in plasma drug levels. The capacity of the liver to metabolize phenytoin is affected by slight changes in the dosage of the drug, not necessarily the length of time the client has been taking the drug. Large increments in dosage will greatly increase plasma levels leading to drug toxicity.
CN: Physiological integrity; CNS: Pharmacological and parenteral therapies; CL: Application

57. 4. Differences in bioavailability exist among different formulations (tablets and capsules) and among the same formulations produced by different manufacturers. Clients shouldn't switch from one formulation to another or from one brand to another without primary health care provider approval and supervision.
CN: Physiological integrity; CNS: Pharmacological and parenteral therapies; CL: Application

58. 1. Because the child with meningitis is already at increased risk of cerebral edema and increased intracranial pressure due to inflammation of the meningeal membranes, the nurse should monitor fluid intake and output to avoid fluid volume overload. Renal failure and cardiogenic shock aren't complications of I.V. therapy. The child with a healthy heart wouldn't be expected to develop left-sided heart failure.
CN: Physiological integrity; CNS: Pharmacological and parenteral therapies; CL: Application

59. 2. Ongoing evaluation of the therapeutic effects can be accomplished by maintaining a seizure frequency chart that indicates the date, time, and nature of all seizure activity. These data may be helpful in making dosage alterations and specific drug selection. Avoidance of hazardous activities and wearing a medical identification bracelet are ways to minimize danger related to seizure activity, but these factors don't affect drug efficacy. Anticonvulsant drugs should never be discontinued abruptly due to the potential for the development of status epilepticus.
CN: Physiological integrity; CNS: Pharmacological and parenteral therapies; CL: Application

60. I.V. administration of phenytoin would be contraindicated if which condition was identified in the preadmission assessment?
1. Episodic nosebleeds
2. History of Stokes-Adams syndrome
3. History of bone marrow depression
4. Attention deficit hyperactivity disorder (ADHD)

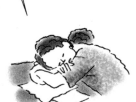

You should be able to answer this question with your eyes closed.

60. 2. I.V. administration of phenytoin can lead to arrhythmia and hypotension and is contraindicated in a history of sinus bradycardia, sinoatrial block, second- or third-degree heart block, or Stokes-Adams syndrome. Phenytoin would be administered cautiously in clients with episodic nosebleeds or bone marrow depression due to its adverse effects of leukopenia, anemia, and thrombocytopenia. Phenytoin has no known effect on ADHD but can interfere with cognitive function in excessive doses.
CN: Physiological integrity; CNS: Pharmacological and parenteral therapies; CL: Analysis

61. The parents of a child newly diagnosed with seizures ask the nurse at what time is seizure activity most likely to occur. Which response by the nurse would be the most accurate?
1. During the rapid eye movement (REM) stage of sleep
2. During long periods of excitement
3. While falling asleep and on awakening
4. While eating, particularly if the client is hurried

61. 3. Falling asleep or awakening from sleep are periods of functional instability of the brain; seizure activity is more likely to occur during these times. Eating quickly, excitement without undue fatigue, and REM sleep haven't been identified as contributing factors.
CN: Physiological integrity; CNS: Physiological adaptation; CL: Application

62. When educating the family of a child with seizures, it's appropriate to tell them to call emergency medical services in the event of a seizure if which complication occurs?
1. Continuous vomiting for 30 minutes after the seizure
2. Stereotypic or automatous body movements during the onset
3. Lack of expression, pallor, or flushing of the face during the seizure
4. Unilateral or bilateral posturing of one or more extremities during the onset

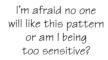

I'm afraid no one will like this pattern or am I being too sensitive?

62. 1. Continuous vomiting after a seizure has ended can be a sign of an acute problem and indicates that the child requires an immediate medical evaluation. All of the other manifestations are normally present in various types of seizure activity and don't indicate a need for immediate medical evaluation.
CN: Physiological integrity; CNS: Reduction of risk potential; CL: Analysis

63. Identifying factors that trigger seizure activity could lead to which alteration in the child's environment or activities of daily living?
1. Avoiding striped wallpaper and ceiling fans
2. Having the child sleep alone to prevent sleep interruption
3. Including extended periods of intense physical activity daily
4. Allowing the child to drink soda only between noon and 5 p.m.

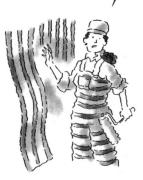

63. 1. Striped wallpaper, ceiling fans, and blinking lights on a Christmas tree can all be triggers to seizure activity if the child is photosensitive. Sleep interruption hasn't been identified as a triggering factor. Avoidance of fatigue can reduce seizure activity; therefore, intense physical activity for extended periods should be avoided. Restricting caffeine intake by using caffeine-free soda is a dietary modification that may prevent seizures.
CN: Physiological integrity; CNS: Physiological adaptation; CL: Application

CN: Client needs category   CNS: Client needs subcategory   CL: Cognitive level

64. Which nursing intervention should be included to support the goal of avoiding injury, respiratory distress, or aspiration during a seizure?
1. Positioning the child with the head hyperextended
2. Placing a hand under the child's head for support
3. Using pillows to prop the child into the sitting position
4. Working a padded tongue blade or small plastic airway between the teeth

65. Which diagnostic measure is the <u>most</u> accurate in detecting neural tube defects?
1. Flat plate of the lower abdomen after the 23rd week of gestation
2. Significant level of alpha-fetoprotein present in the amniotic fluid
3. Amniocentesis for lecithin-sphingomyelin (L/S) ratio
4. Presence of high maternal levels of albumin after 12th week of gestation

66. A nurse is teaching the parents of a child who has been diagnosed with spina bifida. Which statement by the nurse would be the <u>most</u> accurate description of spina bifida?
1. "It has little influence on the intellectual and perceptual abilities of the child."
2. "It's a simple neurologic defect that's completely corrected surgically within 1 to 2 days after birth."
3. "Its presence predisposes that many areas of the central nervous system (CNS) may not develop or function adequately."
4. "It's a complex neurologic disability that involves a collaborative health care team effort for the entire first year of life."

67. Common deformities occurring in the child with spina bifida are related to the muscles of the lower extremities that are active or inactive. These may include which complication?
1. Club feet
2. Hip extension
3. Ankylosis of the knee
4. Abduction and external rotation of the hip

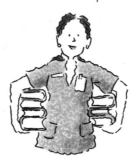

Hang on! You've reached question 65!

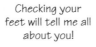

Checking your feet will tell me all about you!

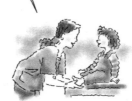

64. 2. Placing a hand or a small cushion or blanket under the child's head will help prevent injury. Position the child with the head in midline, not hyperextended, to promote a good airway and adequate ventilation. Don't attempt to prop the child up into a sitting position, but ease him to the floor to prevent falling and unnecessary injury. Don't put *anything* in the child's mouth because it could cause infection or obstruct the airway.
CN: Physiological integrity; CNS: Reduction of risk potential; CL: Application

65. 2. Significant levels of alpha-fetoprotein have been effective in detecting neural tube defects. Prenatal screening includes a combination of maternal serum and amniotic fluid levels, amniocentesis, amniography, and ultrasonography and has been relatively successful in diagnosing the defect. Flat plate X-rays of the abdomen, L/S ratio, and maternal serum albumin levels aren't diagnostic for the defect.
CN: Health promotion and maintenance; CNS: None; CL: Application

66. 3. When a spinal cord lesion exists at birth, it commonly leads to altered development or function of other areas of the CNS. Spina bifida is a complex neurologic defect that heavily impacts the physical, cognitive, and psychosocial development of the child and involves a collaborative, life-long management due to the chronicity and multiplicity of the problems involved.
CN: Physiological integrity; CNS: Physiological adaptation; CL: Application

67. 1. The type and extent of deformity in the lower extremities depends on the muscles that are active or inactive. Passive positioning *in utero* may result in deformities of the feet such as equinovarus (club foot), knee flexion and extension contractures, hip flexion with adduction and internal rotation leading to subluxation or dislocation of the hip.
CN: Physiological integrity; CNS: Physiological adaptation; CL: Analysis

68. What's the nurse's priority when caring for a 10-month-old infant with meningitis?
1. Maintaining an adequate airway
2. Maintaining fluid and electrolyte balance
3. Controlling seizures
4. Controlling hyperthermia

69. The nurse is caring for an infant with myelomeningocele and notices a change in the assessment which may indicate the infant has a Chiari II malformation. Which change was noted in the assessment?
1. Rapidly progressing scoliosis
2. Changes in urologic functioning
3. Back pain below the site of the sac closure
4. Respiratory stridor

70. A child with myelomeningocele and hydrocephalus may demonstrate problems related to damage of the white matter caused by ventricular enlargement. This damage may manifest itself in which condition?
1. Inability to speak
2. Early hand dominance
3. Impaired intellectual functions
4. Flaccid paralysis of the lower extremities

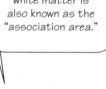

For question 70, it helps to know that my white matter is also known as the "association area."

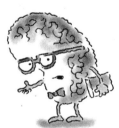

68. 1. Maintaining an adequate airway is always a top priority. Maintaining fluid and electrolyte balance and controlling seizures and hyperthermia are all important but not as important as an adequate airway.
CN: Physiological integrity; CNS: Reduction of risk potential; CL: Application

69. 4. Children with a myelomeningocele have a 90% chance of having a Chiari II malformation. This may lead to a possibility of respiratory function problems, such as respiratory stridor associated with paralysis of the vocal cords, apneic episodes of unknown cause, difficulty swallowing, and an abnormal gag reflex. Urologic function changes and scoliosis occur with myelomeningocele, but these complications aren't specifically related to Chiari II malformation. Lower back pain doesn't occur due to the loss of sensory function related to the cord defect.
CN: Physiological integrity; CNS: Reduction of risk potential; CL: Analysis

70. 3. Damage to the white matter (association area) caused by ventricular enlargement has been linked to impairment of intellectual and perceptual abilities often seen in children with spina bifida. It hasn't been related to hand dominance development, flaccid paralysis of the lower extremities, or the ability to speak, though it may affect the semantics of speech dependent upon the association areas.
CN: Physiological integrity; CNS: Physiological adaptation; CL: Analysis

CN: Client needs category   CNS: Client needs subcategory   CL: Cognitive level

71. The parents of a child newly diagnosed with myelomeningocele ask the nurse why surgical repair needs to be done immediately. Which response would be the most accurate?
1. "It's done for rapid restoration of the neural pathways to the legs."
2. "It's done to decrease the possibility of infection and further cord damage."
3. "It's done to expose the spinal cord defect to individualize the therapeutic strategy."
4. "It's done for removal of excess nerve tissue from the vertebral canal to decrease pressure on the cord."

72. One of the most important aspects of pre-operative care with myelomeningocele is the positioning of the infant. Which position is the most appropriate?
1. Prone position with head turned to the side for feeding
2. Side-lying position with the head at a 30-degree angle to the feet
3. Prone position with a nasogastric (NG) tube inserted for feedings
4. Supported by diaper rolls, both anterior and posterior, in the side-lying position

73. Large body areas of sensory and motor impairment associated with myelomeningocele necessitate which nursing intervention?
1. Gentle stretching of contractures
2. Vigorous active range-of-motion exercises
3. Frequent turning side-to-side and prone-to-supine
4. Keeping skin dry and avoiding the use of emollients and lubricants

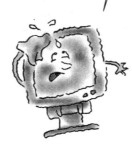

Don't sweat it! Just choose the most appropriate response.

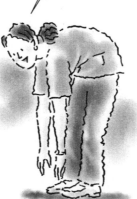

Sometimes it helps to stretch.

71. 2. The myelomeningocele sac presents a dynamic disability and is treated as a life-threatening situation with sac closure taking place within the first 24 to 48 hours after birth. This early management decreases the possibility of infection and further injury to the exposed neural cord. There's complete loss of nervous function below the level of the spinal cord lesion. The aim of surgery is to replace the nerve tissue into the vertebral canal, cover the spinal defect, and achieve a watertight sac closure.
CN: Physiological integrity; CNS: Reduction of risk potential; CL: Application

72. 1. Prone position is used preoperatively because it minimizes tension on the sac and the risk of trauma. The head is turned to one side for feeding. There's no advantage to positioning the body with a 30-degree head elevation. Although feeding can be a problem in the prone position, it can be accomplished without the need for an NG tube. Side-lying or partial side-lying positions are better used *after* the repair has been accomplished unless it permits undesirable hip flexion.
CN: Physiological integrity; CNS: Reduction of risk potential; CL: Application

73. 1. Areas of sensory and motor impairment require meticulous care, including gentle range-of-motion exercises to prevent contractures as well as stretching of contractures when indicated. Vigorous exercise is avoided in contrast to the gentle range of motion that is recommended. Frequent turning is indicated in order to maintain skin integrity, but the supine position shouldn't be used to avoid pressure on the surgical site. Skin should be kept clean and dry, but lubrication can be used to facilitate massage, which increases circulation to the areas involved.
CN: Physiological integrity; CNS: Basic care and comfort; CL: Application

74. Children with spina bifida are at high risk for developing intraoperative anaphylaxis linked to an allergic response to latex. Which risk factor leads to this allergic response?
1. Weakened immune response
2. Need for life-long steroid therapy
3. Need for numerous bladder catheterizations
4. Use of large amounts of adhesive tape to attach sac dressings

74. 3. Children with spina bifida are at high risk for developing a latex allergy because of repeated exposure to latex products during multiple surgeries and from numerous bladder catheterizations related to lack of bladder function. A weakened immune response wouldn't elicit an anaphylactic reaction due to the reduced functioning of the immune response. Steroid therapy isn't indicated in the management of spina bifida and also wouldn't support an anaphylactic reaction. Sac removal is accomplished as quickly as possible after birth, and the sac usually isn't covered with any type of dressing because it may contribute to trauma to the sac.
CN: Physiological integrity; CNS: Reduction of risk potential; CL: Application

> Taking folic acid before conception reduces certain risks in infants.

75. Which explanation about how to avoid the incidence of a second child with spina bifida is most accurate?
1. There's no known way to avoid it; adoption is recommended.
2. A previous pregnancy affected by a neural tube defect isn't a factor.
3. Prepregnancy intake of 4 mg of folic acid daily reduces the recurrence rate.
4. Aerobic exercise in the first trimester to decrease the chances of a positive alpha-fetoprotein (AFP).

75. 3. Studies have shown that women at high risk for having an infant with a neural tube defect, demonstrated by a previously delivered infant or fetus with spina bifida, significantly reduced the recurrence rate by taking supplements of folic acid before conception. The chances of having a second affected child are low (between 1% and 2%), but still greater than the chances of the general population. Aerobic exercise won't decrease the chances of a positive AFP.
CN: Health promotion and maintenance; CNS: None; CL: Analysis

76. A school-age child with a diagnosis of epilepsy is admitted to the pediatric unit of a local hospital for evaluation of his anticonvulsant medications. As a nurse enters the child's room, the child begins to have a seizure. Which nursing action should the nurse do first?
1. Push the call bell and ask for help.
2. Hold the child down so he doesn't injure himself.
3. Loosen any restrictive clothing.
4. Force the jaw open to maintain an open airway.

76. 3. The primary nursing goal during a seizure is to protect the client from physical injury and maintain a patent airway. Loosening clothing will allow free movement and aid in keeping the airway open. After making sure the client is safe from injury, the nurse should push the call bell only if further assistance is needed. The nurse should never forcibly hold a client down and shouldn't force the jaw open; the jaw could be injured or break.
CN: Physiological integrity; CNS: Reduction of risk potential; CL: Application

CN: Client needs category   CNS: Client needs subcategory   CL: Cognitive level

77. When planning care for a 9-year-old boy with Down syndrome, which statement should a nurse keep in mind?
 1. Nursing interventions should be planned at a 9-year-old developmental level.
 2. Nursing interventions should be planned at a 7-year-old developmental level.
 3. The nurse should assess the child's developmental level before planning interventions.
 4. The developmental level of the child is not important in planning care.

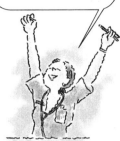

You're almost there and you've done a great job.

77. 3. Before developing a care plan, the nurse should assess the child's developmental level and plan care at that level. The nurse shouldn't plan care geared towards the child's chronological age without first assessing the child. The nurse also shouldn't assume that the child is at a lower developmental level without assessing the child. The child's developmental age is important in planning age-appropriate care and teaching.

CN: Health promotion and maintenance; CNS: None; CL: Application

78. A 6-year-old child is unconscious with a head injury from a bicycle accident. A nurse is assessing him for increased intracranial pressure (ICP). His baseline vital signs are respirations 20 breaths/minute; blood pressure 100/56 mm Hg; pulse 100 beats/minute. Which set of vital signs would indicate increased ICP?
 1. Respirations 12 breaths/minute; blood pressure 90/45 mm Hg; pulse 80 beats/minute
 2. Respirations 14 breaths/minute; blood pressure 130/40 mm Hg; pulse 70 beats/minute
 3. Respirations 30 breaths/minute; blood pressure 80/45 mm Hg; pulse 130 beats/minute
 4. Respirations 14 breaths/minute; blood pressure 70/58 mm Hg; pulse 102 beats/minute

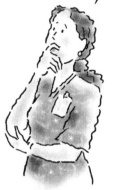

Which vital signs would indicate increased ICP?

78. 2. Classic signs of increased ICP are a decrease in respirations, an increase in blood pressure, and a decrease in pulse rate. Option 1 may indicate normal vital signs. Options 3 and 4 may indicate shock.

CN: Physiological integrity; CNS: Physiological adaptation; CL: Analysis

79. When assessing an infant for changes in intracranial pressure (ICP), it's important to palpate the fontanels. Identify the area where a nurse should palpate to assess the anterior fontanel.

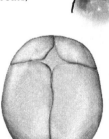

79. The anterior fontanel is formed by the junction of the sagittal, frontal, and coronal sutures. It's shaped like a diamond and normally measures 4 to 5 cm at its widest point. A widened, bulging fontanel is a sign of increased ICP.

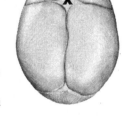

CN: Health promotion and maintenance; CNS: None; CL: Application

80. A nurse is preparing a dose of amoxicillin for a 3-year-old with acute otitis media. The child weighs 33 lb. The dosage prescribed is 50 mg/kg/day in divided doses every 8 hours. The concentration of the drug is 250 mg/5 ml. How many milliliters should the nurse administer? Record your answer using a whole number.

_____ milliliters

81. A nurse is caring for a 3-year-old with viral meningitis. Which signs and symptoms should the nurse expect to find during the initial assessment? Select all that apply:
1. Bulging anterior fontanel
2. Fever
3. Nuchal rigidity
4. Petechiae
5. Irritability
6. Photophobia
7. Hypothermia

82. The nurse is assessing the primitive reflexes of a one-month-old infant. Which of the reflexes shown in the photos below should not be present after the age of 2 months?

1.

2.

3.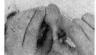

4.

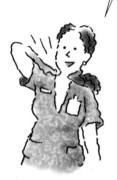

Congratulations! You finished! Give yourself a pat on the back.

80. 5. To calculate the child's weight in kilograms, the nurse should use the following formula: 1 kg/2.2 lb = X kg/33 lb; $2.2X = 33$; $X = 15$ kg. Next, the nurse should calculate the daily dosage for the child: 50 mg/kg/day $\times$ 15 kg = 750 mg/day. To determine divided daily dosage, the nurse should know that "every 8 hours" means 3 times per day. So, she should perform the calculation in this way: Total daily dosage ÷ 3 times per day = divided daily dosage; 750 mg/day ÷ 3 = 250 mg. The drug's concentration is 250 mg/5 ml, so the nurse should administer 5 ml.

CN: Physiological integrity; CNS: Pharmacological and parenteral therapies; CL: Application

81. 2, 3, 5, 6. Common signs and symptoms of viral meningitis include fever, nuchal rigidity, irritability, and photophobia. A bulging anterior fontanel is a sign of hydrocephalus, which isn't likely to occur in a toddler because the anterior fontanel typically closes by age 18 months. A petechial, purpuric rash may be seen with bacterial meningitis. Hypothermia is a common sign of bacterial meningitis in an infant younger than age 3 months.

CN: Physiological integrity; CNS: Physiological adaptation; CL: Application

82. 4. Option 4 shows the tonic neck reflex. Persistence of this reflex beyond 2 months suggests asymmetric central nervous system development. Option 1 shows the palmer grasp reflex. This reflex disappears around age three to four months. Option 2 shows the plantar grasp reflex. This reflex disappears at age six to eight months. Option 3 shows the Moro reflex. This reflex disappears around age four months.

CN: Physiological integrity; CNS: Reduction of risk potential; CL: Analysis

CN: Client needs category   CNS: Client needs subcategory   CL: Cognitive level

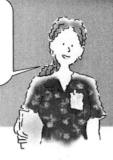

Chapter 18
Musculoskeletal system

1. A nurse is caring for a 10-year-old in Buck's traction for a fractured femur following a bicycle accident. Which intervention should the nurse do first when the child complains of increasing pain 1 hour after receiving an I.V. opioid analgesic?
  1. Tell the child that he needs to give the analgesic time to work.
  2. Perform a neurovascular assessment.
  3. Make sure the weights are hanging freely.
  4. Administer more analgesics.

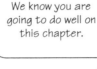

We know you are going to do well on this chapter.

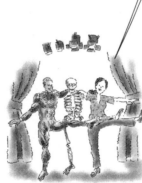

2. Which observation by a nurse indicates that an 18-month-old in Bryant's traction is properly positioned?
  1. The hips are resting on the bed.
  2. The hips are slightly elevated off the bed.
  3. The hips are elevated above the level of the heart.
  4. The hips are resting on a pillow.

3. A mother of a neonate with clubfoot feels guilty because she believes she did something to cause the condition. The nurse should explain that which factor causes clubfoot in neonates?
  1. Unknown
  2. Hereditary
  3. Restricted movement in utero
  4. Anomalous embryonic development

1. 2. Pain, unrelieved by analgesics, in a client with a dressing or cast may be a sign of compartment syndrome if pressure develops within the muscle and its surrounding structures due to the constrictive ace wrap dressing used in Buck's traction. The nurse should immediately perform a neurovascular assessment to detect signs of impaired circulation and nerve function. The findings should then immediately be reported to the physician and the pressure dressing loosened or removed. The child who has received an I.V. opioid should have had pain relief 1 hour after administration. While the weights in Buck's traction should hang freely, the child should be assessed first. More analgesics may be administered as ordered, but only after the neurovascular status is assessed.
CN: Physiological integrity; CNS: Reduction of risk potential; CL: Analysis

2. 2. In Bryant's traction, the child's hips should be slightly elevated off the bed at a 15-degree angle. They shouldn't be resting on the bed or a pillow and shouldn't be elevated above the level of the heart.
CN: Physiological integrity; CNS: Basic care and comfort; CL: Application

3. 1. The definitive cause of clubfoot is unknown. In some families, there's an increased incidence. Some postulate that anomalous embryonic development or restricted fetal movement are the reasons. Currently, there's no way to predict the occurrence of clubfoot.
CN: Psychosocial integrity; CNS: None; CL: Application

CN: Client needs category   CNS: Client needs subcategory   CL: Cognitive level

4. Which nursing diagnosis has the <u>highest priority</u> in a 6-year-old child who had a plaster cast applied 6 hours ago to the left leg for a fracture of the tibia?
1. *Deficient knowledge*
2. *Impaired physical mobility*
3. *Risk for peripheral neurovascular dysfunction*
4. *Dressing self-care deficit*

5. Which statement by the father of an 8-year-old boy with Duchenne's muscular dystrophy indicates that he has realistic expectations about the course of the disease?
1. "My son will gradually lose his ability to walk."
2. "Corticosteroids will help prevent muscle degeneration."
3. "Surgery will help my son walk."
4. "My son will have a normal lifespan."

6. A nurse is teaching the parents of a 3-month-old infant with severe torticollis who has presented with the head rotated to the left and the side bent to the right. Which statement by the parents about which muscle is shortened indicates that the teaching has been effective?
1. "It involves shortening of the left upper trapezius."
2. "It involves shortening of the right middle trapezius."
3. "It involves shortening of the left sterno-cleidomastoid."
4. "It involves shortening of the right sterno-cleidomastoid."

7. A 9-month-old infant has torticollis with rotation of the head to the left and side bending to the right. Placing the infant in which position would be most effective for developing muscle lengthening?
1. Prone
2. Supine
3. Left side-lying
4. Right side-lying

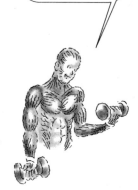

I've heard of muscle strengthening, but what's muscle lengthening?

4. 3. The highest priority in a client with a newly applied cast is to assess for and prevent circulatory complications, which can lead to loss of function. The other nursing diagnoses are important for a client in a cast, but only after adequate circulation has been assured.
CN: Safe, effective care environment; CNS: Management of care; CL: Analysis

5. 1. Duchenne's muscular dystrophy is a progressive muscular degenerative disorder in which children lose their ability to walk independently by age 12. Corticosteroids may slow muscle degeneration, but won't stop its progression. Surgery may be done to correct contractures but it doesn't change the course of the disease. Death occurs by early adulthood, usually from respiratory failure.
CN: Physiological integrity; CNS: Physiological adaptation; CL: Application

6. 4. The right sternocleidomastoid is shortened with the head in this position. The left upper trapezius isn't shortened; the right one is. The middle trapezius isn't affected, and the left sternocleidomastoid is in a lengthened position.
CN: Physiological integrity; CNS: Physiological adaptation; CL: Application

7. 3. The left side-lying position will help assist with lengthening of the muscles because this position will make it easier to stretch the sternocleidomastoid and upper trapezius. No other positions will assist in increasing muscle length.
CN: Physiological integrity; CNS: Reduction of risk potential; CL: Application

CN: Client needs category   CNS: Client needs subcategory   CL: Cognitive level

8. A nurse is teaching a 13-year-old girl diagnosed with scoliosis and her parents how to apply a Milwaukee brace. Which action should the nurse do first?
  1. Refer them to a scoliosis support group.
  2. Ask them to read the brochure that comes with the brace and then answer their questions.
  3. Ask them what they already know about the brace and answer their questions.
  4. Develop learning objectives and then explain them to the parents and teen.

9. A nurse is caring for a child who received a hip-spica cast 24 hours ago for hip dysplasia. Which nursing diagnoses should the nurse give the <u>highest priority</u>?
  1. *Impaired gas exchange*
  2. *Risk for peripheral neurovascular dysfunction*
  3. *Risk for impaired skin integrity*
  4. *Urinary retention*

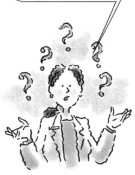

Does this mean the brace was made in Milwaukee?

10. Which intervention is appropriate for a child with a newly applied wet hip-spica cast?
  1. Use the abductor bar to help move the child.
  2. Cover the cast in plastic to keep it clean.
  3. Reposition the child every 1 to 2 hours.
  4. Use the fingertips when handling the cast.

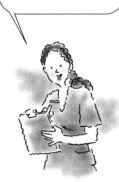

Congratulations! You've finished the first 10 questions!

11. The parents of an infant born with clubfoot express feelings of guilt and anxiety about their child's condition. Which intervention should a nurse do first?
  1. Teach them about their child's condition.
  2. Introduce them to other parents whose children have the same condition.
  3. Ask if they would like to speak with the chaplain.
  4. Encourage discussion of their feelings.

12. The Milwaukee brace is commonly used in the treatment of scoliosis. Which position best describes the placement of the pressure rods?
  1. Laterally on convex portion of the curve
  2. Laterally on concave portion of the curve
  3. Posteriorly on convex portion of the curve
  4. Posteriorly along the spinal column at the exact level of the curve

8. 3. The first step in teaching this teen and her parents is to assess what they already know about the brace and answer their questions. This allows the nurse to clear up misconceptions and address their concerns. A support group is helpful but isn't the initial step the nurse should take. Written instructions should reinforce the teaching done by the nurse, not take the place of the nurse's teaching. Learning objectives should be developed with the teen and her parents.
CN: Health promotion and maintenance; CNS: None; CL: Application

9. 2. After cast application, a client is at risk for peripheral neurovascular dysfunction due to swelling within the confined space of the cast. Impaired gas exchange isn't a high risk since the cast was applied for hip dysplasia and not a fracture of a long bone, which would increase the risk of pulmonary embolism. Risk for impaired skin integrity and urinary retention is important, but neurovascular impairment is a higher priority.
CN: Safe, effective care environment; CNS: Management of care; CL: Analysis

10. 3. The child in a wet hip-spica cast should be turned every 1 to 2 hours to help dry all sides of the cast and prevent skin breakdown. The abductor bar shouldn't be used for turning the child, even with a dry cast. A wet cast shouldn't be covered with plastic because this impairs the drying of the cast. A wet cast should be handled using the palms because fingers may cause indentations and pressure points.
CN: Physiological integrity; CNS: Basic care and comfort; CL: Application

11. 4. While all the options are appropriate interventions for the nurse to implement, the first step is to encourage the parents to verbalize their concerns and feelings about their child's condition. This helps alleviate anxiety and to develop a trusting therapeutic relationship.
CN: Physiological integrity; CNS: None; CL: Analysis

12. 1. Lateral pressure applied to the convex portion of the curve will help best in reducing the curvature. Pressure pads applied posteriorly will help maintain erect posture. Pressure applied to the concave portion of the curve will increase the lordosis.
CN: Physiological integrity; CNS: Reduction of risk potential; CL: Application

13. Strengthening of which muscle group is important in a client diagnosed with talipes equinovarus?

1. Evertors
2. Invertors
3. Plantar flexors
4. Plantar fascia musculature

14. A nurse is caring for a 15-year-old who sustained a fracture of the femur 24 hours ago. Which finding should alert the nurse to an early complication?

1. Pain
2. Local swelling
3. Loss of function
4. Dyspnea

15. Which statement made by an adolescent girl with scoliosis indicates that she understands its treatment?

1. "I will have to wear a brace for several years."
2. "I can put on the brace after I get home from school."
3. "I should avoid any exercise that will stretch my spine."
4. "I can remove the brace at night."

16. A child has just returned to his room with a cast on his leg after open reduction of a fractured femur. What's the most appropriate action for a nurse to take when a 6 cm by 10 cm area of blood is noted on the cast?

1. Tape gauze pads over the bloody area.
2. Mark the bloody drainage and monitor hourly.
3. Assess vital signs.
4. Call the physician.

17. Which observation by a nurse indicates proper fit of crutches in a 9-year-old boy?

1. The crutches fit snugly under the axilla.
2. The crutches end 2″ (5 cm) below the axilla.
3. The elbow is flexed 60 degrees.
4. The elbow is flexed 90 degrees.

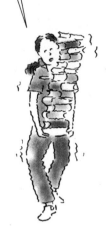

All this studying is strengthening my muscle groups. Oh, goody.

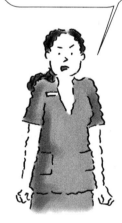

Brace yourself. Question 15 requires a long-term solution.

13. 1. Because the foot is held in inversion, it's important to strengthen the evertors to counter the inversion present in the foot. Inversion is incorrect because the foot is already held in this position. Plantar musculature and plantar flexors aren't important because the foot is already in a plantar flexed position.

CN: Physiological integrity; CNS: Reduction of risk potential; CL: Analysis

14. 4. After the fracture of a long bone, such as the femur, the client is at risk for fat embolism. Clinical manifestations include dyspnea, hypoxia, tachypnea, tachycardia, and chest pain. Pain, local swelling, and loss of function are all typical findings after a fracture.

CN: Physiological integrity; CNS: Reduction of risk potential; CL: Analysis

15. 1. A brace worn to correct scoliosis must be worn for several years to correct the spinal deformity. The child must wear the brace all day, even during school and sleep. Exercises are commonly prescribed to be performed several times per day to stretch and strengthen back muscles. It should only be removed for 1 hour each day while bathing.

CN: Physiological integrity; CNS: Basic care and comfort; CL: Analysis

16. 3. The most appropriate action for the nurse is to assess the client's vital signs for evidence of hemorrhage, such as tachycardia and hypotension. After the nurse has assessed the client, the physician should be notified with the findings. Gauze pads may be placed over the bloody drainage after the client is assessed and the physician notified. The size of the bloody drainage should be monitored after the client is assessed and the physician notified.

CN: Physiological integrity; CNS: Reduction of risk potential; CL: Application

17. 2. The crutches should end 2″ below the axilla and the elbow should be flexed 20 to 30 degrees.

CN: Physiological integrity; CNS: Basic care and comfort; CL: Application

CN: Client needs category   CNS: Client needs subcategory   CL: Cognitive level

18. Which technique may assist a 3-month-old client diagnosed with torticollis?
1. Lying supine
2. Gentle massage
3. Range-of-motion (ROM) exercises
4. Lying on the side

19. A physical therapist has instructed the nursing staff in range-of-motion (ROM) exercises for an infant with torticollis. Which intervention should a nurse perform if she feels uncomfortable performing the stretches that result in crying and grimacing of the client?
1. Check the primary health care provider's orders.
2. Call the primary health care provider.
3. Call the physical therapist.
4. Discontinue the exercises.

20. A client has developed a right torticollis with side-bending to the right and rotation to the left. Which exercises may assist in reduction of the torticollis?
1. Rotation exercises to the right
2. Rotation exercises to the left
3. Cervical extension exercises
4. Cervical flexion exercises

21. Which complication may occur due to severe scoliosis?
1. Increased vital capacity
2. Increased oxygen uptake
3. Diminished vital capacity
4. Decreased residual volume

22. A 4-year-old child is diagnosed with cerebral palsy and resultant thoracic scoliosis. Which condition may be the cause of the scoliosis?
1. Hypotonia
2. Mental retardation
3. Autonomic dysreflexia
4. Increased thoracic kyphosis

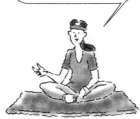

Do you think there's any truth to no pain, no gain?

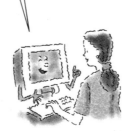

You've done 20 questions already. Great job!!

18. 4. Side-lying opposite the affected side may help elongate shortened muscles. Lying supine won't assist with elongation of muscles. Gentle massage won't assist with elongation of muscles. ROM exercises won't assist with shortened muscles unless in specific patterns and with stretching.
CN: Health promotion and maintenance; CNS: None; CL: Application

19. 3. The only cure for the torticollis is exercise or surgery. The therapist is the expert in exercise and should be called for assistance in this situation. The primary health care provider would be called only if there was concern over the orders written or an abnormal development in the child.
CN: Physiological integrity; CNS: Physiological adaptation; CL: Analysis

20. 1. Performing rotation exercises to the right will help increase the length of the shortened right sternocleidomastoid. Rotation to the left will just add to the torticollis because the head is already rotated in that direction. Cervical extension exercises won't lengthen tightened muscles. Cervical flexion will add to shortening of the muscles.
CN: Physiological integrity; CNS: Reduction of risk potential; CL: Application

21. 3. Scoliosis of greater than 60 degrees can cause shifting of organs and decreased ability for the ribs to expand, thus decreasing vital capacity. An increase in vital capacity also won't occur secondary to a decrease in chest expansion. An increase in oxygen uptake won't occur secondary to a decrease in chest expansion. Residual volume will increase secondary to decreased ability of the lungs to expel air.
CN: Physiological integrity; CNS: Physiological adaptation; CL: Analysis

22. 1. Cerebral palsy is usually associated with some degree of hypotonia or hypertonia. Poor muscle tone may result in scoliosis. Mental retardation isn't a cause of scoliosis. Autonomic dysreflexia is described in spinal cord injury and involves abnormal muscle spasms secondary to abnormal inhibitory neurons present during stretch reflexes. Increased thoracic kyphosis won't result in scoliosis.
CN: Physiological integrity; CNS: Physiological adaptation; CL: Application

23. Which statement by the parents of a child with crutches indicates understanding of how to safely walk down stairs?
  1. "First place the crutches on the lower step."
  2. "Advance the fractured leg first."
  3. "Advance the strong leg first."
  4. "First place the crutch on the fractured side on the lower step."

24. During a scoliosis screening, a school nurse notices a raised iliac crest height. She should suspect which condition?
  1. Forward head posture
  2. Leg length discrepancy
  3. Increased lumbar lordosis
  4. Increased thoracic kyphosis

25. A school nurse is performing a scoliosis screening on a group of students. Which student would most commonly develop this condition?
  1. A 7-year-old girl
  2. A 7-year-old boy
  3. A 13-year-old girl
  4. A 13-year old boy

26. In caring for a child with a Harrington instrumentation rod placement, which symptom should be of <u>greatest concern</u> 2 days postoperatively?
  1. Fever of 99.5° F (37.5° C)
  2. Pain along the incision
  3. Decreased urinary output
  4. Hypoactive bowel sounds

27. Observing which structure will serve a nurse best when screening a child for scoliosis?
  1. Iliac crests
  2. Spinous processes
  3. Acromion processes
  4. Posterior superior iliac spines

28. Which intervention may be a possible treatment choice for talipes equinovarus?
  1. Traction
  2. Serial casting
  3. Short leg braces
  4. Inversion range-of-motion exercises

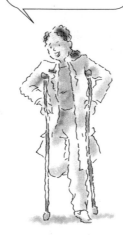

Read question 23 carefully and take it one step at a time.

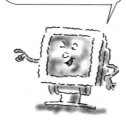

In question 26, you've got to determine the symptom that causes the most concern.

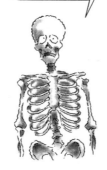

No bones about it. You're doing great!

23. 1. To walk down the stairs with crutches, the crutches are first placed on the lower step. Then the fractured or weaker leg is lowered, followed by the unaffected or stronger leg. This way the arms and unaffected leg share the work of carrying the body weight.
CN: Safe, effective care environment; CNS: Safety and infection control; CL: Application

24. 2. A raised iliac crest may be indicative of a leg length discrepancy or a curvature in the lumbar spine. It isn't indicative of forward head posture, lumbar lordosis, or thoracic kyphosis.
CN: Health promotion and maintenance; CNS: None; CL: Application

25. 3. Scoliosis is eight times more prominent in adolescent girls than boys. Peak incidence is between ages 8 and 15. Therefore, a 13-year-old girl is at the highest risk. Seven-year-old boys and girls are at lower risk.
CN: Health promotion and maintenance; CNS: None; CL: Analysis

26. 3. Because of extensive blood loss during surgery and possible renal hypoperfusion, decreased urinary output could indicate decreased renal function. A fever of 99.5° F is of concern, but it may be due to decreased chest expansion secondary to anesthesia, surgery, and pain. Pain along the incision site is expected. A paralytic ileus is common after this surgery, and the client may have a nasogastric tube for the first 48 hours.
CN: Physiological integrity; CNS: Reduction of risk potential; CL: Analysis

27. 2. Spinous processes are the best bony landmark to identify when attempting to screen for scoliosis because this will show lateral deviation of the column. Abnormalities in the acromion process, iliac crests, and posterior superior iliac spines may not be indicative of scoliosis.
CN: Health promotion and maintenance; CNS: None; CL: Application

28. 2. Serial casting is a treatment choice in attempts to change the length of soft tissue. Traction isn't an option. Corrective shoes are used instead of short leg braces. Inversion exercises won't help; eversion exercise will.
CN: Physiological integrity; CNS: Reduction of risk potential; CL: Application

CN: Client needs category   CNS: Client needs subcategory   CL: Cognitive level

29. When performing stretches with a child who has scoliosis, which technique should be used?
1. Slow and sustained
2. Until a change in muscle length is seen
3. Quick movements to the end range of pain
4. Slow movements for brief, 3- to 4-second periods

30. Which observation by a nurse indicates that the parent of a neonate with developmental dysplasia of the hip understands the discharge teaching?
1. A folded towel is placed between the infant's legs.
2. The infant is wearing three diapers.
3. The infant is tightly swaddled in a blanket.
4. The infant is placed in a prone position to sleep.

31. A nurse is caring for an infant with suspected developmental dysplasia of the hip (DDH). Which information should the nurse give the parents about diagnostic testing?
1. A diagnosis can't be confirmed until the child begins to walk.
2. Diagnostic testing is performed at 6 months if the dysplasia hasn't resolved by then.
3. A radiopaque dye will be injected into the subarachnoid space of the spine.
4. An X-ray confirms the diagnosis.

32. Which hip position should be avoided in an 8-month-old infant who has been diagnosed with developmental dysplasia of the hip?
1. Extension
2. Abduction
3. Internal rotation
4. External rotation

33. Which activity in a client with muscular dystrophy should a nurse anticipate the client having difficulty with <u>first</u>?
1. Breathing
2. Sitting
3. Standing
4. Swallowing

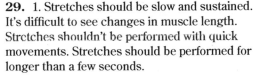

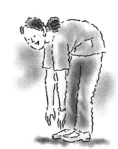

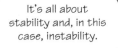

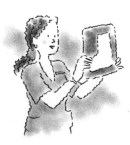

29. 1. Stretches should be slow and sustained. It's difficult to see changes in muscle length. Stretches shouldn't be performed with quick movements. Stretches should be performed for longer than a few seconds.
CN: Health promotion and maintenance; CNS: None; CL: Application

30. 2. Placing several diapers on the infant will keep the hips and knees flexed and the hips abducted. A towel placed between the legs is not enough to keep the hips abducted. Swaddling the infant tightly straightens the legs and doesn't allow the hips to be abducted. Placing the infant in a prone position won't keep the hips abducted and isn't recommended due to the increased risk of sudden infant death syndrome.
CN: Physiological integrity; CNS: Basic care and comfort; CL: Application

31. 4. X-rays show the location of the femur head and a shallow acetabulum, confirming the diagnosis DDH. The diagnosis can be made in the neonate and should be made as soon as possible since it becomes more difficult to correct as the child ages. Myelography is an invasive procedure used to evaluate abnormalities of the spinal canal and cord. It isn't used in the diagnosis of congenital hip dysplasia.
CN: Physiological integrity; CNS: Physiological adaptation; CL: Application

32. 3. Internal rotation of the hip is an unstable position and should be avoided in infants with hip instability. Hip extension is a relatively stable position. Typically, the child is placed in slight abduction while in a hip-spica cast. External rotation isn't necessarily an unstable position, as long as it isn't externally rotated too far.
CN: Physiological integrity; CNS: Reduction of risk potential; CL: Application

33. 3. Muscular dystrophy usually affects postural muscles of the hip and shoulder first. Sitting may be affected, but a client would have difficulty standing before having difficulty sitting. Swallowing and breathing are usually affected last.
CN: Physiological integrity; CNS: Physiological adaptation; CL: Application

34. The nurse would expect her client's suspected developmental dysplasia of the hip (DDH) to be confirmed by which diagnostic technique?
  1. X-ray
  2. Positive Ortolani's signs
  3. Positive Trendelenburg gait
  4. Audible clicking with adduction

35. Which finding should a nurse expect when assessing a neonate with a positive Galeazzi sign?
  1. Raised iliac crest
  2. Pelvic downward tilt on weight bearing
  3. Knees are flexed to 90 degrees, one knee higher
  4. Involved leg flexed to 90 degrees, audible click with external rotation

36. A young child sustains a dislocated hip as well as a subcapital fracture. Which complication is of <u>greatest concern</u>?
  1. Avascular necrosis
  2. Postsurgical infection
  3. Hemorrhage during surgery
  4. Poor postsurgical ambulation

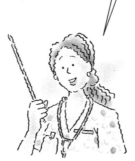

Question 36? Another chance to prioritize.

37. Which position of the femur is accurate in relation to the acetabulum in a child with developmental dysplasia of the hip (DDH)?
  1. Anterior
  2. Inferior
  3. Posterior
  4. Superior

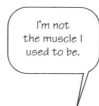

I'm not the muscle I used to be.

38. The nurse is planning to teach the parents of a child with newly diagnosed muscular dystrophy about the disease. Which description accurately describes this condition?
  1. A demyelinating disease
  2. Lesions of the brain cortex
  3. Upper motor neuron lesions
  4. Degeneration of muscle fibers

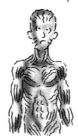

39. When a child is suspected of having muscular dystrophy, a nurse should expect which muscles to be affected <u>first</u>?
  1. Muscles of the hip
  2. Muscles of the foot
  3. Muscles of the hand
  4. Muscles of respiration

34. 1. X-ray will confirm the diagnosis of DDH. All of the options are positive signs of DDH, but only the X-ray will confirm the diagnosis.
CN: Physiological integrity; CNS: Physiological adaptation; CL: Application

35. 3. A positive Galeazzi sign is used to help diagnose hip dislocation. It's exhibited as one knee being higher than the other. Raised iliac crest isn't indicative of specific hip pathology. A downward pelvic tilt with weight bearing is Trendelenburg gait. External rotation of the hip with audible click is Ortolani-Barlow test.
CN: Health promotion and maintenance; CNS: None; CL: Application

36. 1. Avascular necrosis is common with fractures to the subcapital region secondary to possible compromise of blood supply to the femoral head. Postsurgical infection is always a concern but not a priority at first. Hemorrhage shouldn't occur. Poor postsurgical ambulation is of concern but not as much as the possibility of avascular necrosis.
CN: Physiological integrity; CNS: Reduction of risk potential; CL: Application

37. 1. The head of the femur is anterior to the acetabulum in developmental dysplasia of the hip. All other positions are inaccurate.
CN: Physiological integrity; CNS: Physiological adaptation; CL: Application

38. 4. Degeneration of muscle fibers with progressive weakness and wasting best describes muscular dystrophy. Demyelination of myelin sheaths is a description of multiple sclerosis. Lesions within the cortex and in upper motor neurons suggest a neurologic, not a muscular, disease.
CN: Physiological integrity; CNS: Physiological adaptation; CL: Application

39. 1. Positional muscles of the hip and shoulder are affected first. Progression advances to muscles of the foot and hand. Involuntary muscles, such as the muscles of respiration, are affected last.
CN: Physiological integrity; CNS: Physiological adaptation; CL: Application

CN: Client needs category   CNS: Client needs subcategory   CL: Cognitive level

40. Which information should a nurse provide to the parents of child undergoing testing for the diagnosis of muscular dystrophy?
1. The genitals will be covered by a lead apron.
2. A local anesthetic will be used for the test.
3. Electrode wires will be attached to the scalp.
4. A fiber-optic endoscope will be inserted into a joint.

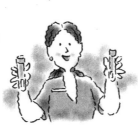

Question 41 asks which lab test helps in diagnosing the condition.

41. The nurse is reviewing the laboratory tests of a child diagnosed with muscular dystrophy. Which laboratory test would aid in the diagnosis of this condition?
1. Bilirubin
2. Creatinine
3. Serum potassium
4. Sodium

42. The nurse is teaching the student nurse about muscular dystrophy. The student nurse asks which form of muscular dystrophy is most common. Which response is most accurate?
1. Duchenne's
2. Becker's
3. Limb girdle
4. Myotonic

43. Which condition would alert the nurse that a child might be suffering from muscular dystrophy?
1. Hypertonia of extremities
2. Increased lumbar lordosis
3. Upper extremity spasticity
4. Hyperactive lower extremity reflexes

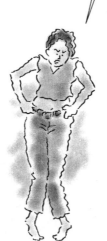

It's all in the jeans...I mean the genes.

44. The parents of a child with Duchenne's muscular dystrophy want to know how it is acquired. The most accurate response by the nurse would be which mechanism?
1. Virus
2. Hereditary
3. Autoimmune factors
4. Environmental toxins

40. 2. A muscle biopsy, used to confirm the diagnosis of muscular dystrophy, shows the degeneration of muscle fibers and infiltration of fatty tissue. It's typically performed using a local anesthetic. Genitals are covered by a lead apron during an X-ray examination which is used to detect osseous, not muscular, problems. Electrode wires are attached to the scalp during EEG to observe brain wave activity. It isn't used to diagnose muscular dystrophy. Arthroscopy involves the insertion of a fiber-optic scope into a joint and isn't used to diagnose muscular dystrophy.
CN: Physiological integrity; CNS: Basic care and comfort; CL: Application

41. 2. Creatinine values would aid in the diagnosis of muscular dystrophy. Creatinine is a by-product of muscle metabolism as it hypertrophies. Bilirubin is a by-product of liver function. Potassium and sodium levels can change due to various factors and aren't indicators of muscular dystrophy.
CN: Health promotion and maintenance; CNS: None; CL: Application

42. 1. Duchenne's, also known as pseudo-hypertrophic, accounts for 50% of all cases of muscular dystrophy. It affects cardiac and respiratory muscles, as well as all voluntary muscles.
CN: Physiological integrity; CNS: Physiological adaptation; CL: Application

43. 2. An increased lumbar lordosis would be seen in a child suffering from muscular dystrophy secondary to paralysis of lower lumbar postural muscles; it also occurs to increase lower extremity support. Hypertonia isn't seen in this disease. Upper extremity spasticity isn't seen because this disease isn't due to upper motor neuron lesions. Hyperactive reflexes aren't indications of muscular dystrophy.
CN: Physiological integrity; CNS: Physiological adaptation; CL: Analysis

44. 2. Muscular dystrophy is hereditary and acquired through a recessive sex-linked trait. Therefore, it isn't viral, autoimmune, or caused by toxins.
CN: Physiological integrity; CNS: Physiological adaptation; CL: Application

45. A client with muscular dystrophy has lost complete control of his lower extremities. He has some strength bilaterally in the upper extremities, but poor trunk control. Which mechanism would be the most important to have on the wheelchair?
  1. Antitip device
  2. Extended breaks
  3. Headrest support
  4. Wheelchair belt

46. A 2-year-old infant has muscular dystrophy. His legs are held together with the knees touching. Which muscles are contracted?
  1. Hip abductors
  2. Hip adductors
  3. Hip extensors
  4. Hip flexors

47. A 12-year-old child diagnosed with muscular dystrophy is hospitalized secondary to a fall. Surgery is necessary as well as skeletal traction. Which complication should be of <u>greatest concern</u> to the nursing staff?
  1. Skin integrity
  2. Infection of pin sites
  3. Respiratory infection
  4. Nonunion healing of the fracture

48. A nurse is talking with a 12-year-old boy and his parents about his osteogenesis imperfecta. Which is the best response by the nurse when the boy reports that he likes to swim?
  1. Tell him that he should also add a weight-bearing exercise.
  2. Tell him that swimming isn't safe since he can slip on the wet area around the pool.
  3. Tell him that he should restrict his exercise to only swimming.
  4. Tell him that any form of exercises isn't safe.

49. Which problem is most commonly encountered by adolescent females with scoliosis?
  1. Respiratory distress
  2. Poor self-esteem
  3. Poor appetite
  4. Renal difficulty

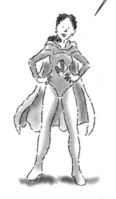

Question 45 tests your ability to ensure the client's safety.

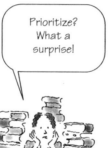

Prioritize? What a surprise!

45. 4. This client has poor trunk control; a belt will prevent him from falling out of the wheelchair. Antitip devices, head rest supports, and extended breaks are all important options but aren't the best choice in this situation.
CN: Safe, effective care environment; CNS: Safety and infection control; CL: Application

46. 2. The hip adductors are in a shortened position. The abductors are in a lengthened position. This position isn't indicative of hip flexor or hip extensor shortening.
CN: Health promotion and maintenance; CNS: None; CL: Application

47. 3. Respiratory infection can be fatal for clients with muscular dystrophy due to poor chest expansion and decreased ability to mobilize secretions. Skin integrity, infection of pin sites, and nonunion healing are important but not as important as prevention of respiratory infection.
CN: Physiological integrity; CNS: Reduction of risk potential; CL: Analysis

48. 1. Swimming is a beneficial form of exercise for people with osteogenesis imperfecta, but since it does little to prevent bone loss, the client should add a weight-bearing exercise. Although wet areas around the pool are a risk for the person with osteogenesis imperfecta, the risk can be minimized by walking carefully and wearing nonskid footwear. In the past, clients with osteogenesis imperfecta were told that exercise increased the risk of bone fractures. Mild forms of exercise are encouraged to promote bone density, cardiovascular conditioning, and to maintain joint mobility.
CN: Health promotion and maintenance; CNS: None; CL: Application

49. 2. Poor self-esteem is a major issue with many adolescents. The use of orthopedic appliances, such as those used to treat scoliosis, make this issue much more significant for adolescents with scoliosis. Although respiratory distress and poor appetite may surface, they aren't as common as self-esteem problems. Renal problems aren't usually an issue in adolescents with scoliosis.
CN: Health promotion and maintenance; CNS: None; CL: Application

CN: Client needs category   CNS: Client needs subcategory   CL: Cognitive level

50. A child has developed difficulty ambulating and tends to walk on his toes. Which surgical technique may benefit the client?
1. Adductor release
2. Hamstring release
3. Plantar fascia release
4. Achilles tendon release

51. The parents of a child with muscular dystrophy ask the nurse what causes this condition. The nurse responds that muscular dystrophy is a result of:
1. gene mutation.
2. chromosomal aberration.
3. unknown nongenetic origin.
4. environmental factors.

52. The nurse is assessing a child suspected of having muscular dystrophy for muscle weakness. At what age would evidence of muscle weakness associated with muscular dystrophy appear?
1. Age 1
2. Age 2
3. Age 3
4. Age 4

53. To promote safe transfers in a client with muscular dystrophy, a nurse should teach exercises to maintain which muscles?
1. Gastrocnemius
2. Gluteus maximus
3. Hamstrings
4. Quadriceps

54. Which of the following strategies would be the <u>first choice</u> in attempting to maximize function in a child with muscular dystrophy?
1. Long leg braces
2. Motorized wheelchair
3. Manual wheelchair
4. Walker

55. A child is having increased difficulty getting out of his chair at school. Which recommendation should the nurse make to assist the child?
1. A seat cushion
2. Long leg braces
3. Powered wheelchair
4. Removable arm rests on wheelchair

Hooray! You've reached question 50!

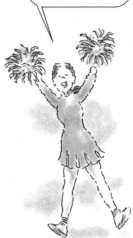

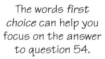

The words *first choice* can help you focus on the answer to question 54.

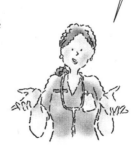

50. 4. A shortened Achilles tendon may cause a child to walk on his toes. A release of the tendon may assist the child in walking. An adductor release is commonly performed if the legs are held together. A plantar fascia release won't help, and a hamstring release is done only when there's a knee flexion contracture.
CN: Physiological integrity; CNS: Reduction of risk potential; CL: Application

51. 1. Muscular dystrophy is a result of a gene mutation. It isn't from a chromosome aberration or environmental factors. It's genetic, and there's a known origin of the disease.
CN: Physiological integrity; CNS: Physiological adaptation; CL: Application

52. 3. Studies have shown that children diagnosed with muscular dystrophy usually show some form of weakness around age 3.
CN: Health promotion and maintenance; CNS: None; CL: Application

53. 2. Gluteus maximus is the strongest muscle in the body and is important for standing as well as for transfers. All of the named muscles are important, but the maintenance of the gluteus maximus will enable maximum function.
CN: Health promotion and maintenance; CNS: None; CL: Application

54. 1. Long leg braces are functional assistive devices that provide increased independence and increased use of upper and lower body strength. Wheelchairs, both motorized and manual, provide less independence and less use of upper and lower body strength. Walkers are functional assistive devices that provide less independence than braces.
CN: Physiological integrity; CNS: Basic care and comfort; CL: Application

55. 1. A seat cushion will put the hip extensors at an advantage and make it somewhat easier to get up. Long leg braces wouldn't be the first choice. A powered wheelchair wouldn't be important in assisting with the transfer. Removable armrests have no bearing on assisting the client.
CN: Physiological integrity; CNS: Basic care and comfort; CL: Application

56. What findings would be expected while palpating the muscles of a child with muscular dystrophy?
1. Soft on palpation
2. Firm or woody on palpation
3. Extremely hard on palpation
4. No muscle consistency on palpation

57. A nurse should instruct a wheelchair-bound client with muscular dystrophy in which exercise to best prevent skin breakdown?
1. Wheelchair push-ups
2. Leaning side-to-side
3. Leaning forward
4. Gluteal sets

58. How would the nurse best describe <u>Gower's sign</u> to the parents of a child with muscular dystrophy?
1. A transfer technique
2. A waddling-type gait
3. The pelvis position during gait
4. Muscle twitching present during a quick stretch

59. A 13-year-old boy admitted with a fractured femur had an open reduction and internal fixation 2 days ago and currently is in traction. He asks the nurse what would happen to him if a terrorist decided to bomb the hospital. What's the nurse's best response?
1. "I wouldn't worry about that. Spend your energy on getting well and going home."
2. "We have plans to call your parents and take care of you if there's a problem."
3. "What do you think might happen if terrorists attack?"
4. "That's silly thinking. Why would anyone bomb a hospital?"

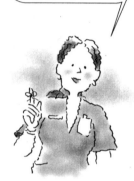

To remember Gower's sign, think going somewhere— that's a description of what the child is trying to do.

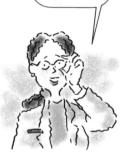

Focus on what response is best.

56. 2. Muscles will commonly be firm on palpation secondary to the infiltration of fatty tissue and connective tissue into the muscle. The muscles won't be soft secondary to the infiltration and won't be hard upon palpation. There's some consistency to the muscle although, in advanced stages, atrophy is present.
CN: Physiological integrity; CNS: Physiological adaptation; CL: Analysis

57. 1. A wheelchair push-up will alleviate the most pressure off the buttocks. Leaning side-to-side and leaning forward will help but not as much as wheelchair push-ups. Gluteal sets won't help with pressure relief.
CN: Health promotion and maintenance; CNS: None; CL: Application

58. 1. Gowers' sign is a description of a transfer technique present during some phases of muscular dystrophy. The child turns on the side or abdomen, extends the knees, and pushes on the torso to an upright position by walking his hands up the legs. Waddling-type gait doesn't describe Gowers' sign. The position of the pelvis during gait isn't described by Gowers' sign. Muscle twitching present after a quick stretch is described as *clonus*.
CN: Physiological integrity; CNS: Physiological adaptation; CL: Analysis

59. 3. Something prompted the child to ask such a question, and the nurse needs to take advantage of this opportunity to further explore his concerns and fears. Option 1 discounts the boy's feelings and may actually increase his anxiety. Although option 2 may be technically correct, it doesn't provide reassurance or help build a therapeutic relationship that can promote health and wellness. Option 4 is dismissive and childes the boy for asking the question.
CN: Physiological integrity; CNS: None; CL: Analysis

CN: Client needs category   CNS: Client needs subcategory   CL: Cognitive level

60. A client with bilateral fractured femurs is scheduled for a double-hip-spica cast. She says to the nurse, "Only 3 more months and I can go home." Further investigation reveals that the client and her family believe she'll be hospitalized until the cast comes off. The nurse should explain to the client and her family that the client:

1. may be hospitalized 2 to 4 months.
2. will go home 2 to 4 days after casting.
3. will go home 1 week after casting.
4. will go home as soon as she can move.

61. Which observation by a nurse indicates that an infant in a hip-spica cast is properly positioned?

1. The infant's upper body and cast are at a 180-degree angle.
2. The infant's hips are higher than the head.
3. The infant's upper body and the cast are at a 45-degree angle.
4. The infant is flat in bed.

62. The nurse receives a report on a child admitted with severe muscular dystrophy. The nurse suspects the child has been diagnosed with the most severe form of the disease, known as:

1. Duchenne's.
2. fascioscapulohumeral.
3. limb girdle.
4. myotonic.

63. Which finding should alert a nurse to a potential complication in a client with a cast following fracture of the radius?

1. Discomfort occurs at the site of the break.
2. Fingers are pink and warm.
3. Swelling is reduced with cast elevation.
4. Pain occurs over a bony prominence.

64. The parents of a child with newly diagnosed developmental dysplasia of the hip (DDH) ask the nurse how their child developed this condition. The nurse explains that the <u>greatest number</u> of cases is caused by which condition?

1. Dislocation
2. Subluxation
3. Acetabular dysplasia
4. Dislocation with fracture

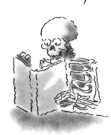

I know all about pain over a bony prominence.

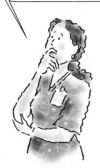

The greatest number of cases? This is getting complicated.

60. 2. The cast will dry fairly rapidly with the use of fiberglass casting material. The time spent in the hospital after casting, typically 2 to 4 days, will be for teaching the client and her family how to care for her at home and evaluating the client's skin integrity and neurovascular status before discharge. The timeframes in the other options given are inaccurate for a double-hip-spica cast.

CN: Health promotion and maintenance; CNS: None; CL: Application

61. 1. The infant's body and cast should be at a 180-degree angle. While the cast should be kept level with the body, it should be on a slant with the head of the bed elevated so that urine and stool can drain downward and not soil the cast.

CN: Physiological integrity; CNS: Basic care and comfort; CL: Application

62. 1. Studies have shown that Duchenne's is the most severe form of muscular dystrophy, affecting all voluntary muscles as well as cardiac and respiratory muscles.

CN: Physiological integrity; CNS: Physiological adaptation; CL: Analysis

63. 4. Pain over a bony prominence, such as in the wrist or elbow, signals an impending pressure ulcer and requires prompt attention. Pain or discomfort at the site of the fracture is expected and is relieved by analgesics. Warm and pink fingers are an expected finding. Swelling may be relieved by elevation of the extremity. Swelling that isn't relieved by elevation of the affected limb should be reported to the physician.

CN: Physiological integrity; CNS: Reduction of risk potential; CL: Application

64. 2. Studies show that subluxation accounts for the greatest number of cases of DDH.

CN: Physiological integrity; CNS: Physiological adaptation; CL: Application

65. Which finding would the nurse expect in a client with developmental dysplasia of the hip (DDH)?
1. Ligamentum teres is shortened.
2. Femoral head loses contact with acetabulum and is displaced inferiorly.
3. Femoral head loses contact with the acetabulum and is displaced posteriorly.
4. Femoral head maintains contact with acetabulum, but there's noted capsular rupture.

66. A toddler is immobilized with traction to the legs. Which play activity would be appropriate for this child?
1. Pounding board
2. Tinker toys
3. Pull toy
4. Board games

67. Which choice is best for handling a client's hip-spica cast that has been soiled?
1. Clean with damp cloth and dry cleanser.
2. Clean with soap and water.
3. Don't do anything.
4. Change the cast.

68. Which position is best for a child in a hip-spica cast who needs to be toileted?
1. Supine
2. Sitting in a toilet chair
3. Shoulder lower than buttocks
4. Buttocks lower than shoulder

69. Which intervention should a nurse perform in a 4-year-old child in Buck's traction?
1. Provide daily pin site care.
2. Release weights for 1 hour each day.
3. Change the child's position every 4 hours.
4. Unwrap the elastic bandage every shift to assess the skin.

Knowing the shape of a hip-spica cast can help answer this question.

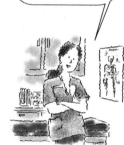

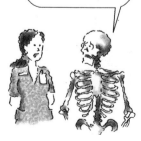

Pulling and pins? This doesn't sound like fun.

65. 3. In DDH, the femoral head loses contact with the acetabulum and is displaced posteriorly, not inferiorly. Ligamentum teres is lengthened.
CN: Physiological integrity; CNS: Physiological adaptation; CL: Application

66. 1. A pounding board is appropriate for an immobilized toddler because it promotes physical development and provides an acceptable energy outlet. Toys with small parts, such as tinker toys, aren't suitable because a toddler may swallow the parts. A pull toy is suitable for most toddlers, but not for one who is immobilized. Board games are usually too advanced for the developmental skills of a toddler.
CN: Health promotion and maintenance; CNS: None; CL: Application

67. 1. A damp cloth is best to use rather than water. Water will break the cast down. If nothing is done, the cast will give off an odor. Changing the cast isn't an option.
CN: Physiological integrity; CNS: Basic care and comfort; CL: Application

68. 4. The buttocks need to be lowered to toilet the child. This will keep the cast from being soiled. Supine will cause soiling of the cast. The child isn't able to use a toilet chair.
CN: Physiological integrity; CNS: Basic care and comfort; CL: Application

69. 1. Buck's traction is a form of skeletal traction which pulls directly on the skeleton using a pin placed into the bone. Pin site care involves cleaning the insertion sites to reduce the risk of infection and observing the site for signs and symptoms of infection. Weights should hang freely and shouldn't be released. The child's position should be changed every 2 hours to prevent skin breakdown. Elastic bandages are used in skin, not skeletal, traction.
CN: Physiological integrity; CNS: Basic care and comfort; CL: Application

CN: Client needs category   CNS: Client needs subcategory   CL: Cognitive level

70. The nurse observes a client who has a positive Trendelenburg gait. Which characteristic would indicate this gait?
1. Pelvis tilts downward upon weight bearing
2. Pelvis tilts upward upon weight bearing
3. Abnormal height of the iliac crests
4. Leg length discrepancy

71. Which complication involving leg length should a nurse anticipate in a client with developmental dysplasia of the hip?
1. Increased hip abduction
2. Increased leg length on the affected side
3. Decreased leg length on the affected side
4. No change in muscle length or leg length

72. A nurse recognizes that the parent of a child with developmental hip dysplasia needs more teaching when the parent places the child in a position that encourages:
1. hip abduction.
2. knee extension.
3. external rotation.
4. internal rotation.

73. Immediately after a spinal fusion, which restriction is usually put on the child's activity?
1. Supine bed rest
2. Non-weight bearing
3. No restriction
4. Limited weight bearing

74. Which intervention should a nurse expect to use to prevent venous stasis after skeletal traction application?
1. Bed rest only
2. Convoluted foam mattress
3. Vigorous pulmonary care
4. Antiembolism stockings or an intermittent compression device

75. A 13-year-old girl is suspected of having structural scoliosis by her school nurse. What should the nurse ask the girl to do to help confirm her suspicion?
1. Bend over and touch her toes while the nurse observes from the back.
2. Stand sideways while the nurse observes her profile.
3. Assume a knee-chest position on the examination table.
4. Arch her back while the nurse observes her from the back.

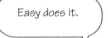
Easy does it.

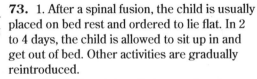

70. 1. The pelvis will tilt downward upon weight bearing secondary to a weakness of the abductors on the affected side. The pelvis doesn't tilt upward. Leg length and iliac crest height aren't indicative of Trendelenburg gait.
CN: Physiological integrity; CNS: Physiological adaptation; CL: Application

71. 3. The internal rotation with subsequent dislocation will cause the leg to be shorter, not longer. There's usually *decreased* abduction as well as muscle and leg length changes.
CN: Physiological integrity; CNS: Physiological adaptation; CL: Analysis

72. 4. Internal rotation increases the risk of hip dislocation. Abduction, external rotation, and knee extension won't increase the risk of dislocation.
CN: Health promotion and maintenance; CNS: None; CL: Application

73. 1. After a spinal fusion, the child is usually placed on bed rest and ordered to lie flat. In 2 to 4 days, the child is allowed to sit up in and get out of bed. Other activities are gradually reintroduced.
CN: Physiological integrity; CNS: Basic care and comfort; CL: Application

74. 4. To prevent venous stasis after skeletal traction application, antiembolism stockings or an intermittent compression device is used on the unaffected leg. Bed rest can *cause* venous stasis. Convoluted foam mattresses and pulmonary care don't prevent venous stasis.
CN: Health promotion and maintenance; CNS: None; CL: Application

75. 1. As the child bends over, the curvature of the spine is more apparent. The scapula on one side becomes more prominent, and the opposite side hollows. The knee-chest position is used for lumbar puncture. Scoliosis can't be properly assessed from the side or the front.
CN: Health promotion and maintenance; CNS: None; CL: Application

76. At the scene of a trauma, which nursing intervention is appropriate for a child with a suspected fracture?
1. Never move the child.
2. Sit the child up to facilitate breathing.
3. Move the child to a safe place immediately.
4. Immobilize the extremity and then move child to a safe place.

77. A nurse is assessing an 18-month-old infant who's in Bryant's traction for a fractured left femur. The infant is properly positioned when:
1. the left leg is extended 90 degrees off the bed.
2. the right leg is extended 90 degrees off the bed.
3. both legs are extended 90 degrees off the bed.
4. both legs are extended at 180 degrees with the upper body.

78. A child in skeletal traction for a fracture of the right femur exhibits a positive Homans' sign, complains of left-sided leg pain, and has edema in the left leg. A nurse should further assess the child for which condition?
1. A fat emboli
2. An infection
3. A pulmonary embolism
4. Deep vein thrombosis (DVT)

79. Nursing care for a client in traction may include which intervention?
1. Assessing pin sites every shift and as needed
2. Ensuring that the rope knots catch on the pulley
3. Adding and removing weights per client's request
4. Placing all joints through range of motion (ROM) every shift

80. After assisting the primary health care provider in applying a cast, a nurse should include which intervention in the immediate cast care?
1. Rest the cast on the bedside table
2. Dispose of the plaster water in the sink
3. Support the cast with her palms
4. Wait until the cast dries before cleaning surrounding skin

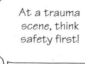

At a trauma scene, think safety first!

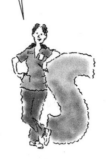

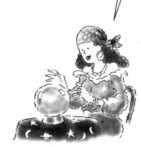

Is Homans' sign an astrological sign?

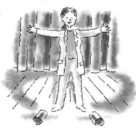

Your performance has been Oscar winning so far. Good luck!!

76. 4. At the scene of a trauma, the nurse should immobilize the extremity of a child with a suspected fracture and then move him to a safe place. If the child is already in a safe place, don't attempt to move him. Never try to sit the child up; this could make the fracture worse.
CN: Safe, effective care environment; CNS: Safety and infection control; CL: Application

77. 3. Bryant's traction, a type of skin traction, is for lower extremity fractures in children younger than age 2 years. Both legs are suspended at 90 degrees off the bed, even though only one is fractured, with the child's body weight providing the countertraction.
CN: Physiological integrity; CNS: Basic care and comfort; CL: Application

78. 4. Unilateral leg pain and edema with a positive Homans' sign (not always present) should lead you to suspect DVT. Symptoms of fat emboli include restlessness, tachypnea, and tachycardia and are more common in long bone injuries. It's unlikely that an infection would occur on the opposite side of the fracture without cause. Tachycardia, chest pain, and shortness of breath may be symptoms of a pulmonary embolism.
CN: Physiological integrity; CNS: Reduction of risk potential; CL: Analysis

79. 1. Nursing care for a client in traction may include assessing pin sites every shift and as needed and ensuring that the knots in the rope don't catch on the pulley. Weights should be added and removed per the primary health care provider's order, and all joints, except those immediately proximal and distal to the fracture, should be placed through ROM every shift.
CN: Physiological integrity; CNS: Basic care and comfort; CL: Application

80. 3. After a cast has been applied, it should be immediately supported with the palms of the nurse's hands. Later, the nurse should dispose of the plaster water in a sink with a plaster trap or in a garbage bag, clean the surrounding skin before the cast dries, and make sure that the cast isn't resting on a hard or sharp surface.
CN: Physiological integrity; CNS: Reduction of risk potential; CL: Application

CN: Client needs category   CNS: Client needs subcategory   CL: Cognitive level

81. A school-age child tells a nurse that he's experiencing intense itching from under his cast. What's the most appropriate response for the nurse to make?

    1. "Toughen up, there's nothing that can be done."

    2. "Place the eraser-end of a new pencil under the cast to scratch."

    3. "Elevate the cast above the level of your heart."

    4. "Aim cool air from a hair dryer under the cast."

82. Which nursing intervention should be taken if, while a cast is drying, the client complains of heat from the cast?

    1. Remove the cast immediately.

    2. Notify the primary health care provider.

    3. Assess the client for other signs of infection.

    4. Explain to the client that this is a normal sensation.

83. Which nursing intervention can be implemented to <u>prevent</u> foot drop in a casted leg?

    1. Encourage bed rest.

    2. Support the foot with 45 degrees of flexion.

    3. Support the foot with 90 degrees of flexion.

    4. Place a stocking on the foot to provide warmth.

84. A client with a hip-spica cast should avoid gas-forming foods for which reason?

    1. To prevent flatus

    2. To prevent diarrhea

    3. To prevent constipation

    4. To prevent abdominal distention

85. A nurse determines that a client with a fractured left femur understands the instructions for touch-down weight bearing when he makes which statement?

    1. "I will place full weight on my left leg."

    2. "I will place about 30% to 50% of my weight on my left leg."

    3. "I will keep my left leg off the floor."

    4. "I will allow my left leg to touch the floor without placing weight on it."

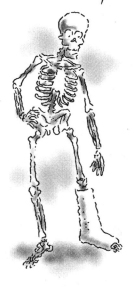

Can you help me prevent foot drop?

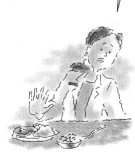

My eyes are bigger than my stomach…or not.

81. 4. Cool air from a hair dryer may soothe the itchiness. Telling the child to toughen up isn't therapeutic, erodes the nurse-client relationship, and isn't true since cool air may relieve itchiness. Nothing should be placed under a cast because this can cause skin irritation and breakdown. Elevating the cast above the heart doesn't relieve itching. This position is used to reduce swelling.

CN: Physiological integrity; CNS: Basic care and comfort; CL: Application

82. 4. Normally, as the cast is drying, the client may complain of heat from the cast. The nurse should offer reassurance but doesn't need to notify the primary health care provider or remove the cast. Heat from the cast isn't a sign of infection.

CN: Physiological integrity; CNS: Reduction of risk potential; CL: Application

83. 3. To prevent foot drop in a casted leg, the foot should be supported with 90 degrees of flexion. Bed rest can cause foot drop. Keeping the extremity warm won't prevent foot drop.

CN: Health promotion and maintenance; CNS: None; CL: Application

84. 4. A client with a hip spica cast should avoid gas-forming foods to prevent abdominal distention. Gas-forming foods may cause flatus, but that isn't a reason to avoid them. Gas-forming foods don't generally cause diarrhea or constipation.

CN: Physiological integrity; CNS: Reduction of risk potential; CL: Application

85. 4. Touch-down weight bearing allows the client to put no weight on the extremity, but the client may touch the floor with the affected extremity. Full weight bearing allows for full weight bearing on the affected extremity. Partial weight bearing allows for only 30% to 50% weight bearing on the affected extremity. Non-weight bearing is no weight on the extremity, and the extremity must remain elevated.

CN: Physiological integrity; CNS: Basic care and comfort; CL: Application

86. Which strategy should a nurse teach an adolescent to prevent sports-related injuries?
1. Warming up
2. Pacing activity
3. Building strength
4. Moderating intensity

87. Which activity may be most helpful for a child who's allowed full activity after repair of a clubfoot?
1. Playing catch
2. Standing
3. Swimming
4. Walking

88. Which statement by the parent of an infant diagnosed with clubfoot indicates understanding of the casting treatment regimen?
1. "The cast will come off in 8 weeks."
2. "The cast will come off in 2 weeks."
3. "The cast will come off when my child starts to walk."
4. "The cast will come off when my child starts to crawl."

89. The X-ray result for a child who experienced a fall on the basketball court indicates a greenstick fracture of the tibia. Which graphic represents a greenstick fracture?

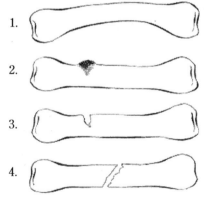

1.
2.
3.
4.

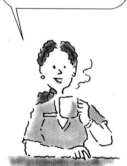

This warming-up activity should keep me awake for the rest of the test.

86. 1. To prevent sports-related injuries, instruct your client that the best prevention is warming up. Pacing activity, building strength, and using moderate intensity are also prevention measures.
CN: Health promotion and maintenance; CNS: None; CL: Application

87. 4. Walking will stimulate all of the involved muscles and help with strengthening. All of the options are good exercises, but walking is the best choice.
CN: Health promotion and maintenance; CNS: None; CL: Application

88. 2. Because an infant grows quickly, a series of casts will be needed as often as every 2 weeks to correct the deformity as the child grows. Eight weeks is too long to leave a cast on the rapidly growing child. Casting should be complete by the time the child is crawling and walking.
CN: Physiological integrity; CNS: Reduction of risk potential; CL: Analysis

89. 3. A greenstick fracture occurs when the bone is bent beyond its limits, causing an incomplete fracture. The first graphic is a plastic deformation or bend, where there is a microscopic fracture line where the bone bends. The second graphic shows a buckle fracture which occurs due to compression of the porous bone, causing a raised area or bulge at the fracture site. The fourth graphic is of a complete fracture in which the bone is broken into separate pieces.
CN: Physiological integrity; CNS: Physiological adaptation; CL: Application

CN: Client needs category   CNS: Client needs subcategory   CL: Cognitive level

90. Which instruction should be included in the teaching plan for a 10-year-old with a fracture of the radial bone?
1. Report capillary refill less than 3 seconds.
2. Report warmth under the cast during the first 24 hours after application.
3. Report foul odors coming from the cast.
4. Report cool fingers that warm within 20 minutes of being covered.

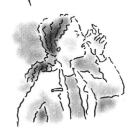

The nose knows the answer to this question.

90. 3. Foul odors from the cast may be a sign of infection and should be reported to the physician immediately. Capillary refill less than 3 seconds is a normal finding. During the first 24 hours, the client may feel warmth under the cast as it dries. After 24 hours, warmth may be a sign of infection and should be reported. Cool fingers that warm up within 20 minutes of being covered is normal; cool fingers that don't warm up after 20 minutes of being covered should be reported because the client may have circulatory impairment under the cast.
CN: Physiological integrity; CNS: Reduction of risk potential; CL: Application

91. Which history finding is the <u>most significant</u> related to developmental dysplasia of the hip (DDH)?
1. Mother's activity during the third trimester
2. Breech presentation at birth
3. Infant's serum calcium level at birth
4. Apgar score of 4 at 1 minute and 6 at 5 minutes

91. 2. Breech presentation is a factor commonly associated with DDH. The mother's activity during the third trimester, the infant's serum calcium level at birth, and Apgar scores have no bearing on DDH.
CN: Health promotion and maintenance; CNS: None; CL: Application

92. A 13-year-old with structural scoliosis has Harrington rods inserted. Which position would be best during the postoperative period?
1. Supine in bed
2. Side-lying
3. Semi-Fowler's
4. High Fowler's

92. 1. After placement of Harrington rods, the client must remain flat in bed. The gatch on a manual bed should be taped, and electric beds should be unplugged to prevent the client from raising the head or foot of the bed. Other positions, such as side-lying, semi-Fowler's, or high Fowler's, could prove damaging because the rods may not be able to maintain the spine in a straight position.
CN: Physiological integrity; CNS: Reduction of risk potential; CL: Application

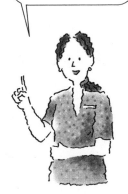

Remember you're looking for the nursing diagnosis with the *highest* priority.

93. A nurse notes dyspnea and calf pain in a 14-year-old client 48 hours after open reduction of a fractured femur. Which nursing diagnosis has the <u>highest priority</u>?
1. *Impaired gas exchange*
2. *Acute pain*
3. *Impaired physical mobility*
4. *Deficient knowledge*

93. 1. Immobility, a fractured femur, and orthopedic surgery all increase the risk of deep vein thrombosis (DVT). The client who complains of calf pain and dyspnea should be promptly assessed for a pulmonary embolism. While all these nursing diagnoses are appropriate, assessing for *Impaired gas exchange* has the highest priority.
CN: Physiological integrity; CNS: Reduction of risk potential; CL: Analysis

94. A 6-month-old male with developmental dysplasia of the hip has been treated for the past 6 weeks with a Frejka splint, which maintains abduction through padding of the diaper area. At his follow-up visit, the child's mother reports that she removes the splint when he gets too fussy and that he settles down and sleeps well for several hours after the padding is removed. Which response by the nurse would be most appropriate?

    1. "I can tell you're concerned about his comfort, but he must wear the padded splint except during the three times per day when you perform range-of-motion exercises on his legs."

    2. "I'm pleased that you recognize that the padding is too thick and have adjusted it so he can sleep comfortably."

    3. "I realize that seeing him uncomfortable is difficult for you, but he needs to keep his splint on except when you bathe him or change his diaper."

    4. "If he seems uncomfortable while wearing the splint, it's important that you call us immediately."

95. A nurse is caring for a 2-year-old child who weighs 25 lb (11.3 kg) and has a simple fracture of his femur. For this client, which <u>initial</u> treatment is <u>most</u> likely?

    1. Setting the fracture with a pin during surgery

    2. Placing the child in skeletal traction

    3. Immediately setting and casting the fractured leg

    4. Putting the child in Bryant's traction

96. A female client, age 15 months, has just had a hip-spica cast applied. Which nursing intervention is a <u>priority</u> for this client?

    1. Limit fluids so she won't urinate often and won't risk getting the cast wet.

    2. Instruct the parents on how to get their child home in the car.

    3. Assess sensation, circulation, and motion of her feet and toes.

    4. Avoid giving her pain medication so she won't become constipated.

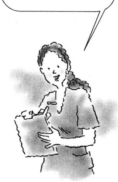

Questions 95 and 96 are asking you to prioritize!

94. 3. Soft abduction devices, such as the Frejka splint, must be worn continually except for diaper changes and skin care. The abduction position must be maintained to establish a deep hip socket. Discomfort is anticipated; appropriate responses including changing position, holding, cuddling, and providing diversion.

CN: Physiological integrity; CNS: Physiological adaptation; CL: Application

95. 4. Bryant's traction is the usual method for treating a child younger than age 3 and weighing less than 35 lb (15.9 kg). Surgery and pin placement is an invasive treatment that isn't usually needed. Skeletal traction is used for older children. For a femur fracture to heal properly, it usually requires traction before casting.

CN: Physiological integrity; CNS: Reduction of risk potential; CL: Application

96. 3. Assessing sensation, circulation, and motion is necessary in all children with a cast. Fluids should be encouraged; careful diapering and padding will keep the cast dry. Instructions about discharge can be shared with the parents at a later date. Children experiencing pain should receive medication as needed.

CN: Safe, effective care environment; CNS: Management of care; CL: Application

97. A male client, age 16, was injured in a motorcycle accident and fractured his left tibia and fibula. He's in a long leg cast and complains of deep pain unrelieved by analgesics. The physician must be notified immediately because the client may be exhibiting the signs and symptoms of which condition?

1. Volkmann's contracture
2. Dupuytren's contracture
3. Compartment syndrome
4. Peroneal nerve compression

98. A 6-year-old boy is admitted to a pediatric unit for treatment of osteomyelitis. The nurse knows that the peak incidence in children is between ages 1 and 12 and that boys are affected two to three times more commonly than girls. Which organism most commonly causes osteomyelitis?

1. *Staphylococcus epidermidis*
2. *Escherichia coli* O157.H7
3. *Pneumocystis carinii*
4. *Staphylococcus aureus*

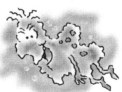

I admit it! I'm the common cause.

99. A 14-year-old girl was recently fitted with a full back brace for scoliosis. Which response by the girl indicates she understands when she must wear the brace.

1. "I can leave the brace off for school parties."
2. "I have to wear the brace all the time, except when bathing."
3. "I can take the brace off for a couple of hours if my back starts to hurt."
4. "I only have to wear the brace for a couple of weeks."

97. 3. Deep pain unrelieved by analgesics is an important sign of compartment syndrome, which may occur with a crush injury or when a fracture is reduced. Compartment syndrome occurs when swelling associated with inflammation reduces blood flow to the affected areas; casting causes additional constriction of blood flow. Volkmann's contracture is a contraction of the fingers and sometimes the wrist that occurs after severe injury or improper use of a tourniquet or cast. Dupuytren's contracture is a flexion deformity of the fingers or toes caused by shortening, thickening, and fibrosis of the palmar or plantar fascia. Peroneal nerve compression is compression of the nerve that innervates the calf and foot.

CN: Physiological integrity; CNS: Physiological adaptation; CL: Analysis

98. 4. *S. aureus* is the most common causative pathogen of osteomyelitis; the usual source of the infection is an upper respiratory infection. *S. epidermidis* is a microorganism found on the skin of healthy individuals. *E. coli* O157.H7, which is in uncooked meat, can cause a severe case of diarrhea. *P. carinii* causes pneumonia in clients with human immunodeficiency virus or acquired immunodeficiency syndrome but doesn't normally cause healthy individuals to become ill.

CN: Physiological integrity; CNS: Physiological adaptation; CL: Application

99. 2. A brace must be worn at all times except for bathing. It can't be removed for other reasons including parties and discomfort. Most braces must be worn for several months to 1 year.

CN: Physiological integrity; CNS: Reduction of risk potential; CL: Analysis

100. A 16-year-old client had a full body cast applied 3 days ago. She's diaphoretic, tachycardic, and tachypneic. Which condition is the client <u>most likely</u> experiencing?
 1. Pneumonia
 2. Compartment syndrome
 3. Anxiety
 4. Decreased intestinal motility

100. 3. The client is exhibiting signs and symptoms of anxiety most likely caused by the feeling of being claustrophobic. Pneumonia usually presents with fever and coughing. A client with compartment syndrome would exhibit signs of intense pain unrelieved by analgesics. Compression of the mesenteric blood supply can cause constipation, but the symptoms don't indicate that constipation is the most likely condition.
CN: Psychological integrity; CNS: Psychological adaptation; CL: Analysis

101. A nurse is preparing to give an I.M. injection into the left leg of a 2-year-old client. Identify the area where the nurse would give the injection.

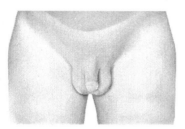

101. The vastus lateralis muscle, located in the thigh, is the muscle into which the nurse should administer an I.M. injection for a toddler. To give the injection, the nurse should first divide the distance between the greater trochanter and the knee joints into quadrants, then inject in the center of the upper quadrant.
CN: Physiological integrity; CNS: Pharmacological and parenteral therapies; CL: Application

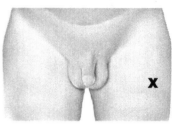

102. A nurse is caring for a 5-year-old client who's in the terminal stages of cancer. Which statements are true? Select all that apply:
 1. The parents may be at different stages in dealing with the child's impending death.
 2. The child is thinking about the future and knows he may not be able to participate.
 3. The dying child may become clingy and act like a toddler.
 4. Whispering in the child's room will help the child cope.
 5. The death of a child may have long-term disruptive effects on the family.
 6. The child doesn't fully understand the concept of death.

102. 1, 3, 5, 6. When dealing with a dying child, parents may be at different stages of grief at different times. The child may regress in his behaviors. The stress of a child's death commonly results in divorce and behavioral problems in siblings. Preschoolers see death as temporary, a type of sleep or separation. They recognize the word "dead" but don't fully understand its meaning. Thinking about the future is typical of an adolescent facing death, not a preschooler. Whispering in front of the child only increases his fear of death.
CN: Psychosocial integrity; CNS: None; CL: Analysis

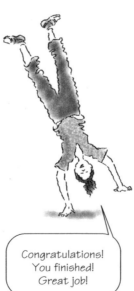

Congratulations! You finished! Great job!

CN: Client needs category   CNS: Client needs subcategory   CL: Cognitive level

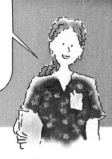

I'll bet that when you started nursing school, you had no idea kids could be subject to so many GI disorders. This chapter tests you on the most common ones. Good luck!

Chapter 19
Gastrointestinal system

1. Which statement by the mother of a child with celiac disease indicates an understanding of a nurse's dietary counseling?
  1. "I won't serve wheat, rye, oats, or barley."
  2. "I will provide a diet high in gluten."
  3. "I won't serve potatoes, rice, or flour."
  4. "I can safely serve any frozen or packaged food."

2. Which goal is <u>most important</u> when teaching the parents of a child diagnosed with celiac disease?
  1. Promote a normal life for the child.
  2. Stress the importance of good health in preventing infection.
  3. Introduce the parents and child to a peer with celiac disease.
  4. Help the parents and child follow the prescribed dietary restrictions.

3. What characteristic stool would a nurse expect to find in a child diagnosed with celiac disease?
  1. Constipated hard stool
  2. Clay-colored stool
  3. Red currant jelly stool
  4. Foul-smelling, fatty, frothy stool

4. A client with celiac disease is being discharged from the hospital. Which food item should be included in his diet?
  1. Oatmeal cereal
  2. Sliced pepperoni
  3. Cheese pizza
  4. Rice

In question 2, the words *most important* guide you to the right answer.

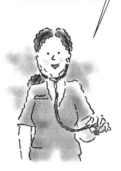

1. 1. The child with celiac disease should consume a gluten-free diet, thus eliminating foods containing wheat, rye, oats, and barley. Foods containing potatoes, rice, and flour are permissible. The mother should read the packages of all foods carefully to ensure that they're gluten-free.
CN: Physiological integrity; CNS: Basic care and comfort; CL: Application

2. 4. It takes a long time to describe the disease process, the specific role of gluten, and the foods that must be restricted. Gluten is added to many foods but is obscurely listed on labels. To avoid hidden sources of gluten, parents need to read labels carefully. Promoting a normal life for the child, stressing good health in preventing infection, and meeting a peer with celiac disease are also important nursing considerations, but they would come after the dietary means of dealing with this chronic disease.
CN: Physiological integrity; CNS: Reduction of risk potential; CL: Analysis

3. 4. Steatorrhea (fatty, foul-smelling frothy, bulky stools) is common because of the inability to absorb fat. Profuse and watery diarrhea, not constipated hard stool, is usually a sign or celiac crisis. Clay-colored stools are characteristic of a decrease or absence of conjugated bilirubin. Red currant jelly type stool is an indication of intussusception.
CN: Physiological integrity; CNS: Physiological adaptation; CL: Application

4. 4. Sources of gluten found in wheat, rye, barley, and oats should be avoided. Rice and corn are suitable substitutes because they don't contain gluten. Pizza, luncheon meat, and cereal contain gluten and, when broken down, can't be digested by people with celiac disease.
CN: Physiological integrity; CNS: Basic care and comfort; CL: Application

CN: Client needs category   CNS: Client needs subcategory   CL: Cognitive level

5. To help promote a normal life for a child with celiac disease, which intervention should his parents use?

    1. Treat the child differently from other siblings.
    2. Focus on restrictions that make him feel different.
    3. Introduce the child to another peer with celiac disease.
    4. Don't allow the child to express doubt in keeping with dietary restrictions.

6. Which assessment should a nurse make to evaluate the effectiveness of nutritional therapy for a child with celiac disease?

    1. Vital signs
    2. Appearance, size, and number of stools
    3. Blood urea nitrogen (BUN) and serum creatinine levels
    4. Intake and output

7. Within 1 or 2 days after starting their prescribed diet, most children with celiac disease show which characteristic?

    1. Diarrhea
    2. Foul-smelling stools
    3. Improved appetite
    4. Weight loss

8. In caring for a neonate with cleft lip and palate, which issue is <u>first</u> encountered by the nurse?

    1. Feeding difficulties
    2. Operative care
    3. Pain management
    4. Parental reaction

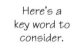

You'll be finished before you know it!

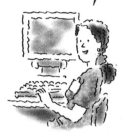

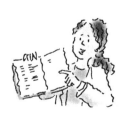

Here's a key word to consider.

5. 3. Introducing the child to another child with celiac disease will let him know he isn't alone. It will show him how other people live a normal life with similar restrictions. Treat the child no differently from other siblings, but stress appropriate limit setting. Instead of focusing on restrictions that make him feel different, the nurse should encourage the parents to focus on ways he can be normal. Allow the child with celiac disease to express his feelings about dietary restrictions.
CN: Psychosocial integrity; CNS: None; CL: Application

6. 2. The fat, bulky, foul-smelling stools should be gone when a child with celiac disease follows a gluten-free diet. Vital signs, BUN and serum creatinine levels, and intake and output aren't affected by a gluten-free diet.
CN: Physiological integrity; CNS: Basic care and comfort; CL: Analysis

7. 3. Within a day or two of starting their diet, most children with celiac disease show improved appetite, disappearance of diarrhea, and weight gain. It takes longer than 2 days for steatorrhea (fatty, oily, foul-smelling stools) to subside.
CN: Physiological integrity; CNS: Physiological adaptation; CL: Application

8. 4. Parents typically show strong negative responses to this deformity. They may mourn the loss of the perfect child. Helping the parents cope with their child's condition is the first step. Feeding issues are important, but parents must first cope with the reality of their neonate's condition. Surgical repair is usually delayed until 6 to 12 weeks of age. This deformity isn't painful.
CN: Psychosocial integrity; CNS: None; CL: Analysis

CN: Client needs category   CNS: Client needs subcategory   CL: Cognitive level

9. To prevent trauma to the suture line of an infant who underwent cleft lip repair, a nurse should perform which intervention?
1. Place mittens on the infant's hands.
2. Maintain arm restraints.
3. Not allow the parents to touch the infant.
4. Remove the lip device from the infant after surgery.

10. To prevent tissue infection and breakdown after cleft palate or lip repair, a nurse should use which intervention?
1. Keep the suture line moist at all times.
2. Allow the infant to suck on his pacifier.
3. Rinse the infant's mouth with water after each feeding.
4. Follow orders from the physician to not feed the infant by mouth.

11. Which nursing intervention has the highest priority in an infant during the first 24 hours after surgery for cleft lip repair?
1. Carefully clean the suture line using sterile technique after feedings to reduce the risk of infection.
2. Position the infant in the prone position after feedings to promote drainage.
3. Allow the infant to cry to promote lung expansion.
4. Encourage the infant to use a pacifier to satisfy the urge to suck.

12. When bottle-feeding an infant with a cleft palate or lip, gentle steady pressure should be applied to the base of the bottle for which reason?
1. To reduce the risk of choking or coughing
2. To prevent further damage to the affected area
3. To decrease the amount of formula lost while eating
4. To decrease the amount of noise the infant makes when eating

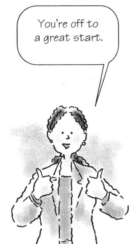

You're off to a great start.

9. 2. Arm restraints are used to prevent the infant from rubbing the sutures. Placing mittens alone won't prevent the infant from rubbing the suture line. Parental contact will increase the infant's comfort. The lip device shouldn't be removed.
CN: Physiological integrity; CNS: Reduction of risk potential; CL: Analysis

10. 3. To prevent formula buildup around the suture line, the mouth is usually rinsed. The sutures should be kept dry at all times. Placing objects in the mouth is generally avoided after surgery. Infants are fed by mouth using the syringe technique.
CN: Physiological integrity; CNS: Physiological adaptation; CL: Analysis

11. 1. The suture line must be cleaned after each feeding to reduce the risk of infection, which could adversely affect the healing and cosmetic results. The incision should be cleaned carefully so the sutures are not disrupted. A sterile solution should be used to reduce the risk of infection. The infant shouldn't be placed on his abdomen in the prone position because this puts pressure on the incision and may affect healing. Anticipatory care should be provided to reduce the risk of the infant crying, which puts pressure on the incision. Pacifiers and other firm objects shouldn't be placed in the infant's mouth because they can disrupt the suture line.
CN: Physiological integrity; CNS: Reduction of risk potential; CL: Application

12. 1. Children with cleft palate or lip have a greater risk of choking while eating, so all measures are used to reduce this risk. Steady pressure creates a seal when the nipple is against the cleft palate or lip, reducing the risk of aspiration. The nurse can't cause more damage to an infant's cleft lip or palate unless proper precautions aren't followed postoperatively. If the nipple is cut correctly and proper procedures are followed, the infant won't lose a lot of formula during a feeding. Infants with cleft palate or lip usually make more noise while eating.
CN: Physiological integrity; CNS: Reduction of risk potential; CL: Application

13. Which nursing intervention should be used when feeding an infant with cleft lip and palate?
1. Burp the infant often.
2. Limit the amount the infant eats.
3. Feed the infant at scheduled times.
4. Remove the nipple if the infant is making loud noises.

14. Which intervention is essential in the nursing care of an infant with cleft lip or palate?
1. Discourage breast-feeding.
2. Hold the infant flat while feeding.
3. Involve the parents as soon as possible.
4. Use a normal nursery nipple for feedings.

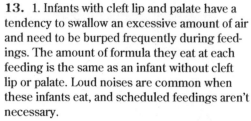

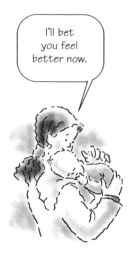

15. The parents of an infant born with cleft lip and palate are seeing the infant for the first time. The nurse caring for the infant should focus on which area?
1. The infant's positive features
2. Irritation with how the infant eats
3. Ambivalence in caring for an infant with this defect
4. Dissatisfaction with the infant's physical appearance

16. Following repair of a cleft lip in a 3-month-old, the mother asks the nurse what would be the most appropriate toy to bring the infant. Which toy should the nurse recommend?
1. A plastic teething ring
2. A stuffed animal
3. A mobile to hang over the crib
4. Children's books

13. 1. Infants with cleft lip and palate have a tendency to swallow an excessive amount of air and need to be burped frequently during feedings. The amount of formula they eat at each feeding is the same as an infant without cleft lip or palate. Loud noises are common when these infants eat, and scheduled feedings aren't necessary.
CN: Physiological integrity; CNS: Physiological adaptation; CL: Application

14. 3. The sooner the parents become involved, the quicker they're able to determine the method of feeding best suited for them and the infant. Breast-feeding, like bottle-feeding, may be difficult but can be facilitated if the mother intends to breast-feed. Feedings are usually given in the upright position to prevent formula from coming through the nose. Various special nipples have been devised for infants with cleft lip or palate; a normal nursery nipple isn't effective. Sometimes, especially if the cleft isn't severe, breast-feeding may be easier because the human nipple conforms to the shape of the infant's mouth.
CN: Physiological integrity; CNS: Physiological adaptation; CL: Application

15. 1. To relieve the parents' anxiety, positive aspects of the infant's physical appearance need to be emphasized. Showing optimism toward surgical correction and showing a photograph of possible cosmetic improvements may be helpful. Because this is the parents' first encounter with the infant, there isn't any indication of irritation, ambivalence, or dissatisfaction.
CN: Psychosocial integrity; CNS: None; CL: Application

16. 3. Given the infant's age, a mobile would be the most appropriate toy because he doesn't have the manual dexterity to play with a stuffed animal. The mobile would provide the infant with visual stimulation. A plastic teething ring and a stuffed animal should be avoided because they can disrupt the suture line if the infant sucks on them. The infant wouldn't be able to understand children's stories but may enjoy the sound of another person's voice. A mobile, however, could be used when no one was around to read.
CN: Physiological integrity; CNS: None; CL: Analysis

CN: Client needs category   CNS: Client needs subcategory   CL: Cognitive level

17. The mother of a neonate born with a cleft lip and palate is preparing to feed him for the first time. Which intervention should the nurse teach the mother <u>first</u>?
1. Burp the neonate.
2. Clean the mouth.
3. Hold the neonate in an upright position.
4. Prepare the bottle using a normal nursery nipple.

18. An infant returns from surgery after repair of a cleft palate. Which nursing intervention should be done first?
1. Offer a pacifier for comfort.
2. Position the infant on his side.
3. Suction the mouth and nose of all secretions.
4. Remove the arm restraints placed on the infant after surgery.

19. A small child has just had surgical repair of a cleft palate. Which instruction should be included in the discharge teaching to his parents?
1. Continue a normal diet.
2. Continue using arm restraints at home.
3. Don't allow the child to drink from a cup.
4. Establish good mouth care and proper brushing.

20. In which position should a nurse place an infant following cleft lip and palate repair to irrigate the mouth after feeding?
1. Supine with the head to the side
2. Fowler's position with the head to the side
3. Upright with the head tilted forward
4. Prone with the head over the side of the bed

21. After an infant with a cleft lip has surgical repair and heals, the nurse would instruct the parents that they may see:
1. a large scar on the lip.
2. an abnormally large upper lip.
3. a distorted jaw.
4. minimal scarring.

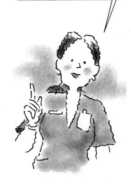

There are many things to teach this mother, so what do you teach her first?

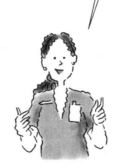

Client teaching includes the family.

17. 3. When neonates are held in the upright position, the formula is less likely to leak out of the nose or mouth. Neonates need to be burped frequently but not before a feeding. There's no need to clean the mouth before eating. After surgical repair, the mouth is cleaned at the suture site to prevent infection. The bottle should be prepared using a special nipple or feeding device.
CN: Physiological integrity; CNS: Physiological adaptation; CL: Application

18. 2. The infant should be positioned on his side to allow oral secretions to drain from the mouth and avoid suctioning. Pacifiers shouldn't be used because they can damage the suture line. Arm restraints should be kept on to protect the suture line. The restraints should be removed periodically to allow for full range of motion during this time. Only one restraint should be removed at a time, and the infant should be closely supervised.
CN: Physiological integrity; CNS: Reduction of risk potential; CL: Analysis

19. 2. Arm restraints are also used at home to keep the child's hands away from the mouth until the palate is healed. A soft diet is recommended; no food harder than mashed potatoes can be eaten. Fluids are best taken from a cup. Proper mouth care is encouraged after the palate is healed.
CN: Physiological integrity; CNS: Physiological adaptation; CL: Application

20. 3. Following repair of a cleft palate, the nurse should irrigate the infant's mouth with the infant in an upright position and head tilted forward to prevent aspiration. A supine or Fowler's position with the head to the side won't prevent aspiration. The prone position isn't appropriate following cleft lip repair because this may put pressure on the suture line.
CN: Physiological integrity; CNS: Reduction of risk potential; CL: Application

21. 4. If there's no trauma or infection to the site, healing occurs with little scar formation. There may be some inflammation right after surgery, but after healing, the lip is a normal size. No jaw malformation occurs with cleft lip repair.
CN: Physiological integrity; CNS: Physiological adaptation; CL: Application

22. The nurse would explain to the parents of a newborn with a cleft lip and palate that they will need to schedule an appointment with which specialist?
1. Cardiologist
2. Neurologist
3. Nutritionist
4. Otolaryngologist

23. Which sign should alert a nurse to dehydration in a neonate with esophageal atresia and tracheoesophageal fistula?
1. Bulging eyeballs
2. Sunken anterior fontanelle
3. Skin that returns briskly when pinched
4. Weight gain

24. Feedings are being withheld in a neonate with esophageal atresia and tracheoesophageal fistula until a gastrostomy tube can be placed. Which nursing action would be most appropriate when the neonate is irritable and crying?
1. Offer him a pacifier.
2. Encourage his parents to talk to him.
3. Encourage his parents to hold him.
4. Distract him by placing a mobile over the crib.

25. Which finding indicates to a nurse that a neonate born with esophageal atresia needs suctioning?
1. Cyanosis
2. Decreased production of saliva
3. Inability to cough
4. Inadequate swallow

26. For a neonate suspected of having esophageal atresia, a definitive diagnostic evaluation would include which factor?
1. Decreased breath sounds
2. Absence of bowel sounds
3. How the neonate tolerates eating
4. Ability to pass a catheter down the esophagus

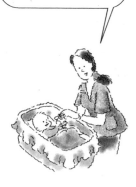

This will help satisfy the infant's need to suck.

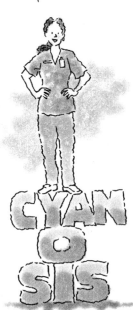

It's time to take action.

22. 4. An otolaryngologist is used because ear infections are common, along with hearing loss. Cardiac and brain function is usually normal. A nutritionist isn't needed unless the neonate becomes malnourished.
CN: Safe, effective care environment; CNS: Management of care; CL: Application

23. 2. A sunken anterior fontanelle is a sign of dehydration in the neonate whose fontanelle hasn't yet closed. Bulging eyeballs and weight gain are signs of overhydration. Skin that returns quickly when pinched is a sign of adequate hydration.
CN: Physiological integrity; CNS: Reduction of risk potential; CL: Application

24. 1. A neonate who's unable to suck to obtain nutrition may be comforted if given a pacifier to satisfy his need to suck. Encouraging his parents to hold and talk to him and placing a mobile over the crib are appropriate interventions but won't satisfy a newborn as much as a pacifier.
CN: Physiological integrity; CNS: Basic care and comfort; CL: Analysis

25. 1. Cyanosis occurs when fluid from the blind pouch is aspirated into the trachea, requiring suctioning. Increased saliva production is common, along with choking, coughing, and sneezing. The ability to swallow isn't affected by this disorder.
CN: Physiological integrity; CNS: Physiological adaptation; CL: Analysis

26. 4. A moderately stiff catheter will meet resistance if the esophagus is blocked and will pass unobstructed if the esophagus is patent. Breath sounds are normal unless aspiration occurs. The intestinal tract isn't affected with this anomaly, so bowel sounds are present. If a neonate doesn't tolerate eating, it doesn't mean he has an esophageal atresia.
CN: Physiological integrity; CNS: Physiological adaptation; CL: Analysis

CN: Client needs category   CNS: Client needs subcategory   CL: Cognitive level

27. For a neonate diagnosed with a tracheo-esophageal fistula, which intervention would be needed?
   1. Start antibiotic therapy.
   2. Keep the neonate lying flat.
   3. Continue feedings.
   4. Remove the diagnostic catheter from the esophagus.

28. When tracheoesophageal fistula or esophageal atresia is suspected, which nursing intervention should be done <u>first</u>?
   1. Give oxygen.
   2. Tell the parents.
   3. Put the neonate in an Isolette or on a radiant warmer.
   4. Report the suspicion to the physician.

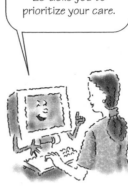

Question 28 asks you to prioritize your care.

29. Which complication may follow the surgical repair of a tracheoesophageal fistula?
   1. Atelectasis
   2. Choking during feeding attempts
   3. Damaged vocal cords
   4. Infection

30. The nurse is caring for an infant suspected of having esophageal atresia and tracheoesophageal fistula. Which sign would the nurse <u>initially</u> observe?
   1. Abdominal distention
   2. Decreased oral secretions
   3. Normal respiratory effort
   4. Scaphoid abdomen

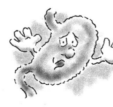

I feel so bloated!

27. 1. Antibiotic therapy is started because aspiration pneumonia is inevitable and appears early. The neonate's head is usually kept in an upright position to prevent aspiration. I.V. fluids are started, and the neonate isn't allowed oral intake. The catheter is left in the upper esophageal pouch to easily remove fluid that collects there.
CN: Physiological integrity; CNS: Pharmacological and parenteral therapies; CL: Analysis

28. 4. The physician needs to be told so that immediate diagnostic tests can be done for a definitive diagnosis and surgical correction. Oxygen should be given only after notifying the physician, except in the case of an emergency. It isn't the nurse's responsibility to inform the parents of the suspected finding. By the time tracheoesophageal fistula or esophageal atresia is suspected, the neonate would have already been placed in an Isolette or a radiant warmer.
CN: Physiological integrity; CNS: Physiological adaptation; CL: Analysis

29. 1. Respiratory complications (atelectasis) are a threat to the neonate's life preoperatively and postoperatively because of the continual risk of aspiration. Choking is more likely to occur preoperatively, although careful attention is paid postoperatively when neonates begin to eat to make sure they can swallow without choking. Vocal cord damage isn't common after this repair. The neonate is generally given antibiotics preoperatively to prevent infection.
CN: Physiological integrity; CNS: Physiological adaptation; CL: Analysis

30. 1. Crying may force air into the stomach, causing distention. Secretions in a client with this condition may be more visible, though normal in quantity, because of the client's inability to swallow effectively. Respiratory effort is usually more difficult. When no distal fistula is present, the abdomen will appear scaphoid.
CN: Physiological integrity; CNS: Physiological adaptation; CL: Application

31. Dietary management in a child diagnosed with ulcerative colitis should include which diet?
1. High-calorie diet
2. High-residue diet
3. Low-protein diet
4. Low-salt diet

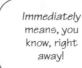

Immediately means, you know, right away!

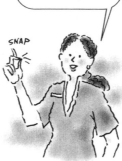

SNAP

32. A neonate comes back from the operating room after surgical repair of a tracheoesophageal fistula and esophageal atresia. Which intervention is done <u>immediately</u>?
1. Maintain a patent airway.
2. Start feedings right away.
3. Let the parents hold the neonate right away.
4. Suction the endotracheal tube, stopping when resistance is met.

33. Which discharge instruction should a nurse give the parents following repair of tracheoesophageal fistula and esophageal atresia in a neonate?
1. Give antibiotics through the feeding tube.
2. Maintain proper care of a chest tube.
3. Maintain proper positioning for feedings.
4. Utilize tips for preventing crying.

34. Which nursing intervention should be done postoperatively for a neonate after repair of tracheoesophageal fistula and esophageal atresia?
1. Withhold mouth care.
2. Offer a pacifier frequently.
3. Decrease tactile stimulation.
4. Use restraints to prevent injury to the repair.

Hmmm. Now I have to think long term.

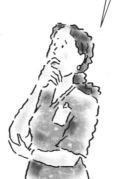

35. A client is admitted with a history of tracheoesophageal fistula and esophageal atresia repair. The nurse should evaluate this client for which potential <u>long-term</u> postoperative complication?
1. Oral aversion
2. Gastroesophageal reflux
3. Inability to tolerate feedings
4. Strictures

31. 1. A high-calorie diet is given to combat weight loss and restore nitrogen balance. A low-residue or residue-free diet is encouraged to decrease bowel irritation. A high-protein diet is also encouraged. Salt reduction isn't a factor in this disease.
CN: Physiological integrity; CNS: Basic care and comfort; CL: Analysis

32. 1. Maintaining a patent airway is essential until sedation from surgery wears off. Feedings usually aren't started for at least 48 hours after surgery. Parents are encouraged to participate in the neonate's care, but not immediately after surgery. The catheter should be measured before suctioning so the tube doesn't meet resistance, which could cause damage.
CN: Safe, effective care environment; CNS: Management of care; CL: Application

33. 3. The neonate should be kept in an upright position after feeding to reduce the risk of refluxed stomach contents and aspiration pneumonia. Although antibiotics are given after surgery, they're discontinued before discharge. Because the chest cavity is entered during surgery, the neonate may have a chest tube inserted that's removed prior to discharge. Because lung expansion is important following chest surgery, vigorous crying helps expand the lungs and shouldn't be discouraged.
CN: Physiological integrity; CNS: Basic care and comfort; CL: Application

34. 2. Meeting the neonate's oral needs, such as by offering him a pacifier, is important because he can't drink from a bottle. The nurse should give mouth care to this neonate. The nurse should provide tactile stimulation. Restraints should be avoided, if possible.
CN: Physiological integrity; CNS: Physiological adaptation; CL: Application

35. 4. Strictures of the anastomosis occur in 40% to 50% of the cases. Oral aversion can be a problem, but it occurs quickly after surgery. Reflux is a common complication but appears when feedings are started. If the neonate is having problems tolerating feedings, it's quickly noted.
CN: Physiological integrity; CNS: Physiological adaptation; CL: Application

CN: Client needs category   CNS: Client needs subcategory   CL: Cognitive level

36. The nurse would suspect which structural defect if she observes that a neonate has excessive salivation and drooling, accompanied by coughing, choking, and sneezing?
1. Cleft lip
2. Cleft palate
3. Gastroschisis
4. Tracheoesophageal fistula and esophageal atresia

37. Which nursing diagnosis takes the highest priority during the first 24 hours following surgical repair of esophageal atresia and tracheoesophageal fistula?
1. *Ineffective airway clearance*
2. *Imbalanced nutrition: Less than body requirements*
3. *Risk for impaired parenting*
4. *Ineffective infant feeding pattern*

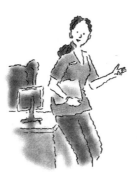

Think surgery for an esophageal disorder, and then prioritize.

38. An infant was born with a portion of an organ protruding through an abnormal opening. The nurse would explain to the parents that this structural defect is which condition?
1. Cleft lip
2. Cleft palate
3. Gastroschisis
4. Tracheoesophageal fistula

39. When an infant is diagnosed with a diaphragmatic hernia on the <u>left side</u>, which abdominal organ may be found in the thorax?
1. Appendix
2. Descending colon
3. Right kidney
4. Spleen

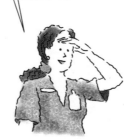

Hmmm, which way did that mediastinum go?

40. In which direction does the mediastinum shift in an infant diagnosed with a diaphragmatic hernia?
1. No shift
2. Shifts to the affected side
3. Shifts to the unaffected side
4. Partial shifts to the affected or unaffected sides

36. 4. Because tracheoesophageal fistula and esophageal atresia cause an ineffective swallow, saliva and secretions appear in the mouth and around the lips. Coughing, choking, and sneezing occur for the same reason and usually after an attempt at eating. Cleft lip and palate don't produce excessive salivation. None of these symptoms occurs with gastroschisis.
CN: Physiological integrity; CNS: Physiological adaptation; CL: Application

37. 1. The priority nursing diagnosis for the first postoperative day is *Ineffective airway clearance.* The nurse must assess the infant's airway for the buildup of mucus and other secretions. The nurse must also perform a respiratory assessment and keep suction equipment, a laryngoscope, and endotracheal suction equipment immediately available. The other nursing diagnoses are all important in the infant in the immediate postoperative period, but assessing and maintaining a patent airway is the greatest priority.
CN: Physiological integrity; CNS: Reduction or risk potential; CL: Analysis

38. 3. Gastroschisis is a herniation of the bowel through an abnormal opening in the abdominal wall. Cleft lip and palate are facial malformations, not herniations. Tracheoesophageal fistula is a malformation of the trachea and esophagus.
CN: Physiological integrity; CNS: Physiological adaptation; CL: Application

39. 4. The spleen has commonly been seen in the thorax of infants with this defect. The appendix and descending colon usually don't protrude into the thorax because of limited space from the other organs present. The right kidney wouldn't be seen with a left-sided defect.
CN: Physiological integrity; CNS: Physiological adaptation; CL: Analysis

40. 3. The increased volume in the chest cavity from the abdominal organs causes the mediastinum to shift to the unaffected side, which causes a partial collapse of that lung. Because of the increased volume on the affected side, the mediastinum can't shift that way.
CN: Physiological integrity; CNS: Physiological adaptation; CL: Analysis

41. Which is the <u>best</u> way to position an infant with a diaphragmatic hernia before surgery?
1. On the affected side
2. On the unaffected side
3. Supine
4. Trendelenburg's position

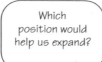

Which position would help us expand?

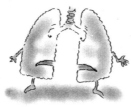

42. Before surgery, which intervention should be used for an infant with a diaphragmatic hernia?
1. Feed the infant.
2. Provide tactile stimulation.
3. Prevent the infant from crying.
4. Place the infant on the unaffected side.

43. Which action by the nurse is essential when caring for a neonate with an omphalocele?
1. Keep the omphalocele dry.
2. Don't let the parents see the omphalocele.
3. Carefully position and handle the omphalocele.
4. Touch the omphalocele often to assess any changes.

44. Which toy would be most appropriate for a nurse to give to an 8-month-old admitted for repair of a diaphragmatic hernia?
1. Large crayons and a coloring book
2. Colorful, plastic, multitextured rattle
3. Black-and-white mobile
4. Colorful pull toys

Shake, rattle, and roll!

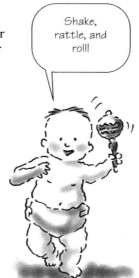

41. 1. Positioning the infant on the affected side lets the lung on the unaffected side expand, making breathing easier. Positioning the infant on the unaffected side or in Trendelenburg's position would further diminish respiration and would increase pressure in the chest cavity, compromising respirations. Supine position doesn't facilitate lung expansion.
CN: Physiological integrity; CNS: Basic care and comfort; CL: Analysis

42. 3. To prevent the intestines from being pulled into the chest cavity by the negative pressure caused by crying, it should be avoided. The stomach and intestine in the chest cavity may also become distended with swallowed air from crying. The infant usually isn't fed until after surgery. Tactile stimulation is limited because it may disturb the infant's fragile condition. The infant is always placed on the affected side.
CN: Physiological integrity; CNS: Physiological adaptation; CL: Application

43. 3. Careful positioning and handling prevent infection and rupture of the omphalocele. The omphalocele is kept moist until the neonate is taken to the operating room. The parents can see the defect if they so choose. Touching it often increases the risk of infection.
CN: Physiological integrity; CNS: Physiological adaptation; CL: Application

44. 2. By 8 months old, an infant can transfer toys and enjoys different textures, making a colorful plastic rattle with different textures an age-appropriate toy. Because infants at this age still put objects in their mouths, crayons wouldn't be appropriate. Newborns enjoy the visual stimulation of black-and-white mobiles. Pull toys are appropriate for the toddler who's walking.
CN: Health promotion and maintenance; CNS: None; CL: Analysis

CN: Client needs category   CNS: Client needs subcategory   CL: Cognitive level

45. Which nursing intervention is most appropriate when an adolescent with a nasogastric (NG) tube in place following surgery for a ruptured appendix reports feeling nauseated?
1. Provide oral hygiene.
2. Measure the gastric drainage.
3. Assess serum electrolytes.
4. Irrigate the tube.

45. 4. When a client with an NG tube complains of nausea, the nurse should first determine the position of the tube and then irrigate it to check for patency. A clogged tube allows contents to accumulate in the stomach, contributing to nausea. Oral hygiene is important to promote comfort but isn't the most appropriate intervention here. Measuring the gastric drainage is important but won't relieve nausea. Serum electrolytes should be monitored in the client with an NG tube. Although an electrolyte imbalance may cause nausea, the tube should first be checked for patency.
CN: Physiological integrity; CNS: Reduction of risk potential; CL: Application

46. Which nursing intervention is most appropriate for a 1-month-old infant with pyloric stenosis who's vomiting?
1. Place the infant in a supine position to sleep.
2. Weigh the infant every 8 hours.
3. Assess for signs of dehydration.
4. Assess vital signs every 8 hours.

46. 3. Because the infant is vomiting, the nurse should assess for signs and symptoms of dehydration. The infant should be placed on the right side to sleep to prevent aspiration of vomitus. The infant should be weighed daily, not every 8 hours. Vital signs should be assessed every 4 hours until stable.
CN: Physiological integrity; CNS: Reduction of risk potential; CL: Application

47. Which sign noted during an admission assessment of a 6-month-old infant admitted for intestinal obstruction should alert the nurse to a potential problem?
1. Moro reflex
2. Playing with feet
3. Eruption of the first tooth
4. Rolling from stomach to back

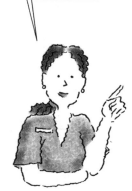

A 6-month-old should have no Moro of this reflex... get it?

47. 1. By 6 months of age, the Moro reflex should no longer be observed. Playing with the feet, eruption of the first tooth, and rolling from stomach to back are all normal for a 6-month-old infant.
CN: Health promotion and maintenance; CNS: None; CL: Analysis

48. The nurse explains to an infant's parents that the pyloric canal narrows in clients with pyloric stenosis at:
1. the stomach and esophagus.
2. the stomach and duodenum.
3. both the stomach and esophagus and the stomach and duodenum.
4. neither the stomach and esophagus nor the stomach and duodenum.

48. 2. The narrowing of the pyloric canal occurs between the stomach and duodenum, where the pyloric sphincter is located. Hyperplasia and hypertrophy cause narrowing and, possibly, obstruction of the circular muscle of the pylorus.
CN: Physiological integrity; CNS: Physiological adaptation; CL: Application

49. The nurse caring for an infant with pyloric stenosis should be alert for which classic sign or symptom?
1. Loss of appetite
2. Chronic diarrhea
3. Projectile vomiting
4. Occasional nonprojectile vomiting

49. 3. The obstruction doesn't allow food to pass through to the duodenum. When the stomach becomes full, the infant vomits for relief. Chronic hunger is commonly seen. There's no diarrhea because food doesn't pass the stomach. Occasional nonprojectile vomiting may occur initially if the obstruction is only partial.
CN: Physiological integrity; CNS: Physiological adaptation; CL: Analysis

50. When assessing a neonate, the nurse notes visible peristaltic waves across the epigastrium. This characteristic is indicative of which disorder?
1. Hypertrophic pyloric stenosis
2. Imperforate anus
3. Intussusception
4. Short-gut syndrome

51. After surgical repair of pyloric stenosis, the nurse should expect an infant's <u>normal</u> feeding regimen to resume after what time frame?
1. 4 to 6 hours after surgery
2. 24 hours after surgery
3. 48 hours after surgery
4. 1 week after surgery

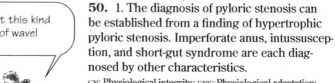

Not this kind of wave!

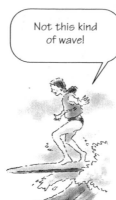

52. A nurse admits an infant diagnosed with pyloric stenosis. Which nursing intervention would most likely be done first?
1. Weigh the infant.
2. Check urine specific gravity.
3. Place an I.V. catheter.
4. Change the infant and weigh the diaper.

53. A nurse is caring for an infant with pyloric stenosis. After feeding the infant, the nurse should place him in which position?
1. Prone in Fowler's position
2. On his back without elevation
3. On the left side in Fowler's position
4. Slightly on the right side in high semi-Fowler's position

Here's that important positioning again!

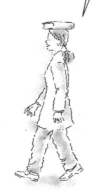

54. When preparing to feed an infant with pyloric stenosis before surgical repair, which intervention is important?
1. Give feedings quickly.
2. Burp the infant frequently.
3. Discourage parental participation.
4. Don't give more feedings if the infant vomits.

50. 1. The diagnosis of pyloric stenosis can be established from a finding of hypertrophic pyloric stenosis. Imperforate anus, intussusception, and short-gut syndrome are each diagnosed by other characteristics.
CN: Physiological integrity; CNS: Physiological adaptation; CL: Analysis

51. 3. Small frequent feedings of clear fluids are usually started 4 to 6 hours after surgery. If clear fluids are tolerated, formula feedings are started 24 hours after surgery, in gradually increasing amounts. It usually takes 48 hours to reach a normal full feeding regimen in this manner. The infant usually goes home on the fourth postoperative day.
CN: Physiological integrity; CNS: Physiological adaptation; CL: Application

52. 1. Weighing the infant would be done first so a baseline weight can be established and weight changes can be assessed. After a baseline weight is obtained, an I.V. catheter can be placed because oral feedings generally aren't given. These infants are usually dehydrated, so although specific gravity and checking the diaper are important tools to help assess their status, they aren't the first priority.
CN: Physiological integrity; CNS: Physiological adaptation; CL: Analysis

53. 4. Positioning the infant slightly on the right side in high semi-Fowler's position will help facilitate gastric emptying. The other positions won't facilitate gastric emptying and may cause the infant to vomit.
CN: Physiological integrity; CNS: Physiological adaptation; CL: Application

54. 2. These infants usually swallow a lot of air from sucking on their hands and fingers because of their intensive hunger (feedings aren't easily tolerated). Burping frequently will lessen gastric distention and increase the likelihood that the infant will retain the feeding. Feedings are given slowly with the infant lying in a semiupright position. Parental participation should be encouraged and allowed to the extent possible. Record the type, amount, and character of the vomit as well as its relation to the feeding. The amount of feeding volume lost is usually refed to the infant.
CN: Physiological adaptation; CNS: Physiological adaptation; CL: Application

CN: Client needs category   CNS: Client needs subcategory   CL: Cognitive level

55. A nurse should expect which finding up to 48 hours after the surgical repair of pyloric stenosis?

1. Dysuria
2. Oral aversion
3. Scaphoid abdomen
4. Vomiting

56. Which intervention will help prevent vomiting in an infant diagnosed with pyloric stenosis?

1. Hold the infant for 1 hour after feeding.
2. Handle the infant minimally after feedings.
3. Space the feedings out, and give them in large amounts.
4. Lay the infant prone with the head of the bed elevated.

57. It's an important nursing function to give support to the parents of an infant diagnosed with pyloric stenosis. Which nursing intervention best serves that purpose?

1. Keep the parents informed of the infant's progress.
2. Provide all care for the infant, even when the parents visit.
3. Tell the parents to minimize handling of the infant at all times.
4. Tell the physician to keep the parents informed of the infant's progress.

58. Which symptom would be likely in an infant diagnosed with pyloric stenosis?

1. Apathy
2. Arrhythmia
3. Dry lips and skin
4. Hypothermia

59. When assessing an infant diagnosed with pyloric stenosis, which finding would the nurse consider <u>normal</u>?

1. Decreased or diminished bowel sounds
2. Heart murmur
3. Normal respiratory effort
4. Positive bowel sounds

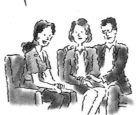

Encourage parents to be involved with their infant's care.

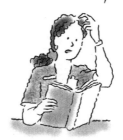

Question 59 asks what's normally found with a disease, not what's normal in a healthy infant.

55. 4. Even with successful surgery, most infants have some vomiting during the first 24 to 48 hours afterward. Dysuria isn't a complication with this surgical procedure. Oral aversion doesn't occur because these infants may be fed up until surgery. Scaphoid abdomen isn't characteristic of this condition; the abdomen may appear distended, not scaphoid.
CN: Physiological integrity; CNS: Physiological adaptation; CL: Application

56. 2. Minimal handling, especially after a feeding, will help prevent vomiting. Holding the infant would provide too much stimulation, which might increase the risk of vomiting. Feedings are given frequently and slowly in small amounts. An infant should be positioned in a semi-Fowler's position and slightly on the right side after a feeding.
CN: Physiological integrity; CNS: Physiological adaptation; CL: Application

57. 1. Keeping the parents informed will decrease their anxiety. The nurse should encourage the parents to be involved with the infant's care. Telling the parents to minimize handling of the infant isn't appropriate because parent-child contact is important. The physician is responsible for updating the parents on the infant's medical condition, and the nurse is responsible for updating the parents on the day-to-day activities of the infant and his improvement with the day's activities.
CN: Psychosocial integrity; CNS: None; CL: Analysis

58. 3. Dry lips and skin are signs of dehydration, which is common in infants with pyloric stenosis. These infants are constantly hungry because of their inability to retain feedings. Apathy, arrhythmias, and hypothermia aren't clinical findings with pyloric stenosis.
CN: Physiological integrity; CNS: Physiological adaptation; CL: Application

59. 1. Bowel sounds decrease because food can't pass into the intestines. Heart murmurs may be present but aren't directly associated with pyloric stenosis. Normal respiratory effort is affected by the abdominal distention that pushes the diaphragm up into the pleural cavity.
CN: Physiological integrity; CNS: Physiological adaptation; CL: Analysis

60. The nurse explains to the parents of a child with hypertrophied pylorus that the defect is located between:

1. the colon and rectum.
2. the stomach and duodenum.
3. the stomach and esophagus.
4. the liver and bile ducts.

61. Which nursing intervention is the <u>most important</u> in dealing with a child who has been poisoned?

1. Stabilize the child.
2. Notify the parents.
3. Identify the poison.
4. Determine when the poisoning took place.

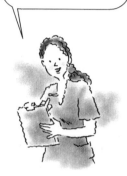

Practice setting priorities because it's part of nursing practice.

62. For a child who has ingested a poisonous substance, the initial step in emergency treatment is to stop the exposure to the substance. Which method would best achieve this?

1. Make the child vomit.
2. Call 911 as soon as possible.
3. Give large amounts of water to flush the system.
4. Empty the mouth of pills, plant parts, or other material.

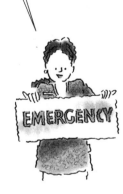

Would you know what to do first in this emergency situation?

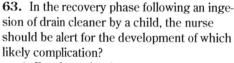

63. In the recovery phase following an ingesion of drain cleaner by a child, the nurse should be alert for the development of which likely complication?

1. Esophageal strictures
2. Esophageal diverticula
3. Tracheal stenosis
4. Tracheal varices

60. 2. This defect occurs at the pyloric sphincter, which is located between the stomach and duodenum. The colon, rectum, esophagus, liver, and bile ducts aren't affected by this obstructive disorder.

CN: Physiological integrity; CNS: Physiological adaptation; CL: Application

61. 1. Stabilization and the initial emergency treatment of the child (such as respiratory assistance, circulatory support, or control of seizures) will prevent further damage to the body from the poison. If the parents didn't bring the child in, they can be notified as soon as the child is stabilized or treated. Identification of the poison is crucial and should begin at the same time as the stabilization of the child, although the initial ABCs (airway, breathing, and circulation) should be assessed first. Determining when the poisoning took place is an important consideration, but emergency stabilization and treatment are priorities.

CN: Physiological integrity; CNS: Physiological adaptation; CL: Analysis

62. 4. Emptying the mouth of pills, plant parts, or other material will stop exposure to the poison. Making the child vomit won't remove exposure to the substance; it's also contraindicated with some poisons. Calling 911 is important, but removing any further sources of the poison would come first. Only small amounts of water are recommended so the poison is confined to the smallest volume. Large amounts of water will let the poison pass the pylorus. The small intestines will then absorb fluid rapidly, increasing the potential toxicity.

CN: Physiological integrity; CNS: Physiological adaptation; CL: Analysis

63. 1. Scar tissue develops as the burn from the drain cleaner ingestion heals, leading to esophageal strictures. The formation of esophageal diverticula is rare. Tracheal stenosis may occur but only if the child vomited and aspirated. Tracheal varices don't commonly occur after drain cleaner ingestion.

CN: Physiological integrity; CNS: Physiological adaptation; CL: Analysis

64. A preschooler is brought to the emergency department after ingesting kerosene. The nurse should be alert for which complication?
1. Pneumonitis
2. Carditis
3. Uremia
4. Hepatitis

65. Which action should a nurse instruct parents to perform first if their child ingests a poison?
1. Administer syrup of ipecac.
2. Call the poison control center.
3. Transport the child to the emergency department.
4. Watch the child for adverse effects.

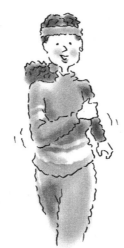

You're moving right along!

66. If a child ingests poisonous hydrocarbons, an important nursing intervention would include which action?
1. Induce vomiting.
2. Keep the child calm and relaxed.
3. Scold the child for the wrongdoing.
4. Keep the parents away from the child.

67. Shock is a complication of several types of poisoning. Which measure would help reduce the risk of shock?
1. Keep the child on his right side.
2. Let the child maintain normal activity as possible.
3. Elevate the head and legs to the level of the heart.
4. Keep the head flat, and raise the legs to the level of the heart.

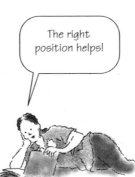

The right position helps!

64. 1. Chemical pneumonitis is the most common complication following ingestion of a hydrocarbon, such as kerosene. The pneumonitis is caused by irritation from the hydrocarbon aspirated into the lungs. The other options aren't complications of kerosene ingestion.
CN: Physiological integrity; CNS: Physiological adaptation; CL: Analysis

65. 2. The first step parents should take if their child has ingested a poisonous substance is to call the poison control center for instructions. Home administration of syrup of ipecac is no longer recommended by the American Academy of Pediatrics. The parents should contact poison control before transporting their child since valuable time may be lost if poison control recommends a specific action to take to remove the poisonous substance from the body. If the child needs to be taken to the emergency department, the parents should call emergency services to transport the child. Poison control may recommend watching the child for adverse effects, but parents shouldn't make this decision without consulting with poison control.
CN: Physiological integrity; CNS: Reduction of risk potential; CL: Analysis

66. 2. Keeping the child calm and relaxed will help prevent vomiting. If vomiting is induced, there's a strong chance the esophagus will be damaged from regurgitation of the gastric poison. Additionally, the risk of chemical pneumonitis exists if vomiting occurs. Scolding the child may upset him. The parents should remain with the child to help keep him calm.
CN: Physiological integrity; CNS: Physiological adaptation; CL: Analysis

67. 3. Elevating the head and legs to the level of the heart will promote venous drainage and decrease the chance of the child going into shock. The child may safely lie on the side he prefers. The child should be encouraged to get plenty of rest.
CN: Physiological integrity; CNS: Physiological adaptation; CL: Application

68. A 7-year-old child ingested several leaves of a poinsettia plant. After arrival in the emergency department, which intervention should be the <u>main</u> nursing function for this client?

1. Begin teaching accident prevention.
2. Provide emotional support to the child.
3. Be prepared for immediate intervention.
4. Provide emotional support to the parents.

69. A child is being admitted through the emergency department with a diagnosis of suspected accidental poisoning by medication. The nurse is aware that which class of medication is the <u>most</u> common cause of accidental poisoning in children?

1. Pain medications
2. Vitamins
3. Laxatives
4. Antibiotics

70. A client is undergoing testing for a diagnosis of ulcerative colitis. Which symptom would the nurse most likely identify during this <u>initial</u> diagnosis?

1. Constipation
2. Diarrhea
3. Vomiting
4. Weight loss

71. A child arrives in the emergency department after ingesting poisonous amounts of salicylates. How soon after ingestion should the nurse look for <u>obvious</u> signs of toxicity?

1. Immediately
2. 2 to 4 hours after ingestion
3. 6 hours after ingestion
4. 18 hours after ingestion

72. The nurse caring for a client with an <u>extreme</u> case of salicylate poisoning should anticipate, or prepare the client for, which treatment?

1. Gastric lavage
2. Hypothermia blankets
3. Peritoneal dialysis
4. Vitamin K injection

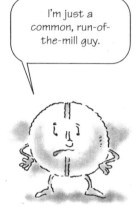

I'm just a common, run-of-the-mill guy.

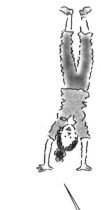

There's more on the next page. Hooray!

68. 3. Time and speed are critical factors in recovery from poisonings. The remaining three answers are important nursing functions but don't require the immediate attention that first stabilizing the child does.
CN: Health promotion and maintenance; CNS: None; CL: Analysis

69. 1. According to the Centers for Disease Control and Prevention, the most common accidentally ingested class of drugs is pain medications. The most common pain medications ingested are acetaminophen-containing (Tylenol-containing) drugs, non-steroidal anti-inflammatory drugs, and opioids. The other classes of drugs are less commonly ingested.
CN: Health promotion and maintenance; CNS: None; CL: Analysis

70. 2. Recurrent or persistent diarrhea is a common feature of ulcerative colitis. Constipation doesn't occur because the bowel becomes smooth and inflexible. Vomiting isn't common in this disease. Weight loss will occur after or during the episode, but not initially.
CN: Physiological integrity; CNS: Physiological adaptation; CL: Analysis

71. 3. There's usually a delay of 6 hours before evidence of toxicity is noted. Toxic evidence is rarely immediate. Aspirin will exert its peak effect in 2 to 4 hours. The effect of aspirin may last as long as 18 hours.
CN: Health promotion and maintenance; CNS: None; CL: Application

72. 3. Peritoneal dialysis is usually reserved for cases of life-threatening salicylism. Gastric lavage is used in the immediate treatment for salicylate poisoning because the stomach contents and salicylates will move from the stomach to the remainder of the GI tract, where vomiting will no longer result in the removal of the poison. Hyperthermia blankets may be used to reduce the possibility of seizures. Vitamin K may be used to decrease bleeding tendencies, but only if evidence of this exists.
CN: Physiological integrity; CNS: Physiological adaptation; CL: Analysis

CN: Client needs category   CNS: Client needs subcategory   CL: Cognitive level

73. When a child has been poisoned, identifying the ingested poison is an important treatment goal. Which action would help determine which poison was ingested?
  1. Call the local poison control center.
  2. Ask the child.
  3. Ask the parents.
  4. Save all evidence of poison.

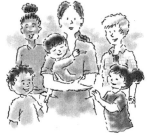

Know your nursing responsibilities.

73. 4. Saving all evidence of poison (container, vomitus, urine) will help determine which drug was ingested and how much. Calling the local poison control center may help get information on specific poisons or if a certain household placed a call, although rarely can they help determine which poison has been ingested. Asking the child may help, but the child may fear punishment and may not be honest about the incident. The parent may be helpful in some instances, although the parent may not have been home or with the child when the ingestion occurred.
CN: Health promotion and maintenance; CNS: None; CL: Analysis

74. One of the most important nursing responsibilities to help prevent salicylate poisoning should include which action?
  1. Identify salicylate overdose.
  2. Teach children the hazards of ingesting nonfood items.
  3. Decrease curiosity; teach parents to keep aspirin and drugs in clear view.
  4. Teach parents to keep large amounts of drugs on hand but out of reach of children.

74. 2. Teaching children the hazards of ingesting nonfood items will help prevent ingestion of poisonous substances. Identifying the overdose won't prevent it from occurring. Aspirin and drugs should be kept out of the sight of children. Parents should be warned about keeping large amounts of drugs on hand.
CN: Health promotion and maintenance; CNS: None; CL: Application

75. In evaluating the effectiveness of therapy with acetylcysteine (Mucomyst) in a child with acetaminophen poisoning, which laboratory value would be the <u>most</u> important for the nurse to monitor?
  1. Serum alanine aminotransferase and aspartate aminotransferase
  2. Serum calcium levels
  3. Prothrombin time (PT)
  4. Serum glucose levels

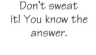

Don't sweat it! You know the answer.

75. 1. Acetaminophen poisoning damages the liver, leading to elevated serum alanine aminotransferase and aspartate aminotransferase levels. After therapy with acetylcysteine is started, these liver enzymes should begin to fall. Serum calcium levels may fall following chelation therapy in clients with lead poisoning. Because PT is elevated and blood glucose levels are reduced with salicylate poisoning, after treatment is initiated the nurse should observe the PT and blood glucose levels return to normal.
CN: Physiological integrity; CNS: Reduction of risk potential; CL: Analysis

76. A client is diagnosed with acetaminophen poisoning. Which sign would the nurse expect when assessing the client 12 to 24 hours after ingestion?
  1. Hyperthermia
  2. Increased urine output
  3. Profuse sweating
  4. Rapid pulse

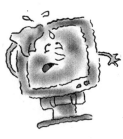

76. 3. During the first 12 to 24 hours, profuse sweating is a significant sign of acetaminophen poisoning. Weak pulse, hypothermia, and decreased urine output are also common findings.
CN: Physiological integrity; CNS: Physiological adaptation; CL: Analysis

77. For a client diagnosed with acetaminophen poisoning who comes to the emergency department 3 hours after ingestion, the most important therapeutic action is to:
1. perform gastric lavage.
2. obtain blood work.
3. give I.V. fluid.
4. use activated charcoal.

78. Which response by a nurse is most appropriate when the mother of a child admitted for ingesting a caustic cleaning product states she feels guilty?
1. "Now you'll know to keep all cleaning products locked up."
2. "Luckily, your child is going to be fine."
3. "You'll need to watch your child more carefully."
4. "Tell me more about your guilty feelings."

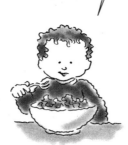

Everything tastes good to me!

79. The ingestion of lead-containing substances is <u>mostly</u> influenced by which risk factor?
1. Child's age
2. Child's gender
3. Child's race
4. A parent with the same habit

80. The nurse explains to the mother of a child with lead poisoning that X-rays are necessary, as lead retained in the body is initially stored in the:
1. bone.
2. brain.
3. kidney.
4. liver.

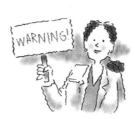

Be aware of the initial signs of lead poisoning.

81. Which condition is one of the <u>initial</u> signs of lead poisoning?
1. Anemia
2. Constipation
3. Anorexia
4. Paralysis

77. 4. If the client is seen within 4 hours, activated charcoal should be given to prevent absorption of acetominophen. Gastric lavage is recommended only if the client is seen within 1 hour of ingestion. Blood work would be obtained but wouldn't be the first priority. I.V. fluids would also be administered, but administering activated charcoal is the priority.
CN: Physiological integrity; CNS: Physiological adaptation; CL: Analysis

78. 4. Encouraging the mother to talk about her feelings shows the nurse accepts the mother's feelings and that she's prepared to listen. This also helps establish a trusting nurse-client relationship. Telling the mother she should keep all cleaning products locked up and that she needs to watch her child more carefully acknowledges that the mother was at fault and may block further communication. Telling the mother that the child will be fine dismisses the mother's feelings and may be giving false reassurances.
CN: Psychosocial integrity; CNS: None; CL: Analysis

79. 1. The highest risk of lead poisoning occurs in young children who have a tendency to put things in their mouth. In older homes that contain lead-based paint, paint chips may be eaten directly by the child or they may cling to toys or hands that are then put into the child's mouth. Poisoning isn't gender-related. African Americans have a higher incidence of lead poisoning, but it can happen in any race. Most parents don't eat lead-based paint on purpose.
CN: Health promotion and maintenance; CNS: None; CL: Application

80. 1. Ingested lead is initially absorbed by bone; X-rays reveal a characteristic "lead line" at the epiphyseal line. If chronic ingestion occurs, then the central nervous, renal, and hematologic systems are affected.
CN: Physiological integrity; CNS: Physiological adaptation; CL: Application

81. 1. Lead is dangerously toxic to the biosynthesis of heme, and the reduced heme molecule in red blood cells causes anemia. Constipation and anorexia are vague, nonspecific symptoms. Paralysis may occur as toxic damage to the brain progresses.
CN: Physiological integrity; CNS: Physiological adaptation; CL: Analysis

CN: Client needs category   CNS: Client needs subcategory   CL: Cognitive level

82. The most serious and irreversible adverse effects of lead intoxication affect which system?
1. Central nervous system (CNS)
2. Hematologic system
3. Renal system
4. Respiratory system

83. A mother of a recently admitted child asks the nurse about the black lines along her child's gums. The nurse would respond that the black lines indicate which of the following types of poisoning?
1. Acetaminophen
2. Lead
3. Plants
4. Salicylates

84. The parents of a child with lead poisoning ask the nurse which procedure is the main treatment for lead poisoning. Which treatment would the nurse describe?
1. Exchange transfusion
2. Bone marrow transplant
3. Chelation therapy
4. Dialysis

85. Which nursing objective should be the most important for a child with lead poisoning who must undergo chelation therapy?
1. Prepare the child for complete bed rest.
2. Prepare the child for I.V. fluid therapy.
3. Prepare the child for an extended hospital stay.
4. Prepare the child for a large number of injections.

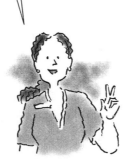

Watch for these two words—most important.

86. Which condition may occur during chelation therapy in a child with lead poisoning?
1. Hypercalcemia
2. Hypocalcemia
3. Hyperglycemia
4. Hypoglycemia

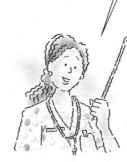

You know the routine; keep on teachin'.

87. Which intervention is the best way to prevent lead poisoning in children?
1. Educate the child.
2. Educate the public.
3. Identify high-risk groups.
4. Provide home chelation kits.

82. 1. Damage that occurs to the CNS is difficult to repair. Damage to the hematologic and renal systems can be reversed if treated early. The respiratory system isn't affected until coma and death occur.
CN: Physiological integrity; CNS: Physiological adaptation; CL: Analysis

83. 2. One diagnostic characteristic of lead poisoning is black lines along the gums. Black lines don't occur along the gums with acetaminophen, plant, or salicylate poisoning.
CN: Physiological integrity; CNS: Physiological adaptation; CL: Application

84. 3. Chelation therapy is the main treatment for lead poisoning and involves the removal of metal by combining it with another substance. Sometimes exchange transfusions are used to rid the blood of lead quickly. Bone marrow transplants usually aren't needed. Dialysis usually isn't part of the treatment.
CN: Physiological integrity; CNS: Physiological adaptation; CL: Application

85. 4. Chelation therapy involves getting a large number of injections in a relatively short period of time. It's traumatic to the majority of children, and they need some preparation for the treatment. The other components of the treatment plan are important but aren't as likely to cause the same anxiety as multiple injections. Allowing adequate rest to not aggravate the painful injection sites is important. Receiving I.V. fluid isn't as traumatizing as multiple injections. Physical activity is usually limited.
CN: Physiological integrity; CNS: Physiological adaptation; CL: Analysis

86. 2. A calcium chelating agent is used for the treatment of lead poisoning, so calcium is removed from the body with the lead. Hypocalcemia, not hypercalcemia, occurs. Hyperglycemia and hypoglycemia don't occur as a result of this therapy.
CN: Physiological integrity; CNS: Physiological adaptation; CL: Analysis

87. 2. By educating others about lead poisoning, including the danger signs, symptoms, and treatment, identification can be determined quickly. Very young children may not understand the dangers of lead poisoning. Identifying high-risk groups will help but won't prevent the poisoning. Home chelation kits currently aren't available.
CN: Health promotion and maintenance; CNS: None; CL: Analysis

88. When planning care for a 14-year-old client following surgical repair of a ruptured appendix, the nurse should plan interventions that:
1. reduce conflict between the client and his parents.
2. promote the development of an identity and independence.
3. encourage the development of trust.
4. confirm plans for the future.

89. Certain forms of pica are caused by a deficiency. Which nutrient is most commonly deficient?
1. Minerals
2. Vitamin B complex
3. Vitamin C
4. Vitamin D

90. Which action should a nurse take when a child with appendicitis reports a sudden cessation of abdominal pain?
1. Prepare the child and parents for discharge.
2. Begin feeding the child, as tolerated.
3. Prepare the child for emergency surgery.
4. Begin ambulation, as tolerated.

91. Which advice should a nurse give over the telephone to the mother of a 7-year-old child with abdominal pain, a low-grade fever, and vomiting?
1. Give prune juice to relieve constipation.
2. Test for rebound tenderness in the left lower quadrant of the abdomen.
3. Encourage fluids to prevent dehydration.
4. Seek immediate emergency medical care.

92. Which symptom is the most common for acute appendicitis?
1. Bradycardia
2. Fever
3. Pain descending to the lower left quadrant
4. Pain radiating down the legs

88. 2. Since adolescents are in Erikson's stage of identity versus role confusion, the nursing care plan should include interventions that promote a sense of identity and independence. During adolescence, conflict is usually intensified, not reduced. Trust is a developmental task of infancy. Plans for the future aren't confirmed at age 14.
CN: Health promotion and maintenance; CNS: None; CL: Analysis

89. 1. Eating clay is related to zinc deficiency; eating chalk, to calcium deficiency. Vitamin deficiencies aren't related to pica.
CN: Health promotion and maintenance; CNS: None; CL: Analysis

90. 3. The sudden cessation of abdominal pain in the client with appendicitis may indicate perforation or infarction of the appendix requiring emergency surgery. Therefore, the child shouldn't be prepared for discharge or given oral feedings. The child with a ruptured appendix should be on complete bed rest and be prepared for surgery.
CN: Physiological integrity; CNS: Reduction of risk potential; CL: Application

91. 4. The client with abdominal pain, fever, and vomiting (the cardinal signs of appendicitis) should seek immediate emergency care to reduce the risk of complications if the appendix should rupture. Prune juice has laxative effects and shouldn't be given because laxatives increase the risk of rupture of the appendix. The nurse shouldn't rely on the mother's findings when testing for rebound tenderness. The client should be given nothing by mouth in case surgery is needed.
CN: Physiological integrity; CNS: Reduction of risk potential; CL: Application

92. 2. Fever, abdominal pain, and tenderness are the first signs of appendicitis. Tachycardia, not bradycardia, is seen. Pain can be generalized or periumbilical. It usually descends to the lower right quadrant, not the left.
CN: Physiological integrity; CNS: Physiological adaptation; CL: Analysis

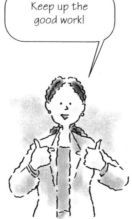

Keep up the good work!

CN: Client needs category CNS: Client needs subcategory CL: Cognitive level

93. Which nursing intervention would be important to preoperatively perform in a child with appendicitis?
1. Give clear fluids.
2. Apply heat to the abdomen.
3. Maintain complete bed rest.
4. Administer an enema, if ordered.

94. Postoperative care of a child with a ruptured appendix should include which treatment or intervention?
1. Liquid diet
2. Oral antibiotics for 7 to 10 days
3. Positioning the child on the left side
4. Parenteral antibiotics for 7 to 10 days

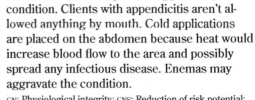

Believe me, position counts.

95. After surgical repair of a ruptured appendix, which position would be the <u>most appropriate</u>?
1. High Fowler's position
2. Left side
3. Semi-Fowler's position
4. Supine

96. Which statement by the parent of a child being treated for pinworms indicates that more teaching is necessary?
1. "I will make my child wash his hands well before meals."
2. "I will tell my child not to share hairbrushes or hats."
3. "I will give my child only one dose of medication."
4. "I will keep my child's nails short."

97. During an initial nursing assessment, a nurse determines that an 8-year-old child has right lower quadrant pain, a low-grade fever, nausea, rebound tenderness, and a positive psoas sign. The nurse suspects that the client has which condition?
1. Appendicitis
2. Gastroenteritis
3. Pancreatitis
4. Cholecystitis

93. 3. Bed rest will prevent aggravating the condition. Clients with appendicitis aren't allowed anything by mouth. Cold applications are placed on the abdomen because heat would increase blood flow to the area and possibly spread any infectious disease. Enemas may aggravate the condition.
CN: Physiological integrity; CNS: Reduction of risk potential; CL: Analysis

94. 4. Parenteral antibiotics are used for 7 to 10 days postoperatively to help prevent the spread of infection. The child is kept on I.V. fluids and isn't allowed anything by mouth. Oral antibiotics may continue after the parenteral antibiotics are discontinued. The child is positioned on the right side after surgery.
CN: Physiological integrity; CNS: Reduction of risk potential; CL: Analysis

95. 3. Using the semi-Fowler's or right side-lying positions will facilitate drainage from the peritoneal cavity and prevent the formation of a subdiaphragmatic abscess. High Fowler's, left side, and prone positions won't facilitate drainage from the peritoneal cavity.
CN: Physiological integrity; CNS: Physiological adaptation; CL: Analysis

96. 2. Sharing hairbrushes and hats reduces the spread of lice, not pinworms. Hands should be washed well before food preparation and eating to avoid ingesting eggs that may be under the fingernails from scratching the itchy, infested perianal area. Only a single dose of medication, such as mebendazole, is needed to treat pinworms. Keeping the fingernails short reduces the risk of carrying the eggs under the nails.
CN: Safe, effective care environment; CNS: Safety and infection control; CL: Application

97. 1. Right lower quadrant pain, a low-grade fever, nausea, rebound tenderness, and a positive psoas sign are all consistent with appendicitis. Gastroenteritis is characterized by generalized abdominal tenderness. Pancreatitis is characterized by pain in the left abdominal quadrant. Cholecystitis is characterized by pain in the right upper abdominal quadrant.
CN: Physiological integrity; CNS: Physiological adaptation; CL: Analysis

98. A neonate has been diagnosed with a unilateral complete cleft lip and cleft palate. The nurse formulating the care plan for this neonate will have which nursing diagnosis as a priority?
 1. *Risk for infection*
 2. *Impaired skin integrity*
 3. *Risk for aspiration*
 4. *Delayed growth and development*

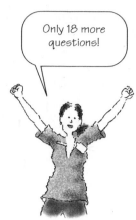

Only 18 more questions!

99. A neonate is suspected of having a tracheoesophageal fistula (type III/C). Which symptom would be seen on the initial assessment?
 1. Excessive drooling
 2. Excessive vomiting
 3. Mottling
 4. Polyhydramnios

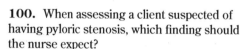

You made it to question 100. Good for you!

100. When assessing a client suspected of having pyloric stenosis, which finding should the nurse expect?
 1. An "olive" mass in the right upper quadrant
 2. An "olive" mass in the left upper quadrant
 3. A "sausage" mass in the right upper quadrant
 4. A "sausage" mass in the left upper quadrant

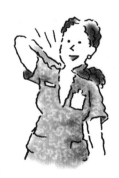

101. A nurse caring for an infant with pyloric stenosis should expect to observe which laboratory values?
 1. pH, 7.30; chloride, 120 mEq/L
 2. pH, 7.38; chloride, 110 mEq/L
 3. pH, 7.43; chloride, 100 mEq/L
 4. pH, 7.49; chloride, 90 mEq/L

98. 3. Although all of these diagnoses are important for the neonate with a cleft lip and cleft palate, the most important diagnosis relates to the airway. Neonates with a cleft lip and a cleft palate may have an excessive amount of saliva and usually have a difficult time with feedings. Special feeding techniques, such as using a flanged nipple, may be necessary to prevent aspiration.
CN: Physiological integrity; CNS: Reduction of risk potential; CL: Analysis

99. 1. In type III/C tracheoesophageal fistula, the proximal end of the esophagus ends in a blind pouch and a fistula connects the distal end of the esophagus to the trachea. Saliva will pool in this pouch and cause the child to drool. Because the distal end of the esophagus is connected to the trachea, the neonate can't vomit, but he can aspirate and stomach acid may go into the lungs through this fistula, causing pneumonitis. Mottling is a netlike, reddish blue discoloration of the skin usually due to vascular contraction in response to hypothermia. The mother of a neonate with tracheoesophageal fistula may have had polyhydramnios.
CN: Physiological integrity; CNS: Reduction of risk potential; CL: Analysis

100. 1. Pyloric stenosis involves hypertrophy of the circular (or olive-shaped) muscle fibers of the pylorus. This hypertrophy is palpable in the right upper quadrant of the abdomen. A "sausage" mass is palpable in the right upper quadrant in children with intussusception. A "sausage" mass in the left upper quadrant wouldn't indicate pyloric stenosis.
CN: Physiological integrity; CNS: Physiological adaptation; CL: Analysis

101. 4. Infants with pyloric stenosis vomit hydrochloric acid. This causes them to become alkalotic and hypochloremic. Normal serum pH is 7.35 to 7.45; levels above 7.45 represent alkalosis. The normal serum chloride level is 99 to 111 mEq/L; levels below 99 mEq/L represent hypochloremia.
CN: Physiological integrity; CNS: Physiological adaptation; CL: Analysis

102. Which nursing diagnosis has the highest priority in a 1-month-old infant admitted with projectile vomiting after feeding?
1. *Deficient fluid volume*
2. *Risk for impaired parenting*
3. *Interrupted breast-feeding*
4. *Risk for infection*

103. Which findings would the nurse assess in a premature neonate who may have necrotizing enterocolitis?
1. Abdominal distention and gastric retention
2. Gastric retention and guaiac-negative stools
3. Metabolic alkalosis and abdominal distention
4. Guaiac-negative stools and metabolic alkalosis

104. An infant has been admitted to the hospital with gastroenteritis. The nursing care plan for this infant will consider which nursing diagnosis first?
1. *Acute pain*
2. *Diarrhea*
3. *Deficient fluid volume*
4. *Imbalanced nutrition: Less than body requirements*

105. Nursing assessments in an infant with gastroenteritis should be directed toward detecting which potential problem?
1. Urinary retention
2. Heart failure
3. Electrolyte imbalance
4. Hyperactive reflexes

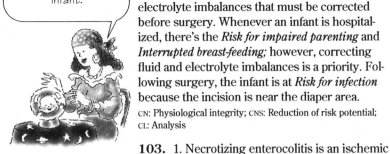

I see the highest priority nursing diagnosis for this infant.

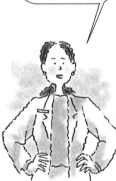

The nursing diagnosis is so important.

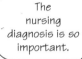

102. 1. Projectile vomiting in an infant is a sign of pyloric stenosis, a condition that requires surgical intervention to correct. Because the infant has been vomiting, he is at risk for fluid and electrolyte imbalances that must be corrected before surgery. Whenever an infant is hospitalized, there's the *Risk for impaired parenting* and *Interrupted breast-feeding;* however, correcting fluid and electrolyte imbalances is a priority. Following surgery, the infant is at *Risk for infection* because the incision is near the diaper area.
CN: Physiological integrity; CNS: Reduction of risk potential; CL: Analysis

103. 1. Necrotizing enterocolitis is an ischemic disorder of the gut. The cause is unknown, but it's more common in premature neonates who had a hypoxic episode. The neonate's intestines become dilated and necrotic, and the abdomen becomes very distended. Paralytic ileus develops, causing the neonate to have gastric retention. These retained gastric contents, along with any passed stool, will be guaiac-positive. The neonate also develops metabolic acidosis.
CN: Physiological integrity; CNS: Physiological adaptation; CL: Analysis

104. 3. Young children with gastroenteritis are at high risk for developing a fluid volume deficit. Their intestinal mucosa allows for more fluid and electrolytes to be lost when they have gastroenteritis. The main goal of the health care team should be to rehydrate the infant. The other nursing diagnoses are important, but deficient fluid volume is more life-threatening.
CN: Physiological integrity; CNS: Physiological adaptation; CL: Application

105. 3. Diarrhea in infants can rapidly lead to dehydration and electrolyte imbalances, especially hyponatremia and hypokalemia. Urinary retention isn't a sign of dehydration; however, it should be distinguished from kidney failure, which may occur with severe dehydration. Heart failure occurs with fluid volume overload, not fluid volume deficit. Reflexes are typically diminished or absent with hypokalemia.
CN: Physiological integrity; CNS: Reduction of risk potential; CL: Application

106. A mother calls the children's clinic, saying that she found her toddler with an open and empty bottle of acetaminophen (Tylenol), and wanting to know what to do. What's the priority intervention for this situation?
1. Ask the mother whether she has any syrup of ipecac.
2. Ask the mother to give the child a large glass of milk.
3. Ask the mother to bring the child to the emergency department (ED).
4. Ask the mother whether she knows cardiopulmonary resuscitation (CPR).

107. Which fact should be emphasized in the teaching plan for the parents of a child with celiac disease?
1. The gluten-free diet alterations must be continued for a lifetime.
2. The diet needs to be free of lactose because the child is intolerant.
3. Diet alterations are necessary when the child reports cramping and bloating.
4. The diet needs to be low in fats because of the malabsorption problem in the intestines.

108. A pediatrician suspects that a child has pinworms and instructs the nurse to assess the child for their presence. Which is the most reliable method of assessing for pinworms?
1. A history of itching at the anal area and of restlessness at night
2. A blood culture
3. Eggs retrieved from the anal edge on a piece of cellophane tape
4. A stool culture

109. An infant age 1 month is brought to the pediatrician's office. His mother states that he's fussy and cries as if in pain. He's tolerating normal amounts of formula, gaining weight, and having episodes of paroxysmal abdominal cramping after feedings. These signs and symptoms indicate that the infant most likely has which condition?
1. Intussusception
2. Meconium ileus
3. Colic
4. Pyloric stenosis

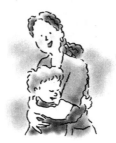

Do you know the priority intervention for this toddler?

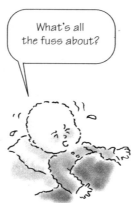

What's all the fuss about?

106. 3. The child should be brought to the ED for evaluation and possible acetyleysteine administration. Home administration of syrup of ipecac is no longer recommended. Milk isn't an antidote for acetaminophen toxicity. Asking about CPR isn't appropriate as the priority intervention; it would distract from the immediate interventions needed.
CN: Safe, effective care environment; CNS: Safety and infection control; CL: Analysis

107. 1. Celiac disease is the inability to digest gluten. The treatment is a gluten-free diet for life. It's important the diet is continued to avoid symptoms and the associated risk of colon cancer. The disease isn't caused by lactose intolerance or a problem digesting fats.
CN: Health promotion and maintenance; CNS: None; CL: Application

108. 3. Cellophane tape placed near the anal edge will capture the eggs. A history of itching and of restlessness aren't enough to definitely diagnosis pinworms. Neither a blood culture nor a stool culture would be helpful.
CN: Physiological integrity; CNS: Reduction of risk potential; CL: Application

109. 3. An infant with colic exhibits symptoms of abdominal cramping after feedings, cries as if in pain, and is fussy. An intussusception begins suddenly and leads to bloody stools and vomiting. A meconium ileus is nonpassage of meconium by 24 hours of age. Signs of pyloric stenosis include projectile vomiting and weight loss.
CN: Physiological integrity; CNS: Physiological adaptation; CL: Analysis

CN: Client needs category   CNS: Client needs subcategory   CL: Cognitive level

110. A 16-year-old African-American student visits a school nurse with complaints of nausea and fatigue. The nurse determines a need to check for jaundice. Which area of the body should the nurse examine?
1. Sclera of the eye
2. Overall skin color
3. Outer ears and back of the neck
4. Tongue and inside the cheek area

111. A mother brings her 4-week-old child to the clinic. She states that he hasn't been eating well and is lethargic when she holds and cuddles him. He has lost 7 oz (198.5 g) since birth. He's otherwise healthy and has no congenital defects. Which condition is the pediatrician most likely to diagnose?
1. Celiac disease
2. Failure to thrive
3. Hirschsprung's disease
4. Imperforate anus

112. A 15-year-old client needs a nasogastric tube inserted because of peritonitis caused by a ruptured appendix. The client is afraid that the procedure will hurt. Which statement would most help decrease the client's anxiety?
1. "Breathe deeply through your mouth and relax. It will be over soon."
2. "This is a simple procedure, and it won't hurt."
3. "You'll feel pressure and be uncomfortable for a few minutes, but it shouldn't be painful."
4. "You're a man now and need to be able to handle pain."

113. A mother brings her 18-month-old child to the emergency department and tells a nurse that he has been ill for the past 2 days. He has a fever of 104° F (40° C), is irritable, has had diarrhea, and hasn't been wetting his diaper much in the past 24 hours. The child is admitted to the pediatric unit for treatment of moderate dehydration and gastroenteritis. I.V. therapy and strict intake and output are ordered. As rehydration occurs, the child is started on oral feedings of a rehydration fluid. When caring for this child during the later stage of rehydration, the nurse should take which action?
1. Force fluids.
2. Allow the client to drink as much as he wants.
3. Monitor the client's intake and output.
4. Monitor the client's ability to retain fluids.

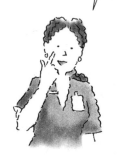
"Eye" think you know the answer to this one.

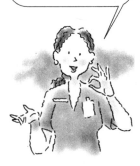
Just a little more to go and you're done with this chapter.

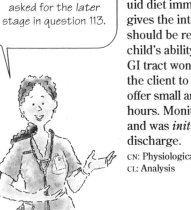
You're being asked for the later stage in question 113.

110. 1. The sclera is the best place to check for jaundice, especially in a person of darker color. The outer ears and back of the neck as well as the tongue and inside of the cheek aren't appropriate places to check for jaundice.
CN: Physiological integrity; CNS: Physiological adaptation; CL: Application

111. 2. These signs and symptoms are classic of the condition failure to thrive. Celiac disease presents with steatorrhea, weight loss, and inability to digest gluten foods. Hirschsprung's disease and imperforate anus present with abdominal distention and absence of stool; no anal opening is present in imperforate anus.
CN: Physiological integrity; CNS: Physiological adaptation; CL: Application

112. 3. Discussing the procedure will help the client understand the extent of discomfort. Breathing deeply will help relieve discomfort, but the statement may also imply that the procedure will be painful and will, thus, increase the client's anxiety. By saying the procedure is simple, the nurse isn't acknowledging the client's concerns. Calling the client a man and telling him that he should be able to handle pain is condescending. No matter what the client's age, he has a right to express his fears and to have those fears acknowledged.
CN: Psychosocial integrity; CNS: None; CL: Analysis

113. 4. The GI tract may not tolerate a full liquid diet immediately. Allowing only clear liquids gives the intestine time to heal, but the fluids should be reintroduced slowly to determine the child's ability to tolerate and retain them. The GI tract won't tolerate forcing fluids. Don't allow the client to drink as much as he wants; instead, offer small amounts of fluid every couple of hours. Monitoring intake and output is important and was *initially* ordered; it will continue until discharge.
CN: Physiological integrity; CNS: Basic care and comfort; CL: Analysis

114. A nurse is conducting an infant nutrition class for parents. Which foods should the nurse tell the parents it's OK to introduce during the first year of life? Select all that apply:

1. Sliced beef
2. Pureed fruits
3. Whole milk
4. Rice cereal
5. Strained vegetables
6. Fruit juice

115. A nurse is teaching a female adolescent with inflammatory bowel disease about treatment with corticosteroids. Which adverse effects are concerns for this client? Select all that apply:

1. Acne
2. Hirsutism
3. Mood swings
4. Osteoporosis
5. Growth spurts
6. Adrenal suppression

116. A mother brings her child to the pediatrician's office for evaluation of chronic stomach pain. The mother states that the pain seems to go away when she tells the child he can stay home from school. The physician diagnoses school phobia. Which other behaviors or symptoms may be present in the child with school phobia? Select all that apply:

1. Nausea
2. Headaches
3. Weight loss
4. Dizziness
5. Fever

114. 2, 4, 5. The first food provided to a neonate is breast milk or formula. Between ages 4 and 6 months, rice cereal can be introduced, followed by pureed or strained fruits and vegetables, then strained or ground meat. Meats must be chopped or ground prior to feeding them to an infant to prevent choking. Infants shouldn't be given whole milk until they're at least 1 year old. Fruit drinks provide no nutritional benefit and shouldn't be encouraged.

CN: Health promotion and maintenance; CNS: None; CL: Application

115. 1, 2, 3, 4, 6. Adverse effects of corticosteroids include acne, hirsutism, mood swings, osteoporosis, and adrenal suppression. Steroid use in children and adolescents may cause delayed growth, not growth spurts.

CN: Physiological integrity; CNS: Pharmacological and parenteral therapies; CL: Application

116. 1, 2, 4. Children with school phobia commonly complain of vague symptoms, such as stomachaches, nausea, headaches, and dizziness, to avoid going to school. Typically, these symptoms don't occur on weekends. A careful history must be taken to identify a pattern of school avoidance. Such signs as weight loss and fever are more likely to have a physiologic cause and are uncommon in the child with school phobia.

CN: Psychosocial integrity; CNS: None; CL: Analysis

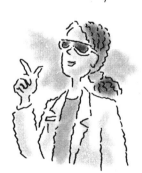

You're done with all those questions? I knew you could do it!

CN: Client needs category   CNS: Client needs subcategory   CL: Cognitive level

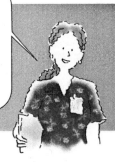

Caring for a child with an endocrine system disorder can be overwhelming. To get started on the right track, check out the Web site of the Juvenile Diabetes Research Foundation International at **www.jdrf.org**. Go for it!

Chapter 20
Endocrine system

1. When explaining the causes of hypothyroidism to the parents of a newly diagnosed infant, a nurse should recognize that further education is needed when the parents ask which question?
1. "Hypothyroidism can be only temporary, right?"
2. "Are you saying that hypothyroidism is caused by a problem in the way the thyroid gland develops?"
3. "Do you mean that hypothyroidism may be caused by a problem in the way the body makes thyroxine?"
4. "Hypothyroidism can be treated by exposing our baby to a special light, right?"

2. An infant with hypothyroidism is receiving oral thyroid hormone. Which assessment findings should alert a nurse to a potential overdose?
1. Tachycardia, irritability, and diaphoresis
2. Bradycardia, excessive sleepiness, and dry scaly skin
3. Bradycardia, irritability, and cool extremities
4. Tachycardia, cool extremities, and irritability

3. When a nurse is teaching the parents of a neonate newly diagnosed with hypothyroidism, which statement should be included?
1. "A large goiter in a neonate doesn't present a problem."
2. "Preterm neonates usually aren't affected by hypothyroidism."
3. "Usually the neonate exhibits obvious signs of hypothyroidism."
4. "The severity of the disorder depends on the amount of thyroid tissue present."

1. 4. Congenital hypothyroidism can be permanent or transient and may result from a defective thyroid gland or an enzymatic defect in thyroxine synthesis. Only the last question, which refers to phototherapy for physiologic jaundice, indicates that the parents need more information.

CN: Health promotion and maintenance; CNS: None; CL: Application

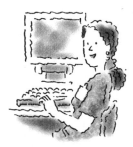

You're off to a good start.

2. 1. Clinical manifestations of thyroid hormone overdose in an infant include tachycardia, irritability, and diaphoresis. Bradycardia, excessive sleepiness, dry scaly skin, and cool extremities are manifestations of hypothyroidism.

CN: Physiological integrity; CNS: Pharmacological and parenteral therapies; CL: Application

3. 4. The severity of the disorder depends on the amount of thyroid tissue present. The more thyroid tissue is present, the less severe the disorder. A large goiter in a neonate could possibly occlude the airway and lead to obstruction. Preterm neonates are usually affected by hypothyroidism due to hypothalamic and pituitary immaturity. Usually the neonate doesn't exhibit obvious signs of the disorder because of maternal circulation.

CN: Health promotion and maintenance; CNS: None; CL: Application

CN: Client needs category   CNS: Client needs subcategory   CL: Cognitive level

4. Which condition is a subtle sign of hypothyroidism?
1. Diarrhea
2. Lethargy
3. Severe jaundice
4. Tachycardia

5. A nurse is assessing a toddler with hypothyroidism. Which signs should alert the nurse to the most serious complication of this condition?
1. Low hemoglobin and hematocrit
2. Cyanosis
3. Bone and muscle dystrophy
4. Mental retardation

6. When counseling the parents of a neonate with congenital hypothyroidism, the nurse understands that the severity of the intellectual deficit is related to which parameter?
1. Duration of condition before treatment
2. Degree of hypothermia
3. Cranial malformations
4. Thyroxine (T_4) level at diagnosis

7. Which statement should be included in an explanation of the diagnostic evaluation of neonates for congenital hypothyroidism?
1. Tests are mandatory in all states.
2. An arterial blood test is preferred.
3. Tests shouldn't be performed until after discharge.
4. Blood tests should be done after the first month of life.

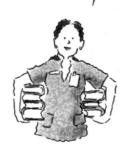

The diagnostic evaluation of a neonate may include tests that are mandated by the state.

4. 2. Subtle signs of this disorder that may be seen shortly after birth include lethargy, poor feeding, prolonged jaundice, respiratory difficulty, cyanosis, constipation, and bradycardia. Diarrhea in the neonate isn't normal and isn't associated with this disorder. Severe jaundice needs immediate attention by the primary health care provider and isn't a subtle sign. Tachycardia typically occurs in hyperthyroidism, not hypothyroidism.
CN: Health promotion and maintenance; CNS: None; CL: Application

5. 4. The most serious consequence of congenital hypothyroidism is delayed development of the central nervous system, which leads to severe mental retardation. The other choices occur but aren't the most serious consequences.
CN: Physiological integrity; CNS: Physiological adaptation; CL: Analysis

6. 1. The severity of the intellectual deficit is related to the degree of hypothyroidism and the duration of the condition before treatment. Cranial malformations don't affect the severity of the intellectual deficit nor does the degree of hypothermia as it relates to hypothyroidism. It isn't the specific T_4 level at diagnosis that affects the intellect but how long the client has been hospitalized.
CN: Health promotion and maintenance; CNS: None; CL: Application

7. 1. Heelstick blood tests are mandatory in all states and are usually performed on neonates between 2 and 6 days of age. Typically, specimens are taken before the neonate is discharged from the hospital; the test is included with other tests that screen the neonate for errors of metabolism.
CN: Health promotion and maintenance; CNS: None; CL: Application

CN: Client needs category   CNS: Client needs subcategory   CL: Cognitive level

8. Which result would indicate to a nurse the possibility that a neonate has congenital hypothyroidism?
1. High level thyroxine (T_4) and low level thyroid-stimulating hormone (TSH)
2. Low level T_4 and high level TSH
3. Normal TSH and high level T_4
4. Normal T_4 and low level TSH

9. A nurse is teaching parents about therapeutic management of their neonate diagnosed with congenital hypothyroidism. Which response by a parent would indicate the need for <u>further teaching</u>?
1. "My baby will need regular measurements of his thyroxine (T_4) levels."
2. "Treatment involves lifelong thyroid hormone replacement therapy."
3. "Treatment should begin as soon as possible after diagnosis is made."
4. "As my baby grows, his thyroid gland will mature and he won't need medications."

10. Which comment made by the mother of a neonate at her 2-week office visit should alert the nurse to suspect congenital hypothyroidism?
1. "My baby is unusually quiet and good."
2. "My baby seems to be a yellowish color."
3. "After feedings, my baby pulls her legs up and cries."
4. "My baby seems to really look at my face during feeding time."

11. Which statement should be included when educating a mother about giving levothyroxine (Synthroid) to her neonate after a diagnosis of hypothyroidism is made?
1. The drug has a bitter taste.
2. The pill shouldn't be crushed.
3. Never put the medication in formula or juice.
4. If a dose is missed, double the dose the next day.

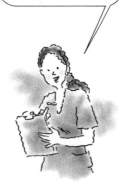

In question 9, the phrase *further teaching* indicates that you're looking for an incorrect statement.

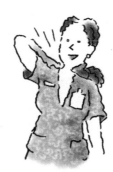

You've finished 10 questions already! Congratulations!

8. 2. Screening results that show a low level of T_4 and a high level of TSH indicate congenital hypothyroidism and the need for further tests to determine the cause of the disease.
CN: Physiological integrity; CNS: Reduction of risk potential; CL: Application

9. 4. Treatment involves lifelong thyroid hormone replacement therapy that begins as soon as possible after diagnosis to abolish all signs of hypothyroidism and to reestablish normal physical and mental development. The drug of choice is synthetic levothyroxine (Synthroid or Levothroid). Regular measurements of T_4 levels are important in ensuring optimum treatment.
CN: Health promotion and maintenance; CNS: None; CL: Application

10. 1. Parental remarks about an unusually "quiet and good" neonate together with any of the early physical manifestations should lead to a suspicion of hypothyroidism, which requires a referral for specific tests. If a neonate begins to look yellow in color, hyperbilirubinemia may be the cause. If the neonate is pulling her legs up and crying after feedings, she might be showing signs of colic. The neonate likes looking at the human face and should show interest in this at age 2 weeks.
CN: Health promotion and maintenance; CNS: None; CL: Application

11. 4. If a dose is missed, twice the dose should be given the next day. The importance of compliance with the drug regimen for the neonate to achieve normal growth and development must be stressed. Because the drug is tasteless, it can be crushed and added to a small amount of water.
CN: Physiological integrity; CNS: Pharmacological and parenteral therapies; CL: Application

12. When teaching parents about signs that indicate levothyroxine (Synthroid) overdose, which comment from a parent indicates the need for <u>further</u> teaching?
  1. "Irritability is a sign of overdose."
  2. "If my baby's heartbeat is fast, I should count it."
  3. "If my baby loses weight, I should be concerned."
  4. "I shouldn't worry if my baby doesn't sleep very much."

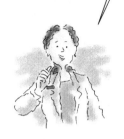

Watch out! Question 12 is another further teaching question.

13. A nurse should recognize that exophthalmos (protruding eyeballs) may occur in children with which condition?
  1. Hypothyroidism
  2. Hyperthyroidism
  3. Hypoparathyroidism
  4. Hyperparathyroidism

14. A nurse is assessing a child with juvenile hypothyroidism. Which common clinical finding would most likely be observed?
  1. Accelerated growth
  2. Diarrhea
  3. Dry skin
  4. Insomnia

15. A nurse is observing an infant with thyroid hormone deficiency. Which signs would the nurse <u>commonly</u> observe?
  1. Tachycardia, profuse perspiration, and diarrhea
  2. Lethargy, feeding difficulties, and constipation
  3. Hypertonia, small fontanels, and moist skin
  4. Dermatitis, dry skin, and round face

Question 16 is asking for the most appropriate behavior. In other words, *prioritize!*

16. When counseling parents of a neonate with congenital hypothyroidism, the nurse should encourage which behavior?
  1. Seeking professional genetic counseling
  2. Retracing the family tree for others born with this condition
  3. Talking to relatives who have gone through a similar experience
  4. Seeking alternative therapies for this condition

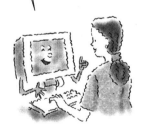

12. 4. Parents need to be aware of signs indicating overdose, such as rapid pulse, dyspnea, irritability, insomnia, fever, sweating, and weight loss. The parents would be given acceptable parameters for the heart rate and weight loss or gain. If the baby is experiencing a heart rate or weight loss outside of the acceptable parameters, the physician should be called.
CN: Physiological integrity; CNS: Pharmacological and parenteral therapies; CL: Analysis

13. 2. Exophthalmos occurs when there's an overproduction of thyroid hormone, or hyperthyroidism. This sign should alert the physician to follow up with further testing.
CN: Health promotion and maintenance; CNS: None; CL: Application

14. 3. Children with hypothyroidism will have dry skin. The other choices aren't evident in children with juvenile hypothyroidism.
CN: Health promotion and maintenance; CNS: None; CL: Application

15. 2. Hypothyroidism results from inadequate thyroid production to meet an infant's needs. Clinical signs include feeding difficulties, prolonged physiologic jaundice, lethargy, and constipation.
CN: Health promotion and maintenance; CNS: None; CL: Analysis

16. 1. Seeking professional genetic counseling is the best option for parents who have a neonate with a genetic disorder. Education about the disorder should occur as soon as the parents are ready, so they'll understand the genetic implications for future children. Retracing the family tree and talking to relatives won't help the parents to become better educated about the disorder. Seeking alternative therapies should be discouraged to prevent possible complications.
CN: Health promotion and maintenance; CNS: None; CL: Application

CN: Client needs category   CNS: Client needs subcategory   CL: Cognitive level

17. While receiving teaching about giving insulin injections, an adolescent questions the nurse about the reuse of disposable needles and syringes. Which response from the nurse is most appropriate?
 1. "This is an unsafe practice."
 2. "This is acceptable for up to 7 days."
 3. "This is acceptable for only 48 hours."
 4. "This is acceptable only if the family has very limited resources."

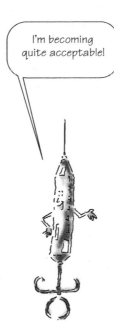

I'm becoming quite acceptable!

18. When children are more physically active, which change in the management of the child with diabetes should the nurse expect?
 1. Increased food intake
 2. Decreased food intake
 3. Decreased risk of insulin shock
 4. Increased risk of hyperglycemia

19. When a nurse is helping an adolescent deal with diabetes, which characteristic of adolescence should be considered?
 1. Wanting to be an individual
 2. Needing to be like peers
 3. Being preoccupied with future plans
 4. Teaching peers that this is a serious disease

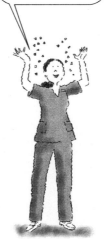

20 questions completed? That's cause for celebration!

20. An adolescent with diabetes tells the community nurse that he has recently started drinking alcohol on the weekends. Which action would initially be most appropriate for the nurse to take?
 1. Recommend referral to counseling.
 2. Make the adolescent promise to stop drinking.
 3. Discuss with the adolescent why he has started drinking.
 4. Teach the adolescent about the effects of alcohol on diabetes.

17. 2. It has become acceptable practice for clients to reuse their own disposable needles and syringes for up to 7 days. Bacteria counts are unaffected, and there are considerable cost savings. If this method is approved, it's imperative to stress the importance of vigorous hand washing before handling equipment as well as capping the syringe immediately after use and storing it in the refrigerator to decrease the growth of organisms.
CN: Safe, effective care environment; CNS: Safety and infection control; CL: Application

18. 1. If a child is more active at one time of the day than another, food or insulin can be altered to meet the activity pattern of the individual. Food should be increased when children are more physically active. The child has an increased risk of insulin shock and a decreased risk of hyperglycemia when he's more physically active.
CN: Physiological integrity; CNS: Reduction of risk potential; CL: Application

19. 2. Adolescents appear to have the most difficulty in adjusting to diabetes. Adolescence is a time when there's much stress on being "perfect" and being like one's peers and, to adolescents, having diabetes is being different.
CN: Health promotion and maintenance; CNS: None; CL: Application

20. 4. Confusion about the effects of alcohol on blood glucose is common. Teenagers may believe that alcohol will increase blood glucose levels, when in fact the opposite occurs. Ingestion of alcohol inhibits the release of glycogen from the liver, resulting in hypoglycemia. Teens who drink alcohol may become hypoglycemic, but they are then treated as if they were intoxicated. Behaviors may be similar, such as shakiness, combativeness, slurred speech, and loss of consciousness. Finding out why the adolescent has started drinking and recommending counseling may be appropriate, but only after education is provided. An adolescent may promise to stop drinking but not follow through.
CN: Health promotion and maintenance; CNS: None; CL: Application

21. A child has experienced symptoms of hypoglycemia and has eaten sugar cubes. A nurse should follow this rapid-releasing sugar with which food?
1. Fruit juices
2. Six glasses of water
3. Foods that are high in protein
4. Complex carbohydrates and protein

21. 4. When a child exhibits signs of hypoglycemia, the majority of cases can be treated with a simple concentrated sugar, such as honey, that can be held in the mouth for a short time. A complex carbohydrate and protein, such as a slice of bread or a cracker spread with peanut butter, should follow the rapid-releasing sugar or the client may become hypoglycemic again.
CN: Health promotion and maintenance; CNS: None; CL: Application

22. The nurse is teaching the parents of a child newly diagnosed with diabetes to identify the signs and symptoms of hypoglycemia. Which response by the parents indicates the teaching has been effective?
1. "Irritability, shakiness, hunger, headache, and dizziness are signs to look for."
2. "Drowsiness, lethargy, and decreased urine output need to be reported."
3. "Abdominal pain, nausea and vomiting, and constipation are the most common findings."
4. "We will report immediately any signs of urinary frequency."

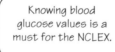

If you know the definitions of hypo and hyper, it can help you with a bunch of questions.

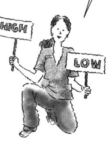

22. 1. Signs of hypoglycemia include irritability, shaky feeling, hunger, headache, and dizziness. Drowsiness, abdominal pain, polyuria, nausea, and vomiting are signs of *hyper*glycemia.
CN: Physiological integrity; CNS: Physiological adaptation; CL: Application

23. The nurse is assessing a child recently admitted with diabetes who has developed ketoacidosis. Which statement is the most accurate?
1. This is a normal outcome of diabetes.
2. This is a life-threatening situation.
3. This is a situation that can easily be treated at home.
4. This is a situation best treated in the pediatrician's office.

23. 2. Diabetic ketoacidosis, the most complete state of insulin deficiency, is a life-threatening situation. The child should be admitted to an intensive care facility for management, which consists of rapid assessment, adequate insulin to reduce the elevated blood glucose level, fluids to overcome dehydration, and electrolyte replacement (especially potassium).
CN: Physiological integrity; CNS: Physiological adaptation; CL: Application

24. Which guideline is appropriate when teaching an 11-year-old child who was recently diagnosed with diabetes about insulin injections?
1. The parents don't need to be involved in learning this procedure.
2. Self-injection techniques aren't usually taught until the child reaches age 16.
3. At age 11, the child should be old enough to give most of his own injections.
4. Self-injection techniques should be taught only when the child can reach all injection sites.

Knowing blood glucose values is a must for the NCLEX.

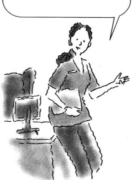

24. 3. The parents must supervise and manage the child's therapeutic program, but the child should assume responsibility for self-management as soon as he's capable. Children can learn to collect their own blood for glucose testing at a relatively young age (4 to 5 years), and most are able to check their blood glucose level and administer insulin at about age 9. Some children may be able to do it earlier.
CN: Health promotion and maintenance; CNS: None; CL: Application

CN: Client needs category   CNS: Client needs subcategory   CL: Cognitive level

25. The nurse suspects a client of having diabetic ketoacidosis. Which blood glucose value would be observed with this condition?
1. 50 mg/dl
2. 90 mg/dl
3. 150 mg/dl
4. 300 mg/dl

26. A 2-year-old child has been admitted with a diagnosis of diabetes mellitus. Which cardinal sign would support this diagnosis?
1. Nausea
2. Seizure
3. Hyperactivity
4. Frequent urination

27. The parent of a child with diabetes asks a nurse why blood glucose monitoring is needed. The nurse should base her reply on which premise?
1. This is an easier method of testing.
2. This is a less expensive method of testing.
3. This allows children the ability to better manage their diabetes.
4. This gives children a greater sense of control over their diabetes.

28. To increase an adolescent's compliance with treatment for diabetes mellitus, the nurse should attempt which strategy?
1. Provide for a special diet in the high school cafeteria.
2. Clarify the adolescent's values to promote involvement in care.
3. Identify energy requirements for participation in sports activities.
4. Educate the adolescent about long-term consequences of poor metabolic control.

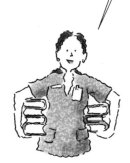

Teaching clients how to help manage their own conditions is a common subject on the NCLEX.

25. 4. Diabetic ketoacidosis is determined by the presence of hyperglycemia (blood glucose measurement of 300 mg/dl or higher), accompanied by acetone breath, dehydration, weak and rapid pulse, and a decreased level of consciousness.
CN: Physiological integrity; CNS: Physiological adaptation; CL: Analysis

26. 4. Polyphagia, polyuria (frequent urination), polydipsia, and weight loss are cardinal signs of diabetes mellitus. Other signs include irritability, shortened attention span, lowered frustration tolerance, fatigue, dry skin, blurred vision, sores that are slow to heal, and flushed skin.
CN: Health promotion and maintenance; CNS: None; CL: Application

27. 3. Blood glucose monitoring improves diabetes management and is used successfully by children from the onset of their diabetes. By testing their own blood, children are able to change their insulin regimen to maintain their glucose level in the normoglycemic range of 80 to 120 mg/dl. This allows them to better manage their diabetes.
CN: Health promotion and maintenance; CNS: None; CL: Application

28. 2. Adolescent compliance with diabetes management may be hampered by dependence versus independence conflicts and ego development. Attempts to have the adolescent clarify personal values promotes involvement in his care and fosters compliance.
CN: Health promotion and maintenance; CNS: None; CL: Application

29. A child with diabetes type 1 tells the nurse he feels shaky. The nurse assesses the child's skin color to be pale and sweaty. Which action should the nurse initiate <u>immediately</u>?
1. Give supplemental insulin.
2. Have the child eat a glucose tablet.
3. Administer glucagon subcutaneously.
4. Offer the child a complex carbohydrate snack.

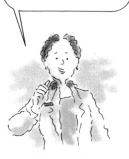

The word *immediately* signals a need for you to prioritize.

30. The parents of a child diagnosed with diabetes ask the nurse about maintaining metabolic control during a minor illness with loss of appetite. Which nursing response is appropriate?
1. "Decrease the child's insulin by half the usual dose during the course of the illness."
2. "Call your physician to arrange hospitalization."
3. "Give increased amounts of clear liquids to prevent dehydration."
4. "Substitute calorie-containing liquids for uneaten solid food."

31. Which criteria should a nurse use to measure good metabolic control in a child with diabetes mellitus?
1. Fewer than eight episodes of severe hyperglycemia in a month
2. Infrequent occurrences of mild hypoglycemic reactions
3. Hemoglobin A values less than 12%
4. Growth below the 15th percentile

It's important for your baby's sake to control your diabetes.

32. The nurse is assessing the neonate of a poorly controlled diabetic mother in the NICU. Which congenital anomaly would likely be observed?
1. Cataracts
2. Low-set ears
3. Cardiac malformations
4. Cleft lip and palate deformities

29. 2. These are symptoms of hypoglycemia. Rapid treatment involves giving the alert child a glucose tablet (4 mg of dextrose) or, if unavailable, a glass of glucose-containing liquid. It would be followed by a complex carbohydrate snack and protein. Giving supplemental insulin would be contraindicated because that would lower the blood glucose even more. Glucagon would be given only if there was a risk of aspiration with oral glucose, such as if the child was semiconscious.
CN: Safe, effective care environment; CNS: Management of care; CL: Application

30. 4. Calorie-containing liquids can help to maintain more normal blood sugar levels as well as decrease the danger of dehydration. The child with diabetes should always take *at least* the usual dose of insulin during an illness based on more frequent blood sugar checks. During an illness where there's vomiting or loss of appetite, NPH insulin may be lowered by 25% to 30% to avoid hyperglycemia, and regular insulin is given according to home glucose monitoring results.
CN: Safe, effective care environment; CNS: Management of care; CL: Application

31. 2. Criteria for good metabolic control generally includes few episodes of hypoglycemia or hyperglycemia, hemoglobin A values less than 8%, and normal growth and development.
CN: Health promotion and maintenance; CNS: None; CL: Application

32. 3. Cardiac and central nervous system anomalies, along with neural tube defects and skeletal and GI anomalies, are most likely to occur in uncontrolled maternal diabetes.
CN: Health promotion and maintenance; CNS: None; CL: Application

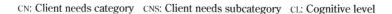

CN: Client needs category   CNS: Client needs subcategory   CL: Cognitive level

33. Which condition could possibly cause <u>hypoglycemia</u>?
1. Too little insulin
2. Mild illness with fever
3. Excessive exercise without a carbohydrate snack
4. Eating ice cream and cake to celebrate a birthday

34. Which assessment factor is the <u>best</u> indicator of a client's diabetic control during the preceding 2 to 3 months?
1. Fasting glucose level
2. Oral glucose tolerance level
3. Glycosylated hemoglobin test
4. A client's record of glucose monitoring

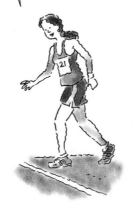

I'm glad I had a snack before I started to race.

35. A client has received diet instruction as part of his treatment plan for diabetes type 1. Which statement by the client indicates to the nurse that he needs <u>additional instructions</u>?
1. "I'll need a bedtime snack because I take an evening dose of NPH insulin."
2. "I can eat whatever I want as long as I cover the calories with sufficient insulin."
3. "I can have an occasional low-calorie drink as long as I include it in my meal plan."
4. "I should eat meals as scheduled, even if I'm not hungry, to prevent hypoglycemia."

36. The nurse suspects a 10-year-old client with diabetes is hyperglycemic. Which symptom would indicate this condition?
1. Rapid heart rate
2. Headache
3. Hunger
4. Thirst

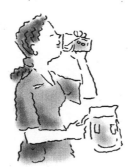

All this studying makes me thirsty.

33. 3. Excessive exercise without a carbohydrate snack could cause hypoglycemia. The other options describe situations that cause *hyper*glycemia.
CN: Health promotion and maintenance; CNS: None; CL: Application

34. 3. A glycosylated hemoglobin level provides an overview of a person's blood glucose level over the previous 2 to 3 months. Glycosylated hemoglobin values are reported as a percentage of the total hemoglobin within an erythrocyte. The time frame is based on the fact that the usual life span of an erythrocyte is 2 to 3 months; a random blood sample, therefore, will theoretically give samples of erythrocytes for this same period. The other options won't indicate a true picture of the person's blood glucose level over the previous 2 to 3 months.
CN: Health promotion and maintenance; CNS: None; CL: Application

35. 2. The goal of diet therapy in diabetes mellitus is to attain and maintain ideal body weight. Each client will be prescribed a specific caloric intake and insulin regimen to help accomplish this goal.
CN: Physiological integrity; CNS: Basic care and comfort; CL: Analysis

36. 4. Thirst (polydipsia) is one of the symptoms of hyperglycemia. Rapid heart rate, headache, and hunger are signs and symptoms of *hypo*glycemia.
CN: Physiological integrity; CNS: Physiological adaptation; CL: Application

37. A client is learning to mix regular insulin and NPH insulin in the same syringe. Which action, if performed by the client, would indicate the need for <u>further teaching</u>?
1. Withdrawing the NPH insulin first
2. Injecting air into the NPH insulin bottle first
3. After drawing up first insulin, removing air bubbles
4. Injecting an amount of air equal to the desired dose of insulin

38. A client is diagnosed with diabetes type 1. The primary health care provider prescribes an insulin regimen of regular insulin and NPH insulin administered subcutaneously each morning. How soon after administration will the onset of regular insulin begin?
1. Within 5 minutes
2. ½ to 1 hour
3. 1 to 1½ hours
4. 4 to 8 hours

39. When assessing a neonate for signs of diabetes insipidus, a nurse should recognize which symptom as a sign of this disorder?
1. Hyponatremia
2. Jaundice
3. Polyuria
4. Hypochloremia

40. Which is an initial symptom of diabetes insipidus in an infant?
1. Dehydration
2. Inability to be aroused
3. Extreme hunger relieved by frequent feedings of milk
4. Irritability relieved with feedings of water but not milk

It's important to know how and when different types of insulin react.

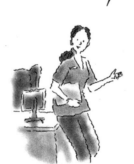

You've reached question 40. How cool is that?

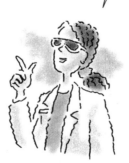

37. 1. Regular insulin is *always* withdrawn first so it won't become contaminated with NPH insulin. The client is instructed to inject air into the NPH insulin bottle equal to the amount of insulin to be withdrawn, because there will be regular insulin in the syringe and he won't be able to inject air when he needs to withdraw the NPH. It's necessary to remove the air bubbles to ensure a correct dosage before drawing up the second insulin.
CN: Physiological integrity; CNS: Pharmacological and parenteral therapies; CL: Application

38. 2. Regular insulin's onset is ½ to 1 hour, peak is 2 to 4 hours, and duration is 3 to 6 hours. Lispro insulin has an onset within 5 minutes. NPH insulin has an onset within 2 to 4 hours, and Ultralente insulin is the longest acting, with an onset of 6 to 10 hours.
CN: Physiological integrity; CNS: Pharmacological and parenteral therapies; CL: Application

39. 3. The cardinal sign of diabetes insipidus is polyuria, along with polydipsia. Hypernatremia, not hyponatremia, occurs with diabetes insipidus. Jaundice occurs because of abnormal bilirubin metabolism, not diabetes insipidus. Hyperchloremia, not hypochloremia, occurs with diabetes insipidus.
CN: Physiological integrity; CNS: Physiological adaptation; CL: Application

40. 4. One initial symptom of diabetes insipidus in an infant is irritability relieved with feedings of water but not milk. Dehydration and the inability to be aroused are late symptoms.
CN: Health promotion and maintenance; CNS: None; CL: Application

CN: Client needs category   CNS: Client needs subcategory   CL: Cognitive level

41. A nurse is helping parents understand when treatments of growth hormone replacement will end. Which statement should be included?

1. The dosage of growth hormone will decrease as the child's age increases.
2. The dosage of growth hormone will increase as the time of epiphyseal closure nears.
3. After giving growth hormone replacement for 1 year, the dose will be tapered down.
4. Growth hormone replacement can't be abruptly stopped; it must be spread out over several months.

42. A nurse is explaining diabetes insipidus to the parents of an infant with the disease. When explaining the diagnostic test that's used, which comment by a parent would indicate an <u>understanding</u> of the diagnostic test?

1. "Fluids will be offered every 2 hours."
2. "My infant's fluid intake will be restricted."
3. "I won't change anything about my infant's intake."
4. "Formula will be restricted, but glucose water is OK."

43. A nurse should anticipate which physiologic response in an infant being tested for diabetes insipidus?

1. Increase in urine output
2. Decrease in urine output
3. No effect on urine output
4. Increase in urine specific gravity

44. An infant has a positive test result for diabetes insipidus. The nurse should anticipate the physician ordering a test dose of which medication?

1. Antidiuretic hormone
2. Biosynthetic growth hormone
3. Adrenocorticotropic hormone
4. Aqueous vasopressin (Pitressin Synthetic)

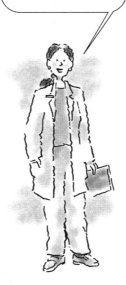

Question 42 asks you to identify a knowledgeable response.

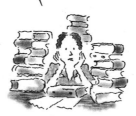

Poly this and poly that. Hypo this and hyper that. I'm confused.

41. 2. Dosage of growth hormone is increased as the time of epiphyseal closure nears, to gain the best advantage of the growth hormone. The medication is then stopped. There's no tapering off of the dose.
CN: Physiological integrity; CNS: Pharmacological and parenteral therapies; CL: Application

42. 2. The simplest test used to diagnose diabetes insipidus is restriction of oral fluids and observation of consequent changes in urine volume and concentration. A weight loss of 3% to 5% indicates severe dehydration, and the test should be terminated at this point. This is done in the hospital, and the infant is watched closely.
CN: Health promotion and maintenance; CNS: None; CL: Application

43. 3. In diabetes insipidus, fluid restriction for diagnostic testing has little or no effect on urine formation but causes weight loss from dehydration.
CN: Physiological integrity; CNS: Physiological adaptation; CL: Application

44. 4. If the fluid restriction test is positive, the child should be given a test dose of injected aqueous vasopressin, which should alleviate the polyuria and polydipsia. Unresponsiveness to exogenous vasopressin usually indicates nephrogenic diabetes insipidus. The other choices are used to determine other types of endocrine disorders.
CN: Physiological integrity; CNS: Pharmacological and parenteral therapies; CL: Application

45. The nurse is teaching the parents of an infant diagnosed with diabetes insipidus. Which treatment would the nurse include in the teaching?
1. Antihypertensive medications
2. The need for blood products
3. Hormone replacement
4. Fluid restrictions

46. When providing information about treatments for diabetes insipidus to parents, a nurse explains the use of nasal spray and injections. Which indication might <u>deter</u> a parent from choosing nasal spray treatment?
1. Applications must be repeated every 8 to 12 hours.
2. Applications must be repeated every 2 to 4 hours.
3. Nasal sprays can't be used in infants.
4. Measurements are too difficult.

47. A nurse is teaching the parents of an infant with diabetes insipidus about an injectable drug used to treat the disorder. Which statement made by a parent would indicate the need for further teaching?
1. "I must hold the medication under warm running water for 10 to 15 minutes before administering it."
2. "The medication must be shaken vigorously before being drawn up into the syringe."
3. "Small brown particles must be seen in the suspension."
4. "I will store this medication in the refrigerator."

48. When teaching parents of an infant newly diagnosed with diabetes insipidus, which statement by a parent indicates a <u>good understanding</u> of this condition?
1. "When my infant stabilizes, I won't have to worry about giving hormone medication."
2. "I don't have to measure the amount of fluid intake that I give my infant."
3. "I realize that treatment for diabetes insipidus is lifelong."
4. "My infant will outgrow this condition."

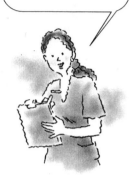

Although the word *deter* sounds like a negative, question 46 actually asks you to identify a *true* characteristic of nasal sprays.

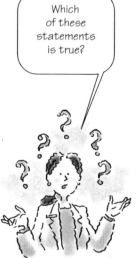

Which of these statements is true?

45. 3. The usual treatment for diabetes insipidus is hormone replacement with vasopressin or desmopressin acetate (DDAVP). No problem with hypertension is associated with this condition, and fluids shouldn't be restricted. Blood products shouldn't be needed.
CN: Health promotion and maintenance; CNS: None; CL: Application

46. 1. Applications of nasal spray used to treat diabetes insipidus must be repeated every 8 to 12 hours; injections last for 48 to 72 hours. The nasal spray must be timed for adequate night sleep. However, the injections are oil-based and quite painful. Nasal sprays have been used in infants with diabetes insipidus and are dispensed in premeasured intranasal inhalers, eliminating the need for measuring doses.
CN: Physiological integrity; CNS: Pharmacological and parenteral therapies CL: Analysis

47. 4. The medication should be stored at room temperature. When giving injectable vasopressin, it must be thoroughly resuspended in the oil by being held under warm running water for 10 to 15 minutes and shaken vigorously before being drawn into the syringe. If this isn't done, the oil may be injected minus the drug. Small brown particles, which indicate drug dispersion, must be seen in the suspension.
CN: Physiological integrity; CNS: Pharmacological and parenteral therapies; CL: Application

48. 3. Diabetes insipidus is a condition that will need lifelong treatment. The amount of fluid intake is very important and must be measured with the infant's output to monitor the medication regime. The infant won't outgrow this condition.
CN: Safe, effective care environment; CNS: Management of care; CL: Application

CN: Client needs category   CNS: Client needs subcategory   CL: Cognitive level

49. A child is admitted with diabetes insipidus. The nurse asks the parents if they know about this condition. Which statement tells the nurse that the parents understand the condition?
1. "We know that our child's thyroid is working too much."
2. "We know that our child's pituitary gland is not working hard enough."
3. "Our child's pituitary gland is working overtime."
4. "Our child's parathyroid gland is not doing a good job. It is acting very lazy."

50. After a nurse has explained the causes of diabetes insipidus to the parents, which statement made by a parent indicates the need for further teaching?
1. "This condition could be familial or congenital."
2. "Drinking alcohol during my pregnancy caused this condition."
3. "My child might have a tumor that's causing these symptoms."
4. "An infection such as meningitis may be the reason my child has diabetes insipidus."

51. Which assessment finding would alert a nurse to <u>change</u> the intranasal route for vasopressin administration?
1. Mucous membrane irritation
2. Severe coughing
3. Nosebleeds
4. Pneumonia

52. A nurse should include which in-home management instruction for a child who's receiving desmopressin acetate (DDAVP) for symptomatic control of diabetes insipidus?
1. Give DDAVP only when urine output begins to decrease.
2. Cleanse skin with alcohol before application of the DDAVP dermal patch.
3. Increase the DDAVP dose if polyuria occurs just before the next scheduled dose.
4. Call the physician for an alternate route of DDAVP when the child has an upper respiratory infection (URI) or allergic rhinitis.

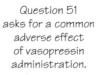

Question 51 asks for a common adverse effect of vasopressin administration.

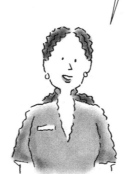

49. 2. The principal disorder of posterior pituitary hypofunction is diabetes insipidus. The disorder results form hyposecretion of antidiuretic hormone, producing a state of uncontrolled diuresis. It is not caused by the thyroid gland or parathyroid gland.
CN: Health promotion and maintenance; CNS: None; CL: Application

50. 2. Drinking alcohol during pregnancy can lead to a neonate born with fetal alcohol syndrome but has no known correlation to diabetes insipidus. The other options are possible causes of diabetes insipidus.
CN: Health promotion and maintenance; CNS: None; CL: Application

51. 1. Mucous membrane irritation caused by a cold or allergy renders the intranasal route unreliable. Severe coughing, pneumonia, or nosebleeds shouldn't interfere with the intranasal route.
CN: Physiological integrity; CNS: Pharmacological and parenteral therapies; CL: Application

52. 4. Excessive nasal mucus associated with URI or allergic rhinitis may interfere with DDAVP absorption because it's given intranasally. Parents should be instructed to contact the physician for advice in altering the hormone dose during times when nasal mucus may be increased. The DDAVP dose should remain unchanged, even if there's polyuria just before the next dose. This is to avoid overmedicating the child.
CN: Safe, effective care environment; CNS: Management of care; CL: Application

53. A nurse is assessing a client with suspected hypopituitarism. Which sign or symptom of this condition would the nurse <u>most</u> commonly observe?
  1. Sleep disturbance
  2. Polyuria
  3. Polydipsia
  4. Short stature

54. Which statement made to a nurse by the parents of a child with idiopathic growth hormone deficiency would indicate the need for <u>further teaching</u>?
  1. "This disorder may be familial."
  2. "There's no genetic basis for this disorder."
  3. "This disorder might be secondary to hypothalamic deficiency."
  4. "There may be other disorders related to pituitary hormone deficiencies."

55. A nurse is teaching health to a class of fifth graders. Which statement related to growth should be included?
  1. "There's nothing that you can do to influence your growth."
  2. "Excessive physical activity that begins before puberty might stunt growth."
  3. "All children who are short in stature also have parents who are short in stature."
  4. "Because this is a time of tremendous growth, being concerned about calorie intake isn't important."

56. While teaching the parents of a child with short stature, the nurse discusses familial short stature. Which statement by the nurse about this condition is the <u>most</u> correct?
  1. "It occurs in children who are members of a very large family with limited resources."
  2. "It occurs in children who have no siblings and who moved a great deal during their early childhood."
  3. "It occurs in children with delayed linear growth and skeletal and sexual maturation that's behind that of age mates."
  4. "It occurs in children who have ancestors with adult height in the lower percentiles and whose height during childhood is appropriate."

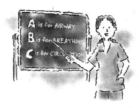

A nurse's responsibility to teach never ends.

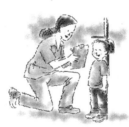

Let's see how you measure up.

53. 4. The most common sign in most instances of hypopituitarism is short stature. Sleep disturbance may indicate thyrotoxicosis. Polydipsia and polyuria may be indications of diabetes mellitus or diabetes insipidus.
CN: Physiological integrity; CNS: Physiological adaptation; CL: Application

54. 2. The cause of idiopathic growth hormone deficiency is unknown. There's a higher-than-average occurrence of the disorder in some families, which indicates a possible genetic cause. The condition is commonly associated with other pituitary hormone deficiencies, such as deficiencies of thyroid-stimulating hormone and corticotropin, and may be secondary to hypothalamic deficiency.
CN: Psychosocial integrity; CNS: None; CL: Application

55. 2. Intensive physical activity (greater than 18 hours per week) that begins before puberty may stunt growth so that the child doesn't reach full adult height. Nutrition and environment influence a child's growth. All children who are short in stature don't necessarily have parents who are short in stature. During the school-age years, growth slows and doesn't accelerate again until adolescence.
CN: Health promotion and maintenance; CNS: None; CL: Application

56. 4. Familial short stature refers to otherwise healthy children who have ancestors with adult height in the lower percentiles and whose height during childhood is appropriate for genetic background. Children who are members of very large families with limited resources or who are only children don't fit the description of familial short stature. Children with delayed linear growth and skeletal and sexual maturation that's behind that of age mates are considered to have constitutional growth delay.
CN: Physiological integrity; CNS: Physiological adaptation; CL: Application

CN: Client needs category   CNS: Client needs subcategory   CL: Cognitive level

57. When assessing a child age 2, which finding would indicate to the nurse the possibility of growth hormone deficiency?
1. The child had normal growth during the first year of life but showed a slowed growth curve below the 3rd percentile for the second year of life.
2. The child fell below the 5th percentile for growth during the first year of life but, at this check-up, falls below only the 50th percentile.
3. There has been a steady decline in growth over the 2 years of this toddler's life that has accelerated during the past 6 months.
4. There was delayed growth below the 5th percentile for the first and second years of life.

58. A nurse is assessing a child with growth hormone deficiency. Which characteristic would the nurse <u>most</u> commonly observe?
1. Decreased weight with no change in height
2. Decreased weight with increased height
3. Increased weight with decreased height
4. Increased weight with increased height

59. A nurse should find which characteristic in her assessment of a child with growth hormone deficiency?
1. Normal skeletal proportions
2. Abnormal skeletal proportions
3. Child's appearing older than his age
4. Longer than normal upper extremities

60. When counseling the parents of a child with growth hormone deficiency, the nurse should <u>encourage</u> which sport?
1. Basketball
2. Field hockey
3. Football
4. Gymnastics

57. 1. Children with growth hormone deficiency generally grow normally during the first year and then follow a slowed growth curve that's below the 3rd percentile. If growth is consistently below the 5th percentile, it may be an indication of failure to thrive.
CN: Health promotion and maintenance; CNS: None; CL: Application

58. 3. Height may be retarded more than weight because, with good nutrition, children with growth hormone deficiency can become overweight or even obese. Their well-nourished appearance is an important diagnostic clue to differentiation from other disorders such as failure to thrive.
CN: Health promotion and maintenance; CNS: None; CL: Application

59. 1. Skeletal proportions are normal for the age, but these children appear younger than their chronological age. However, later in life, premature aging is evident.
CN: Physiological integrity; CNS: Physiological adaptation; CL: Application

60. 4. Children with growth hormone deficiency can be no less active than other children if directed to size-appropriate sports, such as gymnastics, swimming, wrestling, or soccer.
CN: Health promotion and maintenance; CNS: None; CL: Application

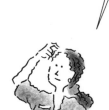

Which of these sports would be best for a child with growth hormone deficiency?

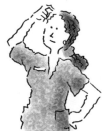

61. In explaining to parents the social behavior of children with hypopituitarism, a nurse should recognize which statement as exhibiting a need for further teaching?

1. "I realize that my child might have school anxiety and a low self-esteem."
2. "Because my child is short in stature, people expect less of him than his peers."
3. "Because of my child's short stature, he may not be pushed to perform at his chronological age by others."
4. "My child's vocabulary is very well developed, so even though he's short in stature, no one will treat him differently."

62. The mother of a child diagnosed with hypopituitarism states to the nurse that she feels guilty because she feels that she should have recognized this disorder. Which statement by the nurse about children with hypopituitarism would be the most helpful?"

1. "They're usually large for gestational age at birth."
2. "They're usually small for gestational age at birth."
3. "They usually exhibit signs of this disorder soon after birth."
4. "They're usually of normal size for gestational age at birth."

63. Which observation when plotting height and weight on a growth chart would indicate that a child age 4 has a growth hormone deficiency?

1. Upward shift of 1 percentile or more
2. Upward shift of 5 percentiles or more
3. Downward shift of 2 percentiles or more
4. Downward shift of 5 percentiles or more

64. When reviewing the results of radiographic examinations of a child with hypopituitarism, which characteristic should the nurse expect to observe?

1. Bone age near normal
2. Epiphyseal maturation normal
3. Epiphyseal maturation retarded
4. Bone maturation greatly retarded

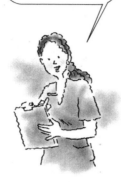

It's important that parents have realistic expectations about their child's disorder.

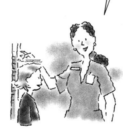

It's important to pay attention to abnormal growth in a child.

61. 4. Height discrepancy has been significantly correlated with emotional adjustment problems and may be a valuable predictor of the extent to which growth hormone–delayed children will have trouble with anxiety, social skills, and positive self-esteem. Also, academic problems aren't uncommon. These children aren't usually pushed to perform at their chronological age but are commonly subjected to juvenilization (related to in an infantile or childish manner).

CN: Psychosocial integrity; CNS: None; CL: Application

62. 4. Children with hypopituitarism are usually of normal size for gestational age at birth. Clinical features develop slowly and vary with the severity of the disorder and the number of deficient hormones.

CN: Psychosocial integrity; CNS: None; CL: Application

63. 3. When the physician evaluates the results of plotting height and weight, upward or downward shifts of 2 percentiles or more in children older than 3 years may indicate a growth abnormality.

CN: Health promotion and maintenance; CNS: None; CL: Analysis

64. 3. Epiphyseal maturation is retarded in hypopituitarism consistent with retardation in height. This is in contrast to hypothyroidism, in which bone maturation is greatly retarded, or Turner syndrome, in which bone age is near normal.

CN: Health promotion and maintenance; CNS: None; CL: Application

CN: Client needs category   CNS: Client needs subcategory   CL: Cognitive level

65. A child has been brought to a pediatrician's office for concerns about growth. The physician suspects hypopituitarism. The mother asks the nurse which test will be done to determine the diagnosis. Which response by the nurse would be most accurate?
　1. Hypersecretion of thyroid hormone
　2. Increased reserves of growth hormone
　3. Hyposecretion of antidiuretic hormone (ADH)
　4. Decreased reserves of growth hormone

66. The parents of a child who's going through testing for hypopituitarism ask the nurse what type of test results they should expect. The nurse's response should be based on which factor?
　1. Measurement of growth hormone will occur only one time.
　2. Growth hormone levels are decreased after strenuous exercise.
　3. There will be increased overnight urine growth hormone concentration.
　4. Growth hormone levels are elevated 45 to 90 minutes following the onset of sleep.

67. Which method is considered the <u>definitive</u> treatment for hypopituitarism due to growth hormone deficiency?
　1. Treatment with desmopressin acetate (DDAVP)
　2. Replacement of antidiuretic hormone (ADH)
　3. Treatment with testosterone or estrogen
　4. Replacement with biosynthetic growth hormone

68. When obtaining information about a child, which comment made by a parent to the nurse would indicate the possibility of hypopituitarism in a child?
　1. "I can pass down my child's clothes to his younger brother."
　2. "Usually my child wears out his clothes before his size changes."
　3. "I have to buy bigger size clothes for my child about every 2 months."
　4. "I have to buy larger shirts more frequently than larger pants for my child."

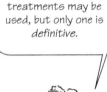

All of these treatments may be used, but only one is definitive.

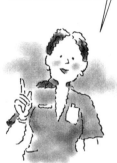

65. 4. Definitive diagnosis is based on absent or subnormal reserves of pituitary growth hormone. ADH and thyroid hormone levels aren't affected.
CN: Health promotion and maintenance; CNS: None; CL: Application

66. 4. Growth hormone levels are elevated 45 to 90 minutes following the onset of sleep. Low growth hormone levels following the onset of sleep would indicate the need for further evaluation. Exercise is a natural and benign stimulus for growth hormone release, and elevated levels can be detected after 20 minutes of strenuous exercise in normal children. Also, growth hormone levels will need to be checked frequently related to the type of therapy instituted.
CN: Physiological integrity; CNS: Physiological adaptation; CL: Application

67. 4. The definitive treatment of growth hormone deficiency is replacement of growth hormone and is successful in 80% of affected children. DDAVP is used to treat diabetes insipidus. ADH deficiency causes diabetes insipidus and isn't related to hypopituitarism. Testosterone or estrogen may be given during adolescence for normal sexual maturation, but neither is the definitive treatment for hypopituitarism.
CN: Physiological integrity; CNS: Pharmacological and parenteral therapies; CL: Application

68. 2. Parents of children with hypopituitarism frequently comment that the child wears out clothes before growing out of them or that, if the clothing fits the body, it's commonly too long in the sleeves or legs.
CN: Health promotion and maintenance; CNS: None; CL: Application

69. In helping parents who are planning to give growth hormone at home, a nurse should explain that optimum dosing is achieved when growth hormone is administered at which time?
  1. At bedtime
  2. After dinner
  3. In the middle of the day
  4. First thing in the morning

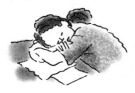

All I can think about is optimum dozing.

69. 1. Optimum dosing is typically achieved when growth hormone is administered at bedtime. Pituitary release of growth hormone occurs during the first 45 to 90 minutes after the onset of sleep, so normal physiologic release is mimicked with bedtime dosing.
CN: Physiological integrity; CNS: Pharmacological and parenteral therapies; CL: Application

70. In educating parents of a child with hypopituitarism about realistic expectations of height for their child who's successfully responding to growth hormone replacement, the nurse should include which statement?
  1. "Your child will never reach a normal adult height."
  2. "Your child will attain his eventual adult height at a faster rate."
  3. "Your child will attain his eventual adult height at a slower rate."
  4. "The rate of your child's growth will be the same as children without this disorder."

70. 3. Even when hormone replacement is successful, these children attain their eventual adult height at a slower rate than their peers do; therefore, they need assistance in setting realistic expectations regarding improvement.
CN: Psychosocial integrity; CNS: None; CL: Application

71. Which statement made by a parent of a child with short stature would indicate to the nurse the need for <u>further teaching</u>?
  1. "Obtaining blood studies won't aid in proper diagnosis."
  2. "A history of my child's growth patterns should be discussed."
  3. "X-rays should be included in my child's diagnostic procedures."
  4. "A family history is important information for me to share with my child's physician."

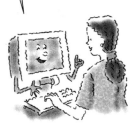

Careful—here's another further teaching question.

71. 1. A complete diagnostic evaluation should include a family history, a history of the child's growth patterns and previous health status, physical examination, physical evaluation, radiographic survey, and endocrine studies that may involve blood samples.
CN: Health promotion and maintenance; CNS: None; CL: Application

72. Which signs and symptoms would the health care team most commonly use as a basis for determining appropriate priorities and interventions for a child with type 1 diabetes mellitus? Select all that apply:
  1. Polyuria
  2. Weakness
  3. Abdominal pain
  4. Weight loss
  5. Postprandial nausea
  6. Orthostatic hypertension

72. 1, 2, 4, 5. Polyuria, weakness, weight loss, and postprandial nausea are commonly seen in diabetes mellitus. The healthcare team would plan care to manage these signs and symptoms. Abdominal pain isn't a symptom in this disease, and orthostatic hypotension rather than orthostatic hypertension would be a significant finding.
CN: Safe, effective care environment; CNS: Management of care; CL: Analysis

CN: Client needs category   CNS: Client needs subcategory   CL: Cognitive level

73. Which metabolic alteration characteristic might be associated with growth hormone deficiency?
1. Galactosemia
2. Homocystinuria
3. Hyperglycemia
4. Hypoglycemia

74. When providing information to the parents of a child who's receiving growth hormone replacement therapy for hypopituitarism, the nurse should include which intervention?
1. Explaining that growth in height and weight won't begin until puberty
2. Teaching how to perform venipuncture for administration of the growth hormone
3. Helping parents recognize the importance of interacting with the child according to age rather than size
4. Advising parents to hold the child back in school until linear growth begins to approximate the normal patterns

75. When assessing a neonate diagnosed with diabetes insipidus, which finding would indicate the need for intervention?
1. Edema
2. Increased head circumference
3. Weight gain
4. Weight loss

76. In a client with diabetes insipidus, a nurse could expect which characteristics of the urine?
1. Pale in color; specific gravity less than 1.006
2. Concentrated; specific gravity less than 1.006
3. Concentrated; specific gravity less than 1.03
4. Pale in color; specific gravity more than 1.03

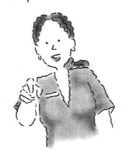

You know the answer to this question. I know you do!

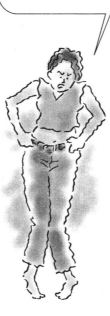

Here's a hint. The answer to question 75 certainly isn't my problem!

73. 4. The development of hypoglycemia is a characteristic finding related to growth hormone deficiency. Galactosemia is a rare autosomal recessive disorder with an inborn error of carbohydrate metabolism. Homocystinuria is an indication of amino acid transport or metabolism problems. Hyperglycemia isn't a problem in hypopituitarism.
CN: Health promotion and maintenance; CNS: None; CL: Application

74. 3. To promote self-esteem and healthy development of a child with growth hormone deficiency, parents should be encouraged to interact with the child according to age, not size. Growth in height and weight will begin soon after treatment with growth hormone begins. Growth hormone administration is subcutaneous, and a child shouldn't be held back in school because of his size.
CN: Psychosocial integrity; CNS: None; CL: Application

75. 4. Diabetes insipidus usually presents gradually. Weight loss from a large loss of fluid occurs. Edema isn't evident in the neonate with diabetes insipidus. There should be an increase in his head circumference with treatment. A normal neonate should gain weight as he grows.
CN: Physiological integrity; CNS: Reduction of risk potential; CL: Application

76. 1. With diabetes insipidus, the client has difficulty with excessive urine output; therefore, the urine will be pale in color and the specific gravity will fall below the low normal of 1.01.
CN: Physiological integrity; CNS: Reduction of risk potential; CL: Analysis

77. Which characteristics would most likely be present in the health history of a child with diabetes insipidus?
  1. Delayed closure of the fontanels, coarse hair, and hypoglycemia in the morning
  2. Gradual onset of personality changes, lethargy, and blurred vision
  3. Vomiting early in the morning, headache, and decreased thirst
  4. Abrupt onset of polyuria, nocturia, and polydipsia

78. Which condition in a client on fluid restriction for diabetes insipidus diagnostic testing would indicate a need for the nurse to discontinue fluid restriction?
  1. Weight gain of 3% to 5%
  2. Weight loss of 3% to 5%
  3. Increase in urine output
  4. Generalized edema

79. When a child with diabetes insipidus has a viral illness that includes congestion, nausea, and vomiting, the nurse should instruct the parents to take which action?
  1. Make no changes in the medication regime.
  2. Give medications only once per day.
  3. Obtain an alternate route for desmopressin acetate (DDAVP) administration.
  4. Give medication 1 hour after vomiting has occurred.

80. A nurse is preparing a child with diabetes insipidus who will be taking injectable vasopressin for hospital discharge. Which action is best for the nurse to take when teaching injection techniques?
  1. Teach injection techniques to the primary caregiver.
  2. Teach injection techniques to anyone who will provide care for the child.
  3. Teach injection techniques to anyone who will provide care for the child as well as to the child if he's old enough to understand.
  4. Provide information about the nearest home health agency so the parents can arrange for the home health nurse to come and give the injection.

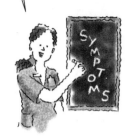

Do you know the symptoms of diabetes insipidus?

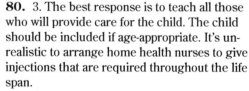

Good work! You're flying through this test!

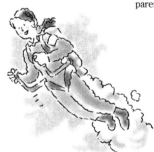

77. 4. Diabetes insipidus is characterized by deficient secretion of antidiuretic hormone leading to diuresis. Most children with this disorder experience an abrupt onset of symptoms, including polyuria, nocturia, and polydipsia. The other choices reflect symptoms of pituitary hyperfunction.
CN: Health promotion and maintenance; CNS: None; CL: Application

78. 2. A weight loss between 3% to 5% indicates significant dehydration and requires termination of the fluid restriction. Weight gain would be a good sign. Generalized edema wouldn't occur with fluid restriction, nor would increased urine output.
CN: Physiological integrity; CNS: Physiological adaptation; CL: Analysis

79. 3. An alternate route for administration of DDAVP would be needed for absorption because of nasal congestion. The other options reflect actions that need to be covered by a physician's order.
CN: Health promotion and maintenance; CNS: None; CL: Application

80. 3. The best response is to teach all those who will provide care for the child. The child should be included if age-appropriate. It's unrealistic to arrange home health nurses to give injections that are required throughout the life span.
CN: Physiological integrity; CNS: Pharmacological and parenteral therapies; CL: Application

CN: Client needs category   CNS: Client needs subcategory   CL: Cognitive level

81. When providing care for a school-age client with diabetes insipidus, the nurse understands that which behavior might be difficult related to this child's growth and development?
1. Taking desmopressin acetate (DDAVP) at school
2. Taking DDAVP before bedtime
3. Letting his mother administer the vasopressin injection
4. Giving himself a vasopressin injection before school starts

82. Which monitoring method would be best for a client newly diagnosed with diabetes insipidus?
1. Measuring abdominal girths every day
2. Measuring intake, output, and urine specific gravity
3. Checking daily weights and measuring intake
4. Checking for pitting edema in the lower extremities

83. A nurse is caring for a neonate with congenital hypothyroidism. Which assessment finding should the nurse anticipate observing in the neonate?
1. Hyperreflexia
2. Long forehead
3. Puffy eyelids
4. Small tongue

84. A child is admitted with complaints of weight loss and lack of energy. The child's ears and cheeks are flushed, and the nurse observes an acetone odor to the child's breath. The child's blood glucose level is 325 mg/dl, his blood pressure is 104/60 mmHg, his pulse is 88 beats/minute, and respirations are 16 breaths/minute. Which does the nurse expect the physician to order first?
1. Subcutaneous administration of glucagon
2. Administration of IV regular insulin by continuous infusion pump
3. Administration of regular insulin subcutaneously every 4 hours as needed by sliding scale insulin
4. Administration of IV fluids in boluses of 20 ml/kg

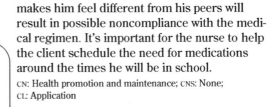

Question 82 asks you to rank monitoring methods for appropriateness. I know you can do it!

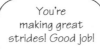

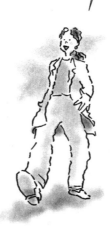

You're making great strides! Good job!

81. 1. Anything that singles a child out and makes him feel different from his peers will result in possible noncompliance with the medical regimen. It's important for the nurse to help the client schedule the need for medications around the times he will be in school.
CN: Health promotion and maintenance; CNS: None; CL: Application

82. 2. Measuring intake and output with related specific gravity results will enable the nurse to closely monitor the client's condition along with daily weights. All of the other options aren't as accurate for a child with diabetes insipidus.
CN: Physiological integrity; CNS: Reduction of risk potential; CL: Application

83. 3. Assessment findings would include depressed nasal bridge, short forehead, puffy eyelids, and large tongue; thick, dry, mottled skin that feels cold to the touch; coarse, dry, lusterless hair; abdominal distention; umbilical hernia; hyporeflexia; bradycardia; hypothermia; hypotension; anemia; and wide cranial sutures.
CN: Physiological integrity; CNS: Physiological adaptation; CL: Application

84. 2. Weight loss, lack of energy, acetone odor to breath, and a blood glucose level of 325 mg/dl indicate diabetic ketoacidosis. Insulin is given IV by continuous infusion pump. Glucagon is administered for mild hypoglycemia. Sliding scale insulin isn't as effective as the administration of insulin by continuous infusion pump. Administration of IV fluids in boluses of 20 ml/kg is recommended for the treatment of shock.
CN: Physiological integrity; CNS: Physiological adaptation; CL: Application

85. Which nursing objective is <u>most important</u> when working with neonates who are suspected of having congenital hypothyroidism?
1. Identifying the disorder early
2. Promoting bonding
3. Allowing rooming in
4. Encouraging fluid intake

86. When the parents of an infant diagnosed with hypothyroidism have been taught to count the pulse, which intervention should the nurse teach them in case they obtain a high pulse rate?
1. Allow the infant to take a nap, and then give the medication.
2. Withhold the medication and give a double dose the next day.
3. Hold the medication and call the physician.
4. Give the medication and then consult the physician.

87. In an infant receiving inadequate treatment for congenital hypothyroidism, the nurse should expect to observe which symptom?
1. Irritability and jitteriness
2. Fatigue and sleepiness
3. Increased appetite
4. Diarrhea

88. When collecting data from a child with Cushing's syndrome, which would the nurse be <u>most</u> likely to find? Select all that apply:
1. Obesity
2. Moon-shaped face
3. Hypotension
4. Emotional instability
5. Quickened healing
6. Loss of hair

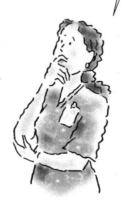

What's the most important nursing objective?

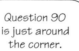

Question 90 is just around the corner.

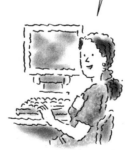

85. 1. The most important nursing objective is early identification of the disorder. Nurses caring for neonates must be certain that screening is performed, especially in neonates who are preterm, discharged early, or born at home. Promoting bonding, allowing rooming in, and encouraging fluid intake are all important but are less important than early identification.
CN: Physiological integrity; CNS: Basic care and comfort; CL: Application

86. 3. If parents have been taught to count the infant's pulse, they should be instructed to withhold the dose and consult their physician if the pulse rate is above a certain value.
CN: Health promotion and maintenance; CNS: None; CL: Application

87. 2. Signs of inadequate treatment are fatigue, sleepiness, decreased appetite, and constipation.
CN: Health promotion and maintenance; CNS: None; CL: Application

88. 1, 2, 4. Cushing's syndrome occurs as a result of excessive cortisol exposure (through corticosteroid medications or production by the adrenal glands). Common findings include obesity, moon-shaped face, and emotional instability. Hypertension, excessive hair growth, and slower healing are additional findings, making the other options incorrect.
CN: Physiological integrity; CNS: Physiological adaptation; CL: Analysis

CN: Client needs category   CNS: Client needs subcategory   CL: Cognitive level

89. Which recommendation for preventing hypoglycemia in an adolescent with diabetes type 1 should the nurse make?
1. Limit participation in planned exercise activities that involve competition.
2. Carry crackers or fruit to eat before or during periods of increased activity.
3. Increase the insulin dosage before planned or unplanned strenuous exercise.
4. Check blood sugar before exercising, and eat a protein snack if the level is elevated.

90. A child with diabetic ketoacidosis is to receive a continuous infusion of insulin for a blood glucose level of 780 mg/dl. Which solution is the most appropriate for the nurse to prepare initially?
1. Normal saline with regular insulin
2. Normal saline with Ultralente insulin
3. 5% dextrose in water with NPH insulin
4. 5% dextrose in water with PZI insulin

91. An adolescent female client is admitted to the hospital with type 1 diabetes and unstable blood glucose levels. Which question is <u>most important</u> to include in her health history?
1. Does she play any team sports?
2. Does she refrigerate her insulin?
3. Is she satisfied with her weight?
4. Does she use recreational drugs?

92. A 14-year-old male client with type 1 diabetes mellitus plans to join the basketball team at his school. The practices are twice a week with games on Saturdays. He calls the nurse at his clinic for advice. The nurse should respond with which statement?
1. "Delay eating a meal until after practice or a game."
2. "Time your insulin to peak at the time of practice and games."
3. "Monitor your blood sugar before, during, and after exercise."
4. "Increase your daily calorie intake by 10% and up your insulin dose by 10%."

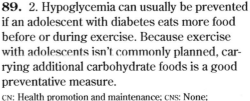

Let's discuss some steps for preventing hypoglycemia.

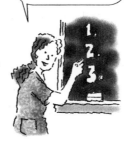

The answer to this question should be a slam dunk.

89. 2. Hypoglycemia can usually be prevented if an adolescent with diabetes eats more food before or during exercise. Because exercise with adolescents isn't commonly planned, carrying additional carbohydrate foods is a good preventative measure.
CN: Health promotion and maintenance; CNS: None; CL: Application

90. 1. Short-acting regular insulin is the only insulin that should be used for insulin infusions. Initially, normal saline is used until blood glucose levels are reduced. Then a dextrose solution may be used to prevent hypoglycemia. Ultralente, NPH, and PZI insulins have a longer duration of action and shouldn't be used for continuous infusions.
CN: Physiological integrity; CNS: Pharmacological and parenteral therapies; CL: Application

91. 3. It's important to ascertain the adolescent's feelings about her body, in particular her weight. Some female adolescents skip their insulin because they know doing so will result in weight loss. The other issues of sports, drug use, and technique of administering insulin are all relevant but not as important as knowing what the client is thinking about her own body.
CN: Psychosocial integrity; CNS: None; CL: Application

92. 3. For increases in activity, a client with type 1 diabetes would require a snack before the activity and increased insulin. The amount of insulin is the most difficult determination. Monitoring is required for accurate regulation before, during, and after the activity. The client shouldn't delay eating until afterward because the body needs the calories to provide energy to the muscles and tissues. Extreme hypoglycemia may occur if the insulin peaks without extra calories. There's no standard of 10% increase in calories and insulin; every person would require individualization of the insulin and calories needed.
CN: Health promotion and maintenance; CNS: None; CL: Application

93. A nurse is collecting a health history from the parents of a 12-month-old infant being evaluated for possible hypopituitarism. Which component of this history is important to establish the diagnosis?
1. Did the mother drink alcohol while pregnant?
2. Does the infant receive multivitamins?
3. What's the infant's growth pattern?
4. Was the infant premature?

94. A nurse has just completed teaching a family about hypothyroidism. Which actions would indicate the parents understand their child's diagnosis?
1. Providing a diet including whole grains, produce, and water
2. Anticipating their child outgrowing hypothyroidism
3. Providing a white diet for their child
4. Providing a diet high in fat for their child to encourage growth

95. A child with diabetes is receiving a continuous insulin infusion for diabetic ketoacidosis. When assessing the child, the nurse should be alert for signs and symptoms of which complication?
1. Hypercalcemia
2. Hyperphosphatemia
3. Hypokalemia
4. Hypernatremia

96. A nurse is caring for a client with pheochromocytoma. Which nursing intervention is appropriate for this client?
1. Promoting an environment free from emotional distress
2. Avoiding analgesia administration
3. Advising a low-calorie, high-nutrient diet
4. Avoiding parents rooming in because they make the client less dependent on staff

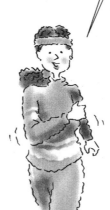

I can see the finish line! You're doing great!

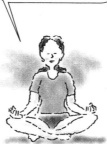

I feel the stress fading away.

93. 3. Hypopituitarism presents with a retarded growth pattern, appearance younger than chronological age, and normal skeletal proportions and intelligence. It's related to tumors, irradiation, infection, and head trauma. Therefore, serial growth patterns will be crucial to the diagnosis process. It isn't related to fetal alcoholism, use of multivitamins, or prematurity.
CN: Physiological integrity; CNS: Physiological adaptation; CL: Application

94. 1. A diet including fruits, vegetables, whole grains, and water will help counteract the trend toward obstinate constipation, the result of a slowed metabolism and hypotonic bowel. Congenital hypothyroidism isn't outgrown, and thyroid replacement is necessary throughout the life span. A white diet involves foods low in fiber, which leads to constipation. Hypothyroid individuals tend to have elevated cholesterol and triglyceride levels; therefore, a diet high in fat is contraindicated.
CN: Health promotion and maintenance; CNS: None; CL: Application

95. 3. Hypokalemia occurs as insulin causes potassium and glucose to move into the cells. Insulin administration doesn't affect calcium or sodium levels. Insulin administration may lead to hypophosphatemia, not hyperphosphatemia, as phosphorus enters the cells with insulin and potassium.
CN: Physiological integrity; CNS: Physiological adaptation; CL: Analysis

96. 1. The child experiencing hyperfunctioning of the adrenal gland, or *pheochromocytoma,* is in a chronic state of "fight or flight" related to excessive exogenous epinephrine. Therefore, the child has an accelerated metabolism. Symptoms include hypertension, headaches, hyperglycemia with weight loss, diaphoresis, and hyperventilation. Through provision of a low-stress environment, analgesia as needed, a high-calorie diet, and supportive parents, the child will be able to prepare for surgery to eliminate the tumor causing the hypersecretion of epinephrine.
CN: Physiological integrity; CNS: Physiological adaptation; CL: Application

CN: Client needs category   CNS: Client needs subcategory   CL: Cognitive level

97. A nurse is instructing parents about promoting the health of their child with diabetes. Which teaching point should be included?
   1. Avoid daily bathing so the skin doesn't become too dry.
   2. Cuts and scratches on the playground are of little concern.
   3. Children with diabetes need few immunizations.
   4. Regular dental care and annual ophthalmologic appointments should be kept.

98. A 10-year-old child monitors and adjusts his own insulin. Which response reflects an understanding of appropriate adjustment of insulin dosage when the child has the flu?
   1. "I withhold all insulin because I'm not eating."
   2. "I'll take my usual dose of regular and NPH insulin."
   3. "I'll perform fingerstick blood sugar testing and adjust my insulin according to results."
   4. "I'll perform fingerstick blood sugar testing and record the results."

99. The nurse is teaching the parents of a child with hypopituitary dwarfism about the diagnosis. Which statement is the most accurate about children with this condition?
   1. They're usually low-birth-weight babies.
   2. Symptoms aren't apparent until puberty.
   3. Symptoms include early primary dentition.
   4. They grow normally the first 2 years and then fall below the 3rd percentile.

100, A client age 10 has been experiencing insatiable thirst and urinating excessively; his serum glucose is <u>normal</u>. Which condition is the client probably experiencing?
   1. Type 2 diabetes mellitus
   2. Type 1 diabetes mellitus
   3. Hyperthyroidism
   4. Diabetes insipidus

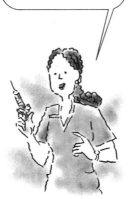

Adjusting insulin reflects that your client understands his disorder.

97. 4. Regular dental care will preserve oral health, and ophthalmologic examinations will ensure visual acuity for reading. Because of their impaired immune system, children with diabetes need to maintain a high level of health to avoid infection. Daily bathing and application of lotion, cleaning minor playground scrapes and applying antibiotic ointments, and keeping immunizations up-to-date are all important.
CN: Health promotion and maintenance; CNS: None; CL: Application

98. 3. Because of the stress of illness, serum glucose will likely be elevated during an episode of the flu. Appropriate adjustment of insulin dosage will help prevent the child from becoming hypoglycemic or ketoacidotic.
CN: Physiological integrity; CNS: Physiological adaptation; CL: Analysis

99. 4. Generally, hypopituitary children are of average birth weight and grow at a normal pace the first 2 or 3 years and then fall behind their peers in height, usually below the 3rd percentile. Dentition of primary teeth is normal; permanent teeth are delayed.
CN: Health promotion and maintenance; CNS: None; CL: Application

100. 4. Polydipsia and polyuria with normal serum glucose may be indicative of diabetes insipidus. Interview and laboratory results can determine whether the origin is neurogenic or nephrogenic. Type 1 or 2 diabetes mellitus requires an elevated serum glucose. A child with hyperthyroidism may present as dehydrated from the excessive sweating and rapid respirations that accompany this hypermetabolic state.
CN: Physiological integrity; CNS: Physiological adaptation; CL: Analysis

101. A client age 4½ with diabetes is ordered to receive 25 ml/hour of I.V. solution. The nurse is using a pediatric microdrip chamber to administer the medication. The microdrip chamber should be set for how many drops per minute? Record your answer using a whole number.

_____ gtt/minute

102. The nurse is preparing to administer I.V. methylprednisolone sodium succinate (Solu-Medrol) to a child who weighs 44 lb. The order is for 0.03 mg/kg I.V. daily. How many milligrams should the nurse prepare? Record your answer using one decimal point.

_____ milligrams

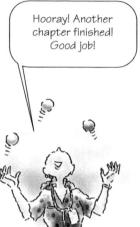

Hooray! Another chapter finished! Good job!

101. 25. When using a pediatric microdrip chamber, the number of milliliters per hour equals the number of drops per minute. If 25 ml/hour is ordered, the I.V. should infuse at 25 drops/minute.

CN: Physiological integrity; CNS: Pharmacological and parenteral therapies; CL: Application

102. 0.6. To perform this dosage calculation, the nurse should first convert the child's weight to kilograms: 44 lb ÷ 2.2 kg/lb = 20 kg. Then she should use this formula to determine the dose: 20 kg × 0.03 mg/kg = X mg. X = 0.6 mg.

CN: Physiological integrity; CNS: Pharmacological and parenteral therapies; CL: Application

CN: Client needs category   CNS: Client needs subcategory   CL: Cognitive level

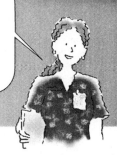

This chapter covers altered patterns of urinary elimination in children and includes glomerulonephritis, hypospadias, and—oh, a whole lot of other conditions. Ready? Let's go!

Chapter 21
Genitourinary system

1. A child with acute glomerulonephritis has a nursing diagnosis of *Impaired urinary elimination* related to fluid retention and impaired glomerular filtration. The child should display which expected outcome?
 1. Exhibits no evidence of infection
 2. Engages in activities appropriate to capabilities
 3. Demonstrates no periorbital, facial, or body edema
 4. Maintains a fluid intake of more than 2,000 ml in 24 hours

2. An important nursing intervention to support the therapeutic management of a child with acute glomerulonephritis should include which action?
 1. Measuring daily weight
 2. Increasing oral fluid intake
 3. Providing sodium supplements
 4. Monitoring the client for signs of hypokalemia

3. A nurse is taking frequent blood pressure readings on a child diagnosed with acute glomerulonephritis. The parents ask the nurse why this is necessary. When implementing nursing care, which teaching statement by the nurse is the <u>most</u> accurate?
 1. "Blood pressure fluctuations are a sign that the condition has become chronic."
 2. "Blood pressure fluctuations are a common adverse effect of antibiotic therapy."
 3. "Hypotension leading to sudden shock can develop at any time."
 4. "Acute hypertension must be anticipated and identified."

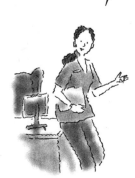

If you're having trouble deciding on an answer, begin by eliminating the ones you *know* are incorrect.

1. 3. The goal of this diagnosis involves interventions, such as decreased fluid and salt intake, designed to minimize or prevent fluid retention and edema. These interventions may be evaluated through observations for edema. The other options are appropriate outcomes for other nursing diagnoses, not the diagnosis in question.
CN: Health promotion and maintenance; CNS: None; CL: Analysis

2. 1. The child with acute glomerulonephritis should be monitored for fluid imbalance, which is done through daily weights. Increasing oral intake, monitoring for hypokalemia, and providing sodium supplements aren't part of the therapeutic management of acute glomerulonephritis.
CN: Physiological integrity; CNS: Basic care and comfort; CL: Application

3. 4. Regular measurement of vital signs, body weight, and intake and output is essential to monitor the progress of the disease and to detect complications that may appear at any time during the course of the disease. Blood pressure fluctuations don't indicate that the condition has become chronic and aren't common adverse reactions to antibiotic therapy. Hypertension is more likely than hypotension to occur with glomerulonephritis.
CN: Physiological integrity; CNS: Physiological adaptation; CL: Application

CN: Client needs category   CNS: Client needs subcategory   CL: Cognitive level

4. A child has been diagnosed with acute glomerulonephritis. Based on the results of the routine urinalysis below, which component is the most consistent with this diagnosis?

Laboratory results	
Urinalysis	
Color:	Straw
Appearance:	Clear
Specific gravity:	1.032
pH:	5.5
Protein:	Negative
Blood:	Negative
RBC casts:	Present
Crystals:	Negative

 1. Specific gravity
 2. Protein
 3. Blood
 4. Red blood cell (RBC) casts

5. When evaluating the urinalysis report of a child with acute glomerulonephritis, the nurse should expect which result?
 1. Proteinuria and decreased specific gravity
 2. Bacteriuria and increased specific gravity
 3. Hematuria and proteinuria
 4. Bacteriuria and hematuria

6. Which statement by a nurse would be the best response to a mother who wants to know the first indication that her child's acute glomerulonephritis is improving?
 1. Urine output will increase.
 2. Urine will be free from protein.
 3. Blood pressure will stabilize.
 4. The child will have more energy.

7. Which statement regarding acute glomerulonephritis indicates that the parents of a child with this diagnosis understand the teaching provided by the nurse?
 1. This disease occurs after a urinary tract infection.
 2. This disease is associated with renal vascular disorders.
 3. This disease occurs after a streptococcal infection.
 4. This disease is associated with structural anomalies of the genitourinary tract.

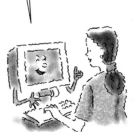

More than one answer may seem correct. It's your job to choose the best answer.

4. 4. Urinalysis findings consistent with acute glomerulonephritis would include a specific gravity less than 1.030, proteinuria, hematuria, and the presence of RBC casts. The presence of crystals in the urine typically indicates a congenital metabolic problem.
CN: Physiological integrity; CNS: Physiological adaptation; CL: Application

5. 3. Urinalysis during the acute phase of this disease characteristically shows hematuria, proteinuria, and increased specific gravity.
CN: Physiological integrity; CNS: Physiological adaptation; CL: Analysis

6. 1. One of the first signs of improvement during the acute phase of glomerulonephritis is an increase in urine output. It will take time for the urine to be free from protein. Antihypertensive drugs may be needed to stabilize the blood pressure. Children generally don't have much energy during the acute phase of this disease.
CN: Health promotion and maintenance; CNS: None; CL: Analysis

7. 3. Acute glomerulonephritis is an immune-complex disease that occurs as a by-product of a streptococcal infection. Certain strains of the infection are usually a beta-hemolytic streptococcus.
CN: Health promotion and maintenance; CNS: None; CL: Analysis

CN: Client needs category   CNS: Client needs subcategory   CL: Cognitive level

8. When obtaining a child's daily weights, the nurse notes that he has lost 6 lb (2.7 kg) after 3 days of hospitalization for acute glomerulonephritis. This is most likely the result of which factor?
1. Poor appetite
2. Reduction of edema
3. Decreased salt intake
4. Restriction to bed rest

9. A nurse should make which dietary recommendation to a client who has been newly diagnosed with acute glomerulonephritis?
1. Decrease calories.
2. Increase potassium.
3. Severely restrict sodium.
4. Moderately restrict sodium.

10. A nurse is evaluating a group of children for acute glomerulonephritis. Which client would be most likely to develop the disease?
1. A client who had pneumonia a month ago
2. A client who was bitten by a brown spider
3. A client who shows no signs of periorbital edema
4. A client who had a streptococcal infection 2 weeks ago

11. A nurse is questioned by a student nurse about which age group has the highest incidence of acute glomerulonephritis. Which response by the nurse is the most accurate?
1. Ages 1 to 2
2. Ages 6 to 7
3. Ages 12 to 13
4. Ages 18 to 20

12. In understanding the recurrence of glomerulonephritis, a nurse should know which characteristic to be true?
1. Second attacks are quite common.
2. A recessive gene transfers this disease.
3. Multiple cases tend to occur in families.
4. Overcrowding in the schoolroom leads to higher incidence.

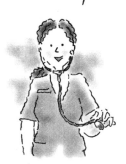

Ten questions down! That's a good start!

8. 2. When there's reduction of edema, the client will lose weight. This should normally occur after treatment for acute glomerulonephritis has been followed for several days. A poor appetite, decreased salt intake, or restriction to bed rest wouldn't lead to such a dramatic weight loss in a child this age.
CN: Physiological integrity; CNS: Basic care and comfort; CL: Application

9. 4. Moderate sodium restriction with a diet that has no added salt after cooking is usually effective. Calorie consumption doesn't need to decrease, and potassium consumption shouldn't increase because of the decrease in urinary output. *Severe* sodium restriction isn't needed and will make it more difficult to ensure adequate nutrition. It will also result in hyponatremia.
CN: Physiological integrity; CNS: Basic care and comfort; CL: Application

10. 4. A latent period of 10 to 14 days occurs between the streptococcal infection of the throat or skin and the onset of clinical manifestations. The peak incidence of disease corresponds to the incidence of streptococcal infections. Pneumonia isn't a precursor to glomerulonephritis, nor is a bite from a brown spider. A sign of periorbital edema would lead the nurse to investigate the possibility of glomerulonephritis, especially if reported to be worse in the morning.
CN: Health promotion and maintenance; CNS: None; CL: Analysis

11. 2. Acute glomerulonephritis can occur at any age, but it primarily affects early school-age children with a peak age of onset of 6 to 7. It's uncommon in children younger than age 2.
CN: Health promotion and maintenance; CNS: None; CL: Application

12. 3. Multiple cases tend to occur in families. Second attacks are rare. Acute glomerulonephritis isn't transmitted through a recessive gene, and overcrowding in the schoolroom should have no influence on this disease.
CN: Health promotion and maintenance; CNS: None; CL: Application

13. When describing enuresis to a child's parents, which statement would the nurse include in the description? Select all that apply:
1. "Your child may experience involuntary urination after age 5."
2. "Episodes primarily occur when your child is awake and playing."
3. "Your child may suffer deep feelings of shame and may withdraw from peers because of ridicule."
4. "The condition may respond to tricyclic antidepressants and antidiuretics."
5. "The condition may become permanent without appropriate intervention."

14. Which comment made by a parent would indicate to the nurse the need for <u>further education</u> about acute glomerulonephritis complications?
1. "Dizziness is expected, and I should have my child lie down when he feels it."
2. "I should let the nurse know every time my child urinates."
3. "I need to ask my child whether he has a headache."
4. "I should encourage quiet play activities."

15. When teaching an 8-year-old child to obtain a clean-catch urine specimen, which technique should be included?
1. Collect the specimen right after a nap.
2. Never use the first voided specimen of the day.
3. Collect the specimen at the beginning of urination.
4. You don't need to wash your perineal area before collecting the specimen.

16. Which therapy should a nurse expect to incorporate into the care of a child with acute glomerulonephritis?
1. Antibiotic therapy
2. Dialysis therapy
3. Diuretic therapy
4. Play therapy

The phrase *further education* indicates that question 14 is looking for an *inaccurate* statement.

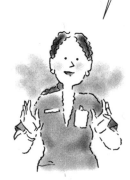

Don't a-void this question. You're doing great!

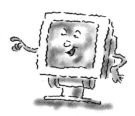

13. 1, 3, 4. Enuresis is a condition in which there's involuntary urination after age 5. It generally occurs while the child is sleeping. There can be long-lasting emotional trauma resulting from peer ridicule and feelings of shame and embarrassment. The condition may be treated with the use of tricyclic antidepressant and antidiuretics. With support and understanding, the condition generally resolves in time.
CN: Physiological integrity; CNS: Physiological adaptation; CL: Analysis

14. 1. Dizziness and headache are signs of encephalopathy and must be reported to the nurse. Hypertensive encephalopathy, acute cardiac decompensation, and acute renal failure are the major complications that tend to develop during the acute phase of glomerulonephritis. In order to maintain an accurate intake and output record, the parent should let the nurse know when the child urinates. Quiet play is encouraged to avoid overstressing the kidneys.
CN: Physiological integrity; CNS: Reduction of risk potential; CL: Application

15. 2. When collecting a clean-catch urine specimen, the first voided specimen of the day should never be used because of urinary stasis; this also applies after a nap. The specimen should be collected midstream, not at the beginning or end of urination. Washing the perineal area before collecting a specimen is very important to make sure there are no contaminants from the skin in the specimen.
CN: Physiological integrity; CNS: Reduction of risk potential; CL: Application

16. 4. Play therapy is an important aspect of care to help the child understand what's happening to him. Unless the child has the ability to express concerns and fears, he may have night terrors and regress in his stage of growth and development. Antibiotic therapy is indicated for an infectious process. Dialysis therapy is appropriate for renal failure. Diuretic therapy is usually ineffective.
CN: Health promotion and maintenance; CNS: None; CL: Application

CN: Client needs category   CNS: Client needs subcategory   CL: Cognitive level

17. In explaining treatment for glomerulonephritis, a nurse should include which statement?
1. All children who have signs of glomerulonephritis are hospitalized for approximately 1 week.
2. Parents should expect children to have a normal energy level during the acute phase.
3. Children who have normal blood pressure and a satisfactory urinary output can generally be treated at home.
4. Children with gross hematuria and significant oliguria should be brought to the physician's office about every 2 days for monitoring.

18. Which action is a nursing priority for a child with acute glomerulonephritis?
1. Assess blood pressure every 4 hours.
2. Check urine specific gravity every 8 hours.
3. Encourage daily fluid intake of 3,500 L.
4. Provide a 2,500-mg sodium diet.

19. Which food should a nurse eliminate from the diet of a child who's diagnosed with acute glomerulonephritis?
1. Turkey sandwich with mayonnaise
2. Hot dog with ketchup and mustard
3. Chocolate cake with white icing
4. Apple with peanut butter

20. A mother of a child with hypospadias asks the nurse what the condition is. The nurse would respond which of the following statements?
1. "It is the absence of a urethral opening."
2. "It is a penis that is shorter than usual for age."
3. "It is an urethral opening along the dorsal surface of the penis."
4. "It is an urethral opening along the ventral surface of the penis."

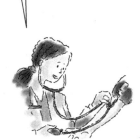

Hypertension is a complication of glomerulonephritis.

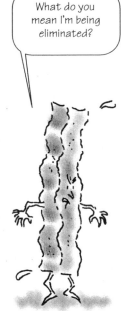

What do you mean I'm being eliminated?

17. 3. Children who have normal blood pressure and a satisfactory urinary output can generally be treated at home. Parents should expect children to have a decrease in energy levels during the acute phase of the disease. Those with gross hematuria and significant oliguria will probably be hospitalized for monitoring.
CN: Health promotion and maintenance; CNS: None; CL: Application

18. 1. Because hypertension is a complication of acute glomerulonephritis, the nurse should check the child's blood pressure every 4 hours. The urine specific gravity should also be monitored, but it isn't as high a priority as monitoring the blood pressure. The child may be placed on fluid or sodium restrictions.
CN: Physiological integrity; CNS: Reduction of risk potential; CL: Application

19. 2. Foods that are high in sodium content, such as hot dogs, should be eliminated from the child's diet. Snacks such as pretzels and potato chips should also be discouraged. Any other foods that the child likes should be encouraged.
CN: Physiological integrity; CNS: Basic care and comfort; CL: Application

20. 4. *Hypospadias* refers to a condition in which the urethral opening is located below the glans penis or anywhere along the ventral surface of the penile shaft.
CN: Health promotion and maintenance; CNS: None; CL: Application

21. After the acute phase of glomerulonephritis is over, which discharge instruction should a nurse include?
1. Every 6 months, a cystogram will be needed for evaluation of progress.
2. Weekly visits to the physician may be needed for evaluation.
3. It will be acceptable to keep the regular yearly check-up appointment for the next evaluation.
4. There's no need to worry about further evaluations by the physician related to this disease.

22. The mother of a newborn tells the nurse that she was told that her infant has chordee. The mother asks the nurse what this condition is. Which response is correct?
1. Ventral curvature of the penis
2. Dorsal curvature of the penis
3. No curvature of the penis
4. Misshapen penis

23. The nurse is caring for an infant with hypospadias. Which anomaly would the nurse assess the infant for that commonly accompanies this condition?
1. Undescended testicles
2. Ambiguous genitalia
3. Umbilical hernias
4. Inguinal hernias

24. Which reason explains why surgical repair of a hypospadias is done as early as possible?
1. To prevent separation anxiety
2. To prevent urinary complications
3. To promote acceptance of hospitalization
4. To promote development of a normal body image

25. A nurse should counsel parents to postpone which action until after their son's hypospadias has been repaired?
1. Circumcising the infant
2. Baptizing the infant
3. Getting hepatitis B vaccine
4. Checking blood for inborn errors of metabolism

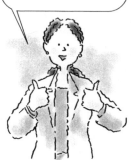

Twenty-one questions done! Keep plugging along!

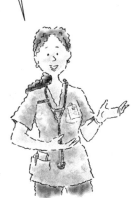

Knowing common accompanying conditions is important for taking the NCLEX.

21. 2. Weekly or monthly visits to the physician will be needed for evaluation of improvement and will usually involve the collection of a urine specimen for urinalysis. A cystogram isn't helpful in determining the progression of this disease; it's used to review the anatomic structures of the urinary tract.
CN: Physiological integrity; CNS: Reduction of risk potential; CL: Application

22. 1. Chordee, or ventral curvature of the penis, results from the replacement of normal skin with a fibrous band of tissue and usually accompanies more severe forms of hypospadias.
CN: Health promotion and maintenance; CNS: None; CL: Application

23. 1. Because undescended testes may also be present, the small penis may appear to be an enlarged clitoris. This shouldn't be mistaken for ambiguous genitalia. If there's any doubt, more tests should be performed. Hernias don't generally accompany hypospadias.
CN: Health promotion and maintenance; CNS: None; CL: Application

24. 4. Whenever there are defects of the genitourinary tact, surgery should be performed early to promote development of a normal body image. A child with normal emotional development shows separation anxiety at 7 to 9 months. Within a few months, he understands the mother's permanence, and separation anxiety diminishes. Hypospadias doesn't put the child at a greater risk for urinary complications.
CN: Health promotion and maintenance; CNS: None; CL: Application

25. 1. Circumcision shouldn't be performed until after the hypospadias has been repaired. The foreskin might be needed to help in the repair of the hypospadias. None of the other choices has any bearing on the repair of the hypospadias.
CN: Health promotion and maintenance; CNS: None; CL: Application

CN: Client needs category   CNS: Client needs subcategory   CL: Cognitive level

26. Which statement made about the principal objective of surgical correction by the parents of a child undergoing hypospadias repair implies a need for <u>further teaching</u>?
   1. "The purpose is to improve the physical appearance of the genitalia for psychological reasons."
   2. "The purpose is to enhance the child's ability to void in the standing position."
   3. "The purpose is to decrease the chance of developing urinary tract infections."
   4. "The purpose is to preserve a sexually adequate organ."

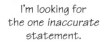

I'm looking for the one inaccurate statement.

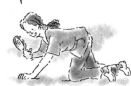

27. Which nursing intervention should be included in the care plan for a male infant following surgical repair of hypospadias?
   1. Sterile dressing changes every 4 hours
   2. Frequent assessment of the tip of the penis
   3. Removal of the suprapubic catheter on the second postoperative day
   4. Urethral catheterization if voiding doesn't occur over an 8-hour period

28. The nurse is explaining to the parents of a child with hypospadias the optimum time for repair of this condition. Which response as to the optimum age of choice would be the most accurate?
   1. 1 week
   2. 6 to 18 months
   3. 2 years
   4. 4 years

29. When providing discharge information to the parents of a child with a hypospadias repair, which instruction would be <u>appropriate</u>?
   1. Care of the circumcision
   2. Techniques for providing tub baths
   3. Care for the indwelling catheter or stent
   4. Encouragement of voiding every 2 hours

You're almost at question 30 and you're doing great.

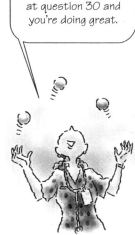

26. 3. A child with hypospadias isn't at greater risk for urinary tract infections. The principal objectives of surgical corrections are to enhance the child's ability to void in the standing position with a straight stream, to improve the physical appearance of the genitalia for psychological reasons, and to preserve a sexually adequate organ.
CN: Health promotion and maintenance; CNS: None; CL: Application

27. 2. Following hypospadias repair, a pressure dressing is applied to the penis to reduce bleeding and tissue swelling. The penile tip should then be assessed frequently for signs of circulatory impairment. The dressing around the penis shouldn't be changed as frequently as every 4 hours. The physician will determine when the suprapubic catheter will be removed. Urethral catheterization should be avoided after repair of hypospadias to prevent injury to the urethra.
CN: Physiological integrity; CNS: Basic care and comfort; CL: Application

28. 2. The preferred time for surgical repair is 6 to 18 months of age, before the child has developed body image and castration anxiety. Surgical repair of hypospadias as early as 3 months old has been successful but with a high incidence of complications.
CN: Health promotion and maintenance; CNS: None; CL: Application

29. 3. Parents are taught to care for the indwelling catheter or stent and irrigation techniques, if indicated. The child with hypospadias shouldn't be circumcised because the foreskin may be needed during surgical repair. A tub bath should be avoided to prevent infection until the stent has been removed. Following surgical repair, the child will have an indwelling urinary catheter, so encouraging the child to void isn't appropriate.
CN: Physiological integrity; CNS: Reduction of risk potential; CL: Analysis

30. When providing discharge instructions to the parents of an older child who has had hypospadias repair, which activity should be encouraged?
1. Riding a bicycle
2. Playing in sandboxes
3. Increased fluid intake
4. Playing with the family pet

31. The mother of a neonate born with hypospadias is sharing her feelings of guilt about this anomaly with a nurse. The nurse should explain which fact about the defect?
1. It occurs around the third month of fetal development.
2. It occurs around the sixth month of fetal development.
3. It's carried by an autosomal recessive gene.
4. It's hereditary.

32. A mother reports that her 6-year-old daughter recently began wetting the bed and running a low-grade fever. A urinalysis is positive for bacteria and protein. A diagnosis of a urinary tract infection (UTI) is made, and the child is prescribed antibiotics. Which interventions are appropriate? Select all that apply:
1. Limit fluids for the next few days to decrease the frequency of urination.
2. Assess the mother's understanding of UTI and its causes.
3. Instruct the mother to administer the antibiotic as prescribed—even if the symptoms diminish.
4. Provide instruction solely to the mother, not the child.
5. Discourage the taking of bubble baths.
6. Advise wiping from back to the front after voiding and defecation.

33. A 3-year-old had a hypospadias repair yesterday; he has a suprapubic catheter in place and an I.V. Which rationale is appropriate for administering propantheline bromide (Pro-Banthine) on an as-needed basis?
1. To decrease the risk of infection at the suture line
2. To decrease the number of organisms in the urine
3. To prevent bladder spasms while the catheter is present
4. To increase urine flow from the kidney to the ureters

30. 3. The family is advised to encourage the child to increase fluid intake. Sandboxes, straddle toys, swimming, and rough activities are avoided until allowed by the surgeon.
CN: Physiological integrity; CNS: Physiological adaptation; CL: Application

31. 1. The defect of hypospadias occurs around the end of the third month of fetal development. Many women don't even know that they're pregnant at this time. This defect isn't hereditary, nor is it carried by an autosomal recessive gene.
CN: Health promotion and maintenance; CNS: None; CL: Application

32. 2, 3, 5. Assessing the mother's understanding of UTI and its causes provides the nurse with a baseline for teaching. The full course of antibiotics must be given to eradicate the organism and prevent recurrence, even if the child's signs and symptoms decrease. Bubble baths can irritate the vulva and urethra and contribute to the development of a UTI. Fluids should be encouraged, not limited, in order to prevent urinary stasis and help flush the organism out of the urinary tract. Instructions should be given to the child at her level of understanding to help her better understand the treatment and promote compliance. The child should wipe from front to the back, not back to front, to minimize the risk of contamination after elimination.
CN: Health promotion and maintenance; CNS: None; CL: Application

33. 3. Propantheline bromide is an antispasmodic that works effectively on children. It isn't an antibiotic and therefore won't decrease the chance of infection or the number of organisms in the urine. The drug has no diuretic effect and won't increase urine flow.
CN: Physiological integrity; CNS: Pharmacological and parenteral therapies; CL: Application

CN: Client needs category   CNS: Client needs subcategory   CL: Cognitive level

34. Which intervention by a nurse would be <u>most helpful</u> when discussing hypospadias with the parents of an infant with this defect?
1. Refer the parents to a counselor.
2. Be there to listen to the parents' concerns.
3. Notify the physician, and have him talk to the parents.
4. Suggest a support group of other parents who have gone through this experience.

35. A nurse should understand that hypospadias defects take the greatest emotional toll on which person?
1. The father
2. The mother
3. The grandfather
4. The grandmother

36. A nurse is questioned by a student nurse about the difference between hypospadias and epispadias. Which response by the nurse is the most accurate?
1. Epispadias defects can only occur in males.
2. The difference between the defects is the length of the urethra.
3. Hypospadias is an abnormal opening on the ventral side of the penis; epispadias is an abnormal opening on the dorsal side.
4. Hypospadias is an abnormal opening on the dorsal side of the penis; epispadias is an abnormal opening on the ventral side.

37. Which nursing diagnosis would be most appropriate for a client with hypospadias?
1. *Deficient fluid volume*
2. *Impaired urinary elimination*
3. *Delayed growth and development*
4. *Risk for infection*

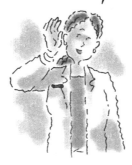

You can almost hear the answer to this question.

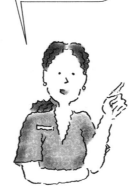

Question 36 is asking you to differentiate between two conditions.

34. 2. The nurse must recognize that parents are going to grieve the loss of the "normal" child when they have a neonate born with a birth defect. Initially, the parents need to have a nurse who will listen to their concerns for their neonate's health. Suggesting a support group or referring the parents to a counselor might be good actions, but not initially. The physician will need to spend time with the parents but, again, the nurse is in the best position to allow the parents to vent their grief and anger.
CN: Psychosocial integrity; CNS: None; CL: Application

35. 1. Because the penis is involved, studies have shown that fathers have a great deal of difficulty dealing with a birth defect like hypospadias.
CN: Psychosocial integrity; CNS: None; CL: Application

36. 3. Hypospadias results from the incomplete closure of the urethral folds along the ventral surface of the developing penis. Epispadias results when the urinary meatus is on the dorsal surface of the penis. Epispadias defects can occur in males and females. The difference is where the opening of the urinary meatus is located, not the length of the urethra.
CN: Health promotion and maintenance; CNS: None; CL: Application

37. 2. The most appropriate diagnosis for a client with hypospadias is *Impaired urinary elimination.* A client with hypospadias should have no problems with the ingestion of fluids. The child's growth and development aren't affected with this defect, and he doesn't have any problem with infection until possibly after a repair of the hypospadias is performed.
CN: Health promotion and maintenance; CNS: None; CL: Analysis

38. When a nurse is teaching a parent how to care for the penis after a hypospadias repair with a skin graft, which statement made by the parent would indicate the need for further teaching?

1. "My infant won't be able to take baths until healing has occurred."
2. "I will change the dressing around the penis daily."
3. "I will make sure I change my infant's diaper often."
4. "If there's a color change in the penis, I will notify my child's physician."

39. A nurse is preparing the parents of an infant with hypospadias for surgery. Which statement made by a parent indicates the need for further teaching?

1. "Skin grafting might be involved in my infant's repair."
2. "After surgery, my infant's penis will look perfectly normal."
3. "Surgical repair may need to be performed in several stages."
4. "My infant will probably be in some pain after the surgery and might need to take some medication for relief."

40. Which piece of assessment data collected by a nurse would indicate to the physician the need for a staged repair of a hypospadias rather than a single repair?

1. There's chordee present with the hypospadias.
2. The urinary meatus opens between the scrotum.
3. The urinary meatus is just below the tip of the penis.
4. The infant had been circumcised before the defect was discovered.

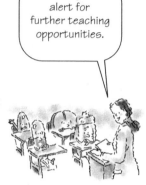

Stay alert for further teaching opportunities.

38. 2. Dressing changes after a hypospadias repair with a skin graft are generally performed by the physician and aren't performed every day because the skin graft needs time to heal and adhere to the penis. Baths aren't given until postoperative healing has taken place. Changing the infant's diapers typically helps keep the penis dry. If the penis color changes, it might be evidence of circulation problems and should be reported.

CN: Health promotion and maintenance; CNS: None; CL: Analysis

39. 2. It's important to stress to the parents that, even after a repair of hypospadias, the outcome isn't a completely "normal-looking" penis. The goals of surgery are to allow the child to void from the tip of his penis, void with a straight stream, and stand up while voiding.

CN: Psychosocial integrity; CNS: None; CL: Application

40. 2. Increased surgical experience and improvements in technique have reduced the number of staged procedures applied to hypospadias defects; however, a staged procedure is indicated in particularly severe defects with marked deficits of available skin for mobilization of flaps. Having a chordee present doesn't require a staged hypospadias repair. If an infant has been circumcised but has a relatively minor hypospadias, the repair can still occur in one stage.

CN: Physiological integrity; CNS: Physiological adaptation; CL: Analysis

CN: Client needs category   CNS: Client needs subcategory   CL: Cognitive level

41. A nurse is planning to teach a female adolescent about pelvic inflammatory disease (PID). Which teaching statement best reflects the focus of preventative teaching needs for this age group?
1. Poor hygiene practices increase the risk of PID.
2. The use of hormonal contraceptives decreases the risk of PID.
3. There are long-term complications related to reproductive tract infections.
4. There are risks of defects in future infants born to adolescents with PID.

42. After a nurse has completed discharge teaching, which statement made by a client treated for a sexually transmitted disease (STD) would indicate that discharge instructions were understood?
1. "I don't need condoms because I'm not allergic to penicillin and I'll come for a shot at the first sign of infection."
2. "I will notify my sex partners and not have unprotected sex from now on."
3. "I will be careful not to have intercourse with someone who has an STD."
4. "If you're going to get it, you're going to get it."

43. Which statement regarding chlamydial infections is correct?
1. The treatment of choice is oral penicillin.
2. The treatment of choice is nystatin or miconazole.
3. Clinical manifestations include dysuria and urethral itching in males.
4. Clinical manifestations include small, painful vesicles on genital areas.

44. Before a client with syphilis can be treated, the nurse must determine which factor?
1. Portal of entry
2. Size of the chancre
3. Names of sexual contacts
4. Existence of medication allergies

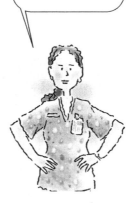

PID untreated can have long-term and serious consequences.

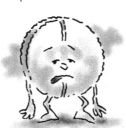

Some people are just hypersensitive—to me, that is.

41. 3. Long-term complications of PID include abscess formation in the fallopian tubes and adhesion formation leading to increased risk of ectopic pregnancy or infertility. It isn't prevented by proper personal hygiene or any form of contraception; some forms of contraception, such as the male or female condom, do help to decrease the incidence of it. PID does not increase the risk of birth defects in infants born to adolescents with PID.
CN: Health promotion and maintenance; CNS: None; CL: Application

42. 2. Goal achievement is indicated by the client's ability to describe preventive behaviors and health practices. The other options indicate that the client doesn't understand the need to take preventive measures.
CN: Health promotion and maintenance; CNS: None; CL: Analysis

43. 3. Clinical manifestations of chlamydia include meatal erythema, tenderness, itching, dysuria, and urethral discharge in the male and mucopurulent cervical exudate with erythema, edema, and congestion in the female. The treatment of choice is doxycycline or azithromycin. Vesicles in the genital area are more consistent with herpes simplex virus.
CN: Health promotion and maintenance; CNS: None; CL: Application

44. 4. The treatment of choice for syphilis is penicillin; clients allergic to penicillin must be given another antibiotic. The other choices aren't necessary before treatment can begin.
CN: Health promotion and maintenance; CNS: None; CL: Application

45. Which technique should a nurse consider when she's discussing sex and sexual activities with adolescents?

1. Break down all the information into scientific terminology.
2. Refer the adolescents to their parents for sexual information.
3. Only answer questions that are asked; don't present any other content.
4. Present sexual information using the proper terminology and in a straightforward manner.

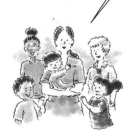

The NCLEX tests your ability to teach clients at different life stages.

46. Without proper treatment, anogenital warts caused by the human papillomavirus (HPV) increases the risk of which illness in adolescent females?

1. Gonorrhea
2. Cervical cancer
3. Chlamydial infections
4. Urinary tract infections (UTIs)

47. Which statement should a nurse include when teaching an adolescent about gonorrhea?

1. It's caused by *Treponema pallidum.*
2. Treatment of sexual partners is an essential part of treatment.
3. It's most commonly treated by multidose administration of penicillin.
4. It may be contracted through contact with a contaminated toilet bowl.

48. When planning sex education and contraceptive teaching for adolescents, which factor should a nurse consider?

1. Neither sexual activity nor contraception requires planning.
2. Most teenagers today are knowledgeable about reproduction.
3. Most teenagers use pregnancy as a way to rebel against their parents.
4. Most teenagers are open about contraception but inconsistently use birth control.

45. 4. Although many adolescents have received sex education from parents and school throughout childhood, they aren't always adequately prepared for the impact of puberty. A large portion of their knowledge is acquired from peers, television, movies, and magazines. Consequently, much of the sex information they have is incomplete, inaccurate, riddled with cultural and moral values, and not very helpful. The public perceives nurses as having authoritative information and being willing to take time with parents. To be effective teachers, nurses need to be honest and open with sexual information.
CN: Health promotion and maintenance; CNS: None; CL: Application

46. 2. All external lesions are treated because of concern regarding the relationship of HPV to cancer. HPV doesn't increase the risk of gonorrhea, chlamydia, or UTIs.
CN: Health promotion and maintenance; CNS: None; CL: Application

47. 2. Adolescents should be taught that treatment is needed for all sexual partners. Gonorrhea is caused by *Neisseria gonorrhoeae.* The medication of choice is a single dose of I.M. ceftriaxone sodium (Rocephin) in males and a single oral dose of cefixime (Suprax) in females. Gonorrhea can't be contracted from a contaminated toilet bowl.
CN: Health promotion and maintenance; CNS: None; CL: Application

48. 4. Most teenagers today are open about discussing contraception and sexuality but may get caught up in the heat of sexuality and forget about birth control measures. Very few teenagers use pregnancy as a way to rebel against their parents. A good deal of the information adolescents have related to reproduction and sexuality may have come from their peers and may not be very reliable.
CN: Health promotion and maintenance; CNS: None; CL: Analysis

CN: Client needs category   CNS: Client needs subcategory   CL: Cognitive level

49. A sexually active teenager seeks counseling from the school nurse about prevention of sexually transmitted diseases (STDs). Which contraceptive measure should the nurse recommend?
1. Rhythm method
2. Withdrawal method
3. Prophylactic antibiotic use
4. Condom and spermicide use

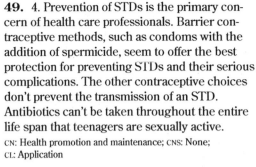

Nice work! You've finished nearly 50 questions already!

50. A nurse understands that which developmental rationale explains risk-taking behavior in adolescents?
1. Adolescents are concrete thinkers and concentrate only on what's happening at the time.
2. Belief in their own invulnerability persuades adolescents that they can take risks safely.
3. Risk of parents' anger and disappointment usually deters adolescents from risky behavior.
4. Peer pressure usually doesn't play an important part in an adolescent's decision to become sexually active.

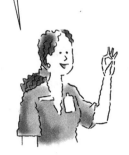

Adolescents may engage in sex as part of risky behavior.

51. Statistics about sexually transmitted diseases (STDs) may not be reliable for which reason?
1. Most adolescents seek out treatment for their STD.
2. Adolescents are usually honest with their parents about their sexual behavior.
3. All sexually transmitted diseases must be reported to the Centers for Disease Control and Prevention (CDC).
4. Chlamydial infections and human papillomavirus (HPV) infections aren't required to be reported to the CDC.

52. It's important for a nurse to include which statement in discharge education for the client who's taking metronidazole (Flagyl) to treat trichomoniasis?
1. Sexual intercourse should stop.
2. Alcohol shouldn't be consumed.
3. Milk products should be avoided.
4. Exposure to sunlight should be limited.

49. 4. Prevention of STDs is the primary concern of health care professionals. Barrier contraceptive methods, such as condoms with the addition of spermicide, seem to offer the best protection for preventing STDs and their serious complications. The other contraceptive choices don't prevent the transmission of an STD. Antibiotics can't be taken throughout the entire life span that teenagers are sexually active.
CN: Health promotion and maintenance; CNS: None; CL: Application

50. 2. Understanding the growth and development of adolescents helps the nurse see that they feel they're invulnerable. Adolescents think about the future and can formally operate in their thought process. Peer pressure plays an important role in risk-taking behaviors; more so than fear of parents' anger or disappointment.
CN: Health promotion and maintenance; CNS: None; CL: Analysis

51. 4. Chlamydial infections and HPV infections aren't required to be reported to the CDC. Most teenagers are afraid to seek out health care for sexual diseases or are unaware of the signs and symptoms of STDs. Teenagers find this a very difficult topic to discuss with their parents and will usually seek out a peer or another adult to obtain information.
CN: Safe, effective care environment; CNS: Safety and infection control; CL: Application

52. 2. While taking metronidazole to treat trichomoniasis, clients shouldn't consume alcohol for at least 48 hours following the last dose. The other choices have no effect on the client taking this medication.
CN: Physiological integrity; CNS: Pharmacological and parenteral therapies; CL: Application

53. Which statement by an adolescent should alert the nurse that <u>more education</u> about sexually transmitted diseases (STDs) is needed?
1. "You always know when you've got gonorrhea."
2. "The most common STD in kids my age is chlamydia infection."
3. "Most of the girls who have *Chlamydia* don't even know it."
4. "If you have symptoms of gonorrhea, they can show up a day or a couple of weeks after you got the infection to begin with."

53. 1. Gonorrhea can occur with or without symptoms. There are four main forms of the disease: asymptomatic, uncomplicated symptomatic, complicated symptomatic, and disseminated disease. All of the other statements are accurate.
CN: Health promotion and maintenance; CNS: None; CL: Application

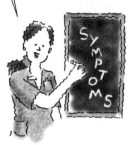

Some sexually transmitted diseases can occur with or without symptoms.

54. Which assessment describes the method of preventing sexually transmitted diseases (STDs) by avoiding exposure?
1. The least accepted and most difficult approach
2. The least expensive and most effective approach
3. The most expensive and least effective approach
4. The most difficult and most time-consuming approach

54. 2. Primary prevention of STDs by avoiding exposure is the least expensive and most effective approach. The nurse can play a role in offering this education to young people before they initiate sexual intercourse.
CN: Safe, effective care environment; CNS: Safety and infection control; CL: Application

55. Which client should a nurse consider to be at greatest risk for developing acquired immunodeficiency syndrome (AIDS)?
1. A client who lives in crowded housing with poor ventilation
2. A young sexually active client with multiple partners
3. An adolescent who's homeless and lives in shelters
4. A young sexually active client with one partner

55. 2. The younger the client when sexual activity begins, the higher the incidence of HIV and AIDS. Also, the more sexual partners he has, the higher the incidence of these diseases. Neither crowded living environments nor homeless environments by themselves lead to an increase in the incidence of AIDS.
CN: Health promotion and maintenance; CNS: None; CL: Analysis

56. When assessing an adolescent for pelvic inflammatory disease (PID), which sign or symptom should the nurse expect to see?
1. A hard, painless, red defined lesion
2. Small vesicles on the genital area with itching
3. Cervical discharge with redness and edema
4. Lower abdominal pain and urinary tract symptoms

Questions about basic assessment skills are common on the NCLEX.

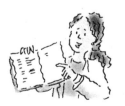

56. 4. PID is an infection of the upper female genital tract most commonly caused by sexually transmitted diseases. Presenting symptoms in the adolescent may be generalized, with fever, abdominal pain, urinary tract symptoms, and vague, influenza-like symptoms. A hard, painless, red defined lesion indicates syphilis. Small vesicles on the genital area with itching indicates herpes genitalis. Cervical discharge with redness and edema indicates chlamydia.
CN: Health promotion and maintenance; CNS: None; CL: Application

CN: Client needs category CNS: Client needs subcategory CL: Cognitive level

57. A nurse should include which fact when teaching an adolescent group about the human immunodeficiency virus (HIV)?
1. The incidence of HIV in the adolescent population has declined since 1995.
2. The virus can be spread through many routes, including sexual contact.
3. Knowledge about HIV spread and transmission has led to a decrease in the spread of the virus among adolescents.
4. About 50% of all new HIV infections in the United States occur in people under age 22.

58. When planning a program to teach adolescents about human immunodeficiency virus infection (HIV), which action might lead to better program success?
1. Surveying the community to evaluate the level of education
2. Obtaining peer educators to provide information about HIV
3. Setting up clinics in community centers and having condoms readily available
4. Having primary health care providers host workshops in community centers

59. After a nurse completes her teaching of an adolescent about syphilis, which statement by the adolescent indicates the need for further teaching?
1. "The disease is divided into four stages: primary, secondary, latent, and tertiary."
2. "Affected persons are most infectious during the first year."
3. "Syphilis is easily treated with penicillin or doxycycline."
4. "Syphilis is rarely transmitted sexually."

60. In teaching a group of parents about monitoring for urinary tract infection (UTI) in preschoolers, which symptom would indicate that a child should be evaluated?
1. Voids only twice in any 6-hour period
2. Exhibits incontinence after being toilet trained
3. Has difficulty sitting still for more than a 30-minute period of time
4. Urine smells strongly of ammonia after standing for more than 2 hours

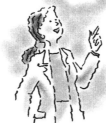

Hey! I think I finally get genitourinary disorders.

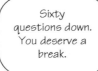
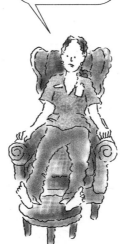

Sixty questions down. You deserve a break.

57. 2. HIV can be spread through many routes, including sexual contact and contact with infected blood or other body fluids. The incidence of HIV in the adolescent population has *increased* since 1995, even though more information about the virus is targeted to reach the adolescent population. Only about 25% of all new HIV infections in the United States occur in people under age 22.
CN: Health promotion and maintenance; CNS: None; CL: Application

58. 2. Peer education programs have noted that teens are more likely to ask questions of peer educators than of adults and that peer education can change personal attitudes and the perception of risk of HIV infection. The other approaches would be helpful but wouldn't necessarily make the outreach program more successful.
CN: Health promotion and maintenance; CNS: None; CL: Analysis

59. 4. About 95% of syphilis cases are transmitted sexually. There are four stages to syphilis, although some people may only experience the first three stages. Affected persons are most contagious in the first year of the disease. The drug of choice for treating syphilis is penicillin or doxycycline.
CN: Health promotion and maintenance; CNS: None; CL: Analysis

60. 2. A child who exhibits incontinence after being toilet trained should be evaluated for UTI. Most urine smells strongly of ammonia after standing for more than 2 hours, so this doesn't necessarily indicate UTI. The other options aren't reasons for parents to suspect problems with their child's urinary system.
CN: Health promotion and maintenance; CNS: None; CL: Application

61. Which instruction should a nurse include in the teaching plan for a client receiving co-trimoxazole (Septra) for a repeated urinary tract infection with *Escherichia coli*?
1. "For the drug to be effective, keep your urine acidic by drinking at least a quart of cranberry juice a day."
2. "Take the medication for 10 days even if your symptoms improve in a few days."
3. "Return to the clinic in 3 days for another urine culture."
4. "Take two of the pills a day now, but keep the rest of the pills to take if the symptoms reappear within 2 weeks."

62. A nurse should include which fact when teaching parents about handling a child with recurrent urinary tract infection (UTI)?
1. Antibiotics should be discontinued 48 hours after symptoms subside.
2. Recurrent symptoms should be treated by renewing the antibiotic prescription.
3. Complicated UTIs are related to poor perineal hygiene practice.
4. Follow-up urine cultures are necessary to detect recurrent infections and antibiotic effectiveness.

63. A nurse is reviewing a child's clean-voided urine specimen results. The nurse understands that which result indicates a urinary tract infection (UTI)?
1. A specific gravity of 1.020
2. Cloudy color without odor
3. A large amount of casts present
4. 100,000 bacterial colonies per milliliter

64. The nurse is teaching the parents of a child with a urinary tract infection. Which factor should the nurse recognize as predisposing the urinary tract to infections?
1. Increased fluid intake
2. Short urethra
3. Ingestion of highly acidic juices
4. Frequent emptying of the bladder

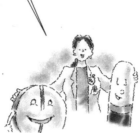

Teaching about medications— that's another common NCLEX subject.

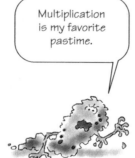

Multiplication is my favorite pastime.

61. 2. Discharge instructions for clients receiving an anti-infective medication should include taking all of the prescribed medication for the prescribed time. Drinking highly acidic juices, such as cranberry juice, may help maintain urinary health but won't get rid of an already present infection. The child won't need to have a culture repeated until the medication is completed.

CN: Physiological integrity; CNS: Pharmacological and parenteral therapies; CL: Application

62. 4. A routine follow-up urine specimen is usually obtained 2 or 3 days after the completion of the antibiotic treatment. All of the antibiotic should be taken as ordered and not stopped when symptoms disappear. If recurrent symptoms appear, a urine culture should be obtained to see whether the infection is resistant to antibiotics. Simple, not complicated, UTIs are generally caused by poor perineal hygiene.

CN: Health promotion and maintenance; CNS: None; CL: Application

63. 4. The diagnosis of UTI is determined by the detection of bacteria in the urine. Infected urine usually contains more than 100,000 colonies/ml, usually of a single organism. The urine is usually cloudy, hazy, and may have strands of mucus. It also has a foul, fishy odor even when fresh. Casts and increased specific gravity aren't specific to UTI.

CN: Physiological integrity; CNS: Reduction of risk potential; CL: Application

64. 2. A short urethra contributes to infection because bacteria have a shorter distance to travel to the urinary tract. The risk of infection is higher in women because women have shorter urethras than men (3/4″ [1.9 cm] in young women, 1″ [3.8 cm] in mature women, 7″ [19.7 cm] in adult men). Increased fluid intake would help flush the urinary tract system and frequent emptying of the bladder would decrease the risk of urinary tract infection. Drinking highly acidic juices, such as cranberry juice, may help maintain urinary health.

CN: Health promotion and maintenance; CNS: None; CL: Application

CN: Client needs category   CNS: Client needs subcategory   CL: Cognitive level

65. A nurse is assessing a child with vesicoureteral reflux. Which condition should the nurse be alert for as a potential complication?
1. Glomerulonephritis
2. Hemolytic uremia syndrome
3. Nephrotic syndrome
4. Renal infection

65. 4. Reflux of urine into the ureters and then back into the bladder after voiding sets up the client for a urinary tract infection. This can lead to renal damage due to scarring of the parenchyma. Glomerulonephritis is an autoimmune reaction to a beta-hemolytic strep infection. Hemolytic uremia syndrome may be the result of genetic factors. Eighty percent of nephrotic syndrome cases are idiopathic.
CN: Health promotion and maintenance; CNS: None; CL: Analysis

66. The mother of a female child asks the nurse why her child seems to have so many urinary tract infections (UTIs). Which response by the nurse would be the most accurate?
1. Vaginal secretions are too acidic.
2. Girls aren't protected by circumcision.
3. The urethra is in close proximity to the anus.
4. Girls touch their genitalia more often than boys do.

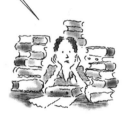

All this studying just to learn that girls are different from boys.

66. 3. Girls are especially at risk for bacterial invasion of the urinary tract because of basic anatomical differences; the urethra is short and in close proximity to the anus. Vaginal secretions are normally acidic, which decreases the risk of infection. Circumcision doesn't protect girls *or* boys from UTIs. There's no documented research that supports that girls touch their genitalia more often than boys do.
CN: Health promotion and maintenance; CNS: None; CL: Application

67. A child has been sent to the school nurse for wetting her pants three times in the past 2 days. The nurse should recommend that this child be evaluated for which complication?
1. School phobia
2. Emotional trauma
3. Urinary tract infection
4. Structural defect of the urinary tract

67. 3. Frequent urinary incontinence should be evaluated by the physician, with the first action being checking the urine for infection. Children exhibit signs of school phobia by complaining of an ailment before school starts and getting better after they're allowed to miss school. After infection, structural defect, and diabetes mellitus have been ruled out, emotional trauma should be investigated.
CN: Health promotion and maintenance; CNS: None; CL: Application

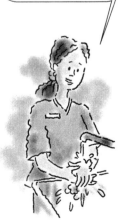

Sometimes simple hygienic habits offer the best preventative measure.

68. When a nurse is teaching parents of children about recurrent urinary tract infections (UTIs), which goal should be included as the most important?
1. Detection
2. Education
3. Prevention
4. Treatment

68. 3. Prevention is the most important goal in teaching about primary and recurrent UTIs; most preventive measures are simple, ordinary hygienic habits that should be a routine part of daily care. Treatment, detection, and education are all important, but none is the most important goal.
CN: Physiological integrity; CNS: Reduction of risk potential; CL: Analysis

69. Which intervention should a nurse recommend to parents of young girls to help prevent urinary tract infections (UTIs)?
1. Limit bathing as much as possible.
2. Increase fluids and decrease salt intake.
3. Have the child wear cotton underpants.
4. Have the child clean her perineum from back to front.

70. A nurse understands that which characteristic is the single most important factor influencing the occurrence of urinary tract infections (UTIs)?
1. Urinary stasis
2. Frequency of baths
3. Uncircumcised penis (in males)
4. Amount of fluid intake

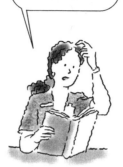

Hmmm... the single most important factor; I need to think about that.

71. When evaluating infants and young toddlers for signs of urinary tract infections (UTIs), a nurse should know that which symptom would be most common?
1. Abdominal pain
2. Feeding problems
3. Frequency
4. Urgency

72. When obtaining a urine specimen for culture and sensitivity, a nurse should understand that which method of collection is best?
1. Bagged urine specimen
2. Clean-catch urine specimen
3. First-voided urine specimen
4. Catheterized urine specimen

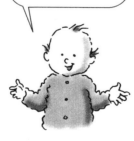

If I'm not eating, something must be wrong!

69. 3. Cotton is a more breathable fabric and allows for dampness to be absorbed from the perineum. Bathing shouldn't be limited; however, the use of bubble bath or whirlpool baths should. However, if the child has frequent UTIs, taking a bath should be discouraged and taking a shower encouraged. Increasing fluids would be helpful, but decreasing salt isn't necessary. The perineum should always be cleaned from front to back.
CN: Health promotion and maintenance; CNS: None; CL: Application

70. 1. Ordinarily, urine is sterile. However, at 98.6° F (37° C), it provides an excellent culture medium. Under normal conditions, the act of completely and repeatedly emptying the bladder flushes away any organisms before they have an opportunity to multiply and invade surrounding tissue. Baths and fluid intake are factors in the development of UTIs, but aren't the most important. There's an increased incidence of UTI in uncircumcised infants under 1 year but not after that age.
CN: Physiological integrity; CNS: Reduction of risk potential; CL: Application

71. 2. In infants and children less than 2 years old, the signs are characteristically nonspecific and feeding problems are usually the first indication. Symptoms more nearly resemble GI tract disorders. Abdominal pain, urgency, and frequency are signs that would be observed in the older child with a UTI.
CN: Physiological integrity; CNS: Physiological adaptation; CL: Application

72. 4. The most accurate tests of bacterial content are suprapubic aspiration (for children less than 2 years old) and properly performed bladder catheterization. The other methods of obtaining a specimen have a high incidence of contamination not related to infection.
CN: Physiological integrity; CNS: Basic care and comfort; CL: Application

CN: Client needs category   CNS: Client needs subcategory   CL: Cognitive level

73. After collecting a urine specimen, which action by a nurse is the <u>most appropriate</u>?
1. Taking the specimen to the laboratory immediately
2. Sending the specimen to the laboratory on the scheduled run
3. Taking the specimen to the laboratory during the nurse's next break
4. Keeping the specimen in the refrigerator until it can be taken to the laboratory

74. When teaching parents of a child with a urinary tract infection (UTI) about fluid intake, which statement by a parent would indicate the need for further teaching?
1. "I should encourage my child to drink about 50 ml per pound of body weight daily."
2. "Clear liquids should be the primary liquids that my child should drink."
3. "I should offer my child carbonated beverages about every 2 hours."
4. "My child should avoid drinking caffeinated beverages."

75. Which treatment should a nurse anticipate in a child who has a history of recurrent urinary tract infections (UTIs)?
1. Frequent catheterizations
2. Prophylactic antibiotics
3. Limited activities
4. Surgical intervention

76. When teaching parents about giving medications to children for recurrent urinary tract infections (UTIs), which instruction should be included?
1. The medication should be given first thing in the morning.
2. The medication should be given right before bedtime.
3. The medication is generally given four times a day.
4. It doesn't matter when the medication is given.

This question calls for immediate action.

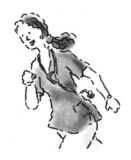

Why do I feel like I'm forgetting something?

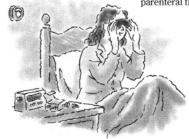

73. 1. Care of urine specimens obtained for culture is an important nursing aspect related to diagnosis. Specimens should be taken to the laboratory for culture immediately. If the culture is delayed, the specimen can be placed in the refrigerator, but storage can result in a loss of formed elements, such as blood cells and casts.
CN: Physiological integrity; CNS: Basic care and comfort; CL: Application

74. 3. Caffeinated or carbonated beverages are avoided because of their potentially irritating effect on the bladder mucosa. Adequate fluid intake is always indicated during an acute UTI. It is recommended that a person drink approximately 50 ml/lb of body weight daily. The client should primarily drink clear liquids.
CN: Physiological integrity; CNS: Basic care and comfort; CL: Analysis

75. 2. Children who experience recurrent UTIs may require antibiotic therapy for months or years. Recurrent UTIs would be investigated for anatomic abnormalities and surgical intervention may be indicated, but the client would also be placed on antibiotics before the tests. The child's activities aren't limited, and frequent catheterization predisposes a child to infection.
CN: Physiological integrity; CNS: Pharmacological and parenteral therapies; CL: Application

76. 2. Medication is commonly administered once a day, and the client and parents are advised to give the antibiotic before sleep because this represents the longest period without voiding.
CN: Physiological integrity; CNS: Pharmacological and parenteral therapies; CL: Application

77. The nurse is providing education to a group of patients about urinary tract infections (UTIs). The nurse knows that teaching has been effective when the patients state that which situation has the <u>greatest</u> impact on the potential for progressive renal injury after UTIs?
1. A school-age child who must get permission to go to the bathroom
2. An adolescent female who has started menstruation
3. Children who compete in competitive sports
4. Young infants and toddlers

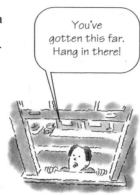

You've gotten this far. Hang in there!

77. 4. The hazard of progressive renal injury is greatest when infection occurs in young children, especially those under 2 years old. The first two options might lead to a simple UTI that would need to be treated. Competitive sports have no bearing on a UTI.
CN: Safe, effective care environment; CNS: Safety and infection control; CL: Application

78. Which statement should a nurse make to help parents understand the recovery period after a child has had surgery to remove a Wilms' tumor?
1. "Children will easily lie in bed and restrict their activities."
2. "Recovery is usually fast in spite of the abdominal incision."
3. "Recovery usually takes a great deal of time because of the large incision."
4. "Parents need to perform activities of daily living for about 2 weeks after surgery."

78. 2. Children generally recover very quickly from surgery to remove a Wilms' tumor, even though they may have a large abdominal incision. Children like to get back into the normalcy of being a child, which is through play. Parents need to encourage their children to do as much for themselves as possible, although some regression is expected.
CN: Psychosocial integrity; CNS: None; CL: Analysis

79. When teaching parents about administering co-trimoxazole (Septra) to a child for treatment of a urinary tract infection (UTI), the nurse should include which instruction?
1. Give the medication with food.
2. Give the medication with water.
3. Give the medication with a cola beverage.
4. Give the medication 2 hours after a meal.

79. 2. When giving co-trimoxazole, the medication should be administered with a full glass of water on an empty stomach. If nausea and vomiting occur, giving the drug with food may decrease gastric distress. Carbonated beverages should be avoided because they irritate the bladder.
CN: Physiological integrity; CNS: Pharmacological and parenteral therapies; CL: Application

80. The nurse is questioned by a student nurse about the incidence of Wilms' tumor. Which response by the nurse is the most accurate?
1. Peak incidence occurs at 10 years of age.
2. It's the least common type of renal cancer.
3. It's the most common type of renal cancer.
4. It has a decreased incidence among siblings.

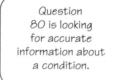

Question 80 is looking for accurate information about a condition.

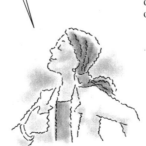

80. 3. Wilms' tumor is the most frequent intra-abdominal tumor of childhood and the most common type of renal cancer. The peak incidence is 3 years, and there's an increased incidence among siblings and identical twins.
CN: Health promotion and maintenance; CNS: None; CL: Application

CN: Client needs category   CNS: Client needs subcategory   CL: Cognitive level

81. Which presenting sign is most common with Wilms' tumor?
1. Pain in the abdomen
2. Fever greater than 104° F (40° C)
3. Decreased blood pressure
4. Swelling within the abdomen

82. When a nurse is explaining the diagnosis of Wilms' tumor to parents, which statement by a parent would indicate the need for further teaching?
1. "Wilms' tumor usually involves both kidneys."
2. "Wilms' tumor occurs slightly more commonly in the left kidney."
3. "Wilms' tumor is staged during surgery for treatment planning."
4. "Wilms' tumor stays encapsulated for an extended period of time."

83. A parent asks a nurse about the prognosis of her child diagnosed with Wilms' tumor. The nurse should base her response on which factor?
1. Usually children with Wilms' tumor need only surgical intervention.
2. Survival rates for Wilms' tumor are the lowest among childhood cancers.
3. Survival rates for Wilms' tumor are the highest among childhood cancers.
4. Children with localized tumor have only a 30% chance of cure with multimodal therapy.

84. If <u>both kidneys</u> are involved in a child with Wilms' tumor, the nurse should understand that treatment prior to surgery might include which method?
1. Peritoneal dialysis
2. Abdominal gavage
3. Radiation and chemotherapy
4. Antibiotics and I.V. fluid therapy

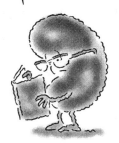

Let me see what I can learn about Wilms' tumor.

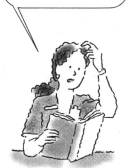

Hmmm, might the treatment for both kidneys differ from that for one?

81. 4. The most common presenting sign is a swelling or mass within the abdomen. The mass is characteristically firm, nontender, confined to one side, and deep within the flank. A high fever isn't a presenting sign for Wilms' tumor. Blood pressure is characteristically increased, not decreased.
CN: Health promotion and maintenance; CNS: None; CL: Application

82. 1. Wilms' tumor usually involves only one kidney and is usually staged during surgery so that an effective course of treatment can be established. Wilms' tumor has a slightly higher occurrence in the left kidney, and it stays encapsulated for an extended period of time.
CN: Health promotion and maintenance; CNS: None; CL: Application

83. 3. Survival rates for Wilms' tumor are the highest among childhood cancers. Usually children with Wilms' tumor who have stage I or II localized tumor have a 90% chance of cure with multimodal therapy.
CN: Health promotion and maintenance; CNS: None; CL: Application

84. 3. If both kidneys are involved, the child may be treated with radiation therapy or chemotherapy preoperatively to shrink the tumor, allowing more conservative therapy. Peritoneal dialysis would be needed only if the kidneys aren't functioning. Abdominal gavage wouldn't be indicated. Antibiotics aren't needed because Wilms' tumor isn't an infection.
CN: Physiological integrity; CNS: Reduction of risk potential; CL: Application

85. When caring for the child with Wilms' tumor <u>preoperatively</u>, which nursing intervention would be most important?

1. Avoid abdominal palpation.
2. Closely monitor arterial blood gas (ABG) levels.
3. Prepare the child and his family for long-term dialysis.
4. Prepare the child and his family for renal transplantation.

86. A child is scheduled for surgery to remove a Wilms' tumor from one kidney. The parents ask the nurse what treatment, if any, they should expect after their child recovers from surgery. Which response would be most accurate?

1. "Chemotherapy may be necessary."
2. "Kidney transplant is indicated eventually."
3. "No additional treatments are usually necessary."
4. "Chemotherapy with or without radiation therapy is indicated."

87. When assessing the abdomen of a child with a potential diagnosis of Wilms' tumor, which factor might lead to a different diagnosis?

1. The mass is on one side of the abdomen.
2. There is a mass on both sides of the abdomen.
3. The mass crosses the midline of the abdomen.
4. There's no pain associated with palpation of the mass.

88. A parent of a child with Wilms' tumor asks the nurse about surgery. Which statement concerning the nature of surgery for Wilms' tumor is the <u>most accurate</u>?

1. Surgery isn't indicated in children with Wilms' tumor.
2. Surgery is usually performed within 24 to 48 hours of admission.
3. Surgery is the least favorable therapy for the treatment of Wilms' tumor.
4. Surgery will be delayed until the client's overall health status improves.

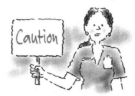

Note the word preoperatively in question 85.

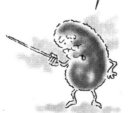

Do you know the preferred treatment for Wilms' tumor?

85. 1. After the diagnosis of Wilms' tumor is made, the abdomen shouldn't be palpated. Palpation of the tumor might lead to rupture, which will cause the cancerous cells to spread throughout the abdomen. ABG levels shouldn't be affected. If surgery is successful, there won't be a need for long-term dialysis or renal transplantation.
CN: Physiological integrity; CNS: Reduction of risk potential; CL: Application

86. 4. Because radiation therapy and chemotherapy are usually begun immediately after surgery, parents need an explanation of what to expect, such as major benefits and adverse effects. Kidney transplant isn't usually necessary.
CN: Physiological integrity; CNS: Physiological adaptation; CL: Application

87. 3. When an abdominal mass crosses the midline, a neuroblastoma should be suspected—not a Wilms' tumor. A Wilms' tumor arises off the kidneys and can be on one side or both sides of the abdomen but doesn't cross the midline. Pain isn't usually associated with Wilms' tumor.
CN: Health promotion and maintenance; CNS: None; CL: Analysis

88. 2. Surgery is the preferred treatment and is scheduled as soon as possible after confirmation of a renal mass, usually within 24 to 48 hours of admission, to be sure the encapsulated tumor remains intact.
CN: Physiological integrity; CNS: Physiological adaptation; CL: Application

CN: Client needs category   CNS: Client needs subcategory   CL: Cognitive level

89. A 3-year-old child has had surgery to remove a Wilms' tumor. Which action should the nurse take first when the mother asks for pain medication for the child?
  1. Get the pain medication ready for administration.
  2. Assess the client's pain using a pain scale of 1 to 10.
  3. Assess the client's pain using a smiley face pain scale.
  4. Check for the last time pain medication was administered.

90. A child has been diagnosed with Wilms' tumor. Because of the parents' religious beliefs, they choose not to treat the child. Which statement by the nurse indicates the need for further discussion?
  1. "I know this is a lot of information in a short period of time."
  2. "I don't think parents have the legal right to make these kinds of decisions."
  3. "These parents just don't understand how easily treated a Wilms' tumor is."
  4. "I think the parents are in shock."

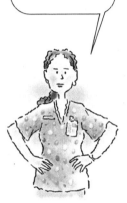

Remember to respect the parents' religious beliefs.

91. A child with a Wilms' tumor has had surgery to remove a kidney and has received chemotherapy. The nurse should include which instruction at discharge?
  1. Avoid contact sports.
  2. Decrease fluid intake.
  3. Decrease sodium intake.
  4. Avoid contact with other children.

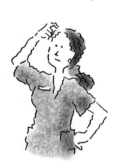

Which finding suggests the need to notify the physician?

92. When caring for a child after removal of a Wilms' tumor, which assessment finding would indicate the need to notify the physician?
  1. Fever of 101° F (38.3° C)
  2. Absence of bowel sounds
  3. Slight congestion in the lungs
  4. Complaints of pain when moving

89. 3. The first action of the nurse should be to assess the client for pain. A 3-year-old child is too young to use a pain scale from 1 to 10 but can easily use the smiley face pain scale. After assessing the pain, the nurse should then investigate the time the pain medication was last given and administer the medication accordingly.
CN: Physiological integrity; CNS: Pharmacological and parenteral therapies; CL: Application

90. 2. Parents *do* have the legal right to make decisions regarding the health issues for their child. Religion plays an important role in many people's lives, and decisions about surgery and treatment for cancer are sometimes made that scientifically don't make sense to the health care provider. The parents are probably in a state of shock because a lot of information has been given and this is a cancer that requires decisions to be made quickly, especially surgical intervention.
CN: Safe, effective care environment; CNS: Management of care; CL: Analysis

91. 1. Because the child is left with only one kidney, certain precautions, such as avoiding contact sports, are recommended to prevent injury to the remaining kidney. Decreasing fluid intake wouldn't be indicated; fluid intake is essential for renal function. The child's sodium intake shouldn't be reduced. Avoiding other children is unnecessary, will make the child feel self-conscious, and may lead to regressive behavior.
CN: Health promotion and maintenance; CNS: None; CL: Application

92. 2. This child is at risk for intestinal obstruction. GI abnormalities require notification of the physician. A slight fever following surgery isn't uncommon, nor are slight congestion in the lungs and complaints of pain.
CN: Physiological integrity; CNS: Reduction of risk potential; CL: Application

93. Because surgery is performed for a Wilms' tumor within 24 to 48 hours of admission, a nurse must prepare a family and child quickly for procedures. Which statement should guide the nurse in her preparation of the family?

1. Because the parents are in a state of shock, they don't need explanations.
2. Explanations should be kept simple and should be repeated often.
3. Scientific terminology should be used with drawings and models.
4. The play therapist is the best person to prepare this family.

94. Which statement made by the physician to the parents of a child who has had a Wilms' tumor removed would be the most difficult for the parents to hear and might require nursing intervention?

1. "We will start chemotherapy within the next 24 to 48 hours."
2. "The tumor was a stage IV, which indicates other organ involvement."
3. "We were able to remove all of the tumor, but we had to take the kidney as well."
4. "The incision is long, and the dressing will need to be changed daily."

95. In providing psychosocial care to a 6-year-old child who has had abdominal surgery for Wilms' tumor, which activity would be the <u>most appropriate</u>?

1. Allowing the child to watch a 2-hour movie without interruptions
2. Giving the child a puzzle with five pieces to encourage him to move while in bed
3. Telling the child that you can give him enough medication so that he feels no pain
4. Providing the child with puppets and supplies and asking him to draw how he feels

96. The nurse is teaching the parents of a child with Wilms' tumor about staging. The nurse knows the teaching has been effective when the parents respond that staging helps determine which parameter?

1. Size of tumor
2. Level of treatment
3. Length of incision
4. Amount of anesthesia

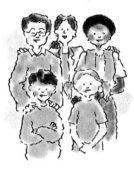

Be sensitive to the needs of a client's family when delivering bad news.

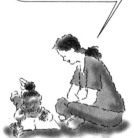

Can you show me how you feel?

93. 2. Decisions are made rapidly after the diagnosis of Wilms' tumor is made. Parents are typically in shock at this time. Explanations should be kept simple and repeated often. The play therapist might become involved with this family, especially postoperatively. There's generally no time to prepare the play therapist for the role of educator in this situation.
CN: Health promotion and maintenance; CNS: None; CL: Application

94. 2. Surgery is an anxiety-producing event to parents. It also marks the confirmation of the stage of the tumor. A stage IV tumor has a poor prognosis because other organs are involved. This statement, above all others, would be the most difficult for the parents to hear.
CN: Psychosocial integrity; CNS: None; CL: Analysis

95. 4. A movie is a good diversion, but giving puppets and encouraging the child to draw his feelings is a better outlet. A puzzle with only five pieces is too basic for a 6-year-old child and wouldn't hold his interest. You probably can't give enough pain medication so that a person who has had surgery will feel no pain.
CN: Psychosocial integrity; CNS: None; CL: Application

96. 2. Staging of the tumor helps to determine the level of treatment because it provides information about the level of involvement. The other choices are insignificant in staging of the tumor.
CN: Health promotion and maintenance; CNS: None; CL: Application

CN: Client needs category   CNS: Client needs subcategory   CL: Cognitive level

97. A nurse is educating parents about Wilms' tumor. Which statement made by a parent would indicate the need for <u>further teaching</u>?
1. "My child could have inherited this disease."
2. "Wilms' tumor can be associated with other congenital anomalies."
3. "This disease could have been a result of trauma to the baby in utero."
4. "There's no method of identification of gene carriers of Wilms' tumor."

98. Which assessment finding will aid in the differentiation of a Wilms' tumor from the liver when doing an abdominal assessment?
1. The liver moves with respiration.
2. The liver is a more encapsulated organ.
3. A Wilms' tumor isn't as deep as the liver.
4. A Wilms' tumor usually isn't well defined.

99. Which action by a nurse would be appropriate to take for a child diagnosed with a Wilms' tumor?
1. Take blood pressure in the right arm only.
2. Offer only clear liquids at room temperature.
3. Post a sign over the bed that reads, "Don't palpate abdomen."
4. Allow the child to participate in group activities in the playroom.

100. Which is the most important instruction for a nurse to tell the parent of a 24-month-old child when the parent asks about starting toilet-training?
1. The child must be developmentally ready.
2. Use a consistent approach.
3. Maintain a positive attitude.
4. Start at the same age siblings were trained.

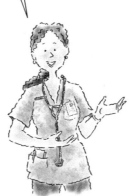

Further teaching is so important that you'll see similar questions more than once.

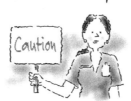

Sometimes you just have to spell it out.

97. 3. Wilms' tumor isn't a result of trauma to the fetus in utero. Wilms' tumor can be genetically inherited and is associated with other congenital anomalies. However, there's no method for identifying gene carriers of Wilms' tumor at this time.
CN: Health promotion and maintenance; CNS: None; CL: Application

98. 1. It's difficult to distinguish a Wilms' tumor from the liver if the tumor is on the right side of the body. One difference is that the liver will move with respirations and a Wilms' tumor won't. A Wilms' tumor is deep in the abdomen and is usually well defined and encapsulated.
CN: Health promotion and maintenance; CNS: None; CL: Application

99. 3. To reinforce the need for caution, it may be necessary to post a sign over the bed that reads, "Don't palpate abdomen." The blood pressure could be taken in any extremity; prior to surgery, there are usually no dietary restrictions. Careful bathing and handling are also important in preventing trauma to the tumor site; thus, group activities should be discouraged.
CN: Health promotion and maintenance; CNS: None; CL: Application

100. 1. Toilet-training should begin when the child is developmentally ready. After training is started, a consistent approach and a positive attitude should be used. Each child's readiness for toilet-training is individual and the child shouldn't be compared to his siblings.
CN: Health promotion and maintenance; CNS: None; CL: Application

101. A previously toilet-trained 4-year-old child begins wetting the bed after being hospitalized. Which statement should a nurse tell the parents?
1. "Children commonly show regressive behavior when hospitalized."
2. "Your child is just acting out to make you feel bad."
3. "Sometimes 4-year-olds still have accidents."
4. "Let's try cutting back on fluids and see whether that helps."

101. 1. Young children may exhibit regressive behaviors when they're under stress, such as occurs with hospitalization. The child may be acting out, but more likely this is not voluntary bed-wetting. Four-year-olds should be fully toilet-trained. Restricting fluids as a first step in a hospitalized child isn't appropriate; other causes of bed-wetting should be considered first.
CN: Physiological integrity; CNS: None; CL: Application

102. A preschooler is scheduled to have a Wilms' tumor removed. Identify the area of the urinary system where this type of tumor is located.

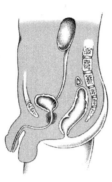

102. Wilms' tumor, also known as *nephroblastoma*, is a tumor located in the kidney. It's most commonly found in children ages 2 to 4.
CN: Physiological integrity; CNS: Physiological adaptation; CL: Application

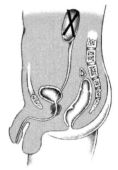

103. A 3-year-old child is to receive 500 ml of dextrose 5% in normal saline solution over 8 hours. At what rate (in ml/hour) should the nurse set the infusion pump? Round your answer to a whole number.

_____ ml/hour

103. 63. To calculate the rate per hour for the infusion, the nurse should divide 500 ml by 8 hours: 500 ml ÷ 8 hours = 62.5 ml/hour, which should be rounded to 63.
CN: Physiological integrity; CNS: Pharmacological and parenteral therapies; CL: Application

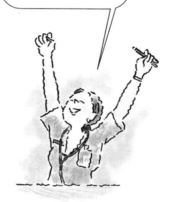

Congratulations! You finished all 103 questions! Fantastic!

CN: Client needs category   CNS: Client needs subcategory   CL: Cognitive level

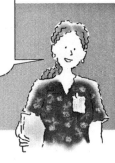

Skin diseases in children and teens are common and varied. This chapter covers common and uncommon skin disorders among these populations.

Chapter 22
Integumentary system

1. A 12-year-old child with burns over 40% of his body is ordered to receive 1,500 ml of I.V. fluid over 6 hours. At what rate should the nurse set the infusion pump?
1. 125 ml/hour
2. 150 ml/hour
3. 175 ml/hour
4. 250 ml/hour

2. Providing adequate nutrition is essential for a burn client. Which statement best describes the nutritional needs of a child who has burns?
1. A child needs 100 cal/kg during hospitalization.
2. The hypermetabolic state after a burn injury leads to poor healing.
3. Caloric needs can be lowered by controlling environmental temperature.
4. Maintaining a hypermetabolic rate will lower the child's risk for infection.

Measuring burns in children is different than measuring burns in adults.

3. A 1-year-old child is treated in the clinic for a burn to the anterior surface of the left hand. Which way to measure burn size would be accurate for this child?
1. The rule of nines
2. Percentage based on the child's weight
3. The child's hand equals 1.25% of the child's body surface area
4. Percentage can't be determined without knowing the type of burn

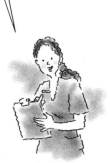

1. 4. 1,500 milliliters divided by 6 hours equals 250 milliliters/hour.

CN: Physiological integrity; CNS: Pharmacological and parenteral therapies; CL: Application

2. 2. A burn injury causes a hypermetabolic state leading to protein and lipid catabolism, which affects wound healing. Caloric intake should be 1½ to 2 times the basal metabolic rate, with a minimum of 1.5 to 2 g/kg of body weight of protein daily. Keeping the temperature within a normal range lets the body function efficiently and use calories for healing and normal physiological processes. If the temperature is too warm or cold, energy must be used for warming or cooling, taking energy away from tissue repair. High metabolic rates increase the risk for infection.

CN: Physiological integrity; CNS: Basic care and comfort; CL: Analysis

3. 3. The anterior surface of a child's hand is equal to 1.25% of that child's body surface. The rule of nines is used for children aged 14 years and older. The child's weight is important to calculate fluid replacement for extensive burns, not to estimate total body surface area. Burn type doesn't determine the percentage of body surface involved.

CN: Physiological integrity; CNS: Physiological adaptation; CL: Application

CN: Client needs category   CNS: Client needs subcategory   CL: Cognitive level

4. An 18-month-old child is admitted to the hospital for full-thickness burns to the anterior chest. The mother asks how the burn will heal. Which statement is accurate about healing for full-thickness burns?

1. Surgical closure and grafting are usually needed.
2. Healing takes 10 to 12 days, with little or no scarring.
3. Pigment in a black client will return to the injured area.
4. Healing can take up to 6 weeks, with a high incidence of scarring.

5. A 9-year-old child is admitted to the hospital with deep partial-thickness burns to 25% of his body. Which assessment finding would the nurse associate with a deep partial-thickness burn?

1. Erythema and pain
2. Minimal damage to the epidermis
3. Necrosis through all layers of skin
4. Tissue necrosis through most of the dermis

6. A 4-year-old child is admitted to the burn unit with a circumferential burn to the left forearm. Which finding should be reported to the physician?

1. Numbness of fingers
2. +2 radial and ulnar pulses
3. Full range of motion (ROM) and no pain
4. Bilateral capillary refill less then 2 seconds

7. Which fact should be given to the parents of a child with fifth disease?

1. There is a possible reappearance of the rash for up to 1 week.
2. Isolation of high-risk contacts should be avoided for 4 to 10 days.
3. Pregnant clients are at risk for fetal death if infected with fifth disease.
4. Children with fifth disease are contagious only while the rash is present.

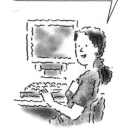

Do you remember what you learned about full-thickness burns?

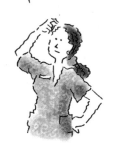

The word circumferential is a clue, right?

4. 1. Full-thickness burns usually need surgical closure and grafting for complete healing. Healing in 10 to 12 days with little or no scarring is associated with superficial partial-thickness burns. With superficial partial-thickness burns, pigment is expected to return to the injured area after healing. Deep partial-thickness burns heal in 6 weeks, with scarring.
CN: Physiological integrity; CNS: Physiological adaptation; CL: Analysis

5. 4. A client with a deep partial-thickness burn will have tissue necrosis to the epidermis and dermis layers. Erythema and pain are characteristic of superficial injury. With deep burns, the nerve fibers are destroyed and the client won't feel pain in the affected area. Superficial burns are characteristic of slight epidermal damage. Necrosis through all skin layers is seen with full-thickness injuries.
CN: Physiological integrity; CNS: Physiological adaptation; CL: Application

6. 1. Circumferential burns can compromise blood flow to an extremity, causing numbness. +2 Pulses indicate normal circulation. Absence of pain and full ROM implies good tissue oxygenation from intact circulation. Capillary refill less then 2 seconds indicates a normal vascular blood flow.
CN: Physiological integrity; CNS: Physiological adaptation; CL: Application

7. 3. There's a 3% to 5% risk for fetal death from hydrops fetalis if a pregnant client is exposed during the first trimester. The cutaneous eruption of fifth disease can reappear for up to 4 months. The child should be isolated from pregnant women, immunocompromised clients, and clients with chronic anemia for up to 2 weeks. A child with fifth disease is contagious during the first stage, when symptoms of headache, body aches, fever, and chills are present, not after the rash.
CN: Safe, effective care environment; CNS: Safety and infection control; CL: Application

CN: Client needs category   CNS: Client needs subcategory   CL: Cognitive level

8. A mother is concerned that her 3-year-old child has been exposed to erythema infectiosum (fifth disease). Which characteristic finding would the nurse incorporate in the response to the mother?

1. A fine, erythematous rash with a sandpaper-like texture
2. Intense redness of both cheeks that may spread to the extremities
3. Low-grade fever, followed by vesicular lesions of the trunk, face, and scalp
4. Three- to 5-day history of sustained fever, followed by a diffuse erythematous maculopapular rash

9. A family that recently went camping brings their child to the clinic with a complaint of a rash after a tick bite. Lyme disease is suspected. Which assessment finding would be seen with Lyme disease?

1. Erythematous rash surrounding a necrotic lesion
2. Bright rash with red outer border circling the bite site
3. Onset of a diffuse rash over the entire body 2 months after exposure
4. A linear rash of papules and vesicles that occur 1 to 3 days after exposure

10. A Mantoux test is ordered for a 6-year-old child. Which action should the nurse take?

1. Read results within 24 hours.
2. Read results 48 to 72 hours later.
3. Use the large muscle of the upper leg.
4. Massage the site to increase absorption.

11. The nurse is teaching the parents of a child with Kawasaki disease. Which statement by the nurse about this condition is the most accurate?

1. "It's a highly contagious condition that requires isolation."
2. "It's an afebrile condition with cardiac involvement."
3. "It usually occurs in children older than 5 years."
4. "Prolonged fever, with peeling of the fingers and toes, is the initial symptom."

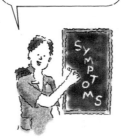

Different symptoms indicate different diagnoses.

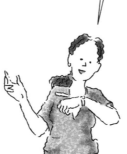

Read the results at the right time!

8. 2. The classic symptoms of erythema infectiosum begin with intense redness of both cheeks. An erythematous rash with a sandpaper-like texture is associated with scarlet fever, which is a bacterial infection. Children with varicella typically have vesicular lesions of the trunk, face, and scalp after a low-grade fever. An erythematous rash after a fever is characteristic of roseola.
CN: Physiological integrity; CNS: Physiological adaptation; CL: Application

9. 2. A bull's eye rash is a classic symptom of Lyme disease. Necrotic, painful rashes are associated with the bite of a brown recluse spider. In Lyme disease, the rash is located primarily at the site of the bite. A linear, papular, vesicular rash indicates exposure to the leaves of poison ivy.
CN: Physiological integrity; CNS: Physiological adaptation; CL: Application

10. 2. The test should be read 48 to 72 hours after placement by measuring the diameter of the induration that develops at the site. The purified protein derivative is injected intradermally on the volar surface of the forearm. Massaging the site could cause leakage from the injection site.
CN: Physiological integrity; CNS: Reduction of risk potential; CL: Application

11. 4. To be diagnosed with Kawasaki syndrome, the child must have a fever for 5 days or more, plus four of the following five symptoms: bilateral conjunctivitis, changes in the oral mucosa, dermatitis of the peripheral extremities, rash, and lymphadenopathy. The syndrome isn't contagious and doesn't require isolation. Kawasaki syndrome is more likely to occur in children aged younger than 5 years.
CN: Physiological integrity; CNS: Physiological adaptation; CL: Application

12. A 22-lb child is diagnosed with Kawasaki syndrome and started on gamma globulin therapy. The physician orders an I.V. infusion of gamma globulin, 2 g/kg, to run over 12 hours. Which dose is correct?
1. 11 g
2. 20 g
3. 22 g
4. 44 g

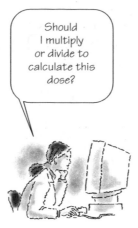

Should I multiply or divide to calculate this dose?

12. 2. First, convert the weight from pounds to kilograms. One kilogram equals 2.2 lb.
Convert the weight using the calculation:
$$22 \text{ (lb)} \div 2.2 = 10 \text{ (kg)}$$
Then, calculate the dose:
$$2 \text{ g} \times 10 = 20 \text{ g}$$

CN: Physiological integrity; CNS: Pharmacological and parenteral therapies; CL: Application

13. A mother is concerned because her child was exposed to varicella in day care. Which statement by the nurse would be the most accurate?
1. "The rash is nonvesicular."
2. "The treatment of choice is aspirin."
3. "Varicella has an incubation period of 5 to 10 days."
4. "A child is no longer contagious once the rash has crusted over."

13. 4. Once every varicella lesion is crusted over, the child is no longer considered contagious. The rash is typically a maculopapular vesicular rash. Use of aspirin has been associated with Reye's syndrome and is contraindicated in varicella. The incubation period is 10 to 20 days.

CN: Physiological integrity; CNS: Physiological adaptation; CL: Application

14. The nurse is discussing with a student nurse the appearance of a rash associated with varicella-zoster virus on a child in the pediatric unit. Which explanation about the rash would be correct?
1. It's diagnostic in the presence of Koplik's spots in the oral mucosa.
2. It's a macular papular rash starting on the scalp and hairline and spreading downward.
3. It's a vesicular macular papular rash that appears abruptly on the trunk, face, and scalp.
4. It appears as yellow ulcers surrounded by red halos on the surface of the hands and feet.

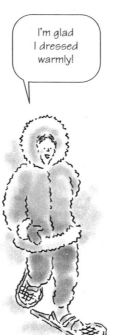

I'm glad I dressed warmly!

14. 3. Teardrop vesicles on an erythematous base generally begin on the trunk, face, and scalp, with minimal involvement of the extremities. Koplik's spots are diagnostic of rubeola. A descending macular papular rash is characteristic of rubeola. Yellow ulcers of the hands and feet are associated with hand-foot-and-mouth disease caused by the coxsackievirus.

CN: Physiological integrity; CNS: Physiological adaptation; CL: Application

15. A child is brought to the emergency department after an extended period of sledding. Frostbite of the hands is suspected. Which assessment finding should the nurse expect to find?
1. The skin is white.
2. The skin looks deeply flushed and red.
3. The skin is cyanotic.
4. The skin is blistered.

15. 1. Signs and symptoms of frostbite include tingling, numbness, burning sensation, and white skin.

CN: Physiological integrity; CNS: Physiological adaptation; CL: Application

CN: Client needs category   CNS: Client needs subcategory   CL: Cognitive level

16. A mother brings her child to the physician's office because he complains of pain, redness, and tenderness of the left index finger. The child is diagnosed with a paronychia. Which organism would the nurse suspect to be the most likely cause of this superficial abscess of the cuticle?
1. *Borrelia burgdorferi*
2. *Escherichia coli*
3. *Pseudomonas* species
4. *Staphylococcus* species

17. Which treatment for paronychia would be the most appropriate?
1. Give warm soaks.
2. Splint and put ice on the affected finger.
3. Allow the infection to resolve without treatment.
4. Admit the child to the hospital for I.V. antibiotic therapy.

18. A mother is concerned that her 9-month-old infant has scabies. Which assessment findings are associated with this infestation?
1. Diffuse pruritic wheals
2. Oval white dots stuck to the hair shafts
3. Pain, erythema, and edema with an embedded stinger
4. Pruritic papules, pustules, and linear burrows of the finger and toe webs

19. After treating her 16-month-old child with permethrin (Elimite) for scabies, the mother is concerned the cream didn't work because the child is still scratching. Which explanation or instruction would be correct?
1. Continue the application daily until the rash disappears.
2. Pruritus caused by secondary reactions of the mites can be present for weeks.
3. Stop treatment because the cream is unsafe for children younger than age 2 years.
4. Pruritus caused by permethrin is usually present in children younger than age 5 years.

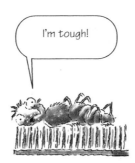

I'm tough!

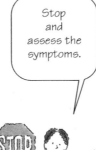

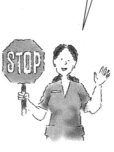

Stop and assess the symptoms.

16. 4. A paronychia is a localized infection of the nail bed caused by either staphylococci or streptococci. *Borrelia burgdorferi* is responsible for Lyme disease. *Escherichia coli* is associated with urinary tract infections. *Pseudomonas* species are associated with ecthyma.
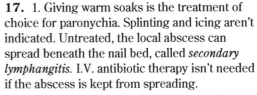
CN: Physiological integrity; CNS: Physiological adaptation; CL: Application

17. 1. Giving warm soaks is the treatment of choice for paronychia. Splinting and icing aren't indicated. Untreated, the local abscess can spread beneath the nail bed, called *secondary lymphangitis*. I.V. antibiotic therapy isn't needed if the abscess is kept from spreading.
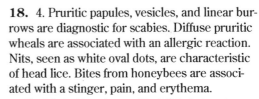
CN: Physiological integrity; CNS: Physiological adaptation; CL: Analysis

18. 4. Pruritic papules, vesicles, and linear burrows are diagnostic for scabies. Diffuse pruritic wheals are associated with an allergic reaction. Nits, seen as white oval dots, are characteristic of head lice. Bites from honeybees are associated with a stinger, pain, and erythema.
CN: Physiological integrity; CNS: Physiological adaptation; CL: Application

19. 2. Sensitization of the host is the cause of the intense itching and can last for weeks. Permethrin is the recommended treatment for scabies in infants as young as 2 months. It can safely be repeated after 2 weeks.
CN: Physiological integrity; CNS: Pharmacological and parenteral therapies; CL: Application

20. A mother of a 5-month-old infant is planning a trip to the beach and asks for advice about sunscreen for her child. Which instruction should the nurse give the mother?
1. The sunscreen protection factor (SPF) of the sunscreen should be at least 10.
2. Apply sunscreen to the exposed areas of the skin.
3. Sunscreen shouldn't be applied to infants younger than 6 months of age.
4. Sunscreen needs to be applied heavily only once one half hour before going out in the sun.

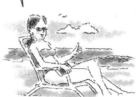

Know the do's and don'ts about sunscreen and its application.

20. 3. Sunscreen isn't recommended for use in infants younger than 6 months of age. These children should be dressed in cool light clothes and kept in the shade. The SPF for children should be 15 or greater. Sunscreen should be applied to all areas of the skin. Sunscreen should be applied evenly throughout the day and each time the child is in the water.
CN: Health promotion and maintenance; CNS: None; CL: Application

21. An infant is being treated with antibiotic therapy for otitis media and develops an erythematous, fine, raised rash in the groin and suprapubic area. Which instruction or explanation will most likely be given to the mother?
1. The infant has candidiasis.
2. Change the brand of diapers.
3. Use an over-the-counter diaper remedy.
4. Stop the antibiotic therapy immediately.

21. 1. Candidiasis, caused by yeast-like fungi, can occur with the use of antibiotics. The treatment for candidiasis is topical nystatin ointment. Changing the brand of diapers or suggesting that the parent use an over-the-counter remedy would be appropriate for treating diaper rash, not candidiasis. Antibiotic therapy shouldn't be stopped.
CN: Physiological integrity; CNS: Physiological adaptation; CL: Analysis

22. The skin in the diaper area of a 6-month-old infant is excoriated and red. Which instructions should the nurse give to the mother?
1. Change the diaper more often.
2. Apply talcum powder with diaper changes.
3. Wash the area vigorously with each diaper change.
4. Decrease the infant's fluid intake to decrease saturating diapers.

Teaching parents helps keep their children healthy.

22. 1. Simply decreasing the amount of time the skin comes in contact with wet soiled diapers will help heal the irritation. Talc is contraindicated in children because of the risks of inhaling the fine powder. Gentle cleaning of the irritated skin should be encouraged. Infants shouldn't have fluid intake restrictions.
CN: Safe, effective care environment; CNS: Safety and infection control; CL: Application

23. A 9-year-old child is being discharged from the hospital after severe urticaria caused by an allergy to nuts. Which instruction would be included in discharge teaching for the child's parents?
1. Use emollient lotions and baths.
2. Apply topical steroids to the lesions as needed.
3. Apply over-the-counter products such as diphenhydramine (Benadryl).
4. Instruct the parents and child on how and when to use an epinephrine administration kit (Epi-Pen).

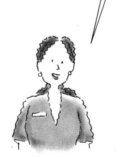

23. 4. Children who have urticaria in response to nuts, seafood, or bee stings should be warned about the possibility of anaphylactic reactions to future exposure. The use of epinephrine pens should be taught to the parents and older children. Other treatment choices, such as diphenhydramine hydrochloride, topical steroids, and emollients, are for the treatment of mild urticaria.
CN: Physiological integrity; CNS: Reduction of risk potential; CL: Application

CN: Client needs category   CNS: Client needs subcategory   CL: Cognitive level

24. When examining a nursery school-age child, the nurse finds multiple contusions over the body. Child abuse is suspected. Which statement indicates which findings should be documented?
1. Contusions confined to one body area are typically suspicious.
2. All lesions, including location, shape, and color, should be documented.
3. Natural injuries usually have straight linear lines, while injuries from abuse have multiple curved lines.
4. The depth, location, and amount of bleeding that initially occurs is constant, but the sequence of color change is variable.

25. A 7-year-old child is diagnosed with head lice. The mother asks what nits are. The nurse states that they represent which part of the louse lifecycle?
1. Adult
2. Empty egg shells
3. Newly laid eggs
4. Nymph

26. The nurse is teaching the mother of a child with lice about treatment options. Which adverse effect would the nurse teach regarding lindane (Kwell) shampoo?
1. Lindane causes alopecia.
2. Lindane causes hypertension.
3. Lindane is associated with seizures.
4. Lindane increases liver function test (LFT) results.

27. Which instruction should be given to the parents about the <u>treatment</u> of head lice?
1. The treatment should be repeated in 7 to 12 days.
2. Treatment should be repeated every day for 1 week.
3. If treated with a shampoo, combing to remove eggs isn't necessary.
4. All contacts with the infested child should be treated even without evidence of infestation.

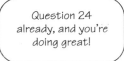

Question 24 already, and you're doing great!

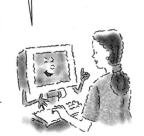

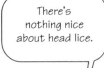

There's nothing nice about head lice.

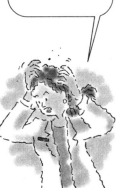

24. 2. An accurate precise examination of all lesions must be properly documented as a legal document. Contusions that result from falls are typically confined to a single body area and are considered a reasonable finding of a child still learning to walk. Injuries from normal falls are usually not linear in nature. The bleeding can cause variations, but the color change is consistent.

CN: Psychosocial integrity; CNS: None; CL: Application

25. 2. The mother is finding empty eggshells in the child's hair. Adults are the last stage of development, living about 30 days. Newly laid eggs are small, translucent, and difficult to see. Nymphs are the newly hatched lice and become adults in 8 to 9 days.

CN: Physiological integrity; CNS: Physiological adaptation; CL: Application

26. 3. Lindane is associated with seizures after absorption with topical use. Alopecia, increased LFT results, and hypertension aren't associated with the use of lindane.

CN: Physiological integrity; CNS: Pharmacological and parenteral therapies; CL: Application

27. 1. Treatment should be repeated in 7 to 12 days to ensure that all eggs are killed. Combing the hair thoroughly is necessary to remove the lice eggs. People exposed to head lice should be examined to assess the presence of infestation before treatment.

CN: Physiological integrity; CNS: Physiological adaptation; CL: Application

28. A mother reports that her 4-year-old child has been scratching at his rectum recently. Which infestation or condition should the nurse suspect?
1. Anal fissure
2. Lice
3. Pinworms
4. Scabies

29. Diagnosing pinworms by the clear cellophane tape test is preferred. How many tests are necessary to detect infestations at virtually 100% accuracy?
1. One
2. Three
3. Five
4. Ten

30. Each member of the family of a child diagnosed with pinworms is prescribed a single dose of pyrantel pamoate (Antiminth). Which statement should the nurse make about pyrantel pamoate?
1. The drug may stain the feces red.
2. The dose may be repeated in 2 weeks.
3. Fever and rash are common adverse effects.
4. The medicine will kill the eggs in about 48 hours.

31. A child received a bite to the hand from a large dog. The nurse would expect to assess which type of injury?
1. Abrasion
2. Crush injury
3. Fracture
4. Puncture wound

32. A nurse knows that bites from dogs are at risk for infection. Which intervention should be done to help prevent infection?
1. Give the rabies vaccine.
2. Give antibiotics immediately.
3. Clean and irrigate the wounds.
4. Nothing; bites from dogs have a low incidence of infection.

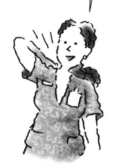

You've finished 30 questions! Good for you!

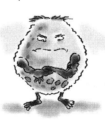

If I come from a dog, grrrr, watch out!

28. 3. The clinical sign of pinworms is perianal itching that increases at night. Anal fissures are associated with rectal bleeding and pain with bowel movements. Lice are infestations of the hair. Scabies are associated with a pruritic rash characterized as linear burrows of the webs of the fingers and toes.
CN: Physiological integrity; CNS: Physiological adaptation; CL: Analysis

29. 3. Detection is virtually 100% accurate with five tests. One test is only 50% accurate. Three tests should detect infestations at about 90% accuracy. Ten tests aren't necessary.
CN: Physiological integrity; CNS: Reduction of risk potential; CL: Application

30. 2. Pyrantel is effective against the adult worms only (not eggs), so treatment can be repeated to eradicate any emerging parasites in 2 weeks. Staining the feces is associated with pyrvinium pamoate. Common adverse effects are headaches and abdominal complaints.
CN: Physiological integrity; CNS: Pharmacological and parenteral therapies; CL: Application

31. 2. Although the bite of a large dog can exert pressure of 150 to 400 pounds per square inch, the bite causes crush injuries, not fractures. Abrasions are associated with friction injuries. Puncture wounds are associated with smaller animals, such as cats.
CN: Physiological integrity; CNS: Physiological adaptation; CL: Application

32. 3. Not every dog bite requires antibiotic therapy, but cleaning the wound is necessary for all injuries involving a break in the skin. Rabies vaccine is used if there is a suspicion the dog has rabies. The infection rate for dog bites has been reported to be as high as 50%.
CN: Physiological integrity; CNS: Reduction of risk potential; CL: Application

CN: Client needs category   CNS: Client needs subcategory   CL: Cognitive level

33. The nurse is reviewing the wound culture report from a child's infected wound caused by a dog bite. Which organism would the nurse suspect to be responsible for the infection?
1. *Escherichia coli*
2. *Francisella tularensis*
3. *Pasteurella multocida*
4. *Rochalimaea henselae*

34. A child is brought to a physician's office for multiple scratches and bites from a kitten. Which symptom is primarily found on assessment with cat-scratch disease?
1. Abdominal pain
2. Adenitis
3. Fever
4. Pruritus

35. The school nurse is discussing giardiasis, a parasitic intestinal infection, with a group of parents. In which population group in the United States is this infection most common?
1. Children riding a school bus
2. Children playing on a playground
3. Children attending a sporting event
4. Children attending group day care or nursery school

36. Which finding should the nurse expect to observe if a child has papules?
1. Palpable elevated masses
2. Loss of the epidermis layer
3. Fluid-filled elevations of the skin
4. Nonpalpable flat changes in skin color

37. A child is diagnosed with impetigo. Pustules are the primary lesions found on this child. Which of the following correctly describes pustules?
1. Lesion filled with pus
2. Superficial area of localized edema
3. Serous-filled lesion less than 0.5 cm
4. Serous-filled lesion greater than 0.5 cm

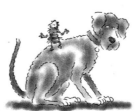

Me and the pooch here are pals.

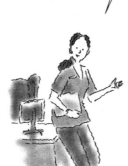

You need to know the correct terms to share information with clients and other health care providers.

33. 3. *Pasteurella multocida* is associated with infection in up to 50% of the bites from dogs. *E. coli* is more likely to cause infections of the urinary tract. *Francisella tularensis* is found in such animals as rabbits, hares, and muskrats. *Rochalimaea henselae*, a gram-negative rickettsial bacterium, is associated with cat-scratch disease.
CN: Physiological integrity; CNS: Physiological adaptation; CL: Application

34. 2. Adenitis is the primary feature of cat-scratch disease. Although low-grade fever has been associated with cat-scratch disease, it's only present 25% of the time. Pruritus and abdominal pain aren't symptoms of cat-scratch disease.
CN: Physiological integrity; CNS: Physiological adaptation; CL: Analysis

35. 4. The most common intestinal parasitic infection in the United States is giardiasis, prevalent among children attending group day care or nursery school. Playgrounds, sporting events, and school buses don't present unusual risk of giardiasis.
CN: Physiological integrity; CNS: Physiological adaptation; CL: Application

36. 1. Papules are elevated up to 0.5 cm. Nodules and tumors are elevated more than 0.5 cm. Erosions are characterized as loss of the epidermis layer. Fluid-filled lesions are vesicles and pustules. Macules and patches are described as nonpalpable flat changes in skin color.
CN: Health promotion and maintenance; CNS: None; CL: Application

37. 1. Pustules are pus-filled lesions, such as acne and impetigo. A wheal is a superficial area of localized edema. Vesicles are serous-filled lesions up to 0.5 cm in diameter. Bullae are serous-filled lesions greater than 0.5 cm in diameter.
CN: Physiological integrity; CNS: Physiological adaptation; CL: Application

38. A 3-month-old infant is noted to have café-au-lait spots on examination. The presence of six or more of these lesions with a diameter greater then 1.5 cm is suggestive of which disorder?
1. Meningococcemia
2. Neurofibromatosis
3. Tinea versicolor
4. Vitiligo

39. A child is brought to the physician's office for treatment of a rash. Many petechiae are seen over his entire body. The nurse would suspect which condition?
1. Bleeding disorder
2. Scabies
3. Varicella
4. Vomiting

40. A child fell at camp and sustained a bruise to his thigh. Which description would accurately describe the bruise after 1 week?
1. Resolved
2. Reddish blue
3. Greenish yellow
4. Dark blue to bluish brown

41. Which factor would lead the nurse to suspect child abuse?
1. Multiple contusions of the shins
2. Contusions of the back and buttocks
3. Contusions at the same stages of healing
4. Large contusion and hematoma of the forehead

42. Which statement would the nurse include when teaching a new mother about salmon patches (stork bites)?
1. They're benign and usually fade in adult life.
2. They're usually associated with syndromes of the neonate.
3. They can cause mild hypertrophy of the muscle associated with the lesion.
4. They're treatable with laser pulse surgery in late adolescence and adulthood.

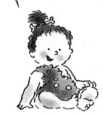

Assessment is an enormously important skill.

38. 2. Six or more uniformly pigmented patches with irregular borders, known as *café-au-lait spots,* with diameters greater then 1.5 cm are associated with neurofibromatosis. Meningowcoccemia has petechiae, not *café-au-lait spots.* Tinea versicolor is a superficial fungus infection. Depigmented areas are signs of vitiligo.
CN: Health promotion and maintenance; CNS: None; CL: Analysis

39. 1. Petechiae are caused by blood outside a vessel, associated with low platelet counts and bleeding disorders. Petechiae aren't found with varicella disease or scabies. Petechiae can be associated with vomiting, but in that case they'd be present on the face, not the entire body.
CN: Physiological integrity; CNS: Physiological adaptation; CL: Analysis

40. 3. After 7 to 10 days, the bruise becomes greenish yellow. Resolution can take up to 2 weeks. Initially after the fall, there's a reddish blue discoloration followed by a dark blue to bluish brown color at days 1 to 3.
CN: Physiological integrity; CNS: Physiological adaptation; CL: Application

41. 2. Contusions of the back and buttocks are highly suspicious of abuse related to punishment. Contusions at various stages of healing are red flags to potential abuse. Contusions of the shins and forehead are usually related to an active toddler falling and bumping into objects.
CN: Psychosocial integrity; CNS: None; CL: Analysis

42. 1. Salmon patches occur over the back of the neck in 40% of neonates and are harmless, needing no intervention. Port wine stains are associated with syndromes of the neonate such as Sturge-Weber syndrome. Port wine stains found on the face or extremities may be associated with soft tissue and bone hypertrophy. Laser pulse surgery isn't recommended for salmon patches because they typically fade on their own in adulthood.
CN: Health promotion and maintenance; CNS: None; CL: Application

CN: Client needs category   CNS: Client needs subcategory   CL: Cognitive level

43. A neonate is born with a blue-black macular lesion over the lower lumbar sacral region. Which term should the nurse use when teaching the parents about this lesion?
1. Café-au-lait spots
2. Mongolian spots
3. Nevis of Ota spot
4. Stork bites

44. Which finding indicates <u>severe</u> dehydration in a child?
1. Gray skin and decreased tears
2. Capillary refill less than 2 seconds
3. Mottling and tenting of the skin
4. Pale skin with dry mucous membranes

45. A client is prescribed isotretinoin (Accutane). Which adverse effect should the nurse include in her teaching?
1. Diarrhea
2. Gram-negative folliculitis
3. Teratogenicity
4. Vaginal candidiasis

46. The nurse is developing a teaching plan for adolescents about acne. The nurse incorporates which characteristic as commonly responsible for the failure of treatment of acne in teenagers?
1. Topical treatment
2. Systemic treatment
3. A dominant parent who wants treatment and a passive teenager who doesn't
4. A dominant teenager who wants treatment and a passive uninterested parent

47. What information should be given to a teenager about acne?
1. Acne is caused by diet.
2. Acne is related to gender.
3. Acne is caused by poor hygiene.
4. Acne is caused by hormonal changes.

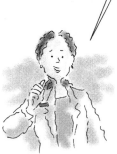

The word severe is a clue to the correct answer.

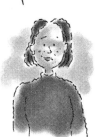

I need to follow the treatment plan.

43. 2. Mongolian spots are large blue-black macular lesions generally located over the lumbosacral areas, buttocks, and limbs. Café-au-lait spots occur between ages 2 and 16 years, not in infancy. Nevis of Ota is found surrounding the eyes. Stork bites or salmon patches occur at the neck and hairline area.
CN: Health promotion and maintenance; CNS: None; CL: Application

44. 3. Severe dehydration is associated with mottling and tenting of the skin. Malnutrition is characterized by gray skin and tenting of the skin. Capillary refill less then 2 seconds is normal. Pale skin with dry mucous membranes is a sign of mild dehydration.
CN: Health promotion and maintenance; CNS: None; CL: Analysis

45. 3. The use of even small amounts of isotretinoin has been associated with severe birth defects. Most female clients taking this medication are prescribed hormonal contraceptives. Cleocin T (clindamycin), another medicine used in the treatment of acne, is associated with both diarrhea and gram-negative folliculitis. Tetracycline (Achromycin) is associated with yeast infections (vaginal candidiasis).
CN: Physiological integrity; CNS: Pharmacological and parenteral therapies; CL: Application

46. 3. The active participation of a teenager is needed for the successful treatment of acne. Systemic and topical therapy are needed in most acne treatment.
CN: Health promotion and maintenance; CNS: None; CL: Application

47. 4. Acne is caused by hormonal changes in sebaceous gland anatomy and the biochemistry of the glands. These changes lead to a blockage in the follicular canal and cause an inflammatory response. Diet, hygiene, and the client's gender don't cause acne.
CN: Health promotion and maintenance; CNS: None; CL: Application

48. When teaching a client about tetracycline (Achromycin) for severe inflammatory acne, which instruction must be given?
1. Take the drug with or without meals.
2. Take the drug with milk and milk products.
3. Take the drug on an empty stomach with small amounts of water.
4. Take the drug 1 hour before or 2 hours after meals with large amounts of water.

49. When advising parents about the prevention of burns to their child from tap water, which instruction should be given?
1. Set the water-heater temperature at 130° F (54.4° C) or less.
2. Run the hot water first, then adjust the temperature with cold water.
3. Before you put your infant in the tub, first test the water with your hand.
4. Supervise an infant in the bathroom, only leaving him for a few seconds, if needed.

50. While caring for a 2-day-old neonate, a nurse notices the left side of the neonate becomes reddened for 2 to 3 minutes. The nurse interprets this finding as suggestive of:
1. contact dermatitis.
2. environmental conditions.
3. harlequin color change.
4. tet spells.

51. A 15-month-old child is diagnosed with pediculosis of the eyebrows. Which intervention is included in the treatment?
1. Use lindane.
2. Use petroleum jelly.
3. Shave the eyebrows.
4. No treatment is needed.

52. A 14-year-old male client is brought to the hospital with smoke inhalation because of a house fire. The nurse's first intervention for this client is to:
1. check the oral mucous membranes.
2. check for any burned areas.
3. obtain a medical history.
4. ensure a patent airway.

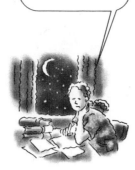

It's hard to study on an empty stomach.

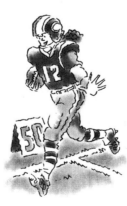

You've reached question 50 and your goal is in sight.

48. 4. Tetracycline must be taken on an empty stomach to increase absorption and with ample water to avoid esophageal irritation. Milk products impede absorption.
CN: Physiological integrity; CNS: Pharmacological and parenteral therapies; CL: Application

49. 3. Instruct the parents to fill the tub with water first and then test all of the water in the tub with their hand for hot spots. Water heaters should be set at 120° F. The cold water should be run first and then adjusted with hot water. Never leave an infant alone in the bathroom, even for a second.
CN: Health promotion and maintenance; CNS: None; CL: Application

50. 3. Harlequin color change is a benign disorder related to the immaturity of hypothalamic centers that control the tone of peripheral blood vessels. A new born who has been lying on its side may appear reddened on the dependent side. The color fades on position change. Contact dermatitis isn't short-lived. Changes in environmental conditions can cause diffuse bilateral mottling of the skin. Tet spells are associated with tetralogy of Fallot and cause cyanotic changes.
CN: Health promotion and maintenance; CNS: None; CL: Analysis

51. 2. Petroleum jelly should be applied twice daily for 8 days, followed by manual removal of nits. Lindane is contraindicated because of the risk for seizures. The eyebrow should never be shaved because of the uncertainty of hair return.
CN: Physiological integrity; CNS: Physiological adaptation; CL: Analysis

52. 4. The nurse's top priority is to make sure the airway is open and the client is breathing. Checking the mucous membranes and burned areas is important but not as vital as maintaining a patent airway. Obtaining a medical history can be pursued after ensuring a patent airway.
CN: Physiological integrity; CNS: Physiological adaptation; CL: Application

CN: Client needs category   CNS: Client needs subcategory   CL: Cognitive level

53. The nurse is assessing a child suspected of having Kawasaki syndrome. Which changes in the mouth would the nurse observe that would indicate this condition?
1. Koplik's spots
2. Tonsillar exudate
3. Vesicular lesions
4. Strawberry tongue

54. A 3-year-old child has palpable purpura of the buttocks and lower extremities. Which condition would the nurse suspect with these symptoms?
1. Child abuse
2. Henoch-Schöenlein purpura (HSP)
3. Idiopathic thrombocytopenic purpura (ITP)
4. Rocky Mountain spotted fever

55. Topical treatment with 2.5% hydrocortisone (Cortane) is prescribed for a 6-month-old infant with eczema. The mother is instructed to use the cream for not longer than 1 week. Why is this time limit appropriate?
1. The drug loses its efficacy after prolonged use.
2. This reduces adverse effects, such as skin atrophy and fragility.
3. If no improvement is seen, a stronger concentration will be prescribed.
4. If no improvement is seen after 1 week, an antibiotic will be prescribed.

56. A 9-year-old child is examined because his mother noticed lesions on his tongue. Painless, slightly depressed, red lesions bordered with white bands are seen on examination. The mother reports the patterns were different yesterday. Which condition would the nurse suspect?
1. Geographic tongue
2. Koplik's spots
3. Scald burns
4. Stomatitis

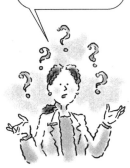

Which symptom goes with which diagnosis?

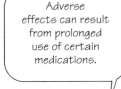

Adverse effects can result from prolonged use of certain medications.

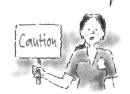

Caution

53. 4. Oral changes associated with Kawasaki syndrome include reddened pharynx, red, dry fissured lips, and strawberry tongue. Koplik's spots are consistent with measles. Tonsillar exudate is consistent with pharyngitis caused by group A beta hemolytic streptococci. Vesicular lesions are associated with coxsackievirus.
CN: Physiological integrity; CNS: Physiological adaptation; CL: Application

54. 2. The rash associated with HSP is believed to occur in every client and allows for a definitive diagnosis. It begins as petechiae and progresses to purpuric lesions of the buttocks and lower extremities. The lesions of child abuse are painful and nonraised. Petechiae or purpura associated with ITP are distributed over the entire body. The rash in Rocky Mountain spotted fever is a nonraised macular papular rash spread over the body.
CN: Physiological integrity; CNS: Physiological adaptation; CL: Application

55. 2. Hydrocortisone cream should be used for brief periods to decrease such adverse effects as atrophy of the skin. The drug doesn't lose efficacy after prolonged use, a stronger concentration may not be prescribed if no improvement is seen, and an antibiotic would be inappropriate in this instance.
CN: Physiological integrity; CNS: Pharmacological and parenteral therapies; CL: Application

56. 1. Geographic tongue is a benign disorder caused by loss of filiform papules. The configuration is known to change from day to day. Koplik's spots and stomatitis lesions don't change patterns. Scald burns are painful lesions from hot liquids.
CN: Physiological integrity; CNS: Physiological adaptation; CL: Application

57. A 4-year-old child had a subungual hemorrhage of the toe after a jar fell on his foot. Electrocautery is performed. The nurse explains to the parents that electrocautery is done to:
1. prevent loss of nail growth.
2. prevent spread of the infection.
3. relieve pain and reduce the risk for infection.
4. prevent permanent discoloration of the nail bed.

58. The nurse is caring for a 12-year-old child with a diagnosis of eczema. Which nursing interventions are appropriate for a child with eczema?
1. Administering antibiotics as prescribed
2. Administering antifungals as ordered
3. Administering tepid baths and patting dry or air drying the affected areas
4. Administering hot baths and using moisturizers immediately after the bath

59. A 9-year-old child is brought to the emergency department with extensive burns received in a restaurant fire. What's the <u>most important</u> aspect of caring for the burned child?
1. Administering antibiotics to prevent superimposed infections
2. Conducting wound management
3. Administering liquids orally to replace fluid
4. Administering frequent small meals to support nutritional requirements

60. A mother of a 4-month-old infant asks about the strawberry hemangioma on his cheek. What information should the nurse provide to the mother?
1. The lesion will continue to grow for 3 years, then need surgical removal.
2. If the lesion continues to enlarge, referral to a pediatric oncologist is warranted.
3. Surgery is indicated before age 12 months if the diameter of the lesion is greater then 3 cm.
4. The lesion will continue to grow until age 1 year, then begin to resolve by age 2 to 3 years.

57. 3. The hematoma is treated with electrocautery to relieve pain and reduce risk for infection. Electrocautery doesn't prevent the loss of the nail. The discoloration seen with subungual hemorrhage is from the collection of blood under the nail bed. It isn't permanent and doesn't affect nail growth.
CN: Physiological integrity; CNS: Physiological adaptation; CL: Application

58. 3. Tepid baths and moisturizers are indicated to keep the infected areas clean and minimize itching. Antibiotics are given only when superimposed infection is present. Antifungals aren't usually administered in the treatment of eczema. Hot baths can exacerbate the condition and increase itching.
CN: Physiological integrity; CNS: Physiological adaptation; CL: Application

59. 2. The most important aspect of caring for a burned child is wound management. The goals of wound care are to speed debridement, protect granulation tissue and new grafts, and conserve body heat and fluids. Antibiotics aren't always administered prophylactically. Fluids are administered I.V. according to the child's body weight to replace volume. Enteral feedings, rather than meals, are initiated within the first 24 hours after the burn to support the child's increased nutritional requirements.
CN: Physiological integrity; CNS: Physiological adaptation; CL: Application

60. 4. These rapidly growing vascular lesions reach maximum growth by age 1 year. The growth period is then followed by an involution period of 6 to 12 months. Lesions show complete involution by age 2 or 3 years. These benign lesions don't need surgical or oncologic referrals.
CN: Health promotion and maintenance; CNS: None; CL: Application

CN: Client needs category   CNS: Client needs subcategory   CL: Cognitive level

61. A 3-year-old child is being discharged from the emergency department after receiving three sutures for a scalp laceration. In how many days should the nurse tell the family to return for suture removal?
1. 1 to 3 days
2. 5 to 7 days
3. 8 to 10 days
4. 10 to 14 days

62. Which symptom is an <u>early sign</u> of infection of a laceration?
1. Fever
2. Copious drainage
3. Excessive discomfort
4. Local nodal enlargement

63. The nurse is teaching a 17-year-old client who'll soon be discharged regarding how to change a sterile dressing on the right leg. During the teaching session, the nurse notices redness, swelling, and induration at the wound site, interpreting these as suggesting:
1. infection.
2. dehiscence.
3. hemorrhage.
4. evisceration.

64. A 6-year-old child is diagnosed with herpes zoster of the left anterior chest. Which assessment finding should the nurse expect to find?
1. Bruising and swelling
2. Papulovesicular eruption with complaints of pain and tenderness of the lesion
3. Linear burrows on the fingers and toes
4. Papulovesicular lesions on the chest, trunk, face, and scalp

65. During an examination of a 5-month-old infant, a flat, dull pink, macular lesion is noted on the infant's forehead. The nurse suspects which condition?
1. Cavernous hemangioma
2. Nevus flammeus
3. Salmon patch
4. Strawberry hemangioma

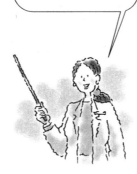

Words with dots under them point to the correct answer.

You made it to question 65. Hang in there.

61. 2. The recommended healing time for this type of laceration is 5 to 7 days. Sutures need longer than 1 to 3 days to form an effective bond. Eight to 10 days is needed for sutures of the fingertips and feet, and 10 to 14 days is the recommended time for extensor surfaces of the knees and elbows.
CN: Physiological integrity; CNS: Physiological adaptation; CL: Application

62. 3. The first sign of infection is usually excessive discomfort. Nodal enlargement, fever, and copious drainage are advanced signs of infection.
CN: Health promotion and maintenance; CNS: None; CL: Analysis

63. 1. Infection produces such signs as redness, swelling, induration, warmth, and possible drainage. Dehiscence may cause unexplained fever and tachycardia, unusual wound pain, prolonged paralytic ileus, and separation of the surgical incision. Hemorrhage can result in increased pulse and respiratory rate, decreased blood pressure, restlessness, thirst, and cold, clammy skin. Evisceration produces visible protrusion of organs, usually through an incision.
CN: Physiological integrity; CNS: Physiological adaptation; CL: Analysis

64. 2. Herpes zoster is caused by the varicella-zoster virus. It has papulovesicular lesions that erupt along a dermatome, usually with hyperesthesia, pain, and tenderness. Contusions are present with bruising and swelling. Scabies appear as linear burrows of the fingers and toes caused by a mite. The papulovesicular lesions of varicella are distributed over the entire trunk, face, and scalp and don't follow a dermatome.
CN: Physiological integrity; CNS: Physiological adaptation; CL: Analysis

65. 3. Salmon patches are common vascular lesions in infants. They appear as flat, dull pink, macular lesions in various regions of the face and head. When they appear on the nape of the neck, they're commonly called "stork bites." These lesions fade by the first year of life. Both strawberry and cavernous hemangiomas are raised lesions. Nevus flammeus, or port wine stains, are reddish-purple lesions that don't fade.
CN: Physiological integrity; CNS: Physiological adaptation; CL: Analysis

66. A young child's parents ask for advice on the use of an insect repellent that contains deet. Which statement would be correct?
1. "Spray the child's clothing instead of the skin."
2. "The repellent works better as the temperature increases."
3. "The repellent isn't effective against the ticks responsible for Lyme disease."
4. "Apply insect repellent as you would sunscreen, with frequent applications during the day."

67. A nurse is teaching a parent about which deet-containing insect repellent to use on his child. Which concentration should she instruct him to use on the child's skin for optimal results?
1. 10%
2. 15%
3. 20%
4. 30%

68. Which statement about warts would the nurse incorporate when assisting with a community health teaching program on common skin problems?
1. Cutting the wart is the preferred treatment for children.
2. No treatment exists that specifically kills the wart virus.
3. Warts are caused by a virus affecting the inner layer of skin.
4. Warts are harmless and usually last 2 to 4 years if untreated.

69. The nurse is assisting with a teaching program for new parents that focuses on oral hygiene promotion. Which factor would the nurse include as causing tooth decay and gum disease when allowed to remain on the teeth for prolonged periods?
1. Breast milk
2. Pacifiers
3. Thumb or other fingers
4. Formula

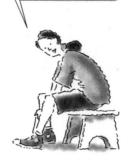

You're almost at question 70. That was quick!

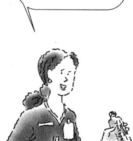

You need to brush those carbs away.

66. 1. Deet spray has been approved for use on children. It should be used sparingly on all skin surfaces. By concentrating spray on clothing and camping equipment, the adverse effects and potential toxic buildup is significantly reduced. Repellent is lost to evaporation, wind, heat, and perspiration. With each 10° F increase in temperature, it leads to as much as a 50% reduction in protection time. Deet is very effective as a tick repellent.
CN: Physiological integrity; CNS: Reduction of risk potential; CL: Application

67. 1. The highest concentration approved by the Food and Drug Administration for children is 10%. Because of thinner skin and greater surface area to mass ratio in children, parents should use deet products sparingly.
CN: Physiological integrity; CNS: Reduction of risk potential; CL: Application

68. 2. The goal of treatment is to kill the skin that contains the wart virus. Cutting the wart is likely to spread the virus. The virus that causes warts affects the outer layer of the skin. Warts are harmless and last 1 to 2 years if untreated.
CN: Health promotion and maintenance; CNS: None; CL: Application

69. 4. Tooth decay and gum disease result when the carbohydrates in formula, cow's milk, and fruit juices are allowed to remain on the teeth for a prolonged period. Studies have shown that breast milk only contributes to dental caries when sugar is already present on the teeth. Breast milk alone actually promotes enamel growth. Pacifiers and fingers don't cause tooth decay and gum disease, although they may contribute to malocclusion.
CN: Health promotion and maintenance; CNS: None; CL: Application

CN: Client needs category   CNS: Client needs subcategory   CL: Cognitive level

70. A child is suspected of having cellulitis. What classic signs should the nurse expect to see in a child?
   1. Pale, irritated, cold to touch
   2. Vesicular blisters at the site of the injury
   3. Fever, edema, tenderness, warmth at the site
   4. Swelling, redness, with well-defined borders

71. A 2-year-old child has cellulitis of the finger. Which organism or condition is the <u>most likely</u> cause of the infection?
   1. Parainfluenza virus
   2. Respiratory syncytial virus
   3. *Escherichia coli*
   4. *Streptococcus*

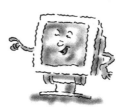

Note that this question asks about the most likely cause, not the only one.

72. A child has a desquamation rash of the hands and feet. Which additional findings should the nurse expect to observe with this rash?
   1. Peeling skin
   2. Thin, reddened layers of epidermis
   3. Thick skin with deep visible burrows
   4. Thinning skin that may appear translucent

73. Which instruction would the nurse include for the parents of a child who is to receive nystatin oral solution?
   1. Give the solution immediately after feedings.
   2. Give the solution immediately before feedings.
   3. Mix the solution with small amounts of the feeding.
   4. Give half the solution before and half the solution after the feeding.

Where are those petechiae?

74. An infant is examined and found to have a petechial rash. The nurse documents a description of this rash as:
   1. a purple macular lesion larger than 1 cm in diameter.
   2. purple to brown bruises, macular or papular, various sizes.
   3. a collection of blood from ruptured blood vessels larger than 1 cm in diameter.
   4. a pinpoint, pink to purple, nonblanching macular lesion 1 to 3 mm in diameter.

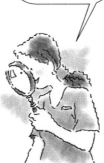

70. 3. Cellulitis is a deep, locally diffuse infection of the skin. It's associated with redness, fever, edema, tenderness, and warmth at the site of the injury. Vesicular blisters suggest impetigo. Cellulitis has no well-defined borders.
CN: Physiological integrity; CNS: Physiological adaptation; CL: Application

71. 4. *Streptococcus* cause most cases of cellulitis. Parainfluenza and respiratory syncytial virus cause infections of the respiratory tract. *E. coli* is a cause of bladder infections.
CN: Physiological integrity; CNS: Physiological adaptation; CL: Analysis

72. 1. Desquamation is characteristic in diseases such as Stevens–Johnson syndrome. Scaling is thin, reddened layers of epidermis. Thickening of the skin with burrows is defined as lichenification. Thinning skin is best described as atrophy of the skin.
CN: Physiological integrity; CNS: Physiological adaptation; CL: Application

73. 1. Nystatin oral solution should be swabbed onto the mouth after feedings to allow for optimal contact with mucous membranes. Before meals and with meals doesn't give the best contact with the mucous membranes.
CN: Physiological integrity; CNS: Pharmacological and parenteral therapies; CL: Application

74. 4. Petechiae are small 1- to 3-mm macular lesions. Purple macular lesions greater than 1 cm are defined as purpura. A bruise is defined as ecchymosis. A hematoma is a collection of blood.
CN: Physiological integrity; CNS: Physiological adaptation; CL: Application

75. When inspecting the <u>palms</u> of a child, with which rash would the nurse expect to find no changes?
1. Coxsackievirus
2. Measles
3. Rocky Mountain spotted fever
4. Syphilis

76. A mother reports that her teenager is losing hair in small round areas on the scalp. The nurse interprets this as suggesting which condition?
1. Alopecia
2. Amblyopia
3. Exotropia
4. Seborrhea dermatitis

77. A topical corticosteroid cream is prescribed for a child with eczema. Which instruction should a nurse give to the mother regarding proper application of the cream?
1. "Apply the cream over the entire body."
2. "Apply the cream in a thin layer to the affected area and rub it in."
3. "Apply the cream to the infected area without washing the area first."
4. "Apply the cream in a thick layer and allow it to absorb."

78. A mother of a toddler diagnosed with atopic dermatitis is concerned about how her child acquired the disease. The nurse should explain that the cause of atopic dermatitis is a:
1. fungal infection.
2. hereditary disorder.
3. sex-linked disorder.
4. viral infection.

79. A mother of a 6-month-old infant with atopic dermatitis asks for advice on bathing the child. Which instruction should be given?
1. Bathe the infant twice daily.
2. Bathe the infant every other day.
3. Use bubble baths to decrease itching.
4. The frequency of the infant's baths isn't important in atopic dermatitis.

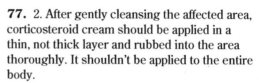

What is the correct term for ready to "pull" your hair out?

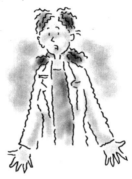

75. 2. The rash in measles occurs on the face, trunk, and extremities. Rocky Mountain spotted fever, syphilis, and coxsackie virus show changes on the palms and soles.
CN: Physiological integrity; CNS: Physiological adaptation; CL: Analysis

76. 1. Alopecia is the correct term for thinning hair loss. Exotropia and amblyopia are eye disorders. Seborrhea dermatitis is cradle cap and occurs in infants.
CN: Physiological integrity; CNS: Physiological adaptation; CL: Application

77. 2. After gently cleansing the affected area, corticosteroid cream should be applied in a thin, not thick layer and rubbed into the area thoroughly. It shouldn't be applied to the entire body.
CN: Physiological integrity; CNS: Pharmacological and parenteral therapies; CL: Analysis

78. 2. Atopic dermatitis is a hereditary disorder that isn't sex-linked and is associated with a family history of asthma, allergic rhinitis, or atopic dermatitis. Viral and fungal infections don't cause atopic dermatitis.
CN: Physiological integrity; CNS: Physiological adaptation; CL: Application

79. 2. Bathing removes lipoprotein complexes that hold water in the stratum corneum and increase water loss. Decreasing bathing to every other day can help prevent the removal of lipoprotein complexes. Soap and bubble bath should be used sparingly while bathing the child.
CN: Physiological integrity; CNS: Basic care and comfort; CL: Application

CN: Client needs category   CNS: Client needs subcategory   CL: Cognitive level

80. Discharge instructions for a child with atopic dermatitis include keeping the fingernails cut short. Which rationale should the nurse give for this intervention?
1. To prevent infection of the nail bed
2. To prevent the spread of the disorder
3. To prevent the child from causing a corneal abrasion
4. To reduce breaks in skin from scratching that may lead to secondary bacterial infections

81. A 10-year-old child being treated for common warts asks about the cause. The nurse would incorporate which virus as the cause?
1. Coxsackievirus
2. Human herpesvirus (HHV)
3. Human immunodeficiency virus (HIV)
4. Human papillomavirus (HPV)

82. The nurse is assessing a 6-year-old child with a spiny projection from the skin suspended from a narrow stalk on the forehead. Which condition would the nurse suspect?
1. Filiform wart
2. Flat wart
3. Plantar wart
4. Venereal warts

83. An adolescent says his feet itch, sweat a lot, and have a foul odor. The nurse suspects which condition?
1. Candidiasis
2. Tinea corporis
3. Tinea pedis
4. Molluscum contagiosum

84. A nurse is explaining treatment to the parents of a child with hypertrophic scarring. Which method would be the <u>best</u> for controlling this condition?
1. Compression garments
2. Moisturizing creams
3. Physiotherapy
4. Splints

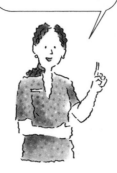

Here's another question pointing out the importance of client teaching.

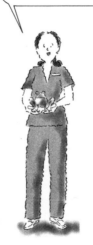

You know what they say about frogs and warts.

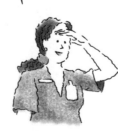

I can almost see the last question.

80. 4. Keeping fingernails cut short will prevent breaks in the skin when a child scratches. Cutting fingernails too short or cutting the skin around the nail can increase the risk of infection. Atopic dermatitis can be found in various areas of the skin, but isn't spread from one area to another. Keeping fingernails short is a good way to reduce corneal abrasions, but doesn't apply to atopic dermatitis.
CN: Physiological integrity; CNS: Physiological adaptation; CL: Application

81. 4. HPV is responsible for various forms of warts. Coxsackievirus is associated with hand-foot-mouth disease. HHV is associated with varicella and herpes zoster. HIV infections aren't associated with epithelial tumors known as warts.
CN: Physiological integrity; CNS: Physiological adaptation; CL: Application

82. 1. Filiform warts are long spiny projections from the skin surface. Flat warts are flat-topped smooth-surfaced lesions. Plantar warts are rough papules, commonly found on the soles of the feet. Venereal warts appear on the genital mucosa and are confluent papules with rough surfaces.
CN: Physiological integrity; CNS: Physiological adaptation; CL: Application

83. 3. Tinea pedis is a superficial fungal infection on the feet, commonly called *athletes' foot.* Candidiasis is a fungal infection of the skin or mucous membranes commonly found in the oral, vaginal, and intestinal mucosal tissue. Tinea corporis, or *ringworm,* is a flat scaling papular lesion with raised borders. Molluscum contagiosum is a viral skin infection with lesions that are small red papules.
CN: Physiological integrity; CNS: Physiological adaptation; CL: Analysis

84. 1. Compression garments are worn for up to 1 year to control hypertrophic scarring. Moisturizing creams help decrease hyperpigmentation. Physiotherapy and splints help keep joints and limbs supple.
CN: Physiological integrity; CNS: Physiological adaptation; CL: Application

85. During a physical examination, a child is noted to have nails with "ice-pick" pits and ridges. The nails are thick and discolored and have splintered hemorrhages easily separated from the nail bed. Which condition would cause this to occur?

1. Paronychia
2. Psoriasis
3. Scabies
4. Seborrhea

86. A neonate is examined and noted to have bruising on the scalp, along with diffuse swelling of the soft tissue that crosses over the suture line. Which assessment is <u>most accurate</u>?

1. Caput succedaneum
2. Cephalhematoma
3. Craniotabes
4. Hydrocephalus

87. A child has a healed wound from a traumatic injury. His mother is concerned because a lesion formed over the wound is pink, thickened, smooth, and rubbery in nature. The nurse should use what term to discuss this condition with the mother?

1. Erosion
2. Fissure
3. Keloids
4. Striae

88. The mother of an infant gives a history of poor feeding for a few days. A complete physical examination shows white plaques in the mouth with an erythematous base. The plaques stick to the mucous membranes tightly and bleed when scraped. The nurse would suspect which condition?

1. Chickenpox
2. Herpes lesions
3. Measles
4. Oral candidiasis

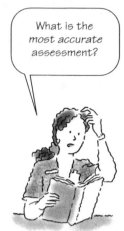

What is the most accurate assessment?

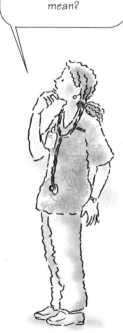

Hmmm, white plaques with an erythematous base. What could that mean?

85. 2. Psoriasis is a chronic skin disorder with an unknown cause that shows these characteristic skin changes. A paronychia is a bacterial infection of the nail bed. Scabies are mites that burrow under the skin, usually between the webbing of the fingers and toes. Seborrhea is a chronic inflammatory dermatitis or cradle cap.
CN: Physiological integrity; CNS: Physiological adaptation; CL: Application

86. 1. Caput succedaneum originates from trauma to the neonate while descending through the birth canal. It's usually a benign injury that spontaneously resolves over time. Cephalhematoma is a collection of blood in the periosteum of the scalp that doesn't cross over the suture line. Craniotabes is the thinning of the bone of the scalp. Hydrocephalus is an increased volume of cerebrospinal fluid (CSF) or the obstruction of the flow of the CSF and isn't related to soft tissue swelling.
CN: Physiological integrity; CNS: Physiological adaptation; CL: Analysis

87. 3. Keloids are an exaggerated connective tissue response to skin injury. An erosion is a depressed vesicular lesion. A fissure is a cleavage in the surface of skin. Striae are linear depressions of the skin.
CN: Physiological integrity; CNS: Physiological adaptation; CL: Application

88. 4. Oral candidiasis, or thrush, is a painful inflammation that can affect the tongue, soft and hard palates, and buccal mucosa. Chickenpox, or varicella, causes open ulcerations of the mucous membranes. Herpes lesions are usually vesicular ulcerations of the oral mucosa around the lips. Measles that form Koplik's spots can be identified as pinpoint white elevated lesions.
CN: Physiological integrity; CNS: Physiological adaptation; CL: Application

CN: Client needs category   CNS: Client needs subcategory   CL: Cognitive level

89. A child was found unconscious at home and brought to the emergency department by the fire and rescue unit. Physical examination showed cherry-red mucous membranes, nail beds, and skin. Which cause is the most likely explanation for the child's condition?
1. Aspirin ingestion
2. Carbon monoxide poisoning
3. Hydrocarbon ingestion
4. Spider bite

90. A 14-year-old diagnosed with acne vulgaris asks what causes it. Which factor should the nurse identify for this client? Select all that apply.
1. Chocolates and sweets
2. Increased hormone levels
3. Growth of anaerobic bacteria
4. Caffeine
5. Heredity
6. Fatty foods

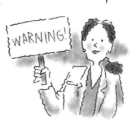

Be careful! There may be more than one correct answer to this question.

91. Which term describes a fungal infection found on the upper arm?
1. Tinea capitis
2. Tinea corporis
3. Tinea cruris
4. Tinea pedis

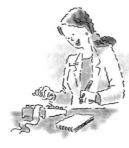

Practice with numbers makes perfect.

92. A 15-kg infant is started on amoxicillin/clavulanate potassium (Augmentin) therapy, 200 mg/5 ml, for cellulitis. The dose is 40 mg/kg over 24 hours given three times daily. How many milliliters would be given for each dose?
1. 2.5 ml
2. 5 ml
3. 15 ml
4. 20 ml

93. A 5-year-old male sustained third-degree burns to the right upper extremity after tipping over a frying pan. Which skin structures would the nurse include when explaining a third-degree burn to the child's mother?
1. Epidermis only
2. Epidermis and dermis
3. All skin layers and nerve endings
4. Skin layers, nerve endings, muscles, tendons, and bones

89. 2. Cherry-red skin changes are seen when a child has been exposed to high levels of carbon monoxide. Nausea and vomiting and pale skin are symptoms of aspirin ingestion. A hydrocarbon or petroleum ingestion usually results in respiratory symptoms and tachycardia. Spider-bite reactions are usually localized to the area of the bite.
CN: Physiological integrity; CNS: Physiological adaptation; CL: Analysis

90. 2, 3, 5. Acne vulgaris is characterized by the appearance of comedones (blackheads and whiteheads). Comedones develop for various reasons, including increased hormone levels, heredity, irritation or application of irritating substances (such as cosmetics), and growth of anaerobic bacteria. A direct relationship between acne vulgaris and consumption of chocolates, caffeine, or fatty foods hasn't been established.
CN: Physiological integrity; CNS: Physiological adaptation; CL: Application

91. 2. *Tinea corporis* describes fungal infections of the body. *Tinea capitis* describes fungal infections of the scalp. *Tinea cruris* is used to describe fungal infections of the inner thigh and inguinal creases. *Tinea pedis* is the term for fungal infections of the foot.
CN: Physiological integrity; CNS: Physiological adaptation; CL: Application

92. 2. 5 ml should be given. The dose is first calculated by multiplying the weight times the milligrams. It's then divided by three even doses. The milligrams are then used to determine the milliliters based on the concentration of the medicine. 40 mg × 15 kg = 600/3 doses = 200 mg/dose. The concentration is 200 mg in every 5 ml.
CN: Physiological integrity; CNS: Pharmacological and parenteral therapies; CL: Application

93. 3. A third-degree burn involves all of the skin layers and the nerve endings. First-degree burns involve only the epidermis. Second-degree burns affect the epidermis and dermis. Fourth-degree burns involve all skin layers, nerve endings, muscles, tendons, and bone.
CN: Physiological integrity; CNS: Physiological adaptation; CL: Application

94. A 4-year-old child has a tick embedded in the scalp. Which method should the nurse use to remove the tick?
1. Burning the tick at the skin surface
2. Surgically removing the tick
3. Grasping the tick with tweezers and applying slow, outward pressure
4. Grasping the tick with tweezers and quickly pulling the tick out

95. A child with hives is prescribed diphenhydramine (Benadryl) 5 mg/kg over 24 hours in divided doses every 6 hours. The child weighs 8 kg. How many milligrams should be given with each dose?
1. 4.5 mg
2. 10 mg
3. 22 mg
4. 40 mg

96. An 8-year-old child arrives at the emergency department with chemical burns to both legs. Which treatment should be performed <u>first</u> on this child?
1. Dilute the burns
2. Apply sterile dressings
3. Apply topical antibiotics
4. Debride and graft the burns

97. A 12-year-old child with full-thickness, circumferential burns to the chest has difficulty breathing. Which procedure will most likely be performed?
1. Chest tube insertion
2. Escharotomy
3. Intubation
4. Needle thoracocentesis

98. A 6-year-old child is evaluated after sustaining burns to his left shoulder. The parents are instructed to use moisturizing cream and protect the burn from sunlight. What's the purpose of this treatment?
1. To avoid keloids
2. To avoid scarring
3. To avoid hypopigmentation
4. To avoid hyperpigmentation

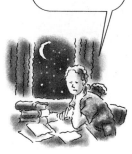

Not another math question!

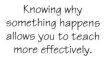

Knowing why something happens allows you to teach more effectively.

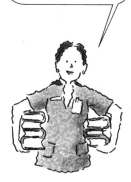

94. 3. Applying gentle outward pressure prevents injury to the skin and the retention of tick parts. Burning the tick and quickly pulling the tick out may cause injury to the skin and should be avoided. Surgical removal is indicated when tick parts have been retained.
CN: Physiological integrity; CNS: Physiological adaptation; CL: Application

95. 2. 10 mg should be given. Multiplying 5 mg by the weight (8 kg) gives the amount of milligrams for 24 hours (40 mg). Divide this by the number of doses per day (4), giving 10 mg/dose. 5 mg × 8 kg = 40 mg/4 doses = 10 mg/dose.
CN: Physiological integrity; CNS: Pharmacological and parenteral therapies; CL: Application

96. 1. Diluting the chemical is the first treatment. It will help remove the chemical and stop the burning process. The remaining treatments are initiated after dilution.
CN: Physiological integrity; CNS: Physiological adaptation; CL: Analysis

97. 2. Escharotomy is a surgical incision used to relieve pressure from edema. It's needed with circumferential burns that prevent chest expansion or cause circulatory compromise. Insertion of a chest tube and needle thoracocentesis are performed to relieve a pneumothorax. Intubation is performed to maintain a patent airway.
CN: Physiological integrity; CNS: Physiological adaptation; CL: Analysis

98. 4. Healed or grafted burns would require creams and protection from the sun to decrease hyperpigmentation. Scarring, hypopigmentation, and keloids aren't treated with moisturizing creams and avoidance of sunlight.
CN: Physiological integrity; CNS: Physiological adaptation; CL: Analysis

CN: Client needs category   CNS: Client needs subcategory   CL: Cognitive level

99. A child arrives in the emergency department 20 minutes after sustaining a major burn injury to 40% of his body. After initiating an I.V. line, which intervention should the nurse perform <u>next</u>?
1. Insert an indwelling catheter.
2. Apply Silvadene cream to the burn.
3. Shave the hair around the burn wound.
4. Obtain cultures from the deepest burn area.

100. A 12-year-old child sustains a moderate burn injury. The mother reports that the child last received a tetanus injection when he was 5 years old. An appropriate nursing intervention would be to administer which immunization?
1. 0.5 ml of tetanus toxoid I.M.
2. 0.5 ml of tetanus toxoid I.V.
3. 250 units of Hyper-Tet I.M.
4. 250 units of Hyper-Tet I.V.

101. A child arrives in the emergency department after sustaining a major burn injury. For which metabolic alterations must the nurse assess during the first 8 hours?
1. Hyponatremia and hypokalemia
2. Hyponatremia and hyperkalemia
3. Hypernatremia and hypokalemia
4. Hypernatremia and hyperkalemia

102. A child weighing 10 kg has a deep partial-thickness burn to 40% of his body surface area. The nurse will titrate this child's I.V. fluids to achieve which hourly urinary outputs?
1. 5 ml
2. 10 ml
3. 30 ml
4. 50 ml

103. A team of nurses is preparing a trauma room for the arrival of a child with partial-thickness burns to both lower extremities and portions of the trunk. Which fluid should be ready for immediate use?
1. Albumin
2. Dextrose 5% and half-normal saline
3. Lactated Ringer's solution
4. Normal saline with 2 mEq KCl/100 ml

What's the magic urinary output number here?

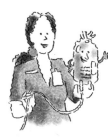

99. 1. I.V. fluids must be started immediately on all children who sustain a major burn injury to prevent the child from going into hypovolemic shock. The fluids are titrated based on urine output. To monitor this output exactly, an indwelling urinary catheter must be inserted. The other interventions will be performed, but not immediately.
CN: Physiological integrity; CNS: Reduction of risk potential; CL: Application

100. 1. Tetanus prophylaxis is given to all clients with moderate to severe burn injuries if it's longer than 5 years since the last immunization or if there is no history of immunization. The correct dosage is 0.5 ml I.M. one time if the child was immunized within 10 years. If it's more than 10 years or the child hasn't received tetanus immunization, the dosage is 250 units of Hyper-Tet one time. There is no I.V. form of tetanus available.
CN: Physiological integrity; CNS: Pharmacological and parenteral therapies; CL: Analysis

101. 2. Capillary permeability increases during the first 48 hours postburn, allowing fluids to shift from the plasma to the interstitial spaces. This fluid is high in sodium, causing the client's serum sodium level to decrease. Potassium also leaks from the cells into the plasma, causing hyperkalemia.
CN: Physiological integrity; CNS: Physiological adaptation; CL: Analysis

102. 2. Fluid resuscitation should be started on all clients with burns over more than 20% of their body surface area. In children, an hourly urine output of 1 to 2 ml/kg of body weight shows adequate kidney perfusion and fluid resuscitation. Adults should have an hourly urine output of 30 to 50 ml.
CN: Physiological integrity; CNS: Physiological adaptation; CL: Application

103. 3. Lactated Ringer's solution is recommended because it replaces the lost sodium and corrects the metabolic acidosis. The use of albumin is controversial. If albumin is given, it's as adjunct therapy and not for primary fluid replacement. The stress from a burn injury affects the glucose metabolism. Dextrose shouldn't be given during the first 24 hours as it can put the client into pseudodiabetes. The client is hyperkalemic from the potassium shift from the intracellular spaces to the plasma, and additional potassium would be detrimental.
CN: Physiological integrity; CNS: Pharmacological and parenteral therapies; CL: Application

104. A mother states that she recently received information that hand-foot-and-mouth disease has been diagnosed in a few of her child's preschool classmates. The nurse should instruct the mother to observe her child for which symptoms?

  1. Low-grade fever, followed by vesicular lesions on the trunk, face, and scalp
  2. Mild, self-limited eruption of vesicles on the buccal mucosa, tongue, soft palate, hands, and feet
  3. Purpuric, maculopapular lesions with GI symptoms and joint pain
  4. Bright red rash with a red outer border circling a bite mark

105. A 27½-lb child is receiving antibiotics for cellulitis. The order reads Pen-Vee K 40 mg/kg/day divided every 6 hours. Which dosage of antibiotics should this child receive with each dose?

  1. 225 mg
  2. 500 mg
  3. 125 mg
  4. 12.5 mg

106. While assessing a 2-year-old child brought into the clinic with an upper respiratory infection, the nurse notes some bruising on his arms, legs, and trunk. Which findings would prompt the nurse to suspect child abuse? Select all that apply:

  1. Superficial scrapes on the lower legs
  2. Welts or bruises in various stages of healing on the trunk
  3. A deep blue-black patch on the buttocks
  4. One large bruise on the thigh
  5. Circular, symmetrical burns on the lower legs
  6. A parent who is hypercritical of the child and pushes the frightened child away

107. A 44-lb preschooler is being treated for inflammation. The physician orders 0.2 mg/kg/day of dexamethasone by mouth to be administered every 6 hours. The elixir comes in a strength of 0.5 mg/5 ml. How many milliliters of dexamethasone should the nurse give this client per dose? Record your answer using a whole number.

_____ milliliters

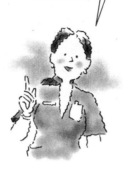

You're being asked about characteristics in question 104.

You did it! You should be on top of the world!

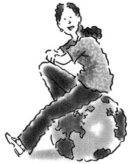

104. 2. Hand-foot-and-mouth disease is caused by coxsackievirus and usually occurs in preschool children. Vesicular lesions accompanied by a low-grade fever are typically signs of varicella. Purpura, GI symptoms, and joint pain are symptoms of Henoch-Schöenlein purpura. A bright-red bull's eye rash is a classic symptom of Lyme disease.

CN: Physiological integrity; CNS: Physiological adaptation; CL: Application

105. 3. The dose is 125 mg. One kilogram equals 2.2 pounds so a 27½-lb child weighs 12.5 kg. 40 mg/kg/day equals a total of 500 mg given every 6 hours or 4 times in 24 hours. 500 mg divided by 4 equals 125 mg.

CN: Physiological integrity; CNS: Pharmacological and parenteral therapies; CL: Application

106. 2, 5, 6. Injuries at various stages of healing in protected or padded areas can be signs of inflicted trauma, leading the nurse to suspect abuse. Burns that are bilateral as well as symmetrical are typical of child abuse. The shape of the burn may resemble the item used to create it, such as a cigarette. Pushing away the child and being hypercritical are typical behaviors of abusive parents. Superficial scrapes and bruises on the lower legs are normal in a healthy, active child. A deep blue-black macular patch on the buttocks is more consistent with a Mongolian spot rather than a traumatic injury.

CN: Psychosocial integrity; CNS: None; CL: Analysis

107. 10. To perform this dosage calculation, convert the child's weight from pounds to kilograms: 44 lb ÷ 2.2 lb/kg = 20 kg. Then calculate the total daily dose: 20 kg × 0.2 mg/kg/day = 4 mg. Next, calculate the amount to be given at each dose: 4 mg ÷ 4 doses = 1 mg/dose. The elixir contains 0.5 mg of drug per 5 ml. To give 1 mg of drug, administer 10 ml to the child at each dose.

CN: Physiological integrity; CNS: Pharmacological and parenteral therapies; CL: Analysis

CN: Client needs category   CNS: Client needs subcategory   CL: Cognitive level

Selected references

Anatomy & Physiology Made Incredibly Easy, 3rd ed. Philadelphia: Lippincott Williams & Wilkins, 2009.

Assessment Made Incredibly Easy, 4th ed. Philadelphia: Lippincott Williams & Wilkins, 2008.

Baranoski, S., and Ayello, E.A. *Wound Care Essentials: Practice Principles,* 2nd ed. Philadelphia: Lippincott Williams & Wilkins, 2008.

Bickley, L.S., and Szilagyi, P.G. *Bates' Guide to Physical Examination and History Taking,* 10th ed. Philadelphia: Lippincott Williams & Wilkins, 2009.

Bowden, V.R., and Greenberg, C.S. *Pediatric Nursing Procedures,* 2nd ed. Philadelphia: Lippincott Williams & Wilkins, 2008.

Boyd, M.A. *Psychiatric Nursing: Contemporary Practice,* 4th ed. Philadelphia: Lippincott Williams & Wilkins, 2008.

Cardiovascular Care Made Incredibly Easy, 2nd ed. Philadelphia: Lippincott Williams & Wilkins, 2009.

ECG Interpretation Made Incredibly Easy, 5th ed. Philadelphia: Lippincott Williams & Wilkins, 2011.

Fauci, A., et al. *Harrison's Principles of Internal Medicine,* 17th ed. New York: McGraw-Hill, 2009.

Fischbach, F., & Dunning, M.B., eds. *A Manual of Laboratory and Diagnostic Tests,* 8th ed. Philadelphia: Lippincott Williams & Wilkins, 2009.

Hockenberry, M.J., and Wilson, D. *Wong's Nursing Care of Infants and Children,* 8th ed. St. Louis: Mosby–Year Book, Inc., 2007.

Ignatavicius, D.D., and Workman, M.L. *Medical-Surgical Nursing: Patient-Centered Collaborative Care,* 6th ed. Philadelphia: Elsevier, 2010.

Judge, N.L. "Neurovascular Assessment," *Nursing Standard* 21(45):39-44, July 2007.

Karch, A.M. *Focus on Nursing Pharmacology,* 5th ed. Philadelphia: Lippincott Williams & Wilkins, 2010.

Kyle, T. *Essentials of Pediatric Nursing.* Philadelphia: Lippincott Williams & Wilkins, 2008.

Lippincott's Nursing Procedures, 5th ed. Philadelphia: Lippincott Williams & Wilkins, 2008.

Nettina, S.M. *Lippincott Manual of Nursing Practice,* 9th ed. Philadelphia: Lippincott Williams & Wilkins, 2010.

Nursing 2010 Drug Handbook. Philadelphia: Lippincott Williams & Wilkins, 2010.

Pillitteri, A. *Maternal & Child Health Nursing: Care of the Childbearing and Childrearing Family,* 6th ed. Philadelphia: Lippincott Williams & Wilkins, 2010.

Porth, C.M., and Matfin, G. *Pathophysiology: Concepts of Altered Health States,* 8th ed. Philadelphia: Lippincott Williams & Wilkins, 2009.

Professional Guide to Diseases, 9th ed. Philadelphia: Lippincott Williams & Wilkins, 2009.

Smeltzer, S.C., et al. *Brunner & Suddarth's Textbook of Medical-Surgical Nursing,* 12th ed. Philadelphia: Lippincott Williams & Wilkins, 2010.

Taylor, C.R., et al. *Fundamentals of Nursing: The Art and Science of Nursing Care,* 6th ed. Philadelphia: Lippincott Williams & Wilkins, 2008.

Townsend, M.C., and Pedersen, D.D. *Essentials of Psychiatric Mental Health Nursing: Concepts of Care in Evidence-Based Practice.* Philadelphia: F.A. Davis Company, 2008.

Wilson, D., and Hockenberry, M.J. *Wong's Clinical Manual of Pediatric Nursing,* 7th ed. St. Louis: Mosby–Year Book, Inc., 2008.

Index

i refers to an illustration; t refers to a table.

i refers to an illustration; t refers to a table.